trautiDung
. 29/3/86
PÂQUES86

BY THE EDITORS OF
CONSUMER GUIDE®
AND NICOLA GIACONA, PHARM. D.

PRESCRIPTION
DRUGS

D1387583

All rights reserved under International and Pan American copyright conventions. Copyright© 1985 Publications International, Ltd. This publication may not be reproduced or quoted in whole or in part by mimeograph or any other printed means, or for presentation on radio, television, videotape, or film without written permission from Louis Weber, President of Publications International, Ltd. Permission is never granted for commercial purposes. PRINTED IN CANADA

Contents

Introduction 5

Filling Your Prescription 7
Reading Your Prescription • Talking to Your Pharmacist •
Over-the-Counter Drugs • Generic Drugs • How Much
to Buy • Storing Your Drugs

Administering Medication Correctly 18
Liquids • Capsules, Tablets, and Oral Powders •
Sublingual Tablets • Eye Drops and Eye Ointments •
Eardrops • Nose Drops and Sprays • Rectal Suppositories •
Vaginal Ointments and Creams • Vaginal Tablets and
Suppositories • Throat Lozenges and Discs • Throat
Sprays • Topical Ointments and Creams • Aerosol Sprays •
Transdermal Patches

Coping with Side Effects 27
Obvious Side Effects • Subtle Side Effects • Drug Use
During Pregnancy and Breastfeeding • Management of
Side Effects

How Drugs Work 35
Cardiovascular Drugs • Drugs for the Ears • Drugs for the
Eyes • Gastrointestinal Drugs • Hormones • Anti-Infectives
• Anti-Neoplastics • Topical Drugs • Central Nervous
System Drugs • Respiratory Drugs • Vitamins and Minerals

Drug Profiles 51

Canadian Brand Names 1158

Glossary 1163

Drug Type Index 1172

Note: Neither the Editors of CONSUMER GUIDE and PUBLICATIONS INTERNATIONAL, LTD. nor the consultant or publisher take responsibility for any possible consequences from any treatment, action, or application of medication or preparation by any person reading or following the information in this book. The publication of this book does not constitute the practice of medicine, and this book does not attempt to replace your physician or your pharmacist. The consultant and publisher advise the reader to check with a physician before administering or consuming any medication or using any health care device.

Every effort has been made to assure that the information in this book is accurate and current at time of printing. However, new developments occur almost daily in drug research, and the consultant and publisher suggest that the reader consult a physician or pharmacist for the latest available data on specific products. All trade names of drugs used in the text of this book are capitalized.

Introduction

The right drug for the right patient in the right dose by the right route at the right time. This rule sums up the decisions made when your doctor gives you a prescription. You've helped make those decisions by giving a complete medical history; you've informed your doctor of any previous allergic reactions you've suffered to drugs, foods, or dyes; of any other drugs you may be taking; of any chronic health problems you may have; and whether you are pregnant or breastfeeding an infant. Once you leave your doctor's office, prescription in hand, you have still more to do as a responsible patient.

You must know how to administer the medication you will be taking. You must understand and comply with your dosage schedule. You must know what to do should side effects occur. You must recognize the signals that indicate the need to call your doctor. All too often, patients leave their doctors' offices without a full understanding of the drug therapy they're about to start, with the result that they do not comply fully with their doctor's prescription. They may stop taking the medication too soon because it doesn't seem to work, or because they feel better, or because it causes bothersome side effects. They may take the drug improperly or at the wrong time or too often. They may continue drinking alcohol or taking other drugs, perhaps not even realizing that such things as cold pills, oral contraceptives, aspirin, and vitamins can affect the action of the prescribed drug. The end result may be that they do not get better; perhaps they will get worse, or they may suffer a dangerous overdose.

PRESCRIPTION DRUGS provides the information you need to take drugs safely. Along with general information on reading a prescription and buying, storing, and using drugs, it provides an introduction to the action of drugs —how drugs work to stop infection, to lower blood pressure, or to relieve pain. It provides detailed information on hundreds of the most commonly prescribed drugs and several over-the-counter products, including how to alleviate certain side effects, whether you should take the drug on an empty stomach or with meals, whether the drug is likely to affect your ability to drive a car, and whether you can substitute a less expensive, generic drug for a prescribed trade name medication. You will discover which side effects are common to some medications and which are danger signals that require immediate attention from your physician.

Of course, this book is not a substitute for consulting your doctor and pharmacist. They are your primary reference sources on the use of drugs. But to assure that you receive the best health care possible, you too must be informed and knowledgeable about the drugs you use.

Filling Your Prescription

While you're having your prescription filled, you should make sure you understand your dosage schedule, what kinds of precautions to take to prevent or reduce side effects, whether you should restrict your diet or drinking habits while taking the drug, which side effects are expected or unavoidable, and which side effects signal a need for a doctor's attention. Your first step in filling your prescription is reading what your doctor has written.

READING YOUR PRESCRIPTION

Prescriptions are not mysterious—they contain no secret messages. Many of the symbols and phrases doctors use on prescriptions are abbreviated Latin or Greek words; they are holdovers from the days when doctors actually wrote in Latin. For example, "gtts" comes from the Latin word *guttae*, which means drops, and "bid" is a shortened version of *bis in die*, Latin for twice a day.

You do not have to be a doctor, nurse, or pharmacist to read a prescription. YOU need to learn how—after all, the prescription describes the drug you will be taking. You should understand what your doctor has written on the prescription blank to be sure the label on the drug container you receive from your pharmacist coincides with your prescription.

The accompanying chart lists the most common prescription symbols and abbreviations. Use it as a guide to read the sample prescriptions that follow.

Common Abbreviations and Symbols
Used in Writing Prescriptions

Abbreviation	Meaning	Derivation and Notes
A₂	both ears	*auris* (Latin)
aa	of each	*ana* (Greek)
ac	before meals	*ante cibum* (Latin)
AD	right ear	*auris dextra* (Latin)
AL	left ear	*auris laeva* (Latin)
AM	morning	*ante meridiem* (Latin)
AS	left ear	*auris sinistra* (Latin)
bid	twice a day	*bis in die* (Latin)
c̄	with	*cum* (Latin)
cap	capsule	—
cc or cm³	cubic centimeter	30 cc equals one ounce
disp	dispense	—
dtd#	give this number	*dentur tales doses* (Latin)
ea	each	
ext	for external use	—
gtts	drops	*guttae* (Latin)
gutta	drop	*gutta* (Latin)
h	hour	*hora* (Latin)
HS	bedtime	*hora somni* (Latin)
M ft	make	*misce fiat* (Latin)
mitt#	give this number	*mitte* (Latin)
ml	milliliter	30 ml equals one ounce
O	pint	*octarius* (Latin)
O₂	both eyes	*oculus* (Latin)
OD	right eye	*oculus dexter* (Latin)
OJ	orange juice	—
OL	left eye	*oculus laevus* (Latin)
OS	left eye	*oculus sinister* (Latin)
OU	each eye	*oculus uterque* (Latin)
pc	after meals	*post cibum* (Latin)

Abbreviation	Meaning	Derivation and Notes
PM	evening	*post meridiem* (Latin)
po	by mouth	*per os* (Latin)
prn	as needed	*pro re nata* (Latin)
q̄	every	*quaqua* (Latin)
qd	once a day	*quaqua die* (Latin)
qid	four times a day	*quater in die* (Latin)
qod	every other day	—
s̄	without	*sine* (Latin)
Sig	label as follows	*signetur* (Latin)
sl	under the tongue	*sub lingua* (Latin)
SOB	shortness of breath	—
sol	solution	—
ss	half-unit	*semis* (Latin)
stat	at once, first dose	*statim* (Latin)
susp	suspension	—
tab	tablet	—
tid	three times a day	*ter in die* (Latin)
top	apply topically	—
ung or ungt	ointment	*unguentum* (Latin)
UT	under the tongue	—
ut dict	as directed	*ut dictum* (Latin)
x	times	—

The first sample prescription is for Darvon Compound-65 (Darvon cpd-65). The prescription tells the pharmacist to give you 24 capsules (#24), and it tells you to take one capsule (cap i) every four hours (q̄4h) as needed (prn) for pain. The prescription indicates that you may receive five refills (5x) and that the label on the drug container should state the name of the drug (yes).

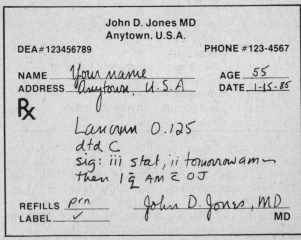

John D. Jones MD
Anytown, U.S.A.

DEA # 123456789   PHONE # 123-4567

NAME _Your name_   AGE _25_
ADDRESS _Anytown, U.S.A_   DATE _1-15-85_

Rx   Darvon cpd - 65
          # 24
          sig: cap ī q̄ 4h prn pain

REFILLS _5X_   _John D. Jones, MD_
LABEL _yes_   **MD**

Look at the second prescription. It shows that you will receive 100 (dtd C) tablets of Lanoxin, 0.125 mg. You will take three tablets at once (iii stat), then two (ii) tomorrow morning (AM), and one (i) every ($\bar{q}$) morning (AM) thereafter with ($\bar{c}$) orange juice (OJ). You may receive refills as needed (prn), and the name of the drug will be on the package ($\sqrt{}$).

John D. Jones MD
Anytown, U.S.A.

DEA # 123456789   PHONE # 123-4567

NAME _Your name_   AGE _55_
ADDRESS _Anytown, U.S.A_   DATE _1-15-85_

Rx
          Lanoxin 0.125
          dtd C
          sig: iii stat, ii tomorrow am
          then 1 q̄ AM c̄ OJ

REFILLS _prn_   _John D. Jones, MD_
LABEL _✓_   **MD**

Do remember to check the label on the drug container. If the information on the label is not the same as on the prescription, question your pharmacist. Make doubly sure that you are receiving the right medication and the correct instructions for taking it.

TALKING TO YOUR PHARMACIST

Once you have read the prescription, its directions may seem clear enough, but will they seem clear when you get home? For example, the prescription for Darvon Compound-65 tells you to take one capsule every four hours as needed. How many capsules can you take each day—four, six, more? The phrase "as needed" is not clear, and unless you understand what it means, you don't know how much medication you can take per day. What if your prescription instructs you to take "one tablet four times a day"? What does four times a day mean? For some antibiotics, it may mean one tablet every six hours around the clock. For other medications, it may mean one tablet in the morning, one at noon, one in the early evening, and one at bedtime. For still others, it may mean one tablet every hour for the first four hours after you get up in the morning. Don't leave the pharmacy with unanswered questions; ask your pharmacist for an explanation of any confusing terms on your prescription.

Your pharmacist is a valuable resource in your health care. He or she should have a record of ALL the prescription drugs you receive, in order to detect any possible life-threatening drug interactions. It is therefore a good idea to purchase your medications through one pharmacy—choose one that maintains careful records.

The pharmacist will be able to tell you if your therapy may be affected by smoking tobacco, eating certain foods, or drinking alcohol, and if the drugs you are taking can cause drowsiness or nausea. He or she can tell you what to expect from the medication and about how long you will have to take it. Of course, people's treatments vary tremendously, but you should ask whether you will have to take medication for five to ten days (for example, to treat a mild respiratory infection) or for a few months (for example, to treat a kidney infection).

Your pharmacist should advise you of possible side

effects and describe their symptoms in terms you can understand. The pharmacist should also tell you which side effects require prompt attention from your physician. For example, one of the major side effects of the drug phenylbutazone is a blood disorder. One of the early symptoms of a blood disorder is a sore throat. Your pharmacist should tell you to consult your physician if you develop a sore throat.

Your pharmacist should also explain how to take your medicine. You should know whether to take the drug before or after a meal or along with it. The timing of doses of a drug can make a big difference, and the effectiveness of each drug depends on following the directions for its use. Your pharmacist should describe what "as needed," "as directed," and "take with fluid" mean. You may take water, but not milk, with some drugs. With other drugs, you should drink milk. Your pharmacist should tell you how many refills you may have and whether you may need them.

OVER-THE-COUNTER DRUGS

Drugs that can be purchased without a prescription are referred to as over-the-counter (OTC) drugs. They are sold in a wide variety of settings, such as drug stores, grocery stores, and hotel lobbies. There are no legal requirements or limitations on who may buy or sell them.

Products sold OTC contain amounts of active ingredients considered to be safe for self-treatment by consumers, when labeling instructions are followed.

Many people visit a doctor for ailments that can be treated effectively by taking non-prescription drugs. Actually, prescriptions are sometimes written for such drugs. Your pharmacist will be able to recommend appropriate use of OTC drugs.

If your pharmacist recommends that you not take certain OTC drugs, follow the advice. OTC drugs may affect the way your body reacts to the prescription drugs you are taking. For instance, people taking tetracycline should avoid taking antacids or other iron-containing products at the same time; their use should be separated by at least two hours. Antacids and iron interfere with the body's absorption of tetracycline, thereby decreasing its effectiveness. Be sure you know what you are taking. If you are unsure of the type or contents of your medications, ask your doctor or pharmacist.

GENERIC DRUGS

One way your pharmacist can help you save money is by dispensing generic drugs. "Generic" means not protected by trademark registration. The generic name of a drug is usually a shortened form of its chemical name. Any manufacturer can use the generic name when marketing a drug. Thus, many manufacturers make a drug called tetracycline.

Usually, a manufacturer uses a trade name as well as a generic name for a drug. A trade name is registered, and only the manufacturer who holds the trademark can use the trade name when marketing a drug. For example, only Lederle Laboratories can call their tetracycline product Achromycin, and only The Upjohn Company can use the trade name Panmycin for tetracycline. Most trade names are easy to remember, are capitalized in print, and usually include the register symbol ® after them. It is important that you know both the generic name and the trade name of every drug you are taking.

Many people think that drugs with trade names are made by large manufacturers and generic drugs are made by small manufacturers. But, in fact, a manufacturer may market large quantities of a drug under a trade name; the same manufacturer may sell the base chemical to several other companies, some of which sell the drug generically and some of which sell it under their own trade names. For example, the antibiotic ampicillin is the base for over 200 different products. However, all ampicillin is produced by only a few dozen drug companies.

Generic drugs are generally priced lower than their trademarked equivalents, largely because they are not as widely advertised. Not every drug is available generically, and not every generic is significantly less expensive than its trademarked equivalent. However, consumers may be able to save as much as 75 percent by purchasing a generic product. For example, 100 capsules of Darvon Compound-65 may cost $19 to $22. One hundred capsules of the generic equivalent can cost as little as $9—a savings of $10 to $13. Pavabid may cost $24 per 100 capsules. If bought generically, the drug may cost only $10 per 100 capsules—a savings of about $14 per prescription.

For certain drugs, however, it's inadvisable to "shop around" for a generic equivalent. Although the Food and Drug Administration has stated that there is no evidence to suspect serious differences between trade name drugs and generic drugs, differences have been shown to exist between brands of certain drugs. The tablets or capsules from different manufacturers may not dissolve in the stomach at the same rate or to the same extent, because of variations in the way they are made or the fillers (non-active ingredients) that are used. This is especially true for the various generic digoxin and phenytoin products. It is therefore important to discuss with your doctor or pharmacist the advantages or disadvantages of any particular generic product.

In most states substitution laws allow pharmacists to fill prescriptions with the least expensive equivalent product. If such a substitution law is not yet legal in your state (contact your state pharmacy association to find out), ask your doctor to prescribe your medications by their generic names. However, you should be aware that there are sometimes differences, and your doctor may have good reason for being specific.

HOW MUCH TO BUY

On a prescription, your doctor specifies exactly how many tablets or capsules or how much liquid medication you will receive. But if you must take a drug for a long time, or if you are very sensitive to drugs, you may want to purchase a different quantity.

The amount of medication to buy depends on several factors. The most obvious is how much money you have, or, for those who have a comprehensive insurance program, how much the insurance company will pay for each purchase. These factors may help you decide how much medication to buy, but you must also consider the kind of medication you will be taking (for example, how long it keeps).

Medications to treat heart disease, high blood pressure,

diabetes, or a thyroid condition may be purchased in large quantity. Patients with such chronic conditions take medication for prolonged periods. Chances are, they will pay less per tablet or capsule by purchasing large quantities of drugs. Generally, the price per dose decreases with the amount of the drug purchased. In other words, a drug that usually costs six cents per tablet may cost four or five cents per tablet if you buy 100 at a time.

Many doctors prescribe only a month's supply of drugs, even those that will be taken for a long time. If you wish to buy more, check with your pharmacist. It is also important to make sure that you have enough medication on hand to cover vacation travel and long holidays. Serious side effects could occur if you miss even a few doses of such drugs as propranolol, prednisone, or clonidine.

On the other hand, if you have been plagued with annoying side effects or have had allergic reactions to some drugs, ask your pharmacist to dispense only enough medication on initial prescriptions for a few days or a week, to determine how your body reacts to the drug. Pharmacists cannot take back prescription drugs once they have left the pharmacy. You may have to pay more by asking the pharmacist to give you a small quantity of the drug, but at least you will not be paying for a supply of medication you cannot take. But be sure you can get the remainder of the prescribed amount of the drug if no serious or intolerable side effects occur. With some drugs, after you have received part of the intended amount, you cannot receive more without obtaining another prescription.

STORING YOUR DRUGS

Before you leave the pharmacy, find out how you should store your medication. If drugs are stored in containers that do not protect them from heat or moisture, they may lose potency.

All medications should be kept in their original containers. Different medications should not be mixed in one container, in order to prevent confusion about which drug is being taken. In addition, some drugs may lose their potency when stored with other medications. Never remove the label from the prescription vial. It contains your prescription number (for refills), the name of the medication, and directions for proper use.

You can safely store most prescription drugs at room temperature and out of direct sunlight. Even those drugs dispensed in colored bottles or containers that reflect light should be kept out of direct sunlight.

Some drugs require storage in the refrigerator; other medications should not be refrigerated. For example, some liquid cough suppressants thicken as they become cold, and will not pour from the bottle. Some people keep nitroglycerin tablets in the refrigerator because they believe the drug will be more stable when kept cold. Nitroglycerin, however, should not be stored in the refrigerator.

Even if the label on your medication states "keep refrigerated," this does NOT mean that you can keep the drug in the freezer. If frozen and thawed, coated tablets may crack, and some liquid medications may separate into layers that cannot be remixed.

Many people keep prescription drugs and other medications in the bathroom medicine cabinet, but this is one of the worst places to keep drugs. Small children can easily climb onto the sink and reach drugs stored above it. Also, the temperature and humidity changes in the bathroom may adversely affect the stability of prescription and non-prescription drugs.

Definitions of Ideal Storage Temperatures

Cold	Any temperature under 46°F (8°C)
Refrigerator	Any cold place where the temperature is between 36°–46°F (2°–8°C)
Cool	Any temperature between 46°–59°F (8°–15°C)
Room temperature	Temperature usually between 59°–86°F (15°–30°C)
Excessive heat	Any temperature above 104°F (40°C)

It is required by law that all prescription medications for oral use be dispensed in child-proof containers. If you find the container difficult to open AND if there are no small children in your home, you can request that your pharmacist dispense your medication in a non-child-proof container.

KEEP ALL DRUGS AWAY FROM CHILDREN, and do not keep unused prescription medications. Flush any left-over medication down the toilet or pour it down the sink, and wash and destroy the empty container. Regularly clean out your medicine cabinet and discard all the drugs you are no longer using and drugs that have expired (the expiration date is often listed on the prescription label). These drugs can be dangerous to your children, and you might be tempted to take them in the future if you develop similar symptoms. Though similar, the symptoms may not be due to the same disease, and you may complicate your condition by taking the wrong medication.

If a child accidentally swallows medication or receives too much of a prescribed medication, IMMEDIATELY CALL YOUR DOCTOR, A POISON CONTROL CENTER, OR THE NEAREST EMERGENCY ROOM for instructions and recommendations. These phone numbers should be written down in a readily accessible place. You should also keep a bottle of ipecac syrup (available over the counter) for each child under five years of age in your home (in case the doctor, poison control center, or emergency room recommends that you induce vomiting in the child).

Administering Medication Correctly

You must use medication correctly to obtain its full benefit. If you administer drugs improperly, you may not receive their full therapeutic effects. Furthermore, improper administration can be dangerous. Some drugs may become toxic if used incorrectly.

LIQUIDS

Liquid medication forms are used in several different ways. Some are intended to be used externally on the skin; some are placed into the eye, ear, nose, or throat; still others may be taken internally. Before taking or using any liquid medication, look at the label to see if there are specific directions.

If a liquid product contains particles that settle to the bottom of the container, it must be shaken before you use the medication. If you don't shake it well each time, you may not get the correct amount of the active ingredient —as the amount of liquid remaining in the bottle becomes smaller, the drug becomes more concentrated. You will be getting more of the active ingredient with each dose. The concentration may even reach toxic levels.

When opening the bottle, point it away from you. Some liquid medications build up pressure inside the bottle; the liquid could spurt out and stain your clothing.

If the medication is intended for application to the skin, pour a small quantity onto a cotton pad or a piece of gauze. Do not use a large piece of cotton or gauze, as it will absorb the liquid and much will be wasted. Don't pour the medication into your cupped hand; you may spill some of it. If you're using it on only a small area, you can spread the medication with your finger or a cotton-tipped applicator. Never dip cotton-tipped applicators or pieces of cotton or gauze into the bottle of liquid, since this might contaminate the rest of the medication.

Liquid medications that are to be swallowed must be measured accurately. When your doctor prescribes one teaspoonful of medication, he or she is thinking of a 5 ml (milliliter) medical teaspoon. The teaspoons you have at home can hold anywhere from 2 to 10 ml of liquid. If you use one of these to measure your medication, you may get too little or too much drug with each dose. Ask your pharmacist for a medical teaspoon or for one of the other plastic devices for accurately measuring liquid medications. Most of these cost only a few cents, and they are well worth their cost in assuring accurate dosage. Such plastic measuring devices have another advantage. While many children balk at medication taken from a teaspoon, they often seem to enjoy taking it from a "special" spoon.

CAPSULES, TABLETS, AND ORAL POWDERS

Many people find it hard to swallow a tablet or capsule. If tablets or capsules tend to catch in your throat, rinse your mouth with water, or at least wet your mouth, before taking one. Place the tablet or capsule on the back of your tongue, take a drink, and swallow. If it is too large, or still "sticks" in your throat, empty the capsule or crush the tablet into a spoon and mix it with applesauce, soup, or even chocolate syrup. But BE SURE TO CHECK WITH YOUR PHARMACIST FIRST. Some tablets and capsules must be swallowed whole—your pharmacist can tell you which ones they are.

If you have trouble swallowing a tablet or capsule and do not wish to mix the medication with food, ask your doctor to prescribe a liquid drug preparation or a chewable tablet instead, if one is available.

Occasionally, medications come in oral powder form (i.e., cholestyramine, colestipol). Such medications should be carefully mixed with liquids, then swallowed. These medications should NOT be swallowed dry.

SUBLINGUAL TABLETS

Some drugs, such as nitroglycerin, are prepared as tablets that must be placed under the tongue. Such medications are more rapidly or more completely absorbed into the bloodstream from the lining of the mouth than they are from the stomach and intestinal tract.

To take a sublingual tablet properly, place the tablet under your tongue, close your mouth, and hold the saliva in your mouth and under your tongue as long as you can before swallowing (until the tablet completely dissolves). If you have a bitter taste in your mouth after five minutes, the drug has not been completely absorbed. Wait at least five more minutes before drinking water. Drinking too soon may wash the medication into the stomach before it has been absorbed thoroughly. Do not smoke, eat, or chew gum while the medication is dissolving.

EYEDROPS AND EYE OINTMENTS

Before administering eyedrops or ointments, wash your hands. Then lie down or sit down, and tilt your head back. Using your thumb and forefinger, gently and carefully pull your lower eyelid down to form a pouch.

If you're applying eyedrops, lay your second finger alongside your nose and apply gentle pressure to your nose. This closes off the duct that drains fluid from the surface of the eye into the nose and throat canal. If you don't close off this duct, the drops are likely to drain away too soon. Hold the dropper close to the eyelid WITHOUT TOUCHING IT. Place the prescribed number of drops into the pouch. Do not place the drops directly on the eyeball; you might blink and lose the medication. Close your eye and keep it shut for a few moments. Do not wash or wipe the dropper before replacing it in the bottle — you might accidentally contaminate the rest of the medication. Tightly close the bottle to keep out moisture.

To administer an eye ointment, squeeze a one-quarter to one-half inch line of ointment into the pouch formed as above, and close your eye. Roll your eye a few times to spread the ointment.

Be sure the drops or ointments you use are intended for use in the eye (all products manufactured for use in the eye must be sterilized to prevent eye infections). Also, check the expiration date on the label or container of the medication. Do not use a drug product after the specified date, and never use any eye product that has changed color. If you find that the medication contains particles that weren't there when you bought it, do not use it.

EARDROPS

Eardrops must be administered so that they fill the ear canal. To administer eardrops properly, tilt your head to one side, turning the affected ear upward. Grasp the earlobe and gently pull it upward and back to straighten the ear canal. When administering eardrops to a child, GENTLY pull the child's earlobe downward and back. Fill the dropper and place the prescribed number of drops (usually a dropperful) into the ear, but be careful to avoid touching the ear canal. The dropper can easily become contaminated by contact with the ear canal.

Keep the ear tilted upward for five to ten seconds while continuing to hold the earlobe. Then gently insert a small piece of clean cotton into the ear to ensure that the drops do not escape. Do not wash or wipe the dropper after use; replace it in the bottle and tightly close the bottle to keep out moisture.

Before administering the medication, you may warm the bottle of eardrops by rolling the bottle back and forth between your hands to bring the solution to body temperature. DO NOT place the bottle in boiling water. The eardrops may become so hot that they will cause pain when placed in the ear. Also, boiling water can loosen or peel off the label, and might even destroy the medication.

NOSE DROPS AND SPRAYS

Before using nose drops or sprays, gently blow your nose if you can. To administer nose drops, fill the dropper, tilt your head back, and place the prescribed number of drops into your nose. Do not touch the dropper to the nasal membranes, to prevent contamination of the rest of the medicine when the dropper is returned to the container. Keep your head tilted for five to ten seconds and sniff gently two or three times.

Do not tilt your head back when using a nasal spray. Insert the sprayer into the nose, but try to avoid touching the inner nasal membranes. Sniff and squeeze the sprayer at the same time. Do not release your grip on the sprayer until you have withdrawn it from your nose (to prevent nasal mucus and bacteria from entering the plastic bottle and contaminating its contents). After you have sprayed the prescribed number of times in one or both nostrils, gently sniff two or three times.

Unless your doctor has told you otherwise, you should not use nose drops or sprays for more than two or three days at a time. If they have been prescribed for a longer period, do not administer nose drops or sprays from the same container for more than one week. Bacteria from your nose can easily enter the container and contaminate the solution. If you must take medication for more than a week, purchase a new container. NEVER allow anyone else to use your nose drops or spray.

RECTAL SUPPOSITORIES

Rectal suppositories are used to deliver various types of medication. They may be used as a laxative, sleeping aid, or tranquilizer, or to relieve the itching, swelling, and pain of hemorrhoids. Regardless of the reason for their use, all rectal suppositories are inserted in the same way.

In extremely hot weather, a suppository may become too soft to handle properly. If this happens, place the suppository inside the refrigerator, in a glass of cool water, or under running cold water until it becomes firm. A few minutes is usually sufficient. Before inserting a suppository, remove any aluminum wrappings. Rubber finger coverings or disposable rubber gloves may be worn when inserting a suppository, but they are not necessary unless your fingernails are extremely long and sharp.

To insert a suppository, lie on your left side with your right knee bent. Push the suppository, pointed end first, into the rectum as far as is comfortable. You may feel like defecating, but lie still for 20 to 30 minutes, until the urge has passed. If you cannot insert a suppository, or if the process is painful, you can coat the suppository with a thin layer of petroleum jelly or mineral oil to make insertion easier.

Manufacturers of many suppositories that are used in the treatment of hemorrhoids suggest that the suppositories be stored in the refrigerator. Be sure to ask your pharmacist if the suppositories you have purchased should be stored in the refrigerator.

VAGINAL OINTMENTS AND CREAMS

Most vaginal products are packaged with complete instructions for use. If a woman is not sure how to administer vaginal medication, she should ask her pharmacist.

Before using any vaginal ointment or cream, read the directions. They will probably tell you to attach the applicator to the top of the tube and to squeeze the tube from the bottom until the applicator is completely filled. Then lie on your back with your knees drawn up. Hold the applicator horizontally or pointed slightly downward, and insert it into the vagina as far as it will comfortably go. Press the plunger down to empty the cream or ointment into the vagina. Withdraw the plunger and wash it in warm, soapy water. Rinse it thoroughly and allow it to dry completely. Once it is dry, return the plunger to its package.

VAGINAL TABLETS AND SUPPOSITORIES

Most packages of vaginal tablets or suppositories include complete directions for use, but you may wish to review general instructions.

Remove any foil wrapping. Place the tablet or suppository in the applicator that is provided. Lie on your back with your knees drawn up. Hold the applicator horizontally or tilted slightly downward, and insert it into the vagina as far as it will comfortably go. Depress the plunger slowly to release the tablet or suppository into the vagina. Withdraw the applicator and wash it in warm, soapy water. Rinse it and let it dry completely. Once it is dry, return the applicator to its package.

Unless your doctor has told you otherwise, do not douche two to three weeks before or after you use vaginal tablets or suppositories. Be sure to ask your doctor for specific recommendations on douching.

THROAT LOZENGES AND DISCS

Lozenges are made with crystalline sugar; discs are not. Both contain medication that is released in the mouth to soothe a sore throat to reduce coughing, or to treat laryngitis. Neither should be chewed; they should be allowed to dissolve in the mouth. After the lozenge or disc has dissolved, try not to swallow or drink any fluids for awhile.

THROAT SPRAYS

To administer a throat spray, open your mouth wide and spray the medication as far back as possible. Try not to swallow—hold the spray in your mouth as long as you can, and do not drink any fluids for several minutes. This gives the medication a greater opportunity to work. Swallowing a throat spray is not harmful, but if you find that your throat spray upsets your stomach, don't swallow it; simply spit it out.

TOPICAL OINTMENTS AND CREAMS

Most ointments and creams exert only local effects—that is, they affect only the area on which they are applied. Most creams and ointments are expensive (especially steroid products, such as betamethasone valerate, fluocinolone, fluocinonide, hydrocortisone, and triamcinolone), and should be applied to the skin as thinly as possible. A thin layer is as effective as (but less costly than) a thick layer; and some steroid-containing creams and ointments can cause toxic side effects if applied too heavily.

Before applying the medication, moisten the skin by immersing it in water or by dabbing the area with a clean, wet cloth. Blot the skin almost dry and apply the medication as directed. Gently massage it into the skin until it disappears. You should feel no greasiness after applying a cream. After an ointment is applied, the skin will feel slightly greasy.

If your doctor has not indicated whether you should receive a cream or an ointment, ask your pharmacist for the one you prefer. Creams are greaseless and do not stain your clothing. Creams are best to use on the scalp or other hairy areas of the body. However, if your skin is dry, ask for an ointment. Ointments help keep the skin soft for a longer period of time.

If your doctor tells you to place a wrap on top of the skin after the cream or ointment has been applied, you may use a wrap of transparent plastic film like that used for wrapping food. A wrap holds the medication close to the skin and helps to keep the skin moist so that the drug can be absorbed. To use a wrap correctly, apply the cream or ointment as directed, then wrap the area with a layer of transparent plastic film. Be careful to follow your doctor's directions EXACTLY. If he or she tells you to leave the wrap in place for a certain length of time, do not leave it in place longer. If you keep a wrap on the skin too long, too much of the drug may be absorbed, which may lead to increased side effects. Do not use such a wrap without your doctor's approval, and never use one on a weeping lesion.

AEROSOL SPRAYS

Many topical (used on the surface of the skin) items are packaged as pressurized aerosol sprays. These sprays usually cost more than the cream or ointment form of the same medication. On the other hand, they are useful on very tender or hairy areas of the body, where it is difficult to apply a cream or ointment. Aerosols can provide a cooling effect on burns or rashes.

Before using an aerosol, shake the can to evenly disperse the particles of medication. Hold the container upright, four to six inches from the skin. Press the nozzle for a few seconds, then release.

Never use an aerosol around the face or eyes. If your doctor tells you to use the spray on a part of your face, apply it to your hand and then rub it into the area. If you get it into your eyes or on a mucous membrane, it can be very painful and it may even damage the eyes.

Aerosol sprays may feel cold when they are applied. If this sensation bothers you, ask your pharmacist or doctor whether another form of the same product is available.

TRANSDERMAL PATCHES

Transdermal patches allow for controlled, continuous release of medication. They are convenient and easy to use. For best results, apply the patch to a hairless or clean-shaven area of skin, avoiding scars and wounds. Choose a site (such as the chest or upper arm) that is not subject to excessive movement. It is all right to bathe or shower with a patch in place. In the event that the patch becomes dislodged, discard and replace it. Replace a patch by applying a new unit before removing the old one. This allows for uninterrupted drug therapy; and since you change the site each time, skin irritation is minimized.

If redness or irritation develops at the application site, consult your physician. Some people are sensitive to the materials used to make the patches.

Coping with Side Effects

Drugs have certain desirable effects—that's why they are taken. The desirable effects of a drug are known as the drug's activity or therapeutic effects. Drugs, however, have undesirable effects as well. Undesirable effects are called side effects, adverse reactions, or, in some cases, lethal effects. An adverse reaction is any undesirable effect of a drug. It can range from minor side effects to toxic or lethal reactions.

Even if you experience minor side effects, it is very important that you take your medication exactly as it was prescribed. You should take the full dose at the appropriate times throughout the day for the length of time prescribed by your doctor. Taking a lesser amount of medication to avoid side effects or because your condition appears to be improving is NOT appropriate. A smaller dose may not provide any benefit whatsoever; that is, half of the dose may not provide half of the therapeutic effects.

Some side effects are expected and unavoidable, but others may surprise the doctor as well as the patient. Unexpected reactions may be due to a person's individual response to the drug.

Side effects generally fall into one of two major groups—those that are obvious and those that cannot be detected without laboratory testing. Discussion between you and your doctor about your medication should not be restricted to easily recognized side effects; other, less obvious side effects may also be harmful.

If you know a particular side effect is expected from a particular drug, you can relax a little. Most expected side effects are temporary and need not cause alarm. You'll merely experience discomfort or inconvenience for a short time. For example, you may become drowsy after taking an antihistamine, or develop a stuffy nose after taking reserpine or certain other drugs that lower blood pressure. Of course, if you find minor side effects especially bothersome, you should discuss them with your doctor, who may be able to prescribe another drug or at least assure you that the benefits of the drug far outweigh its side effects. Sometimes side effects can be minimized or eliminated by changing your dosage schedule or taking the drug with meals. Consult your doctor or pharmacist before making such a change.

Many side effects, however, signal a serious, perhaps dangerous, problem. If these side effects appear, you should consult your doctor immediately. The following discussion should help you determine whether your side effects require attention from your physician.

OBVIOUS SIDE EFFECTS

Some side effects are obvious to the patient; others can be discerned only through laboratory testing. We have divided our discussion according to the body parts affected by the side effects.

Ear

Although a few drugs may cause loss of hearing if taken in large quantities, hearing loss is uncommon. Drugs that are used to treat problems of the ear may cause dizziness, and many drugs produce tinnitus, a sensation of ringing, buzzing, thumping, or hollowness in the ears. Discuss with your doctor any problem with your hearing or your ears if it persists.

Eye

Blurred vision is a common side effect of many drugs. Medications such as digoxin may cause you to see a "halo" around a lighted object (a television screen or a traffic light), and other drugs may cause night blindness. Chlordiazepoxide and clidinium combination makes it difficult to accurately judge distance while driving, and makes the eyes sensitive to sunlight. While the effects on the eye caused by digoxin are danger signs of toxicity, the effects caused by chlordiazepoxide and clidinium combination are to be expected. In any case, if you have difficulty seeing while taking drugs, contact your doctor.

Gastrointestinal System

The gastrointestinal system includes the mouth, esophagus, stomach, small and large intestines, and rectum. A side effect that affects the gastrointestinal system can be expected from almost any drug. Many drugs produce dry mouth, mouth sores, difficulty swallowing, heartburn, nausea, vomiting, diarrhea, constipation, loss of appetite, or abnormal cramping. Other drugs cause bloating and gas, and some cause rectal itching.

Diarrhea can be expected after taking many drugs. Drugs can create localized reactions in intestinal tissue—usually a more rapid rate of contraction, which leads to diarrhea. Diarrhea caused by most drugs is temporary and self-limiting; that is, it should stop within three days. During this time, do not take any diarrhea remedy; drink liquids to replace the fluid you are losing. If the diarrhea lasts more than three days, call your doctor.

Diarrhea sometimes signals a problem. For example, some antibiotics can cause severe diarrhea. When diarrhea is severe, the intestine may become ulcerated and begin to bleed. If you develop severe diarrhea (diarrhea that lasts for several days, or stools that contain blood, pus, or mucus) while taking antibiotics, contact your doctor.

As a side effect of drug use, constipation is less serious and more common than diarrhea. It occurs when a drug slows down the activity of the bowel. Medications such as chlorpromazine or chlordiazepoxide and clidinium combination slow bowel activity. Constipation also occurs when drugs cause moisture to be absorbed from the bowel, resulting in a more solid stool. It may also occur if a drug acts on the nervous system to decrease nerve impulses to the intestine—an effect produced, for example, by a drug such as methyldopa. Constipation produced by a drug can last several days. You may help relieve it by drinking eight to ten glasses of water a day (unless your doctor directs you to do otherwise). Do not take laxatives unless your doctor directs you to do so. If constipation continues for more than three days, call your doctor.

Circulatory System

Drugs may speed up or slow down the heartbeat. If a drug slows the heartbeat, you may feel drowsy and tired, or even dizzy. If a drug accelerates the heartbeat, you probably will experience palpitations (thumping in the chest). You may feel as though your heart is skipping a beat occasionally. For most people, none of these symptoms indicates a serious problem. However, if they bother you, consult your doctor, who may adjust your drug dosage or prescribe other medication.

Some drugs cause edema (fluid retention)—fluid from the blood collects outside the blood vessels. Ordinarily, edema is not serious. But if you are steadily gaining weight or have gained more than three pounds within a week, talk to your doctor.

Drugs may either increase or decrease blood pressure. When blood pressure decreases, you may feel drowsy or tired; you may become dizzy, or even faint, especially when you rise suddenly from a sitting or reclining position. If a medication makes you dizzy or light-headed, sit or lie down awhile. To avoid light-headedness when you stand, contract and relax the muscles of your legs for a few moments before rising. Do this by pushing one foot against the floor while raising the other foot slightly, alternating feet so that you are "pumping" your legs in a pedaling motion. Get up slowly, and be especially careful on stairs. When blood pressure increases, you may feel dizzy, have a headache or blurred vision, hear a ringing or buzzing in your ears, or experience frequent nosebleeds. If you develop any of these symptoms, call your doctor.

Nervous System

Drugs that act on the nervous system may cause drowsiness or stimulation. If a drug causes drowsiness, you may become dizzy or your coordination may become impaired. If a drug causes stimulation, you may become nervous or have insomnia or tremors. Neither drowsiness nor stimulation is cause for concern for most people. When you are drowsy, however, you should be careful around machinery and should avoid driving. Some drugs cause throbbing headaches, and others produce tingling in the fingers or toes. These symptoms are generally expected and should disappear in a few days to a week. If they don't, call your doctor.

Respiratory System

Side effects common to the respiratory system include stuffy nose, dry throat, shortness of breath, and slowed breathing. A stuffy nose and dry throat usually disappear several days after starting a medication. If these side effects are bothersome, you may use nose drops (consult your doctor first) or throat lozenges, or gargle with warm salt water, to relieve them. Shortness of breath is a characteristic side effect of some drugs (for example, propranolol). If shortness of breath continues, check with your doctor. It may be a sign of a serious side effect, or you may simply be over-exercising. Barbiturates (drugs that promote sleep) may retard respiration. Slowed breathing is expected, and you should not be concerned, as long as your doctor knows about it. However, if your breathing becomes labored, contact your doctor immediately.

Skin

Skin reactions include rash, swelling, itching, and sweating. Itching, swelling, and rash frequently indicate a drug allergy. You should NOT continue to take a drug if you develop an allergy to it, but consult your doctor before stopping the drug.

Some drugs increase sweating; others decrease it. Drugs that decrease sweating may cause problems during exercise or hot weather, when your body needs to sweat to reduce body temperature.

If you have a minor skin reaction not diagnosed as an allergy, ask your pharmacist for a soothing cream. Your pharmacist may also suggest that you take frequent baths or dust the sensitive area with a suitable powder.

Another type of skin reaction is photosensitivity (also called phototoxicity or sun toxicity)—that is, unusual sensitivity to the sun. Tetracyclines can cause photosensitivity. If, while taking such a drug, you are exposed to the sun for even a brief period of time, say 10 or 15 minutes, you may receive a severe sunburn. You do not have to stay indoors while taking these drugs, but you should be fully clothed while outside and you should not remain in the sun too long. Furthermore, you should use a protective sunscreen while in the sun—ask your pharmacist to help you choose one. Since medications may remain in your bloodstream after you stop taking them, you should continue to follow these precautions for two days after treatment with these drugs is complete.

SUBTLE SIDE EFFECTS

Some side effects are difficult to detect. You may not notice any symptoms at all, or you may notice only slight ones. Therefore, your doctor may want you to have periodic blood tests or eye examinations to assure that no subtle damage is occurring to any of your organ systems while you are on certain medications.

Kidneys

If one of the side effects of a drug is to reduce the kidneys' ability to remove chemicals and other substances from the blood, these substances begin to accumulate in body tissues. Over a period of time, this accumulation may cause vague symptoms such as swelling, fluid retention, nausea, headache, or weakness. Obvious symptoms, especially pain, are rare.

Liver

Drug-induced liver damage may result in fat accumulation within the liver. Since the liver is responsible for converting many drugs and body chemicals into compounds that can be eliminated by other organs of the body (kidneys, lungs, gastrointestinal tract), drug-induced liver damage can result in a buildup of these substances. Because liver damage may be quite advanced before it produces any symptoms, periodic blood tests of liver function are recommended during therapy with certain drugs.

Blood

A great many drugs affect the blood and the circulatory system but do not produce noticeable symptoms for some time. Some drugs decrease the number of red blood cells—the cells responsible for carrying oxygen and nutrients throughout the body. If you have too few red blood cells, you become anemic; you appear pale and feel tired, weak, dizzy, and perhaps hungry. Other drugs decrease the number of white blood cells—the cells responsible for combating bacteria. Having too few white blood cells increases susceptibility to infection and may prolong illness. If a sore throat or a fever begins after you start taking a drug and continues for a few days, you may have an infection and too few white blood cells to fight it. Call your doctor.

DRUG USE DURING PREGNANCY AND BREASTFEEDING

Before taking ANY medication, it is very important to tell your doctor if you are pregnant or planning to become pregnant, or are breastfeeding an infant. For most drugs, complete information on safety during pregnancy and while breastfeeding is lacking. This is not due to negligence on the part of regulatory agencies or lack of concern, but to the mere fact that it would be unethical to conduct drug experiments on pregnant and nursing women. With this in mind, you should therefore discuss with your doctor the risks versus the benefits of taking any medications during pregnancy or while nursing.

MANAGEMENT OF SIDE EFFECTS

Consult the drug profiles to determine whether the side effects you are experiencing are minor (relatively common and usually not serious) or major (signs that something is amiss in your drug therapy). If your side effects are minor, you may be able to compensate for them simply (see the following table for suggestions). However, consult your doctor if you find minor side effects persistent or particularly bothersome.

If you experience any major side effects, contact your doctor immediately. Your dosage may need adjustment, or you may have developed a sensitivity to the drug. Your doctor may want you to switch to an alternative medication to treat your disorder. Never stop taking a prescribed medication unless you first discuss it with your doctor.

Common Minor Side Effects

Side Effect	Management
Blurred vision	Avoid operating machinery
Constipation	Increase the amount of fiber in your diet, drink plenty of fluids*; exercise*
Decreased sweating	Avoid working or exercising in the sun
Diarrhea	Drink lots of water; if diarrhea lasts longer than 3 days, call your doctor
Dizziness	Avoid operating machinery
Drowsiness	Avoid operating machinery
Dry mouth	Suck on candy or ice chips, or chew gum
Dry nose and throat	Use a humidifier or vaporizer
Fluid retention	Avoid adding salt to foods; keep legs raised, if possible
Headache	Remain quiet; take aspirin or acetaminophen*
Insomnia	Take the last dose of the drug earlier in the day*; drink a glass of warm milk at bedtime; ask your doctor about an exercise program
Itching	Take frequent baths or showers, or use wet soaks
Nasal congestion	If necessary, use nose drops*
Palpitations (mild)	Rest often; avoid tension; do not drink coffee, tea, or cola; stop smoking
Upset stomach	Take the drug with milk or food*

*Consult your doctor first.

How Drugs Work

Prescription drugs fall into a number of groups according to the conditions they are prescribed for. In the following pages we will provide you with a better understanding of the types of medications that are prescribed for different medical conditions. We'll describe the intended actions of drugs and the therapeutic effects you can expect from the various types of medications.

CARDIOVASCULAR DRUGS

Anti-Anginals

Since the heart is a muscle that must work continually, it requires a constant supply of nutrients and oxygen. The chest pain known as angina occurs when there is an insufficient supply of blood, and consequently of oxygen, to the heart. There are several types of anti-angina drugs. These include vasodilators (nitroglycerin, isosorbide dinitrate); calcium channel blockers (diltiazem, nifedipine, verapamil); and beta-blockers (atenolol, metoprolol, nadolol, pindolol, propranolol, timolol). All of these drugs act by increasing the amount of oxygen that reaches the heart muscle.

Anti-Arrhythmics

If the heart does not beat rhythmically or smoothly (a condition called arrhythmia), its rate of contraction must be regulated. Anti-arrhythmic drugs, including disopyramide, procainamide, propranolol, and quinidine, prevent or alleviate cardiac arrhythmias by altering nerve impulses within the heart. Phenytoin, most frequently used as an anti-convulsant in the treatment of epilepsy, can also act as an anti-arrhythmic agent when it is injected intravenously.

Anti-Hypertensives

Briefly, high blood pressure is a condition in which the pressure of the blood against the walls of the blood vessels is higher than what is considered normal. High blood pressure, or hypertension, is controllable. If you have been prescribed a medication for high blood pressure, it is very important that you continue to take it regularly, even if you don't notice any symptoms of hypertension. If hypertension is controlled, other diseases can be prevented. Drugs that counteract or reduce high blood pressure can effectively prolong a hypertensive patient's life.

Several different drug actions produce an anti-hypertensive effect. Some drugs block nerve impulses that cause arteries to constrict; others slow the heart rate and decrease its force of contraction; still others reduce the amount of a certain hormone (aldosterone) in the blood that causes blood pressure to rise. The effect of any of these is to reduce blood pressure. The mainstay of anti-hypertensive therapy is often a diuretic, a drug that reduces body fluids (see below). Examples of additional anti-hypertensive drugs include clonidine, hydralazine, methyldopa, prazosin, and reserpine.

Diuretics

Diuretic drugs, such as chlorothiazide, chlorthalidone, furosemide, hydrochlorothiazide, methyclothiazide, and spironolactone, promote the loss of water and salt from the body (this is why they are sometimes called "water pills"). They also lower blood pressure by increasing the diameter of blood vessels. Because many anti-hypertensive drugs cause the body to retain sodium and water, they are often used concurrently with diuretics. Most diuretics act directly on the kidneys, but there are different types of diuretics, each with different actions. Thus, therapy for high blood pressure can be individualized for each patient's specific needs.

Thiazide diuretics are the most commonly prescribed water pills available today. They are generally well tolerated, and can be taken once or twice a day. Since patients do not develop a tolerance to their anti-hypertensive effect, they can be taken for prolonged periods. However, a major drawback to thiazide diuretics is that they often deplete the body of potassium. This depletion can be compensated for with a potassium supplement. Potassium-rich foods and liquids, such as bananas, apricots, or orange juice, can also be used to help correct the potassium deficiency. Salt substitutes are another source of potassium.

Loop diuretics, such as furosemide, act more vigorously than thiazide diuretics. They promote more water loss, but also deplete more potassium.

To remove excess water from the body but retain its store of potassium, manufacturers developed potassium-sparing diuretics. Drugs such as spironolactone and amiloride are effective in treating potassium loss, heart failure, and hypertension. Potassium-sparing diuretics have been combined with thiazide diuretics in medications such as spironolactone and hydrochlorothiazide combination, triamterene and hydrochlorothiazide combination, and amiloride and hydrochlorothiazide combination. Such combinations enhance the anti-hypertensive effect and reduce the loss of potassium. They are now among the most commonly used anti-hypertensive agents.

Cardiac Glycosides

Cardiac glycosides include drugs that are derived from digitalis (for example, digoxin, digitoxin). They affect the heart rate, but are not strictly anti-arrhythmics. This type of drug slows the rate of the heart but increases its force of contraction. Cardiac glycosides therefore act as both heart depressants and stimulants, and may be used to regulate erratic heart rhythm or to increase heart output in heart failure.

Anti-Coagulants

Drugs that prevent blood clotting are called anti-coagulants (blood thinners). Anti-coagulants fall into two categories.

The first category contains only one drug, heparin. Heparin must be given by injection, so its use is generally restricted to hospitalized patients.

The second category includes oral anti-coagulants, principally derivatives of the drug warfarin. Warfarin may be used in the treatment of conditions such as stroke, heart disease, or abnormal blood clotting. It is also used to prevent the movement of a clot, which could cause serious problems. It acts by preventing the liver from manufacturing the proteins responsible for blood clot formation.

Persons taking warfarin must avoid using many other drugs (including aspirin), because their interaction with the anti-coagulant could cause internal bleeding. Patients taking warfarin should check with their pharmacist or physician before using any other medications, including over-the-counter products for coughs or colds. In addition, they must have blood samples checked frequently by their physician, to ensure that the drug is maintaining the correct degree of blood thinning.

Anti-Hyperlipidemics

Drugs used to treat atherosclerosis (arteriosclerosis, hardening of the arteries) act to reduce the cholesterol and triglycerides (fats) that form plaques (deposits) on the walls of arteries. Some anti-hyperlipidemics, such as cholestyramine and colestipol, bind to bile acids in the gastrointestinal tract, thereby decreasing the body's production of cholesterol. Clofibrate and probucol also decrease the body's production of cholesterol. Use of these drugs is in question; following a special low-fat diet and a good exercise program may be just as beneficial.

Vasodilators

Vasodilating drugs cause the blood vessels to widen. Some of the anti-hypertensive agents, such as hydralazine and prazosin, lower blood pressure by dilating the arteries or veins. Other vasodilators are used in the treatment of stroke and diseases characterized by poor circulation. Ergoloid mesylates, used to reduce the symptoms of senility, and papaverine, used in therapy after a stroke, are additional examples of vasodilating drugs.

Beta-Blockers

Beta-blocking drugs block the response of the heart

and blood vessels to nerve stimulation, in order to slow the heart rate and reduce high blood pressure. They are used in the treatment of angina, hypertension, and arrhythmias. Propranolol and metoprolol are two examples of beta-blockers.

Calcium Channel Blockers

Calcium channel blockers (diltiazem, nifedipine, verapamil) are used for the prevention of angina (chest pain). Verapamil is also useful in correcting certain arrhythmias (heartbeat irregularities). This group of drugs is thought to prevent angina or arrhythmias by blocking the effects of calcium on nerve transmission. This effect results in vasodilation and greater oxygen delivery to the heart muscle.

DRUGS FOR THE EARS

For an ear infection, a physician usually prescribes an antibiotic and a steroid, or a medication that contains a combination of these. The antibiotic attacks the infecting bacteria, and the steroid reduces the inflammation and pain. Often, a local anesthetic, such as benzocaine or lidocaine, may also be prescribed to relieve pain.

DRUGS FOR THE EYES

Almost all drugs that are used to treat eye problems can be used to treat disorders of other parts of the body as well.

Glaucoma is one of the major disorders of the eye, especially in people over 40 years of age. It is caused by increased pressure within the eyeball. Although sometimes treated surgically, the pressure in the eye can usually be reduced, and blindness prevented, through the use of eyedrops. Two drops frequently used are epinephrine and pilocarpine.

Pilocarpine is a cholinergic drug. Cholinergic drugs act by stimulating the body's parasympathetic nerve endings. These are nerve endings that assist in the control of the heart, lungs, bowels, and eyes. When used in the eyes, pilocarpine causes constriction of the pupils and increases the flow of fluid (aqueous humor) out of the eye, thereby reducing the pressure.

Epinephrine is an adrenergic agent. Drugs with adrenergic properties have actions similar to those of adrenalin. Adrenalin is a chemical that is secreted in the body when one must flee from danger, resist attack, or combat stress. Adrenalin increases the amount of sugar in the blood, accelerates the heartbeat, and dilates the pupils. The mechanism by which epinephrine lowers eye pressure is not completely understood, but it appears to involve both a decrease in production of aqueous humor, and an increase in the outflow of this fluid from the eye.

Antibiotics are used to treat bacterial eye infections. Steroids can also be used to treat non-infectious eye inflammations, as long as these medications are not used for too long a period of time. Pharmacists carefully monitor requests for eyedrop refills, particularly for drops that contain steroids, and may refuse to refill such medication until you have revisited your doctor, because these products can cause further eye problems with long-term use.

GASTROINTESTINAL DRUGS

Anti-Nauseants

Anti-nauseants reduce the urge to vomit. Perhaps the most effective anti-nauseant is a phenothiazine derivative such as prochlorperazine. This medication acts on the vomiting center in the brain. It is often administered rectally, and usually alleviates nausea and vomiting within a few minutes to an hour. Antihistamines are also commonly used to prevent nausea and vomiting, especially when those symptoms are due to motion sickness. This type of medication may also work at the vomiting center in the brain.

Anti-Cholinergics

Anti-cholinergic drugs—for example, dicyclomine— slow the action of the bowel and reduce the amount of stomach acid. Because these drugs slow the action of the bowel by relaxing the muscles and relieving spasms, they are said to have an anti-spasmodic action.

Anti-Ulcer Medications

Anti-ulcer medications are prescribed to relieve symptoms and to promote healing of peptic ulcers. The anti-secretory ulcer medications, cimetidine and ranitidine, work by suppressing the production of excess stomach acid. Another anti-ulcer drug, sucralfate, works by forming a chemical barrier over an exposed ulcer—rather like a "bandage"—thereby protecting the ulcer from stomach acid. These medications provide sustained relief from ulcer pain and promote healing.

Anti-Diarrheals

Diarrhea may be caused by many conditions, including influenza and ulcerative colitis, and can sometimes occur as a side effect of drug therapy. Narcotics and anti-cholinergics are used in the treatment of diarrhea because they slow the action of the bowel, alleviating diarrhea. A medication such as diphenoxylate and atropine contains both a narcotic and an anti-cholinergic.

HORMONES

A hormone is a substance produced and secreted by a gland. Hormones stimulate and regulate body functions. Hormone drugs are given to mimic the effects of naturally produced hormones.

Hormone drugs are prescribed to treat various conditions. Most often, they are used to replace naturally occurring hormones that are not being produced in amounts sufficient to regulate specific body functions. This category of medication also includes oral contraceptives and certain types of drugs that are used to combat inflammatory reactions.

Thyroid Drugs

Thyroid hormone was one of the first hormone drugs to be produced synthetically. Originally, thyroid preparations were made by drying and pulverizing the thyroid glands of animals, then forming them into tablets. Such preparations are still used today in the treatment of patients who have reduced levels of thyroid hormone production. However, a synthetic thyroid hormone (levothyroxine) is also available.

Anti-Diabetic Drugs

Insulin, which is secreted by the pancreas, regulates the level of sugar in the blood, as well as metabolism of carbohydrates and fats. Insulin's counterpart, glucagon, stimulates the liver to produce glucose (sugar). Both insulin and glucagon must be present in the right amounts to maintain proper blood sugar levels.

Treatment of diabetes (the condition in which the body is unable to produce and/or utilize insulin) may involve an adjustment of diet and/or the administration of insulin or oral anti-diabetic drugs. Glucagon is given only in emergencies (for example, insulin shock, when blood sugar levels must be raised quickly).

Oral anti-diabetic drugs induce the pancreas to secrete more insulin by acting on small groups of cells within the pancreas that make and store insulin. Oral anti-diabetic medications are prescribed for diabetic patients who are unable, by diet modification alone, to regulate their blood sugar levels. These drugs cannot be used by insulin-dependent (juvenile-onset, or Type I) diabetics—those diabetics who can control their blood sugar levels only with injections of insulin.

Steroids

The pituitary gland secretes adrenocorticotropic hormone (ACTH), which directs the adrenal glands to produce adrenocorticosteroids (for example, cortisone). Oral steroid preparations (for example, methylprednisolone) may be used to treat inflammatory diseases such as arthritis, or to treat poison ivy, hay fever, or insect bites. How these drugs relieve inflammation is currently unknown.

Steroids may also be applied to the skin to treat certain inflammatory skin conditions. Fluocinonide, hydrocortisone and iodochlorhydroxyquin combination, and triamcinolone are steroid hormone creams or ointments.

Sex Hormones

Although the adrenal glands secrete small amounts of sex hormones, these hormones are produced mainly by the sex glands. Estrogens are the female hormones responsible for secondary sex characteristics such as development of the breasts, maintenance of the lining of the uterus, and enlargement of the hips at puberty. Testosterone (also called androgen) is the corresponding male hormone. It is responsible for secondary sex characteristics such as beards and enlarged muscles. Progesterone is produced in females—it prepares the uterus for pregnancy.

Testesterone reduces elimination of protein from the body, thereby producing an increase in muscle size. Athletes sometimes take drugs called anabolic steroids (chemicals similar to testosterone) for this effect; but such use of these drugs is dangerous. Anabolic steroids can adversely affect the heart, nervous system, and kidneys.

Most oral contraceptives (birth control pills) combine estrogen and progesterone, but some contain only progesterone. The estrogen in birth control pills prevents egg production. Progesterone aids in preventing ovulation, alters the lining of the uterus, and thickens cervical mucus—processes that help to prevent conception and implantation. Oral contraceptives, while still used regularly, have many side effects, so their use should be discussed with a doctor.

Conjugated estrogens are used as replacement therapy to treat symptoms of menopause in women who are no longer producing sufficient amounts of estrogen. Medroxyprogesterone is used to treat uterine bleeding and menstrual problems. It prevents uterine bleeding by inducing and maintaining a lining in the uterus that resembles the lining produced during pregnancy. In addition, it suppresses the release of the pituitary gland hormone that initiates ovulation.

ANTI-INFECTIVES

Antibiotics

Antibiotics are used to treat a wide variety of bacterial infections. They are usually derived from molds or are produced synthetically. Antibiotics slow the growth of bacteria by interfering with their production of necessary nutrients, or by damaging their cell walls. The body's natural defenses then have a much easier time eliminating the infection.

When used properly, antibiotics are usually effective. To adequately treat an infection, antibiotics must be taken regularly for a specific period of time. If you do not take an antibiotic for the prescribed period, microorganisms resistant to the antibiotic are given the opportunity to continue growing, and your infection could recur. Aminoglycosides, cephalosporins, erythromycins, penicillins (including ampicillin and amoxicillin), and tetracyclines are some examples of antibiotics.

Antibiotics do not counteract viruses, such as those causing the common cold, so their use in cold therapy is irrational.

Anti-Virals

Anti-viral drugs are used to combat viral infections. A new anti-viral drug called acyclovir is being used in the management of herpes. Acyclovir reduces the reproduction of the herpes virus in initial outbreaks, lessens the number of recurring outbreaks, and speeds the healing of herpes blisters. However, this anti-viral drug does not cure herpes.

Vaccines

Vaccines were used long before antibiotics became available. A vaccine contains weakened or dead disease-causing microorganisms, which activate the body's immune system to produce a natural defense against a particular disease (such as polio or measles). A vaccine may be used to alleviate or treat an infectious disease, but most commonly it is used to prevent a specific disease.

Other Anti-Infectives

Drugs called anthelmintics are used to treat worm infestations. Fungal infections are treated with anti-fungals (such as nystatin)—drugs that destroy and prevent the growth of fungi.

A pediculocide is a drug used to treat a person infested with lice, and a scabicide is a preparation used to treat a person with scabies.

ANTI-NEOPLASTICS

Anti-neoplastic drugs are used in the treatment of cancer. Most of the drugs in this category prevent the growth of rapidly dividing cells, such as cancer cells. Anti-neoplastics are, without exception, extremely toxic, and can cause serious side effects. But for many cancer victims, the benefits received from chemotherapy with anti-neoplastic drugs far outweigh the risks involved

TOPICAL DRUGS

Drugs are often applied topically (locally to the skin) to treat skin disorders with minimal systemic (throughout the body) side effects. Antibiotic creams or ointments are used to treat skin infections; and adrenocorticosteroids are used to treat inflammatory skin conditions. Another common dermatologic (skin) problem is acne. Acne can be—and often is—treated with over-the-counter drugs, but it sometimes requires prescription medication. Antibiotics such as tetracycline, erythromycin, or clindamycin are used orally or applied topically to slow the growth of the bacteria responsible for acne pustules. Keratolytics, agents that soften the skin and cause the outer cells to slough off, are also sometimes prescribed.

Some drugs applied to the skin do have effects within the body. For example, nitroglycerin is absorbed into the bloodstream from ointment or patches placed on the skin. The absorbed nitroglycerin dilates blood vessels and prevents anginal pain.

CENTRAL NERVOUS SYSTEM DRUGS

Sedatives

Medications used in the treatment of anxiety or insomnia selectively reduce activity in the central nervous system (brain and spinal cord). Drugs that have a calming effect include barbiturates, chlordiazepoxide, clorazepate, diazepam, doxepin, hydroxyzine, meprobamate, and oxazepam. Drugs to induce sleep in insomniacs include butabarbital, flurazepam, temazepam, and triazolam.

Tranquilizers

Psychotics are usually prescribed major tranquilizers or anti-psychotic agents. These drugs calm certain areas of the brain but permit the rest of the brain to function normally. They act as a screen that allows transmission of some nerve impulses but restricts others. The drugs most frequently used are phenothiazines (such as chlorpromazine, thioridazine, and trifluoperazine). Haloperidol, a butyrophenone, has the same effect as chlorpromazine.

Psychotic patients sometimes become depressed. In such cases tricyclic (or tetracyclic) anti-depressants, such as amitriptyline, or monoamine oxidase (MAO) inhibitors are used to combat the depression.

Anti-depressants may produce dangerous side effects; they can interact with other drugs and even with foods. For example, monoamine oxidase (MAO) inhibitors can greatly increase blood pressure when taken with certain kinds of cheese or other foods or beverages, so they should be used very carefully.

Amphetamines

Amphetamines or adrenergic drugs are commonly used as anorectics, a category of drugs that are used to reduce the appetite. These drugs temporarily quiet the part of the brain that causes hunger, but they also keep people awake, speed up the heart, and raise blood pressure. After two to three weeks, these medications lose their effectiveness as appetite suppressants.

Amphetamines stimulate most people, but they have the opposite effect on a special group of people, hyperkinetic children. Hyperkinesis (the condition of being highly overactive) is difficult to diagnose or define, and requires a specialist to treat. When hyperkinetic children take amphetamines or the adrenergic methylphenidate, their activity slows down. Why amphetamines affect hyperkinetic children in this way is unknown. Most likely, they quiet these youngsters by selectively stimulating parts of the brain that ordinarily provide control of activity.

Anti-Convulsants

Drugs such as phenytoin and phenobarbital can effectively control most symptoms of epilepsy. They selectively reduce excessive stimulation in the brain.

Anti-Parkinson Agents

Parkinson's disease is a progressive disease that is due to a chemical imbalance in the brain. Victims of Parkinson's disease have uncontrollable tremors, develop a characteristic stoop, and eventually become unable to walk. Drugs such as benztropine, trihexyphenidyl, levodopa, and bromocriptine are used to correct the chemical imbalance, thereby relieving the symptoms of the disease. These drugs are also used to relieve tremors caused by other medications.

Analgesics

Pain is not a disease, but a symptom. Drugs used to relieve pain are called analgesics. These drugs form a rather diverse group. We do not fully understand how most analgesics work. Whether they all act on the brain, or whether some act outside the brain, is not known. Analgesics fall into two categories: they may either be narcotic or non-narcotic.

Narcotics are derived from the opium poppy. They act on the brain to cause deep analgesia and often drowsiness. Some narcotics relieve coughing spasms and are used in many cough syrups. Narcotics relieve pain and also give the patient a feeling of well-being. They are also addictive. Manufacturers have attempted to produce non-addictive synthetic narcotic derivatives, but have not yet been successful.

Many non-narcotic pain relievers are commonly used. Salicylates are the most commonly used pain relievers in the United States today. The most widely used salicylate is aspirin. While aspirin does not require a prescription, many doctors may prescribe it to treat such diseases as arthritis.

The aspirin substitute acetaminophen may be used in place of aspirin to relieve pain. It cannot, however, be

used to reduce inflammation (such as that caused by arthritis).

A number of analgesics contain codeine or other narcotics combined with non-narcotic analgesics (such as
aspirin or acetaminophen). These analgesics are not as
potent as pure narcotics, but frequently they are as effective. Because these medications contain narcotics, they
have the potential for abuse, and must therefore be used
with caution.

Anti-Inflammatory Drugs

Inflammation is the body's response to injury. It causes
swelling, pain, fever, redness, and itching. Aspirin is one
of the most effective anti-inflammatory drugs. Other
drugs—fenoprofen, ibuprofen, indomethacin, naproxen,
and tolmetin—relieve inflammation, and may be more
effective than aspirin in certain individuals. Steroids (see
above) are also used to treat inflammatory diseases.

When sore muscles tense they cause pain and inflammation. Skeletal muscle relaxants (such as orphenadrine,
aspirin, and caffeine combination; meprobamate and
aspirin combination; and chlorzoxazone and acetaminophen combination) can relieve the symptoms of inflammation. Skeletal muscle relaxants are often given in
combination with an anti-inflammatory drug such as aspirin. Some doctors believe that aspirin and rest are better
at alleviating the pain and inflammation of muscle strain
than are skeletal muscle relaxants.

RESPIRATORY DRUGS

Antitussives

Antitussives control coughs. There are numerous over-
the-counter (non-prescription) antitussives available.
Codeine is a narcotic antitussive that is an ingredient in
many prescription cough medications. These cough syrups must be absorbed into the blood, and must circulate
and act on the brain before they relieve a cough; they do
not "coat" the throat.

Expectorants

Expectorants are used to change a non-productive

cough to a productive one (one that brings up phlegm). Expectorants are supposed to increase the amount of mucus produced. However, no expectorant has been proven effective. Drinking water or using a vaporizer or humidifier is probably more effective in increasing mucus production. Popular expectorant products include ammonium chloride, bromdiphenhydramine, diphenhydramine, codeine, and potassium guaiacolsulfonate combination; and promethazine, potassium guaiacolsulfonate, and codeine combination.

Decongestants

Decongestants constrict the blood vessels in the nose and sinuses to open up air passages. Decongestants can be taken orally or as nose drops or spray. Oral decongestants are slow-acting, but do not interfere with the production of mucus or the movement of the cilia (special hair-like structures) of the respiratory tract. They can, however, increase blood pressure, so they should be used cautiously by patients with high blood pressure. Topical decongestants (nose drops or spray) provide almost immediate relief. They do not increase blood pressure as much as oral decongestants, but they do slow the movement of the cilia.

People who use these products may also develop a tolerance for them. Tolerance can be described as a need for ever-increasing dosages to achieve the same beneficial effect—while at the same time developing an ever-increasing risk of side effects. Consequently, topical decongestants should not be used for more than a few days at a time.

Bronchodilators

Bronchodilators (agents that open airways in the lungs) and smooth muscle relaxants (agents that relax smooth muscle tissue—such as that in the lungs) are used to improve breathing. Theophylline and aminophylline are commonly used to relieve the symptoms of asthma and pulmonary emphysema.

Anti-Allergy Medications

Histamine is a body chemical that, when released in

the body, typically causes swelling and itching. Antihistamines counteract these symptoms of allergy by blocking the effects of histamine. For mild respiratory allergies, such as hay fever, antihistamines can be used. Diphenhydramine and other antihistamines are relatively slow-acting. Severe allergic reactions sometimes require the use of epinephrine; in its injectable form it is very fast-acting.

VITAMINS AND MINERALS

Vitamins and minerals are chemical substances vital to the maintenance of normal body function. Some people have vitamin deficiencies, but most people obtain enough vitamins and minerals in their diet. Serious nutritional deficiencies lead to diseases such as pellagra and beri-beri, which must be treated by a physician. People who have an inadequate or restricted diet, those with certain disorders or debilitating illnesses, women who are pregnant or breastfeeding, and some others may benefit from taking supplemental vitamins and minerals. However, even these people should consult a doctor to see if a true vitamin deficiency exists.

Drug Profiles

On the following pages are drug profiles for the most commonly prescribed drugs, as well as a few selected over-the-counter medications. These profiles are arranged alphabetically according to generic name.

A drug profile summarizes the most important information about a particular drug. By studying a drug profile, you will learn what to expect from your medication, when to be concerned about possible side effects, which drugs interact with the drug you are taking, and how to take the drug to achieve its maximum benefit. Each profile includes the following information:

generic name

The drugs profiled in this book are listed by generic names. You should know both the generic and trade names of ALL of the medications you are taking. If you don't know the contents of your medication, check with your pharmacist.

BRAND NAMES (Manufacturers)
The most common trade names of each generic product are listed, along with the manufacturer's name. Not every available trade name is included, but as many as possible have been listed. "Various manufacturers" is listed for some of the generic names—this indicates that there are generic products available.

TYPE OF DRUG
The chemical or pharmacological class or pharmacological effect is listed for each generic drug.

INGREDIENTS
The components of each drug product are itemized. Many drugs contain several active chemical components; all are included under this category.

DOSAGE FORMS
The most common forms (i.e., tablets, capsules, liquid, or suppository) of each profiled drug are listed. Strengths or concentrations are also provided.

STORAGE
Storage requirements for each of the dosage forms listed are discussed. These directions should be followed carefully, in order to ensure the potency of your medications.

USES
It is important that you understand why you are taking each of your medications. This category includes the most important and most common clinical uses for each drug profiled. Your doctor may prescribe a drug for a reason that does not appear in this list. The exclusion does not mean that your doctor has made an error. However, if the use for which you are taking a drug does not appear in this category, and if you have any questions concerning the reason for which the drug was prescribed, consult your doctor. A description of how the drug is thought to work is also provided in this section.

TREATMENT
Instructions are provided on how to take each profiled medication, in order to obtain its maximum benefit. Information can be found on whether or not the drug can be taken with food; how to apply the ointment, cream, ear drops, or eye drops; how to insert suppositories; and recommendations for what to do if you miss a dose of your medication.

SIDE EFFECTS
Minor. The most common and least serious reactions to a drug are listed in this section. Most of these side effects, if they occur, disappear in a day or two. Do not expect to experience these side effects, but if they occur and are particularly annoying, do not hesitate to seek medical advice.

Suggestions for how to prevent or relieve some of these side effects are also provided.

Major. Major side effects are less common than minor side effects, and you will probably never experience them. However, should any of the reactions listed under this section occur, you should call your doctor. These reactions indicate that something may be going wrong with your drug therapy. You may have developed an allergy to the drug, or some other problem could have occurred. If you experience a major side effect, it may be necessary to adjust your dosage or to substitute a different medication in your treatment.

Keep in mind that new side effects are being reported daily. If you experience a reaction that is bothersome or severe, consult your doctor immediately, even if the side effect is not listed.

INTERACTIONS

This category lists the medications (both prescription and over-the-counter drugs) and foods that can interact with the profiled drug. Certain drugs are safe when used alone, but may cause serious reactions when taken in combination with other drugs or chemicals, or with certain foods. A description of how the profiled drug interacts with other drugs or foods, and what to expect if the two are taken together, is also provided. Keep in mind that not all possible drug combinations have been tested. It is therefore important that your doctors and pharmacist be aware of ALL of the drugs you are taking (both prescription and over-the-counter).

WARNINGS

This section lists the precautions necessary for safe use of the profiled drug. It provides information on drugs that should be avoided if you have had a previous allergy or severe drug reaction, and the conditions or disease states that require close monitoring while this drug is being taken.

In this section you will also find out whether the profiled drug is likely to affect your driving ability, whether you are likely to become tolerant to its effects, if it is dangerous to stop the drug abruptly, and if you should discuss with your doctor stopping the drug before having surgery.

Certain individuals are allergic to F.D. & C. Yellow Dye No. 5 (tartrazine). This section provides information on the tartrazine content of the various dosage forms.

Other information included in this category might concern supplemental therapy—drinking extra fluids while treating a urinary tract infection, or wearing cotton panties while treating a vaginal infection.

A discussion of the known risks of this drug during pregnancy or while breastfeeding an infant is provided. It should be kept in mind that for the majority of drugs available, the risks to a fetus or to a nursing infant are not known. Experiments are not usually conducted on pregnant women and infants (for ethical reasons). You should therefore discuss the risks and benefits of any particular drug therapy with your doctor if you are pregnant or planning to become pregnant, or are nursing an infant.

Accutane—see isotretinoin

Aceta with Codeine—see acetaminophen and codeine combination

---

acetaminophen and codeine combination

BRAND NAMES (Manufacturers)
acetaminophen with codeine (various manufacturers)
Aceta with Codeine (Century)
Anacin-3 with Codeine (Ayerst)
Bayapap with Codeine (Bay)
Capital with Codeine (Carnick)
Codap (Reid-Provident)
Empracet with Codeine (Burroughs Wellcome)
Panadol with Codeine (Winthrop)
Phenaphen with Codeine (Robins)
Proval (Reid-Provident)
SK-APAP with Codeine (Smith Kline & French)
Tylenol with Codeine (McNeil)
Ty-Tab (Major)
   Note that, on the label of the vial of tablets or capsules, the name of this drug is followed by a number. This number refers to the amount of codeine present. Hence, #1 contains ⅛ grain (gr) or 7.5 mg codeine; #2 has ¼ grain (15 mg); #3 has ½ grain (30 mg); and #4 contains 1 grain (60 mg) of codeine.

TYPE OF DRUG
Analgesic combination (pain reliever)

INGREDIENTS
acetaminophen and codeine as the phosphate salt

DOSAGE FORMS
Tablets (300 mg acetaminophen with 7.5 mg, 15 mg, 30 mg, or 60 mg codeine; 325 mg acetaminophen with 15 mg, 30 mg, or 60 mg codeine; and 650 mg acetaminophen with 30 mg codeine)
Capsules (300 mg acetaminophen with 30 mg or 60 mg codeine)

Oral elixir (120 mg acetaminophen and 12 mg codeine
    per 5 ml teaspoonful with 7% alcohol)
STORAGE
Acetaminophen and codeine tablets, capsules, and oral
elixir should be stored at room temperature. This medication should never be frozen.

USES
Acetaminophen and codeine is used to relieve mild to
severe pain (formulations with higher codeine contents
are used to relieve more severe pain). Codeine is a narcotic analgesic that acts on the central nervous system
(brain and spinal cord) to relieve pain.

TREATMENT
In order to avoid stomach upset, you can take this medication with food or milk.
    This medication works most effectively if you take it at
the onset of pain, rather than waiting until the pain becomes intense.
    Measure the dose of the liquid form of this medication
carefully, with a specially designed, 5 ml measuring
spoon. An ordinary kitchen teaspoon is not accurate
enough.
    If you are taking this medication on a regular schedule
and you miss a dose, take the missed dose as soon as
possible, unless it is almost time for the next dose. In that
case, don't take the missed dose at all; just return to your
regular dosing schedule. Do not double the next dose.

SIDE EFFECTS
Minor. Constipation; dizziness; drowsiness; dry mouth;
false sense of well-being; flushing; light-headedness; loss
of appetite; nausea; rash; sweating; and painful or difficult urination. These side effects should disappear in
several days, as your body adjusts to the medication.
    If you are constipated, increase the amount of fiber
in your diet (raw vegetables, fruits, salads, bran, and
whole-grain breads) and drink more water (unless your
doctor directs you to do otherwise).
    Chew sugarless gum, or suck on ice chips or a piece of
hard candy to reduce mouth dryness.

If you feel dizzy, light-headed, or nauseated, sit or lie down awhile; get up from a sitting or lying position slowly, and be careful on stairs.

Major. Tell your doctor about any side effects that are persistent or particularly bothersome. IT IS ESPECIALLY IMPORTANT TO TELL YOUR DOCTOR about anxiety; unusual bleeding or bruising; difficulty breathing; excitation; fatigue; palpitations; restlessness; sore throat and fever; tremors; weakness; or yellowing of the eyes or skin

INTERACTIONS

This medication interacts with several other types of drugs.

1. Concurrent use of it with other central nervous system depressants (drugs that slow the activity of the nervous system), such as antihistamines, barbiturates, benzodiazepine tranquilizers, muscle relaxants, phenothiazine tranquilizers, and alcohol, or with tricyclic anti-depressants can cause extreme drowsiness.

2. A monoamine oxidase (MAO) inhibitor taken within 14 days of this medication can lead to unpredictable and severe side effects.

3. Long-term use and high doses of the acetaminophen portion of this medication can increase the effects of oral anti-coagulants (blood thinners, such as warfarin); this combination may lead to bleeding complications.

4. Anti-convulsants (anti-seizure medications), barbiturates, and alcohol can increase the liver toxicity caused by large doses of the acetaminophen portion of this medication.

TELL YOUR DOCTOR if you are currently taking any of the medications listed above.

WARNINGS

• Tell your doctor about unusual or allergic reactions you have had to any medications, especially to acetaminophen, codeine, or other narcotic analgesics (such as hydrocodone, hydromorphone, meperidine, methadone, morphine, oxycodone, or propoxyphene).

• Tell your doctor if you now have, or if you have ever had, acute abdominal conditions, asthma, blood disorders, brain disease, colitis, epilepsy, gallstones or gall-bladder disease, head injuries, heart disease, kidney disease, liver disease, lung disease, mental illness, prostate disease, thyroid disease, or urethral strictures.

• If this drug makes you dizzy or drowsy, do not take part in any activity that requires alertness, such as driving a car or operating potentially dangerous equipment.

• Before having any surgery or other medical or dental treatment, be sure to tell your doctor or dentist that you are taking this medication.

• Because this product contains codeine, it has the potential for abuse, and must be used with caution. Usually, it should not be taken on a regular schedule for longer than ten days at a time. Tolerance develops quickly; do not increase the dosage or stop taking the drug abruptly, unless you first consult your doctor. If you have been taking large amounts of this medication for long periods, you may experience a withdrawal reaction (muscle aches, diarrhea, gooseflesh, runny nose, nausea, vomiting, shivering, trembling, stomach cramps, sleep disorders, irritability, weakness, yawning, and sweating). Your doctor may therefore want to reduce the dosage gradually.

• Be sure to tell your doctor if you are pregnant. The effects of this medication during pregnancy have not yet been thoroughly studied in humans. Codeine, used regularly in large doses during pregnancy, can result in addiction of the fetus, leading to withdrawal symptoms (irritability, excessive crying, tremors, fever, vomiting, diarrhea, sneezing, and yawning) at birth. Also, tell your doctor if you are breastfeeding an infant. Small amounts of this medication may pass into breast milk and cause excessive drowsiness in the nursing infant.

---

acetaminophen and hydrocodone combination

BRAND NAMES (Manufacturers)
Amacodone (Trimen)
Bancap HC (O'Neal)

Co-Gesic (Central)
Dolo-Pap (T.E. Williams)
Duradyne DHC (O'Neal)
Hycodaphen (Ascher)
Hydrogesic (Edwards)
Lortab (Russ)
Norcet (Holloway)
T-Gesic Forte (T.E. Williams)
Vicodin (Knoll)

TYPE OF DRUG

Analgesic combination (pain reliever)

INGREDIENTS

acetaminophen and hydrocodone as the bitartrate salt

DOSAGE FORMS

Tablets (500 mg acetaminophen with 5 mg or 7 mg hydrocodone; 650 mg acetaminophen with 7.5 mg hydrocodone; and 1000 mg acetaminophen with 7.5 mg hydrocodone)

Capsules (500 mg acetaminophen with 5 mg hydrocodone)

STORAGE

Acetaminophen and hydrocodone tablets and capsules should be stored at room temperature in tightly closed, light-resistant containers.

USES

This medication is used to relieve moderate to severe pain. Hydrocodone is a narcotic analgesic that acts on the central nervous system (brain and spinal cord) to relieve pain.

TREATMENT

In order to avoid stomach upset, you can take this medication with food or milk.

This medication works most effectively if you take it at the onset of pain, rather than waiting until the pain becomes intense.

If you are taking this medication on a regular schedule and you miss a dose, take the missed dose as soon as possible, unless it is almost time for your next dose. In that case, don't take the missed dose at all; just return to your regular dosing schedule. Do not double the next dose.

SIDE EFFECTS

Minor. Constipation; dizziness; dry mouth; false sense of well-being; flushing; light-headedness; loss of appetite; nausea; rash; sweating; and painful or difficult urination. These side effects should disappear in several days, as your body adjusts to the medication.

If you are constipated, increase the amount of fiber in your diet (raw vegetables, fruits, salads, bran, and whole-grain breads) and drink more water (unless your doctor directs you to do otherwise).

Chew sugarless gum, or suck on ice chips or a piece of hard candy to reduce mouth dryness.

If you feel dizzy, light-headed, or nauseated, sit or lie down awhile; get up from a sitting or lying position slowly, and be careful on stairs.

Major. Tell your doctor about any side effects that are persistent or particularly bothersome. IT IS ESPECIALLY IMPORTANT TO TELL YOUR DOCTOR about anxiety; unusual bleeding or bruising; difficulty breathing; excitation; fatigue; palpitations; restlessness; sore throat and fever; tremors; weakness; or yellowing of the eyes or skin.

INTERACTIONS

This medication interacts with several other drugs.

1. Concurrent use of this medication with other central nervous system depressants (drugs that slow the activity of the nervous system), such as antihistamines, barbiturates, benzodiazepine tranquilizers, muscle relaxants, phenothiazine tranquilizers, and alcohol, or with tricyclic anti-depressants can cause extreme drowsiness.

2. A monoamine oxidase (MAO) inhibitor taken within 14 days of this medication can lead to unpredictable and severe side effects.

3. Long-term use and high doses of the acetaminophen portion of this medication can increase the effects of oral anti-coagulants (blood thinners, such as warfarin); this combination may lead to bleeding complications.

4. Anti-convulsants (anti-seizure medications), barbiturates, and alcohol can increase the liver toxicity caused by large doses of the acetaminophen portion of this medication.

TELL YOUR DOCTOR if you are currently taking any of the medications listed above.

WARNINGS

• Tell your doctor about unusual or allergic reactions you have had to any medications, especially to acetaminophen, hydrocodone, or other narcotic analgesics (such as codeine, hydromorphone, meperidine, methadone, morphine, oxycodone, or propoxyphene).

• Tell your doctor if you now have, or if you have ever had, acute abdominal conditions, asthma, blood disorders, brain disease, colitis, epilepsy, gallstones or gallbladder disease, head injuries, heart disease, kidney disease, liver disease, lung disease, mental illness, prostate disease, thyroid disease, or urethral strictures.

• If this drug makes you dizzy or drowsy, do not take part in any activity that requires alertness, such as driving a car or operating potentially dangerous equipment.

• Before having any surgery or other medical or dental treatment, be sure to tell your doctor or dentist that you are taking this medication.

• Because this product contains hydrocodone, it has the potential for abuse, and must be used with caution. Usually, it should not be taken on a regular schedule for longer than ten days at a time. Tolerance develops quickly; do not increase the dosage or stop taking the drug abruptly, unless you first consult your doctor. If you have been taking large amounts of this medication for long periods, you may experience a withdrawal reaction (muscle aches, diarrhea, gooseflesh, runny nose, nausea, vomiting, shivering, trembling, stomach cramps, sleep disorders, irritability, weakness, yawning, and sweating). Your doctor may therefore want to reduce the dosage gradually.

• Be sure to tell your doctor if you are pregnant. The effects of this medication during pregnancy have not yet been thoroughly studied in humans. Hydrocodone, used regularly in large doses during pregnancy, can result in addiction of the fetus, leading to withdrawal symptoms (irritability, excessive crying, tremors, fever, vomiting, diarrhea, sneezing, and yawning) at birth. Also, tell your doctor if you are breastfeeding an infant. Small amounts of this medication may pass into breast milk and cause excessive drowsiness in the nursing infant.

---

acetaminophen and oxycodone combination

BRAND NAMES (Manufacturers)
oxycodone hydrochloride with acetaminophen (various manufacturers)
Percocet-5 (Endo)
SK-Oxycodone with Acetaminophen (Smith Kline & French)
Tylox (McNeil)
TYPE OF DRUG
Analgesic combination (pain reliever)
INGREDIENTS
acetaminophen and oxycodone as the hydrochloride or terephthalate salt
DOSAGE FORM
Tablets (325 mg acetaminophen and 5 mg oxycodone; 325 mg acetaminophen, 4.5 mg oxycodone hydrochloride, and 0.38 mg oxycodone terephthalate)
STORAGE
Acetaminophen and oxycodone tablets should be stored at room temperature in a tightly closed container

USES
This medication is used to relieve moderate to severe pain. Oxycodone is a narcotic analgesic that acts on the central nervous system (brain and spinal cord) to relieve pain.

TREATMENT
In order to avoid stomach upset, you can take this medication with food or milk.

This medication works most effectively if you take it at the onset of pain, rather than waiting until the pain becomes intense.

If you are taking this medication on a regular schedule and you miss a dose, take the missed dose as soon as possible, unless it is close to the time for your next dose. In that case, don't take the missed dose at all; just return to your regular dosing schedule. Do not double the next dose.

SIDE EFFECTS

Minor. Constipation; dizziness; drowsiness; dry mouth; false sense of well-being; flushing; light-headedness; loss of appetite; nausea; rash; sweating; and painful or difficult urination. These side effects should disappear in several days, as your body adjusts to the medication.

If you are constipated, increase the amount of fiber in your diet (raw vegetables, fruits, salads, bran, and whole-grain breads) and drink more water (unless your doctor directs you to do otherwise).

Chew sugarless gum, or suck on ice chips or a piece of hard candy, to reduce mouth dryness.

If you feel dizzy, light-headed, or nauseated, sit or lie down awhile; get up from a sitting or lying position slowly, and be careful on stairs.

Major. Tell your doctor about any side effects that are persistent or particularly bothersome. IT IS ESPECIALLY IMPORTANT TO TELL YOUR DOCTOR about anxiety; unusual bleeding or bruising; difficulty breathing; excitation; fatigue; palpitations; restlessness; sore throat and fever; tremors; weakness; or yellowing of the eyes or skin.

INTERACTIONS

This medication interacts with several other types of drugs.

1. Concurrent use of this medication with other central nervous system depressants (drugs that slow the activity of the nervous system), such as antihistamines, barbiturates, benzodiazepine tranquilizers, muscle relaxants, phenothiazine tranquilizers, and alcohol, or with tricyclic anti-depressants can cause extreme drowsiness.

2. A monoamine oxidase (MAO) inhibitor taken within 14 days of this medication can lead to unpredictable and severe side effects.

3. Long-term use and high doses of the acetaminophen portion of this medication can increase the effects of oral anti-coagulants (blood thinners, such as warfarin); this combination may lead to bleeding complications.

4. Anti-convulsants (anti-seizure medications), barbiturates, and alcohol can increase the liver toxicity caused by large doses of the acetaminophen portion of this medication.

TELL YOUR DOCTOR if you are currently taking any of the medications listed above.

WARNINGS

• Tell your doctor about unusual or allergic reactions you have had to any medications, especially to acetaminophen, oxycodone, or other narcotic analgesics (such as codeine, hydrocodone, hydromorphone, meperidine, methadone, morphine, or propoxyphene).

• Tell your doctor if you now have, or if you have ever had, acute abdominal conditions, asthma, blood disorders, brain disease, colitis, epilepsy, gallstones or gallbladder disease, head injuries, heart disease, kidney disease, liver disease, lung disease, mental illness, prostate disease, thyroid disease, or urethral strictures.

• If this drug makes you dizzy or drowsy, do not take part in any activity that requires alertness, such as driving a car or operating potentially dangerous equipment.

• Before having any surgery or other medical or dental treatment, be sure to tell your doctor or dentist that you are taking this medication.

• Because this product contains oxycodone, it has the potential for abuse, and must be used with caution. Usually, it should not be taken on a regular schedule for longer than ten days at a time. Tolerance develops quickly; do not increase the dosage or stop taking the drug abruptly, unless you first consult your doctor. If you have been taking large amounts of this medication for long periods, you may experience a withdrawal reaction (muscle aches, diarrhea, gooseflesh, runny nose, nausea, vomiting, shivering, trembling, stomach cramps, sleep disorders, irritability, weakness, yawning, and sweating). Your doctor may therefore want to reduce the dosage gradually.

• Be sure to tell your doctor if you are pregnant. The effects of this medication during pregnancy have not yet been thoroughly studied in humans. Oxycodone, used regularly in large doses during pregnancy, can result in addiction of the fetus, leading to withdrawal symptoms (irritability, excessive crying, tremors, fever, vomiting, diarrhea, sneezing, and yawning) at birth. Also, tell your doctor if you are breastfeeding an infant. Small amounts of this medication may pass into breast milk and cause excessive drowsiness in the nursing infant.

---

acetaminophen and propoxyphene combination

BRAND NAMES (Manufacturers)
Darvocet-N (Lilly)
Dolacet (Hauck)
Dolene AP-65 (Lederle)
propoxyphene hydrochloride with acetaminophen (various manufacturers)
SK-65 APAP (Smith Kline & French)
Wygesic (Wyeth)

TYPE OF DRUG
Analgesic combination (pain reliever)

INGREDIENTS
acetaminophen and propoxyphene as the hydrochloride or napsylate salt

DOSAGE FORMS
Tablets (325 mg acetaminophen with 50 mg or 100 mg propoxyphene napsylate; 650 mg acetaminophen with 100 mg propoxyphene napsylate; 650 mg acetaminophen with 65 mg propoxyphene hydrochloride)
Capsules (650 mg acetaminophen with 65 mg propoxyphene hydrochloride)

STORAGE
Acetaminophen and propoxyphene tablets and capsules should be stored at room temperature in tightly closed containers.

USES
This medication is used to relieve moderate to severe

pain. Propoxyphene is a narcotic analgesic that acts on the central nervous system (brain and spinal cord) to relieve pain.

TREATMENT

In order to avoid stomach upset, you can take this medication with food or milk.

This medication works most effectively if you take it at the onset of pain, rather than waiting until the pain becomes intense.

SIDE EFFECTS

Minor. Constipation; dizziness; drowsiness; dry mouth; false sense of well-being; flushing; light-headedness; loss of appetite; nausea; rash; sweating; and painful or difficult urination. These side effects should disappear in several days, as your body adjusts to the medication.

If you are constipated, increase the amount of fiber in your diet (raw vegetables, fruits, salads, bran, and whole-grain breads) and drink more water (unless your doctor directs you to do otherwise).

Chew sugarless gum, or suck on ice chips or a piece of hard candy to reduce mouth dryness.

If you feel dizzy, light-headed, or nauseated, sit or lie down awhile; get up from a sitting or lying position slowly, and be careful on stairs.

Major. Tell your doctor about any side effects that are persistent or particularly bothersome. IT IS ESPECIALLY IMPORTANT TO TELL YOUR DOCTOR about anxiety; unusual bleeding or bruising; difficulty breathing; excitation; fatigue; palpitations; restlessness; sore throat and fever; tremors; weakness; or yellowing of the eyes or skin.

INTERACTIONS

This medication interacts with several other types of drugs.

1. Concurrent use of this medication with other central nervous system depressants (drugs that slow the activity of the nervous system), such as antihistamines, barbiturates, benzodiazepine tranquilizers, muscle relaxants, phenothiazine tranquilizers, and alcohol, or with tricyclic anti-depressants can cause extreme drowsiness.

2. A monoamine oxidase (MAO) inhibitor taken within 14 days of this medication can lead to unpredictable and severe side effects.

3. Long-term use and high doses of the acetaminophen portion of this medication can increase the effects of oral anti-coagulants (blood thinners, such as warfarin); this combination may lead to bleeding complications.

4. Anti-convulsants (anti-seizure medication), barbiturates, and alcohol can increase the liver toxicity caused by large doses of the acetaminophen portion of this medication.

5. The propoxyphene portion of this medication decreases the elimination of carbamazepine from the body, which can lead to an increase in side effects.

TELL YOUR DOCTOR if you are currently taking any of the medications listed above.

WARNINGS

• Tell your doctor about unusual or allergic reactions you have had to any medications, especially to acetaminophen, propoxyphene, or other narcotic analgesics (such as codeine, hydrocodone, hydromorphone, meperidine, methadone, morphine, or oxycodone).

• Tell your doctor if you now have, or if you have ever had, acute abdominal conditions, asthma, blood disorders, brain disease, colitis, epilepsy, gallstones or gallbladder disease, head injuries, heart disease, kidney disease, liver disease, lung disease, mental illness, prostate disease, thyroid disease, or urethral strictures.

• If this drug makes you dizzy or drowsy, do not take part in any activity that requires alertness, such as driving a car or operating potentially dangerous equipment.

• Before having any surgery or other medical or dental treatment, be sure to tell your doctor or dentist that you are taking this medication.

• Because this product contains propoxyphene, it has the potential for abuse, and must be used with caution. Usually, it should not be taken on a regular schedule for longer than ten days at a time. Tolerance develops quickly; do not increase the dosage or stop taking the drug abruptly, unless you first consult your doctor. If you have been taking large amounts of this medication for long periods, you may experience a withdrawal reaction (muscle aches, diarrhea, gooseflesh, runny nose, nausea, vomiting, shivering, trembling, stomach cramps, sleep disorders, irritability, weakness, yawning, and sweating). Your doctor may therefore want to reduce the dosage gradually.

• Be sure to tell your doctor if you are pregnant. The effects of this medication during pregnancy have not yet been thoroughly studied in humans. Propoxyphene, used regularly in large doses during pregnancy, can result in addiction of the fetus, leading to withdrawal symptoms (irritability, excessive crying, tremors, fever, vomiting, diarrhea, sneezing, and yawning) at birth. Also, tell your doctor if you are breastfeeding an infant. Small amounts of this medication may pass into breast milk and cause excessive drowsiness in the nursing infant.

acetohexamide

BRAND NAME (Manufacturer)
Dymelor (Lilly)
TYPE OF DRUG
Oral anti-diabetic
INGREDIENT
acetohexamide
DOSAGE FORM
Tablets (250 mg and 500 mg)
STORAGE
This medication should be stored at room temperature in a tightly closed container.

USES

Acetohexamide is used for the treatment of diabetes mellitus (sugar diabetes) that appears in adulthood and cannot be managed by control of diet alone. This type of diabetes is known as noninsulin-dependent diabetes (sometimes called maturity-onset or Type II diabetes). Acetohexamide lowers blood sugar by increasing the release of insulin from the pancreas.

TREATMENT

In order for this medication to work correctly, it must be taken as directed by your doctor. It is best to take this medicine at the same time each day, in order to maintain a constant blood sugar level. It is important, therefore, to try not to miss any doses of this medication. If you do miss a dose, take it as soon as possible, unless it is almost time for the next dose. In that case, do not take the missed dose at all; just return to your regular dosing schedule. Do not double the next dose. Tell your doctor if you feel any side effects from missing a dose of this drug.

Diabetics who are taking oral anti-diabetic medication may need to be switched to insulin if they develop diabetic coma, have a severe infection, are scheduled for major surgery, or are pregnant.

SIDE EFFECTS

Minor. Diarrhea; headache; heartburn; loss of appetite; nausea; vomiting; or stomach pain or discomfort. These side effects usually disappear during treatment, as your body adjusts to this medication.

Major. If any side effects are persistent or particularly bothersome, it is important to notify your doctor. IT IS ESPECIALLY IMPORTANT TO TELL YOUR DOCTOR about dark urine; fatigue; itching of the skin; light-colored stools; sore throat and fever; unusual bleeding or bruising; or yellowing of the eyes or skin.

INTERACTIONS

Acetohexamide interacts with other medications.

1. Chloramphenicol; guanethidine; insulin; monoamine oxidase (MAO) inhibitors; oxyphenbutazone; oxytetracycline; phenylbutazone; probenecid; aspirin or other salicylates; and sulfonamide antibiotics, when combined with acetohexamide, can lower blood sugar levels—sometimes to dangerously low levels.

2. Thyroid hormones; dextrothyroxine; epinephrine; phenytoin; thiazide diuretics (water pills); and cortisone-like medications (dexamethasone, hydrocortisone, prednisone) combined with acetohexamide can actually increase blood sugar levels—just what you are trying to avoid.

3. Oral anti-diabetic medications can increase the effects of warfarin, which can lead to bleeding complications.

4. Beta-blocking medications (such as atenolol, metoprolol, nadolol, pindolol, propranolol, and timolol) combined with acetohexamide can result in either high or low blood sugar levels. Beta-blockers can also mask the symptoms of low blood sugar, which can be dangerous.

BE SURE TO TELL YOUR DOCTOR if you are already taking any of the medications listed above

WARNINGS

- It is important to tell your doctor if you have ever had an unusual or allergic reaction to this medicine or to any sulfa medication [sulfonamide antibiotics, diuretics (water pills), or other oral anti-diabetics].

- It is also important to tell your doctor if you now have, or have ever had, kidney disease, liver disease, severe infection, or thyroid disease.

- It is important to follow the special diet that your doctor gave you. This is an important part of controlling your blood sugar and is necessary in order for this medicine to work properly.

- Avoid drinking alcoholic beverages while taking this medication (unless otherwise directed by your doctor). Some patients who take this medicine suffer nausea; vomiting; dizziness; stomach pain; pounding headache; sweating; and redness of the face and skin when they drink alcohol. Also, large amounts of alcohol can lower blood sugar to dangerously low levels.

- Be sure to tell your doctor or dentist that you are taking this medicine, before having surgery or any other medical or dental treatment.

- Test for sugar in your urine as directed by your doctor. It is a convenient way to determine whether or not your diabetes is being controlled by this medicine.

- Acetohexamide may increase your sensitivity to sunlight. It is therefore important to use caution during exposure to the sun. You may want to wear protective clothing and sunglasses. Use an effective sunscreen, and avoid exposure to sunlamps.

• Eat or drink something containing sugar right away if you experience any symptoms of low blood sugar (such as anxiety; chills; cold sweats; cool or pale skin; drowsiness; excessive hunger; headache; nausea; nervousness; rapid heartbeat; or shakiness, unusual tiredness, or weakness). It is important that your family and friends know the symptoms of low blood sugar and what to do if they observe any of these symptoms in you.

Check with your doctor—even if these symptoms are corrected by the sugar, it is important to contact your doctor as soon as possible. The blood-sugar-lowering effects of this medicine can last for hours, and the symptoms may return during this period. Good sources of sugar are orange juice, corn syrup, honey, sugar cubes, and table sugar. You are at greatest risk of developing low blood sugar if you skip or delay meals, exercise more than usual, cannot eat because of nausea or vomiting, or drink large amounts of alcohol.

• Be sure to tell your doctor if you are pregnant. Studies in animals have shown that this type of medicine can cause birth defects. Studies have not yet been completed in humans. It is also important to tell your doctor if you are breastfeeding an infant. Small amounts of acetohexamide may pass into breast milk.

Achromycin V—see tetracycline

Acillin—see ampicillin

Actacin-C—see pseudoephedrine, tripolidine, guaifenesin, and codeine combination

Actamine-C—see pseudoephedrine, tripolidine, guaifenesin, and codeine combination

Acticort 100—see hydrocortisone (topical)

Actifed-C—see pseudoephedrine, tripolidine, guaifenesin, and codeine combination

Actrapid—see insulin

acyclovir

BRAND NAME (Manufacturer)
Zovirax (Burroughs Wellcome)
TYPE OF DRUG
Anti-viral
INGREDIENT
acyclovir
DOSAGE FORM
Ointment (5%)
STORAGE
Acyclovir ointment should be stored in a cool, dry place

USES

Acyclovir is used to treat genital herpes and herpes infections of the skin. Acyclovir prevents the growth and multiplication of the *Herpes* virus. This drug does not cure a herpes infection, but may relieve the pain associated with the viral infection, and may shorten its duration.

TREATMENT

Wash the infected area with soap and water, then allow it to dry. Apply acyclovir as soon as possible after the symptoms of a herpes infection begin. In order to avoid spreading the infection, use a rubber glove or a finger cot to apply the ointment. Apply enough acyclovir to cover the entire area of the infection.

Be sure to complete the full course of therapy (usually about ten days), even if your symptoms disappear before the end of this period.

If you miss a dose of this medication, apply the missed dose as soon as possible. However, if you do not remember until it is almost time for the next dose, do not apply the missed dose at all; just return to your regular dosing schedule. Do not use a double dose of the medication at the next application.

SIDE EFFECTS

Minor. You may experience temporary pain, burning, stinging, itching, or rash when this medication is applied. This sensation should disappear in several days, as your body adjusts to the medication.

Major. Tell your doctor about any side effects that are persistent or particularly bothersome.

INTERACTIONS
Acyclovir does not interact with other medications, if it is used according to directions.

WARNINGS
• Tell your doctor about unusual or allergic reactions you have had to any medications, especially to acyclovir.
• Acyclovir ointment is intended for use on the skin only; it should not be used in the eyes.
• Try to avoid sexual activity while you have signs or symptoms of genital herpes; this medication does not prevent the transmission of herpes to other individuals, nor does it prevent recurrences.
• This medication has been prescribed for your current infection only. Another infection later on, or one that someone else has, may require a different medication. Therefore, you should not give your medicine to other people, or use it for other infections, unless your doctor specifically directs you to do so.
• BE SURE TO TELL YOUR DOCTOR IF YOU ARE PREGNANT. Although this drug appears to be safe in animals, extensive studies in humans during pregnancy have not yet been completed. Also, tell your doctor if you are breastfeeding an infant. It is not known whether or not acyclovir passes into breast milk.

Adapin—see doxepin

Adipex-P—see phentermine

Adipost—see phendimetrazine

Adphen—see phendimetrazine

Adsorbocarpine—see pilocarpine (ophthalmic)

Aerolate—see theophylline

Aeroseb-HC—see hydrocortisone (topical)

Akarpine—see pilocarpine (ophthalmic)

AK-Sporin—see neomycin, bacitracin, polymyxin B, and gramicidin combination (ophthalmic)

AK-Sporin H.C. Otic—see hydrocortisone, polymyxin B, and neomycin combination (otic)

AK-Sulf—see sodium sulfacetamide (ophthalmic)

Alatone—see spironolactone

Alazide—see spironolactone and hydrochlorothiazide combination

---

albuterol

BRAND NAMES (Manufacturers)
Proventil (Schering)
Ventolin (Glaxo)
TYPE OF DRUG
Bronchodilator (relaxes breathing tubes)
INGREDIENT
albuterol
DOSAGE FORMS
Tablets (2 mg and 4 mg)
Inhalation aerosol (each spray delivers 90 mcg)
STORAGE
Albuterol tablets should be stored at room temperature in a tightly closed, light-resistant container. The inhalation aerosol should be stored at room temperature, away from excessive heat—the contents are pressurized and can explode if heated.

USES

Albuterol is used to relieve wheezing and shortness of breath caused by lung diseases such as asthma, bronchitis, and emphysema. This drug acts directly on the muscles of the bronchi (breathing tubes) to relieve bronchospasm (muscle contractions of the bronchi), which in turn reduces airway resistance and allows air to move more freely to and from the lungs—making breathing easier.

TREATMENT

In order to lessen stomach upset, you can take albuterol tablets with food (unless your doctor directs you to do otherwise).

The inhalation aerosol form of this medication is usually packaged with an instruction sheet. Read the directions carefully before using this medication. The container should be shaken well just before each use. The contents tend to settle on the bottom, so it is necessary to shake the bottle in order to evenly distribute the ingredients and equalize the doses. If more than one inhalation is necessary, wait at least one full minute between doses, in order to receive the full benefit of the first dose.

If you miss a dose of this medication and remember within an hour of the scheduled time, take the missed dose immediately; then follow your regular dosing schedule for the next dose. If you miss the dose by more than an hour or so, just wait until the next scheduled dose. Do not double the dose.

SIDE EFFECTS

Minor. Anxiety; dizziness; headache; flushing; irritability; insomnia; loss of appetite; muscle cramps; nausea; nervousness; restlessness; sweating; tremors; vomiting; weakness; and dryness or irritation of your mouth or throat (from the inhalation aerosol). These side effects should disappear in several days, as your body adjusts to the medication.

To help prevent dryness or irritation of the mouth or throat, rinse your mouth with water after each dose of the inhalation aerosol.

In order to avoid difficulty in falling asleep, check with your doctor to see if you can take the last dose of this medication several hours before bedtime each day.

If you feel dizzy, sit or lie down awhile; get up from a sitting or lying position slowly, and be careful on stairs.

Major. Tell your doctor about any side effects that are persistent or particularly bothersome. IT IS ESPECIALLY IMPORTANT TO TELL YOUR DOCTOR about chest pain; difficult or painful urination; or palpitations.

INTERACTIONS

Albuterol can interact with several other types of medication.

1. The beta-blockers (atenolol, metoprolol, nadolol, pindolol, propranolol, timolol) antagonize (act against) this medication, decreasing its effectiveness.

2. Monoamine oxidase (MAO) inhibitors, tricyclic antidepressants, antihistamines, levothyroxine, and over-the-counter (non-prescription) cough, cold, asthma, allergy, diet, or sinus medications may increase the side effects of this medication.

3. There may be a change in the dosage requirements of insulin or oral anti-diabetic medications when albuterol is started.

4. The blood-pressure-lowering effects of guanethidine may be decreased by this medication.

TELL YOUR DOCTOR if you are already taking any of the medications listed above.

WARNINGS

• Tell your doctor about unusual or allergic reactions you have had to medications, especially to albuterol or any related drug (metaproterenol, amphetamines, ephedrine, epinephrine, isoproterenol, norepinephrine, phenylephrine, phenylpropanolamine, pseudoephedrine, or terbutaline).

• Tell your doctor if you now have, or if you have ever had, diabetes, glaucoma, high blood pressure, epilepsy, heart disease, an enlarged prostate gland, or thyroid disease.

• This medication can cause dizziness. Your ability to perform hazardous tasks, such as driving a car or operating potentially dangerous machinery, may be decreased. Appropriate caution should therefore be taken.

• Before having any surgery or other medical or dental treatment, be sure to tell the doctor or dentist that you are taking this medication.

• Do not exceed the recommended dosage of this medication; excessive use may lead to an increase in side effects or a loss of effectiveness.

- Try to avoid contact of the aerosol inhalation with your eyes.
- Do not puncture, break, or burn the aerosol inhalation container. The contents are under pressure and may explode.
- Contact your doctor if you do not respond to the usual dose of this medication. It may be a sign of worsening asthma, which may require additional therapy.
- Be sure to tell your doctor if you are pregnant. The effects of this medication during pregnancy have not yet been thoroughly studied in humans, but it has caused side effects in offspring of animals who received large doses during pregnancy. Also, tell your doctor if you are breastfeeding an infant. It is not known whether or not albuterol passes into breast milk.

Aldactazide—see spironolactone and hydrochlorothiazide combination

Aldactone—see spironolactone

Aldomet—see methyldopa

Aldoril—see methyldopa and hydrochlorothiazide combination

Allerfed C—see pseudoephedrine, tripolidine, guaifenesin, and codeine combination

Allerfrin with Codeine—see pseudoephedrine, tripolidine, guaifenesin, and codeine combination

Allergine Modified—see phenylpropanolamine and chlorpheniramine combination

Allerid-O.D.—see chlorpheniramine

allopurinol

BRAND NAMES (Manufacturers)
allopurinol (various manufacturers)

Lopurin (Boots)
Zyloprim (Burroughs Wellcome)
TYPE OF DRUG
Anti-gout
INGREDIENT
allopurinol
DOSAGE FORM
Tablets (100 mg and 300 mg)
STORAGE
Allopurinol tablets should be stored at room temperature in a tightly closed container.

USES

This medication is used to treat gout, and to lower blood uric acid levels. Allopurinol blocks the body's production of uric acid.

TREATMENT

In order to avoid stomach irritation, you can take allopurinol with food or with a full glass of water or milk. It may take at least a week before the full effects of this medication are observed.

Drink at least ten to 12 glasses (8 ounces each) of fluids per day while taking this medication, in order to prevent the formation of kidney stones.

If you miss a dose of this medication, take the missed dose as soon as possible, unless it is almost time for the next dose. In that case, do not take the missed dose at all; just return to your regular dosing schedule. Do not double the next dose.

SIDE EFFECTS

Minor. Diarrhea; drowsiness; nausea; stomach upset; and vomiting. These side effects should disappear in several days, as your body adjusts to the medication.
Major. Tell your doctor about any side effects that are persistent or particularly bothersome. IT IS ESPECIALLY IMPORTANT TO TELL YOUR DOCTOR about unusual bleeding or bruising; blurred vision; chills; difficult or painful urination; fatigue; fever; loss of hair; muscle aches; numbness or tingling sensations; paleness; rash; sore throat; or yellowing of the eyes or skin.

INTERACTIONS

Allopurinol interacts with several other types of medications.

1. Alcohol, diuretics (water pills), and pyrazinamide can increase blood uric acid levels, thus decreasing the effectiveness of allopurinol.

2. Allopurinol can increase the body stores of iron salts, which can lead to iron toxicity.

3. When combined with allopurinol, ampicillin can increase the chance of skin rash; thiazide diuretics can increase the chance of allergic reactions; and cyclophosphamide can increase the chance of blood disorders. Allopurinol can also increase the blood levels and side effects of mercaptopurine, azathioprine, oral anticoagulants (blood thinners, such as warfarin), and theophylline.

4. Vitamin C can make the urine acidic, which can increase the risk of kidney stone formation.

Before starting to take allopurinol, BE SURE TO TELL YOUR DOCTOR if you are already taking any of the medications listed above.

WARNINGS

• Tell your doctor about unusual or allergic reactions you have had to any medications, especially to allopurinol.

• Tell your doctor if you now have, or if you have ever had, blood disorders, kidney disease, or liver disease. Also, tell your doctor if you have a relative with idiopathic hemochromatosis.

• If this drug makes you dizzy or drowsy, do not take part in any activity that requires alertness, such as driving a car or operating potentially dangerous equipment.

• Be sure to tell your doctor if you are pregnant. Although this drug appears to be safe in animals, extensive studies in pregnant women have not yet been completed. Also, tell your doctor if you are breastfeeding an infant. It is not known whether or not allopurinol passes into breast milk.

Almocarpine—see pilocarpine (ophthalmic)

Alpen—see ampicillin

alprazolam

BRAND NAME (Manufacturer)
Xanax (Upjohn)
TYPE OF DRUG
Sedative/hypnotic (anti-anxiety medication)
INGREDIENT
alprazolam
DOSAGE FORM
Tablets (0.25 mg, 0.5 mg, and 1 mg)
STORAGE
This medication should be stored at room temperature in a tightly closed, light-resistant container.

USES

Alprazolam is prescribed to treat symptoms of anxiety, and anxiety associated with depression. It is not clear exactly how this medicine works, but it may relieve anxiety by acting as a depressant of the central nervous system. This drug is currently used by many people to relieve nervousness. It is effective for this purpose for short periods, but it is important to try to remove the cause of the anxiety as well.

TREATMENT

This medication should be taken exactly as directed by your doctor. It can be taken with food or a full glass of water if stomach upset occurs. Do not take this medication with antacids, since they may retard its absorption from the gastrointestinal tract.

If you are taking this medication regularly and you miss a dose, take the missed dose immediately, if you remember within an hour of the scheduled time. If more than an hour has passed, skip the dose you missed and wait for the next scheduled time. Do not double the dose.

SIDE EFFECTS

Minor. Bitter taste in mouth; constipation; depression; diarrhea; dizziness; drowsiness (after a night's sleep); dry mouth; fatigue; flushing; headache; heartburn; excess saliva; loss of appetite; nausea; nervousness; sweating; and vomiting. As your body adjusts to the medicine, these side effects should disappear.

If you feel dizzy, sit or lie down awhile; get up slowly, and be careful on stairs.

Major. Tell your doctor about any side effects that are persistent or particularly bothersome. IT IS ESPECIALLY IMPORTANT TO TELL YOUR DOCTOR about blurred vision; chest pain; severe depression; difficulty urinating; double vision; fainting; falling; fever; joint pain; hallucinations; mouth sores; nightmares; palpitations; rash; shortness of breath; slurred speech; sore throat; uncoordinated movements; unusual excitement; unusual tiredness; or yellowing of the eyes or skin.

INTERACTIONS

Alprazolam interacts with several other medications.

1. To prevent over-sedation, this drug should not be taken with alcohol, other sedative drugs, or central nervous system depressants (such as antihistamines, barbiturates, muscle relaxants, pain medicines, narcotics, medicines for seizures, phenothiazine tranquilizers), or with antidepressants.

2. This medication may decrease the effectiveness of carbamazepine, levodopa, and oral anti-coagulants (blood thinners), and may increase the side effects of phenytoin

3. Disulfiram, isoniazid, and cimetidine can increase the blood levels of alprazolam, which can lead to toxic effects.

4. Concurrent use of rifampin may decrease the effectiveness of alprazolam.

If you are currently taking any of the medications listed above, CONSULT YOUR DOCTOR about their use.

WARNINGS

• Tell your doctor about unusual or allergic reactions you have had to any medications, especially to alprazolam or other benzodiazepine tranquilizers.

• Tell your doctor if you now have, or if you have ever had, liver disease, kidney disease, epilepsy, lung disease, myasthenia gravis, narrow-angle glaucoma, porphyria, mental depression, or mental illness.

• This medicine can cause drowsiness. Avoid tasks that

require mental alertness, such as driving a car or using potentially dangerous machinery.
• This medication has the potential for abuse and must be used with caution. Tolerance may develop quickly; do not increase the dose of the drug without first consulting your doctor. It is also important not to stop this drug suddenly if you have been taking it in large amounts or if you have used it for several weeks. Your doctor may want to reduce the dosage gradually.
• This is a safe drug when used properly. When it is combined with other sedative drugs or alcohol, however, serious side effects can develop.
• Be sure to tell your doctor if you are pregnant. This medicine may increase the chance of birth defects if it is taken during the first three months of pregnancy. In addition, too much use of this medicine during the last six months of pregnancy may result in addiction of the fetus —leading to withdrawal side effects in the newborn. Also, use of this medicine during the last weeks of pregnancy may cause drowsiness, slowed heartbeat, and breathing difficulties in the infant. Tell your doctor if you are breastfeeding an infant. This medicine can pass into breast milk and cause drowsiness, slowed heartbeat, and breathing difficulties in nursing infants.

Alupent—see metaproterenol

Amacodone—see acetaminophen and hydrocodone combination

amantadine

BRAND NAME (Manufacturer)
Symmetrel (Endo)
TYPE OF DRUG
Anti-parkinson and anti-viral
INGREDIENT
amantadine as the hydrochloride salt
DOSAGE FORMS
Capsules (100 mg)
Oral syrup (50 mg per 5 ml teaspoonful)

STORAGE
Amantadine capsules and oral syrup should be stored at room temperature, in tightly closed containers. This medication should never be frozen.

USES
Amantadine is used to treat the symptoms of Parkinson's disease and to prevent or treat respiratory tract infections caused by influenza A virus. It is thought to relieve the symptoms of Parkinson's disease by increasing the levels of dopamine, an important chemical in the brain, which is lacking in these patients. Amantadine is also an antiviral agent that slows the growth of the influenza virus.

TREATMENT
Amantadine can be taken on an empty stomach or with food or milk.

Each dose of the oral syrup form of this medication should be measured carefully, with a specially designed, 5 ml measuring spoon. An ordinary kitchen teaspoon is not accurate enough.

If you are taking amantadine to treat a viral infection, you should start taking it as soon as possible after exposure to the infection. It is important to continue to take this medication for the entire time prescribed by your doctor (usually seven to 14 days), even if your symptoms of infection disappear before the end of that period. If you stop taking the drug too soon, the virus is given a chance to continue growing and the infection could recur.

Amantadine works best when the level of medicine in your bloodstream is kept constant. It is best, therefore, to take the doses at evenly spaced intervals, day and night. For example, if you are to take two doses a day, the doses should be spaced 12 hours apart.

If you are taking amantadine to treat Parkinson's disease, you should know that the full effects of this medication may not be apparent for several weeks.

If you miss a dose of this medication, take the missed dose as soon as possible, unless it is almost time for the next dose. In that case, don't take the missed dose at all; just return to your regular dosing schedule. Do not double the next dose.

SIDE EFFECTS

Minor. Anxiety; confusion; constipation; dizziness; dry mouth; fatigue; headache; insomnia; loss of appetite; nausea; and vomiting. These side effects should disappear in several days, as you adjust to the medication.

To relieve constipation, increase the amount of fiber in your diet (bran, salads, fresh fruits and vegetables, and whole-grain breads), exercise, and drink more water (unless your doctor directs you to do otherwise).

If you feel dizzy, sit or lie down awhile; get up slowly, and be careful on stairs.

To relieve mouth dryness, chew sugarless gum, or suck on ice chips or a piece of hard candy.

Major. Tell your doctor about any side effects that are persistent or particularly bothersome. IT IS ESPECIALLY IMPORTANT TO TELL YOUR DOCTOR about convulsions; depression; fluid retention; hallucinations; purplish-red spots on skin; shortness of breath; skin rash; slurred speech; or visual disturbances.

INTERACTIONS

Amantadine interacts with several other drugs.

1. Concurrent use of amantadine and alcohol can lead to dizziness, fainting, and confusion.

2. Phenothiazine tranquilizers and tricyclic antidepressants, in combination with amantadine, can lead to confusion, hallucinations, and nightmares.

BE SURE TO TELL YOUR DOCTOR if you are already taking any of these medications.

WARNINGS

• Tell your doctor about unusual or allergic reactions you have had to any medications, especially to amantadine.

• Before starting to take amantadine, tell your doctor if you now have, or if you have ever had, epilepsy, heart or blood vessel disease, kidney disease, mental disorders, or stomach ulcers.

• If this drug makes you dizzy, avoid taking part in any activity that requires alertness, such as driving a car or operating potentially dangerous equipment.

• If you are taking amantadine to treat Parkinson's disease, do not stop taking the medication unless you first consult your doctor. Stopping the drug abruptly may lead to a worsening of your disease. Your doctor may therefore want to reduce your dosage gradually. In addition, tolerance can develop in several months. If you notice a lack of effectiveness, CONTACT YOUR DOCTOR.

• Be sure to tell your doctor if you are pregnant. Although amantadine appears to be safe in humans, birth defects have been reported in animals whose mothers received large doses during pregnancy. Also, tell your doctor if you are breastfeeding an infant. Small amounts of amantadine pass into breast milk and can cause side effects in nursing infants.

Amaril D Spantab—see phenylpropanolamine, phenylephrine, chlorpheniramine, and phenyltoloxamine combination

Ambay—see ammonium chloride, bromodiphenhydramine, diphenhydramine, codeine, and potassium guaiacolsulfonate combination

Ambenyl—see ammonium chloride, bromodiphenhydramine, diphenhydramine, codeine, and potassium guaiacolsulfonate combination

Amcap—see ampicillin

Amcill—see ampicillin

Amen—see medroxyprogesterone

---

amiloride

BRAND NAME (Manufacturer)
Midamor (Merck Sharp & Dohme)
TYPE OF DRUG
Diuretic (water pill) and anti-hypertensive
INGREDIENT
amiloride

DOSAGE FORM
Tablets (5 mg)
STORAGE
Amiloride should be stored at room temperature in a
tightly closed container.

USES

Amiloride is prescribed to treat high blood pressure. It is
also used to reduce fluid accumulation in the body
caused by conditions such as heart failure, cirrhosis of the
liver, kidney disease, and the long-term use of some
medications. Amiloride reduces fluid accumulation by
increasing the elimination of sodium and water through
the kidneys. It may also be used in combination with
other diuretics to prevent potassium loss.

TREATMENT

To decrease stomach irritation, you can take amiloride
with a glass of milk or with a meal (unless your doctor
directs you to do otherwise). Try to take it at the same time
every day. Avoid taking a dose after 6:00 P.M.—this will
prevent you from having to get up during the night to
urinate.

If you miss a dose of this medication, take the missed
dose as soon as possible, unless it is almost time for the
next one. In that case, do not take the missed dose at all;
just wait until the next scheduled dose. Do not double the
dose.

This medication does not cure high blood pressure, but
it will help to control the condition, as long as you continue to take it.

SIDE EFFECTS

Minor. Constipation; diarrhea; dizziness; dry mouth;
gas; headache; heartburn; loss of appetite; mild skin
rash; nasal congestion; nausea; sleeping problems;
stomach upset; and vomiting. These side effects should
disappear as your body adjusts to the medication.

To avoid dizziness or light-headedness when you
stand, contract and relax the muscles of your legs for a few
moments before rising. Do this by pushing one foot
against the floor while raising the other foot slightly, alter-

nating feet so that you are "pumping" your legs in a pedaling motion.

Major. Tell your doctor about any side effects that are persistent or particularly bothersome. IT IS ESPECIALLY IMPORTANT TO TELL YOUR DOCTOR about black, tarry stools; chest pain; cough; mental depression; confusion; hair loss; impotence; muscle cramps; muscle aches; joint pain; palpitations; itching; nervousness; ringing in the ears; shakiness; shortness of breath; tingling in the fingers or toes; visual disturbances; extreme weakness; or yellowing of the eyes or skin.

INTERACTIONS

Amiloride interacts with several other types of medications and certain foods.

1. Concurrent use with spironolactone, triamterene, potassium salts, low-salt milk, salt substitutes, captopril, or laxatives can cause serious side effects from hyperkalemia (high levels of potassium in the blood).

2. Amiloride may increase the side effects of lithium and digoxin.

BE SURE TO TELL YOUR DOCTOR if you are already taking any of the medications listed above.

WARNINGS

• Be sure to tell your doctor if you have ever had unusual or allergic reactions to medications, especially to amiloride or any other diuretic.

• Tell your doctor if you now have, or if you have ever had, kidney disease or urination problems; hyperkalemia (high levels of potassium in the blood); diabetes mellitus (sugar diabetes); liver disease; or acidosis.

• Amiloride can cause hyperkalemia (high levels of potassium in the blood). Signs of hyperkalemia include palpitations; confusion; numbness or tingling in your hands, feet, or lips; anxiety; or unusual tiredness or weakness. In order to avoid this problem, do not alter your diet and do not use salt substitutes unless you first consult your doctor.

• While taking this medication, limit your intake of alcoholic beverages, in order to prevent dizziness.

• If you have high blood pressure, do not take any over-the-counter (non-prescription) medication for weight control, or for cough, cold, allergy, asthma, or sinus problems, unless you first check with your doctor.

● To prevent severe water loss (dehydration) while taking this medication, check with your doctor if you have any illness that causes severe or continuous nausea, vomiting, or diarrhea.

● Be sure to tell your doctor if you are pregnant. This drug crosses the placenta. Although studies in humans have not been completed, animal studies have shown that there are adverse effects on the fetus if large doses of this drug are given to the mother during pregnancy. Also, tell your doctor if you are breastfeeding an infant. Small amounts of this drug will pass into breast milk.

---

amiloride and hydrochlorothiazide combination

BRAND NAME (Manufacturer)
Moduretic (Merck Sharp & Dohme)
TYPE OF DRUG
Diuretic (water pill) and anti-hypertensive
INGREDIENTS
amiloride and hydrochlorothiazide
DOSAGE FORM
Tablets (5 mg amiloride and 50 mg hydrochlorothiazide)
STORAGE
Amiloride and hydrochlorothiazide should be stored at room temperature, in a tightly closed container.

USES

Amiloride and hydrochlorothiazide is prescribed to treat high blood pressure. It is also used to reduce fluid accumulation in the body caused by conditions such as heart failure, cirrhosis of the liver, kidney disease, and the long-term use of some medications. This medication reduces fluid accumulation by increasing the elimination of sodium and water through the kidneys. Amiloride is combined with hydrochlorothiazide to prevent potassium loss from the body.

TREATMENT

To avoid stomach upset, you can take this medication with food or with a full glass of milk or water (unless your doctor directs you to do otherwise). Try to take it at the same time every day. Avoid taking a dose after 6:00 P.M.—this will prevent you from having to get up during the night to urinate.

If you miss a dose of this medication, take the missed dose as soon as possible, unless it is almost time for the next one. In that case, do not take the missed dose at all; just wait until the next scheduled dose. Do not double the dose.

This medication does not cure high blood pressure, but it will help to control the condition, as long as you continue to take it.

SIDE EFFECTS

Minor. Constipation; cramps; diarrhea; dizziness; drowsiness; headache; heartburn; itching; loss of appetite; nausea; restlessness; upset stomach; vomiting. As your body adjusts to this medication, these side effects should disappear.

This medication can cause increased sensitivity to sunlight. It is important, therefore, to avoid prolonged exposure to sunlight and sunlamps. Wear protective clothing and use an effective sunscreen.

To avoid dizziness or light-headedness when you stand, contract and relax the muscles of your legs for a few moments before rising. Do this by pushing one foot against the floor while raising the other foot slightly, alternating feet so that you are "pumping" your legs in a pedaling motion.

Major. Tell your doctor about any side effects that are persistent or particularly bothersome. IT IS ESPECIALLY IMPORTANT TO TELL YOUR DOCTOR about unusual bleeding; blurred vision; bruising; confusion; difficulty breathing; dry mouth; fever; impotence; joint pain; mood changes; muscle spasms; nervousness; palpitations; skin rash; excessive thirst; sore throat; tingling in your fingers or toes; excessive weakness; or yellowing of the eyes or skin.

INTERACTIONS

Amiloride and hydrochlorothiazide interacts with several other types of medication and certain foods.

1. Concurrent use with triamterene, spironolactone, potassium salts, low-salt milk, salt substitutes, captopril, or laxatives can cause serious side effects from hyperkalemia (high levels of potassium in the blood).

2. This drug may decrease the effectiveness of oral anticoagulants, anti-gout medications, insulin, oral antidiabetic medicines, and methenamine.

3. Indomethacin may decrease the blood-pressure-lowering effects of this medication.

4. Fenfluramine may increase the blood-pressure-lowering effects of this drug (which can be dangerous).

5. Cholestyramine and colestipol can decrease the absorption of amiloride and hydrochlorothiazide from the gastrointestinal tract. Therefore, this drug should be taken one hour before or four hours after a dose of cholestyramine or colestipol.

6. The side effects of amphotericin B, calcium, cortisone-like steroids (such as cortisone, dexamethasone, hydrocortisone, prednisone, prednisolone), digoxin, digitalis, lithium, quinidine, sulfonamide antibiotics, and vitamin D may be increased when taken concurrently with amiloride and hydrochlorothiazide.

Before taking amiloride and hydrochlorothiazide, BE SURE TO TELL YOUR DOCTOR if you are taking any of the medications listed above.

WARNINGS

• Tell your doctor about unusual or allergic reactions you have had to medications, especially to amiloride, hydrochlorothiazide, or any other diuretic, oral anti-diabetic medications, or sulfonamide antibiotics.

• Tell your doctor if you have, or if you have ever had, kidney disease or problems with urination; diabetes mellitus (sugar diabetes); gout; liver disease; asthma; pancreas disease; systemic lupus erythematosus (SLE); acidosis; or hyperkalemia.

• This drug can occasionally cause potassium loss from the body. Signs of potassium loss include dry mouth; thirst; weakness; muscle pain or cramps; nausea; and vomiting. If you experience any of these symptoms, call your doctor.

• Amiloride can cause hyperkalemia (high levels of potassium in the blood). Signs of hyperkalemia include palpitations; confusion; numbness or tingling in the hands, feet, or lips; anxiety; and unusual tiredness or weakness. In order to avoid this problem, do not alter your diet and do not use salt substitutes, unless your doctor tells you to do so.

• While taking this medication, limit your intake of alcoholic beverages, in order to prevent dizziness and light-headedness.

• If you have high blood pressure, do not take any over-the counter (non-prescription) medication for weight control, or for cough, cold, asthma, allergy, or sinus problems, unless you first check with your doctor.

• To prevent severe water loss (dehydration) while taking this medication, check with your doctor if you have any illness that causes severe nausea, vomiting, or diarrhea.

• This medication can raise blood sugar in diabetic patients. Therefore, blood sugar levels should be monitored carefully with blood or urine tests when this medication is started.

• Be sure to tell your doctor if you are pregnant. This drug crosses the placenta. Although studies in humans have not been completed, animal studies have shown adverse effects on the fetuses of animals who received large doses of this drug during pregnancy. Also, tell your doctor if you are breastfeeding an infant. Small amounts of this drug pass into breast milk.

Aminodur—see aminophylline

---

aminophylline

BRAND NAMES (Manufacturers)
Aminodur (Berlex)
aminophylline (various manufacturers)
Amoline (Major)
Lixaminol (Ferndale)

Phyllocontin (Purdue Frederick)
Somophyllin (Fisons)
Truphylline (G & W)
TYPE OF DRUG
Bronchodilator
INGREDIENT
aminophylline (theophylline as tne etnylenediamine salt)
DOSAGE FORMS
Tablets (100 mg and 200 mg)
Sustained-release tablets (225 mg and 300 mg)
Oral liquid (105 mg per 5 ml teaspoonful)
Oral elixir (250 mg per 15 ml tablespoonful)
Suppositories (250 mg and 500 mg)
Rectal solution (300 mg per 5 ml)
STORAGE
Aminophylline tablets, liquid, elixir, and rectal solution
should be stored at room temperature, in tightly closed
containers. This medication should never be frozen. The
suppositories should be stored in a cool place. They can
be refrigerated if they become too soft.

USES
Aminophylline is prescribed to treat breathing problems
(wheezing and shortness of breath) caused by asthma,
bronchitis, or emphysema. It relaxes the smooth muscles
of the bronchial airways (breathing tubes), thus opening
the air passages to the lungs, and allowing air to move in
and out more easily.

TREATMENT
Aminophylline should be taken on an empty stomach, 30
to 60 minutes before a meal, or two hours after a meal. If
this medication causes stomach irritation, however, you
can take it with food or with a full glass of water or milk
(unless your doctor directs you to do otherwise).

Aminophylline works best when the level of medicine
in your bloodstream is kept constant. It is best, therefore,
to take it at evenly spaced intervals, day and night. For
example, if you are to take four doses a day, the doses
should be spaced six hours apart.

The sustained-release tablets should be swallowed
whole (if the tablet is scored for breaking, you can break it

along these lines). Chewing, crushing, or crumbling the tablets destroys their sustained-release activity, and possibly increases the side effects.

Doses of the oral liquid or elixir should be measured carefully, with a specially designed, 5 ml measuring spoon or a cup designed for that purpose. Ordinary kitchen spoons are not accurate enough.

To use the suppository form of this medication, remove the foil wrapper and moisten the suppository with water (if it is too soft to insert, refrigerate it for half an hour or run cold water over it before removing the wrapper). Lie on your left side with your right knee bent. Push the suppository into the rectum, pointed end first. Lie still for a few minutes. Try to avoid having a bowel movement for at least an hour.

Aminophylline suppositories can be irritating to rectal tissue—they should not be used for prolonged periods.

Aminophylline rectal solution is packaged with detailed patient instructions. Be sure to read the instructions before using this medication. If crystals appear in the solution, re-dissolve the crystals by partially immersing the bottle in warm water. The syringe should be washed after each application. To prevent irritation to the rectum, this solution should not be used continuously for longer than 24 to 36 hours.

Try not to miss any doses of this medication. If you do miss a dose, take the missed dose as soon as possible, unless it is almost time for the next dose. In that case, do not take the missed dose at all; just return to your regular dosing schedule. Do not double the next dose.

SIDE EFFECTS

Minor. Diarrhea; dizziness; feeling faint; flushing; headache; heartburn; increased urination; insomnia; irritability; loss of appetite; nausea; nervousness; stomach pain; and vomiting. These side effects should disappear in several days, as your body adjusts to the medication.

If you feel dizzy or light-headed, sit or lie down awhile; get up slowly, and be careful on stairs.

Major. Tell your doctor about any side effects that are persistent or particularly bothersome. IT IS ESPECIALLY IMPORTANT TO TELL YOUR DOCTOR about black, tarry stools; confusion; convulsions; difficulty breathing; muscle twitches; palpitations; rash; severe abdominal pain; or unusual weakness.

INTERACTIONS

Aminophylline interacts with several other medications.

1. It can increase the effects (diuresis) of furosemide.

2. Reserpine in combination with aminophylline can cause a rapid heart rate.

3. Beta-blockers (atenolol, metoprolol, nadolol, pindolol, propranolol, and timolol) can decrease the effectiveness of aminophylline.

4. Aminophylline can increase the side effects of the following products: over-the-counter (non-prescription) sinus, cough, cold, asthma, allergy, and diet preparations; digoxin; and oral anti-coagulants (blood thinners).

5. Aminophylline can decrease the effectiveness of phenytoin and lithium.

6. Phenobarbital can increase the elimination of aminophylline from the body, decreasing its effectiveness.

7. Cimetidine, erythromycin, troleandomycin, allopurinol, and thiabendazole can decrease the elimination of aminophylline from the body, increasing its side effects.

8. Anti-diarrhea medications prevent the absorption of aminophylline. Therefore, at least one hour should separate doses of these two types of medications.

BE SURE TO TELL YOUR DOCTOR if you are taking any of the medications listed above.

WARNINGS

• Tell your doctor about any unusual or allergic reactions you have had to medications, especially to aminophylline, theophylline, caffeine, dyphylline, oxtriphylline, or theobromine.

• Tell your doctor if you now have, or if you have ever had, an enlarged prostate gland, fibrocystic breast disease, heart disease, kidney disease, low or high blood pressure, liver disease, stomach ulcers, or thyroid disease.

• Cigarette or marijuana smoking may affect this drug's action. BE SURE TO TELL YOUR DOCTOR if you smoke.

Also, do not suddenly stop smoking without informing your doctor.

• High fever, diarrhea, the flu, and influenza vaccinations can also affect the action of this drug. You should tell your doctor about episodes of high fever or prolonged diarrhea. Before having any vaccinations, especially those to prevent the flu, be sure to TELL YOUR DOCTOR that you are taking this medication.

• Avoid drinking large amounts of caffeine-containing beverages (coffee, cocoa, tea, and cola drinks) and avoid eating large amounts of chocolate. These products may increase the side effects of aminophylline.

• Do not change your diet without first consulting your doctor. Char-broiled foods or a high-protein, low-carbohydrate diet can affect the action of this drug.

• Before having any surgery or other medical or dental treatment, be sure to tell your doctor or dentist that you are taking this medication.

• Before taking any over-the-counter (non-prescription) asthma, allergy, cough, cold, sinus, or diet preparation, ask your doctor or pharmacist. These products may add to the side effects of aminophylline.

• Be sure to tell your doctor if you are pregnant. Although aminophylline appears to be safe during pregnancy, extensive studies in humans have not yet been completed. Birth defects have been observed in the offspring of animals who received large doses of this drug during pregnancy. Also, tell your doctor if you are breastfeeding an infant. Small amounts of aminophylline pass into breast milk and may cause irritability, fretfulness, or insomnia in nursing infants.

Amitid—see amitriptyline

Amitril—see amitriptyline

amitriptyline

BRAND NAMES (Manufacturers)
Amitid (Squibb)
Amitril (Parke-Davis)

amitriptyline hydrochloride (various manufacturers)
Elavil (Merck Sharp & Dohme)
Emitrip (Major)
Endep (Roche)
SK-Amitriptyline (Smith Kline & French)

TYPE OF DRUG
Tricyclic anti-depressant (mood elevator)

INGREDIENT
amitriptyline as the hydrochloride salt

DOSAGE FORM
Tablets (10 mg, 25 mg, 50 mg, 75 mg, 100 mg, and
150 mg)

STORAGE
This medication should be stored at room temperature in
a tightly closed container.

USES

Amitriptyline is used to relieve the symptoms of mental
depression. This medication belongs to a group of drugs
referred to as the tricyclic anti-depressants. These
medicines are thought to relieve depression by increasing
the concentration of certain chemicals necessary for
nerve transmission in the brain.

TREATMENT

This medication should be taken exactly as your doctor
prescribes. It can be taken with water or with food to
lessen the chance of stomach irritation, unless your doctor tells you to do otherwise.

If you miss a dose of this medication, take the missed
dose as soon as possible, then return to your regular dosing schedule. However, if the dose you missed was a
once-a-day bedtime dose, do not take that dose in the
morning; check with your doctor instead. If the dose is
taken in the morning, it may cause some unwanted side
effects. Never double the dose.

The effects of therapy with this medication may not
become apparent for two or three weeks.

SIDE EFFECTS

Minor. Agitation; anxiety; blurred vision; confusion;
constipation; cramps; diarrhea; dizziness; drowsiness;

dry mouth; fatigue; heartburn; insomnia; loss of appetite; nausea; peculiar tastes in the mouth; restlessness; sweating; vomiting; weakness; or weight gain or loss. As your body adjusts to the medication, these side effects should disappear.

Dry mouth can be relieved by chewing sugarless gum or by sucking on ice chips or a piece of hard candy.

To relieve constipation, increase the amount of fiber (bran, salads, fresh vegetables and fruits, and whole-grain breads) in your diet, and drink more water (unless your doctor directs you to do otherwise).

To avoid dizziness or light-headedness when you stand, contract and relax the muscles of your legs for a few moments before rising. Do this by pushing one foot against the floor while raising the other foot slightly, alternating feet so that you are "pumping" your legs in a pedaling motion.

This medication may cause increased sensitivity to sunlight. You should therefore avoid prolonged exposure to sunlight and sunlamps. Wear protective clothing, and use an effective sunscreen.

Amitriptyline may cause your urine to turn blue-green; this effect is harmless.

Major. Tell your doctor about any side effects that are persistent or particularly bothersome. IT IS ESPECIALLY IMPORTANT TO TELL YOUR DOCTOR about chest pain; convulsions; difficulty urinating; enlarged or painful breasts (in both sexes); fainting; fever; fluid retention; hair loss; hallucinations; headaches; impotence; mood changes; mouth sores; nervousness; nightmares; numbness in the fingers or toes; palpitations; ringing in the ears; seizures; skin rash; sleep disorders; sore throat; tremors; uncoordinated movements or balance problems; unusual bleeding or bruising; or yellowing of the eyes or skin.

INTERACTIONS

Amitriptyline interacts with a number of other medications.

1. Extreme drowsiness can occur when this medicine is taken with other central nervous system depressants (medicines that slow the activity of the nervous system), including alcohol, antihistamines, barbiturates, benzodiazepine tranquilizers, muscle relaxants, narcotics, pain medications, phenothiazine tranquilizers, and sleeping medications.

2. Amitriptyline may decrease the effectiveness of anti-seizure medications and block the blood-pressure-lowering effects of clonidine and guanethidine.

3. Oral contraceptives (estrogens) can increase the side effects and reduce the effectiveness of the tricyclic anti-depressants (including amitriptyline).

4. Tricyclic anti-depressants may increase the side ef-fects of thyroid medication and over-the-counter (non-prescription) cough, cold, allergy, asthma, sinus, and diet medications.

5. The concurrent use of tricyclic anti-depressants and monoamine oxidase (MAO) inhibitors should be under-taken very carefully, because the combination may result in fever, convulsions, or high blood pressure.

Before starting to take amitriptyline, BE SURE TO TELL YOUR DOCTOR if you are already taking any of the medications listed above.

WARNINGS

• Tell your doctor if you have had unusual or allergic reactions to medications, especially to amitriptyline or any of the other tricyclic anti-depressants (imipramine, doxepin, trimipramine, amoxapine, protriptyline, desi-pramine, maprotiline, or nortriptyline).

• Tell your doctor if you now have, or if you have ever had, asthma, high blood pressure, liver or kidney disease, heart disease, a recent heart attack, circulatory disease, stomach problems, intestinal problems, alcoholism, dif-ficulty urinating, enlarged prostate gland, epilepsy, glau-coma, thyroid disease, mental illness, or electroshock therapy.

• If this drug makes you dizzy or drowsy, do not take part in any activity that requires alertness, such as driving a car or operating potentially dangerous equipment.

• Before having any surgery or other medical or dental treatment, be sure to tell your doctor or dentist that you are taking this medication.

ammonium chloride, bromodiphenhydramine,   **99**
diphenhydramine, codeine, and potassium
guaiacolsulfonate combination

- Do not stop taking this drug suddenly. Abruptly stopping it can cause nausea, headache, stomach upset, fatigue, or a worsening of your condition. Your doctor may want to reduce the dosage gradually.
- The effects of this medication may last as long as seven days after you have stopped taking it, so continue to observe all precautions during that period.
- Be sure to tell your doctor if you are pregnant. Problems in humans have not been reported; however, studies have shown that this medication can cause side effects to the fetuses of animals who were given large doses of this drug during pregnancy. Also, tell your doctor if you are breastfeeding an infant. Small amounts of this drug can pass into breast milk and may cause unwanted side effects, such as irritability or sleeping problems, in nursing infants.

amitriptyline hydrochloride—see amitriptyline

---

ammonium chloride, bromodiphenhydramine, diphenhydramine, codeine, and potassium guaiacolsulfonate combination

BRAND NAMES (Manufacturers)
Ambay (Bay)
Ambenyl (Marion)
A-Nil (Vangard)
Bromanyl (various manufacturers)
Bromotuss with Codeine (Rugby)
TYPE OF DRUG
Antihistamine, expectorant, and cough suppressant
  combination

100   ammonium chloride, bromodiphenhydramine,
        diphenhydramine, codeine, and potassium
        guaiacolsulfonate combination

INGREDIENTS
Ammonium chloride, bromodiphenhydramine as the hydrochloride salt, diphenhydramine as the hydrochloride salt, codeine, and potassium guaiacolsulfonate

DOSAGE FORM
Oral liquid (80 mg ammonium chloride, 3.75 mg bromodiphenhydramine, 8.75 mg diphenhydramine, 10 mg codeine, 80 mg potassium guaiacolsulfonate, and 5% alcohol per 5 ml teaspoonful)

STORAGE
This drug combination should be stored at room temperature, in a tightly closed container. This medication should never be frozen.

USES
This combination is used to provide symptomatic relief of coughs due to colds, minor upper respiratory infections, or allergy.

Bromodiphenhydramine and diphenhydramine belong to a group of drugs known as antihistamines (antihistamines block the actions of histamine, a chemical released by the body during an allergic reaction). They are used to relieve and prevent symptoms of allergy.

Ammonium chloride and potassium guaiacolsulfonate are expectorants; they loosen lung secretions.

Codeine is a narcotic cough suppressant, which acts at the cough reflex center in the brain.

TREATMENT
To avoid stomach upset, you can take this medication with food or with a full glass of milk or water (unless your doctor directs you to do otherwise).

The oral liquid should be measured out carefully, with a specially designed, 5 ml measuring spoon. An ordinary kitchen teaspoon is not accurate enough.

If you miss a dose of this medication, take the missed dose as soon as possible, unless it is close to the time for your next dose. In that case, don't take the missed dose at all; just return to your regular dosing schedule. Do not double the next dose.

ammonium chloride, bromodiphenhydramine,   **101**
diphenhydramine, codeine, and potassium
guaiacolsulfonate combination

SIDE EFFECTS

Minor. Blurred vision; confusion; constipation; diarrhea; difficult or painful urination; dizziness; dry mouth, throat, or nose; irritability; loss of appetite; nausea; restlessness; ringing or buzzing in the ears; rash; stomach upset; or unusual increase in sweating. These side effects should disappear in several days, as your body adjusts to the medication.

If you are constipated, increase the amount of fiber in your diet (raw vegetables, fruits, salads, bran, and whole-grain breads), drink more water, and exercise (unless your doctor tells you not to do so).

Chew sugarless gum, or suck on ice chips or a piece of hard candy, to reduce mouth dryness.

This medication can cause increased sensitivity to sunlight. It is therefore important to avoid prolonged exposure to sunlight and sunlamps. Wear protective clothing and use an effective sunscreen.

If you feel dizzy or light-headed, sit or lie down awhile; get up from a sitting or lying position slowly, and be careful on stairs.

Major. Tell your doctor about any side effects that are persistent or particularly bothersome. IT IS ESPECIALLY IMPORTANT TO TELL YOUR DOCTOR about unusual bleeding or bruising; chest pain; feeling faint; headaches; palpitations; severe abdominal pain; or sore throat.

INTERACTIONS

This drug combination interacts with several other types of medications.

1. Concurrent use of this medication with alcohol, other central nervous system depressants (drugs that slow the activity of the nervous system), such as barbiturates, benzodiazepine tranquilizers, muscle relaxants, narcotics, pain medications, and phenothiazine tranquilizers, or with tricyclic anti-depressants can cause extreme drowsiness.

2. Monoamine oxidase (MAO) inhibitors (isocarboxazid, pargyline, phenelzine, tranylcypromine) and tricyclic anti-depressants can increase the side effects of this medication.

3. The blood-pressure-lowering effects of guanethidine, methyldopa, and reserpine may be decreased by this medication.

TELL YOUR DOCTOR if you are currently taking any of the medications listed above.

WARNINGS

• Tell your doctor about unusual or allergic reactions you have had to any medications, especially to bromodiphenhydramine, diphenhydramine, or other antihistamines (azatadine, carbinoxamine, clemastine, cyproheptadine, chlorpheniramine, dexbrompheniramine, dimenhydrinate, dimethindene, diphenylpyraline, doxylamine, hydroxyzine, promethazine, pyrilamine, trimeprazine, tripelennamine, tripolidine); to ammonium chloride; potassium guaiacolsulfonate; or to codeine or any other narcotic cough suppressant or pain medication.

• Tell your doctor if you now have, or if you have ever had, asthma, brain disease, blockage of the urinary or digestive tract, diabetes mellitus (sugar diabetes), colitis, gallbladder disease, glaucoma, heart or blood vessel disease, high blood pressure, kidney disease, liver disease, lung disease, peptic ulcers, enlarged prostate gland, or thyroid disease.

• This medication can cause drowsiness. Your ability to perform tasks that require alertness, such as driving a car or operating potentially dangerous machinery, may be decreased. Appropriate caution should therefore be taken.

• While you are taking this medication, drink at least eight glasses of water a day to help loosen lung secretions.

• Because this product contains codeine, there is potential for abuse, so it must be used with caution. It usually should not be taken for longer than ten days at a time. Tolerance may develop quickly; do not increase the dosage unless you first consult your doctor.

• Before having surgery or any other medical or dental treatment, be sure to tell your doctor or dentist that you

are taking this medication.
• Be sure to tell your doctor if you are pregnant. The effects of this medication during pregnancy have not yet been thoroughly studied in humans. Codeine, used regularly during pregnancy, may lead to addiction of the fetus, resulting in withdrawal symptoms (irritability, excessive crying, tremors, fever, vomiting, diarrhea, sneezing, and yawning) in the newborn infant. Also, tell your doctor if you are breastfeeding an infant. Small amounts of this medication pass into breast milk and may cause unusual excitement or irritability in nursing infants.

Amoline—see aminophylline

---

amoxapine

BRAND NAME (Manufacturer)
Asendin (Lederle)
TYPE OF DRUG
Tricyclic anti-depressant (mood elevator)
INGREDIENT
amoxapine
DOSAGE FORM
Tablets (25 mg, 50 mg, 100 mg, and 150 mg)
STORAGE
This medication should be stored at room temperature in a tightly closed container.

USES

Amoxapine is used to relieve the symptoms of mental depression. This medication belongs to a group of drugs referred to as the tricyclic anti-depressants. These medicines are thought to relieve depression by increasing the concentration of certain chemicals necessary for nerve transmission in the brain.

TREATMENT

This medication should be taken exactly as your doctor prescribes. It can be taken with water or with food to lessen the chance of stomach irritation, unless your doctor tells you to do otherwise.

If you miss a dose of this medication, take the missed dose as soon as possible, then return to your regular dosing schedule. However, if the dose you missed was a once-a-day bedtime dose, do not take that dose in the morning; check with your doctor instead. If the dose is taken in the morning, it may cause some unwanted side effects. Never double the dose.

The effects of therapy with this medication may not become apparent for two or three weeks.

SIDE EFFECTS

Minor. Agitation; anxiety; blurred vision; confusion; constipation; cramps; diarrhea; dizziness; drowsiness; dry mouth; fatigue; heartburn; loss of appetite; nausea; peculiar tastes in the mouth; restlessness; sweating; vomiting; weakness; or weight gain or loss. As your body adjusts to the medication, these side effects should disappear.

Dry mouth can be relieved by chewing sugarless gum or by sucking on ice chips or a piece of hard candy.

To relieve constipation, increase the amount of fiber (bran, salads, fresh vegetables and fruits, and whole-grain breads) in your diet, and drink more water (unless your doctor directs you to do otherwise).

To avoid dizziness or light-headedness when you stand, contract and relax the muscles of your legs for a few moments before rising. Do this by pushing one foot against the floor while raising the other foot slightly, alternating feet so that you are "pumping" your legs in a pedaling motion.

This medication may cause increased sensitivity to sunlight. You should therefore avoid prolonged exposure to sunlight and sunlamps. Wear protective clothing, and use an effective sunscreen.

Major. Tell your doctor about any side effects that are persistent or particularly bothersome. IT IS ESPECIALLY IMPORTANT TO TELL YOUR DOCTOR about unusual bleeding; chest pains; convulsions; difficulty urinating; enlarged or painful breasts (in both sexes); fainting; fever; fluid retention; hair loss; hallucinations; headaches; impotence; mood changes; mouth sores; nervousness; nightmares; numbness in the fingers or toes; palpitations; ringing in the ears; seizures; skin rash; sleep disorders; sore throat; tremors; uncoordinated movements or balance problems; or yellowing of the eyes or skin.

INTERACTIONS

Amoxapine interacts with a number of other medications.

1. Extreme drowsiness can occur when this medicine is taken with central nervous system depressants (medicines that slow the activity of the nervous system), including alcohol, antihistamines, barbiturates, benzodiazepine tranquilizers, muscle relaxants narcotics, pain medications, phenothiazine tranquilizers, and sleeping medications.

2. Amoxapine may decrease the effectiveness of anti-seizure medications and block the blood-pressure-lowering effects of clonidine and guanethidine.

3. Oral contraceptives (estrogens) can increase the side effects and reduce the effectiveness of the tricyclic anti-depressants (including amoxapine).

4. Tricyclic anti-depressants may increase the side effects of thyroid medication and over-the-counter (non-prescription) cough, cold, allergy, asthma, sinus, and diet medications.

5. The concurrent use of tricyclic anti-depressants and monoamine oxidase (MAO) inhibitors should be undertaken very carefully, because the combination may result in fever, convulsions, or high blood pressure.

Before starting to take amoxapine, BE SURE TO TELL YOUR DOCTOR if you are already taking any of the medications listed above.

WARNINGS

• Tell your doctor if you have had unusual or allergic reactions to medications, especially to amoxapine or any of the other tricyclic anti-depressants (amitriptyline, imipramine, doxepin, trimipramine, protriptyline, desipramine, maprotiline, or nortriptyline).

• Tell your doctor if you now have, or if you have ever had, asthma, high blood pressure, liver or kidney disease, heart disease, a recent heart attack, circulatory disease, stomach problems, intestinal problems, alcoholism, difficult urination, enlarged prostate, epilepsy, glaucoma, thyroid disease, mental illness, or electroshock therapy.

• If this drug makes you dizzy or drowsy, do not take part in any activity that requires alertness, such as driving a car or operating potentially dangerous equipment.

• Before having any surgery or other medical or dental treatment, be sure to tell your doctor or dentist that you are taking this medication.

• Do not stop taking this drug suddenly. Abruptly stopping it can cause nausea, headache, stomach upset, fatigue, or a worsening of your condition. Your doctor may want to reduce the dosage gradually.

• The effects of this medication may last as long as seven days after you have stopped taking it, so continue to observe all precautions during that period.

• Be sure to tell your doctor if you are pregnant. Problems in humans have not been reported; however, studies in animals have shown that this type of medication can cause side effects to the fetus when large doses are given to the mother during pregnancy. Also, tell your doctor if you are breastfeeding an infant. Small amounts of this drug can pass into breast milk and may cause unwanted effects, such as irritability or sleeping problems, in nursing infants.

---

amoxicillin

BRAND NAMES (Manufacturers)
amoxicillin (various manufacturers)
Amoxil (Beecham)
Larotid (Beecham)
Polymox (Bristol)
Sumox (Reid-Provident)
Trimox (Squibb)
Utimox (Parke-Davis)
Wymox (Wyeth)
TYPE OF DRUG
Antibiotic (infection fighter)
INGREDIENT
amoxicillin

DOSAGE FORMS
Capsules (250 mg and 500 mg)
Chewable tablets (125 mg and 250 mg)
Oral suspension (50 mg, 125 mg, and 250 mg per 5 ml teaspoonful)

STORAGE
Amoxicillin tablets and capsules should be stored at room temperature in tightly closed containers. The oral suspension should be stored in the refrigerator in a tightly closed container. Any unused portion of the suspension should be discarded after 14 days, because the drug loses its potency after that time. This medication should never be frozen.

USES
Amoxicillin is used to treat a wide variety of bacterial infections, including infections in the middle ear, upper and lower respiratory tracts, and the urinary tract. It acts by severely injuring the cell walls of the infecting bacteria, thereby preventing them from growing and multiplying.

Amoxicillin kills susceptible bacteria, but is not effective against viruses, parasites, or fungi.

TREATMENT
Amoxicillin can be taken either on an empty stomach or with food or milk (in order to prevent stomach upset).

The suspension form of this medication should be shaken well, just before measuring each dose. The contents tend to settle on the bottom of the bottle, so it is necessary to shake the container to evenly distribute the ingredients and equalize the doses. Each dose should then be measured carefully with a specially designed, 5 ml measuring spoon. An ordinary kitchen teaspoon is not accurate enough.

It is important to continue to take this medication for the entire time prescribed by your doctor (usually seven to 14 days)—even if the symptoms of infection disappear before the end of that period. If you stop taking the drug too soon, resistant bacteria are given the chance to continue growing, and the infection could recur.

Amoxicillin works best when the level of medicine in

your bloodstream is kept constant. It is best therefore to take the doses at evenly spaced intervals, day and night. For example, if you are to take four doses a day, the doses should be spaced six hours apart.

If you miss a dose of this medication, take the missed dose immediately. However, if you do not remember to take the missed dose until it is almost time for your next dose, take it; then space the next dose about halfway through the regular interval between doses. Then return to your regular schedule. Try not to skip any doses.

SIDE EFFECTS

Minor. Diarrhea; heartburn; nausea; and vomiting. These side effects should disappear in several days, as your body adjusts to this medication.

Major. Tell your doctor about any side effects that are persistent or particularly bothersome. IT IS ESPECIALLY IMPORTANT TO TELL YOUR DOCTOR about bloating; chills; cough; difficulty breathing; fever; irritation of the mouth; muscle aches; rash; rectal or vaginal itching; severe diarrhea; sore throat; or darkened tongue. Also, if your symptoms of infection seem to be getting worse rather than improving, you should contact your doctor.

INTERACTIONS

Amoxicillin interacts with other medications.

1. Probenecid can increase the blood concentrations of this medication.

2. Amoxicillin may decrease the effectiveness of oral contraceptives (birth control pills), and pregnancy could result. You should therefore use another form of birth control while taking this medication. Discuss this with your doctor.

TELL YOUR DOCTOR if you are currently taking any of the medications listed above.

WARNINGS

• Tell your doctor about unusual or allergic reactions you have had to any medications, especially to amoxicillin or penicillin, or to cephalosporin antibiotics, penicillamine or griseofulvin.

• Tell your doctor if you now have, or if you have ever

had, kidney disease, asthma, or allergies.

• This medication has been prescribed for your current infection only. Another infection later on, or one that someone else has, may require a different medicine. You should not give your medicine to other people or use it for other infections, unless your doctor specifically directs you to do so.

• Diabetics taking amoxicillin should know that this drug can cause a false-positive sugar reaction with a Clinitest urine glucose test. To avoid this problem, while taking amoxicillin you should switch to Clinistix or Tes-Tape to test your urine sugar.

• Be sure to tell your doctor if you are pregnant. Although amoxicillin appears to be safe during pregnancy, extensive studies in humans have not yet been completed. Also, tell your doctor if you are breastfeeding an infant. Small amounts of this medication pass into breast milk and may temporarily alter the bacteria in the intestinal tract of the nursing infant and result in diarrhea.

Amoxil — see amoxicillin

---

amphetamine

Brand Name (Manufacturer)
Amphetamine Sulfate (Lannett)
TYPE OF DRUG
Amphetamine (central nervous system stimulant)
INGREDIENT
amphetamine as the sulfate salt
DOSAGE FORM
Tablets (5 mg and 10 mg)
STORAGE
Amphetamine tablets should be stored at room temperature in a tightly closed container.

USES

This medication is a central nervous system stimulant that increases mental alertness and decreases fatigue. It is used to treat narcolepsy (problems in staying awake) and abnormal behavioral syndrome in children (hyperkinetic syndrome or attention deficit disorder). The way this medication acts to control abnormal behavioral syndrome in children is not clearly understood.

Amphetamine is also used as an appetite suppressant during the first few weeks of dieting (while you are trying to establish new eating habits). It is thought to relieve hunger by altering nerve impulses to the appetite control center in the brain. Its effectiveness as an appetite suppressant lasts only for short periods (three to 12 weeks).

TREATMENT

In order to avoid stomach upset, you can take amphetamine with food or with a full glass of milk or water (unless your doctor directs you to do otherwise).

If this medication is being used to treat narcolepsy or abnormal behavioral syndrome in children, the first dose each day should be taken soon after awakening. Subsequent doses should be spaced at four- to six-hour intervals.

If this medication has been prescribed as a diet aid, it should be taken one hour before each meal.

In order to avoid difficulty in falling asleep, the last dose of this medication each day should be taken four to six hours before bedtime.

If you miss a dose of this medication, take the missed dose as soon as possible, unless it is close to the time for your next dose. In that case, don't take the missed dose at all; just return to your regular dosing schedule. Do not double the next dose.

SIDE EFFECTS

Minor. Abdominal cramps; constipation; diarrhea; dry mouth; false sense of well-being; dizziness; insomnia; loss of appetite; irritability; nausea; overstimulation; restlessness; unpleasant taste in the mouth; and vomiting. These side effects should disappear in several days, as your body adjusts to the medication.

In order to prevent constipation, increase the amount of fiber in your diet (bran, fresh fruits and vegetables, salads, whole-grain cereals and breads), drink more water, and increase your exercise (unless your doctor directs you to do otherwise).

Dry mouth can be relieved by sucking on ice chips or a piece of hard candy, or by chewing sugarless gum.

If you feel dizzy, sit or lie down awhile; get up from a sitting or lying postion slowly, and be careful on stairs.

Major. Tell your doctor about any side effects that are persistent or particularly bothersome. IT IS ESPECIALLY IMPORTANT TO TELL YOUR DOCTOR about blurred vision; confusion; fatigue; headaches; impotence; mental depression; palpitations; rash; sweating; tightness in the chest; tremors; uncoordinated movements; or unusual bleeding or bruising.

INTERACTIONS

Amphetamine interacts with several other types of medications.

1. Use of this medication within 14 days of a monoamine oxidase (MAO) inhibitor (isocarboxazid, pargyline, phenelzine, tranylcypromine) can result in high blood pressure and other side effects.

2. Barbiturate medications, phenothiazine tranquilizers (especially chlorpromazine), and tricyclic anti-depressants can antagonize (act against) this medication.

3. Amphetamine can decrease the blood-pressure-lowering effects of anti-hypertensive medications (especially guanethidine), and may alter insulin and oral anti-diabetic medication dosage requirements in diabetic patients.

4. The side effects of other central nervous system stimulants, such as caffeine, over-the-counter (non-prescription) appetite suppressants, and cough, cold, allergy, asthma, or sinus preparations, may be increased by amphetamine.

5. Acetazolamide and sodium bicarbonate can decrease the elimination and prolong the duration of action of the amphetamines.

TELL YOUR DOCTOR if you are currently taking any of the medications listed above.

WARNINGS

• Tell your doctor about unusual or allergic reactions you have had to any medications, especially to amphetamine or other central nervous system stimulants (albuterol, dextroamphetamine, ephedrine, epinephrine, isoproterenol, metaproterenol, norepinephrine, phenylephrine, phenylpropanolamine, pseudoephedrine, or terbutaline).

• Tell your doctor if you have a history of drug abuse, or if you have ever had problems with agitation, diabetes mellitus (sugar diabetes), glaucoma, heart or blood vessel disease, high blood pressure, or thyroid disease.

• Amphetamine can mask the symptoms of extreme fatigue and can cause dizziness. Your ability to perform hazardous tasks, such as driving a car or operating potentially dangerous machinery, may be decreased. Appropriate caution should therefore be taken.

• Before having any surgery or other medical or dental treatment, be sure to tell your doctor or dentist that you are taking this medication.

• Amphetamine may be habit-forming when taken for long periods of time (both physical and psychological dependence can occur). Therefore, you should not increase the dose of this medication or take it for longer than 12 weeks, unless you first consult your doctor. It is also important that you not stop taking this medication abruptly—fatigue, sleep disorders, mental depression, nausea, vomiting, stomach cramps, or pain can occur. Your doctor may therefore want to decrease the dose gradually in order to prevent these side effects.

• Be sure to tell your doctor if you are pregnant. Although side effects in humans have not yet been studied, some of the amphetamines can cause heart, brain, and biliary tract abnormalities in the fetuses of animals who receive large doses of these drugs during pregnancy. Also, tell your doctor if you are breastfeeding an infant. Small amounts of this drug pass into breast milk.

Amphetamine Sulfate—see amphetamine

---

ampicillin

BRAND NAMES (Manufacturers)
Acillin (ICN)
Alpen (Lederle)

Amcap (Circle)
Amcill (Parke-Davis)
Ampi-Co (Coastal)
Omnipen (Wyeth)
Penbritin (Ayerst)
Pensyn (Upjohn)
Pfizerpen A (Pfipharmecs)
Polycillin (Bristol)
Principen (Squibb)
SK-Ampicillin (Smith Kline & French)
Supen (Reid-Provident)
Totacillin (Beecham)

TYPE OF DRUG
Antibiotic (infection fighter)

INGREDIENT
ampicillin

DOSAGE FORMS
Capsules (250 mg and 500 mg)
Liquid suspension (125 mg and 250 mg per teaspoonful)
Drops for children (50 mg per ml)

STORAGE
Ampicillin capsules can be stored at room temperature;
liquid suspensions and drops should be refrigerated (DO
NOT FREEZE). Do not keep these medications beyond the
expiration date written on the container. Close containers
tightly to keep out moisture.

USES

Ampicillin is used to treat a wide variety of bacterial infections, including middle ear infections in children, and
infections of the respiratory, urinary, and gastrointestinal
tracts. It acts by severely injuring the cell walls of the
infecting bacteria—thereby preventing them from growing and multiplying.

TREATMENT

Usually ampicillin is taken every six hours, even through
the night. It is best to take this drug on an empty stomach
(one hour before or two hours after a meal) with a full
glass of water (not juice or soda pop).

If you have been prescribed the liquid suspension form
of this drug, be sure to shake the bottle well. The contents

tend to settle on the bottom of the bottle, so it is necessary to shake the container to evenly distribute the ingredients and equalize the doses. Be sure to use specially marked droppers or spoons to accurately measure the correct amount of liquid. Household teaspoons vary in size and may not give you the correct dosage.

Ampicillin works best when the level of medicine in your bloodstream is kept constant. So if you miss a dose, take it as soon as possible. If it is already time for the next dose, take it; space the next two doses at half the normal time interval (for example, if you were supposed to take one tablet every six hours, take your next two doses every three hours); then resume your normal dosage schedule.

It is very important to continue to take this medication for the entire time prescribed by your doctor (usually ten days), even if the symptoms disappear before the end of that period. If you stop taking the drug too soon, resistant bacteria are given a chance to continue growing and the infection could recur.

SIDE EFFECTS

Minor. Diarrhea; nausea; vomiting.

Major. Difficulty breathing; darkened tongue; fever; joint pain; mouth sores; rash; rectal or vaginal itching; severe diarrhea; sore throat. BE SURE TO CONTACT YOUR DOCTOR if you have any of these symptoms. Also, if your symptoms of infection seem to be getting worse rather than improving, you should contact your doctor.

INTERACTIONS

1. Ampicillin interacts with several types of drugs, including allopurinol, chloramphenicol, erythromycin, paromycin, tetracycline, and troleandomycin.

2. Ampicillin may decrease the effectiveness of oral contraceptives (birth control pills), and pregnancy could result. You should therefore use another form of birth control while taking ampicillin.

BE SURE TO TELL YOUR DOCTOR if you are already taking one of these medications.

WARNINGS

• Tell your doctor about unusual or allergic reactions you have had to any medications, especially to ampicillin, amoxicillin, or penicillin, or to cephalosporin antibiotics, penicillamine, or griseofulvin.

• Tell your doctor if you now have, or if you have ever had, liver disease, kidney disease, asthma, hay fever, or other allergies.

• This medication has been prescribed for your current infection only. Another infection later on, or one that someone else has, may require a different medicine. You should not give your medicine to other people or use it for other infections, unless your doctor specifically directs you to do so.

• Diabetics taking ampicillin should know that this drug can cause a false-positive sugar reaction with a Clinitest urine glucose test. To avoid this problem, while taking ampicillin you should switch to Clinistix or Tes-Tape to test your urine sugar.

• Be sure to tell your doctor if you are pregnant. Although ampicillin appears to be safe during pregnancy, extensive studies in humans have not yet been completed. Also, tell your doctor if you are breastfeeding an infant. Small amounts of this medication pass into breast milk and may temporarily alter the bacteria in the intestinal tract of the nursing infant and result in diarrhea.

Ampi-Co—see ampicillin

Anacin-3 with Codeine—see acetaminophen and codeine combination

Anadrol-50—see oxymetholone

Anafed—see pseudoephedrine and chlorpheniramine combination

Anamine T.D.—see pseudoephedrine and chlorpheniramine combination

Anaprox—see naproxen

Anavar—see oxandrolone

Android—see methyltestosterone

Ang-O-Span—see nitroglycerin (systemic)

Anhydron—see cyclothiazide

Anorex—see phendimetrazine

Anspor—see cephradine

Antabuse—see disulfiram

Antivert—see meclizine

Anturane—see sulfinpyrazone

Anxanil—see hydroxyzine

A-Nil—see ammonium chloride, bromodiphenhydramine, diphenhydramine, codeine, and potassium guaiacolsulfonate combination

Anugard-HC—see hydrocortisone, benzyl benzoate, bismuth resorcin compound, bismuth subgallate, and Peruvian balsam combination (topical)

Anusol HC—see hydrocortisone, benzyl benzoate, bismuth resorcin compound, bismuth subgallate, and Peruvian balsam combination (topical)

Aphen—see trihexyphenidyl

A-poxide—see chlordiazepoxide

Apresoline—see hydralazine

Aquachloral Supprettes—see chloral hydrate

Aquaphylline—see theophylline

Aquatag — see benzthiazide

Aquatensen — see methyclothiazide

Aquazide — see trichlormethiazide

Aquazide H — see hydrochlorothiazide

Aristocort — see triamcinolone (systemic)

Aristocort — see triamcinolone (topical)

Aristocort A — see triamcinolone (topical)

Arm-A-Med — see isoetharine

Armour Thyroid — see thyroid hormone

Artane — see trihexyphenidyl

Artane Sequels — see trihexyphenidyl

Asendin — see amoxapine

Asmalix — see theophylline

---

aspirin

BRAND NAMES (Manufacturers)
Arthritis Bayer* (Glenbrook)
A.S.A. Enseals* (Lilly)
aspirin* (various manufacturers)
Bayer* (Glenbrook)
Bayer Children's* (Glenbrook)
Cosprin* (Glenbrook)
Easprin (Parke-Davis)
Ecotrin* (Menley & James)
Empirin* (Burroughs Wellcome)
Hipirin* (Blaine)
Measurin* (Breon)
St. Joseph Children's* (Plough)

Zorprin (Boots)
* Note that most of the products listed above are available
   over-the-counter (non-prescription).
TYPE OF DRUG
Analgesic (pain reliever) and anti-inflammatory
INGREDIENT
aspirin
DOSAGE FORMS
Tablets (65 mg, 81 mg, 325 mg, 487.5 mg, 500 mg, and
   650 mg)
Chewable tablets (81 mg)
Enteric-coated tablets (325 mg, 487.5 mg, 500 mg, 650
   mg, and 975 mg)
Sustained-release tablets (650 mg and 800 mg)
Capsules (325 mg and 500 mg)
Suppositories (60 mg, 130 mg, 195 mg, 300 mg, 325 mg,
   600 mg, 650 mg, and 1.2 g)
STORAGE
Aspirin tablets, capsules, and suppositories should be
stored at room temperature in tightly closed containers.
Moisture causes aspirin to decompose.

USES

Aspirin is used to treat mild to moderate pain; fever; and
inflammatory conditions such as rheumatic fever,
rheumatoid arthritis, and osteoarthritis. Because it prevents the formation of blood clots, aspirin has also been
shown to be effective in reducing the risk of transient
ischemic attacks (small strokes), and to have a protective
effect against heart attacks in men with angina (chest
pain).
   Aspirin is a useful medication that is utilized in the
treament of a wide variety of diseases. Because it is so
common and so readily available, you may not think of it
as "real medicine." This is a common misconception;
aspirin certainly is "real medicine." It has been shown to
be effective in the treatment of numerous disorders (for
example, arthritis and stroke). If your doctor prescribes or
recommends aspirin for your condition, it is for good reason. FOLLOW YOUR DOCTOR'S DIRECTIONS CARE-
FULLY!

TREATMENT

To avoid stomach irritation, you should take aspirin with food, or with a full glass of water or milk.

Chewable aspirin tablets may be chewed, dissolved in fluid, or swallowed whole.

Sustained-release or enteric-coated tablets should be swallowed whole. Crushing, chewing, or breaking these tablets destroys their sustained-release activity, and increases the side effects.

To use the suppository form of aspirin, remove the foil wrapper and moisten the suppository with water (if the suppository is too soft to insert, refrigerate the suppository for half an hour or run cold water over it before you remove the wrapper). Lie on your left side with your right knee bent. Push the suppository into the rectum, pointed end first. Lie still for a few minutes. Try to avoid having a bowel movement for at least an hour to give the medication time to be absorbed.

If you are using aspirin to treat an inflammatory condition, it may take two or three weeks until the full benefits are observed.

If you are taking aspirin on a regular schedule and you miss a dose, take the missed dose as soon as possible, unless it is almost time for the next dose. In that case, do not take the missed dose at all; just return to your regular dosing schedule. Do not double the next dose.

SIDE EFFECTS

Minor. Heartburn; nausea; and vomiting. These side effects should disappear in several days, as your body adjusts to the medication.

Major. Tell your doctor about any side effects that are persistent or particularly bothersome. IT IS ESPECIALLY IMPORTANT TO TELL YOUR DOCTOR about any loss of hearing; confusion; dizziness; difficult or painful urination; difficulty breathing; bloody or black, tarry stools; severe stomach pain; skin rash; or unusual weakness.

INTERACTIONS

Aspirin interacts with a number of other medications.

1. It can increase the effects of anti-coagulants (blood thinners, such as warfarin), leading to bleeding complications

2. The anti-gout effects of probenecid and sulfinpyrazone may be blocked by aspirin.

3. Aspirin can increase the gastrointestinal side effects of non-steroidal anti-flammatory drugs, alcohol, phenylbutazone, and adrenocorticosteroids (cortisone-like medicines).

4. Ammonium chloride, methionine, and furosemide can increase the side effects of aspirin.

5. Acetazolamide, methazolamide, antacids, and phenobarbital can decrease the effectiveness of aspirin.

6. Aspirin can increase the effects of methotrexate, penicillin, thyroid hormone, phenytoin, sulfinpyrazone, naproxen, valproic acid, insulin, and oral anti-diabetic medications, and can decrease the effects of spironolactone.

Before starting to take aspirin, BE SURE TO TELL YOUR DOCTOR if you are already taking any of the medications listed above.

WARNINGS

• Tell your doctor about unusual or allergic reactions you have had to any medications, especially to aspirin, methyl salicylate (oil of wintergreen), tartrazine, fenoprofen, ibuprofen, indomethacin, meclofenamate, mefenamic acid, naproxen, sulindac, or tolmetin.

• Before starting to take aspirin, be sure to tell your doctor if you now have, or if you have ever had, asthma, bleeding disorders, congestive heart failure, diabetes, glucose-6-phosphate dehydrogenase (G6PD) deficiency, gout, hemophilia, high blood pressure, kidney disease, liver disease, nasal polyps, peptic ulcers, or thyroid disease.

• Before having any surgery or other medical or dental treatment, be sure to tell your doctor or dentist that you are taking aspirin. Aspirin is usually discontinued five to seven days before surgery, in order to prevent bleeding complications.

• The use of aspirin in children with the flu or chicken pox has been associated with a rare, life-threatening condition called Reye's syndrome. Aspirin should therefore not be given to children with signs of an infection.

• Large doses of aspirin (greater than eight 325 mg tablets per day) can cause false urine glucose test results. Diabetics should therefore check with their doctor before changing insulin doses while taking this medication.

• Be sure to tell your doctor if you are pregnant. Aspirin has been shown to cause birth defects in animals whose mothers received large doses during pregnancy. Large doses of aspirin given to pregnant women close to term can prolong labor and cause bleeding complications in the mother and heart problems in the infant. Also, tell your doctor if you are breastfeeding an infant. Small amounts of aspirin pass into breast milk.

---

aspirin and codeine combination

BRAND NAMES (Manufacturers)
Emcodeine (Major)
Empirin with Codeine (Burroughs Wellcome)
TYPE OF DRUG
Analgesic combination (pain reliever)
INGREDIENTS
aspirin and codeine
DOSAGE FORM
Tablets (325 mg aspirin with 15 mg, 30 mg, or 60 mg of codeine)

Note that on the label of the vial of tablets the name of this drug is followed by a number. This number refers to the amount of codeine present. Hence, #2 contains ¼ grain or 15 mg codeine; #3 has ½ grain (30 mg); and #4 contains 1 grain (60 mg) of codeine.
STORAGE
Aspirin and codeine tablets should be stored at room temperature in a tightly closed container. Moisture causes the aspirin in this product to decompose.

USES
This combination medication is used to relieve tension

headaches and mild to severe pain. Codeine is a narcotic analgesic that acts on the central nervous system to relieve pain.

TREATMENT

In order to avoid stomach upset, you can take this medication with food or milk.

This medication works most effectively if you take it at the onset of pain, rather than waiting until the pain becomes intense.

If you are taking this medication on a regular schedule and you miss a dose, take the missed dose as soon as possible, unless it is close to the time for your next dose. In that case, don't take the missed dose at all; just return to your regular dosing schedule. Do not double the next dose.

SIDE EFFECTS

Minor. Constipation; dizziness; drowsiness; dry mouth; false sense of well-being; flushing; indigestion; itching; light-headedness; loss of appetite; nausea; sweating; and vomiting. These side effects should disappear in several days, as your body adjusts to the medication.

If you are constipated, increase the amount of fiber in your diet (raw vegetables, fruits, salads, bran, and whole-grain breads), drink more water, and exercise (unless your doctor directs you to do otherwise).

Chew sugarless gum, or suck on ice chips or a piece of hard candy, to reduce mouth dryness.

If you feel dizzy, light-headed, or nauseated, sit or lie down awhile; get up from a sitting or lying position slowly, and be careful on stairs.

Major. Tell your doctor about any side effects that are persistent or particularly bothersome. IT IS ESPECIALLY IMPORTANT TO TELL YOUR DOCTOR about severe abdominal pain; bloody or black, tarry stools; chest tightness; difficulty breathing; difficult or painful urination; fatigue; palpitations; rash; ringing in the ears; tremors; or yellowing of the eyes or skin.

INTERACTIONS

This medication interacts with several other drugs.

1. Concurrent use of this medication with other central nervous system depressants (drugs that slow the activity of the nervous system), such as antihistamines, barbiturates, benzodiazepine tranquilizers, muscle relaxants, phenothiazine tranquilizers, and alcohol, or with tricyclic anti-depressants can cause extreme drowsiness.

2. A monoamine oxidase (MAO) inhibitor taken within 14 days of this medication can lead to unpredictable and severe side effects.

3. Alcohol and anti-inflammation medication can increase the gastrointestinal side effects of this medication.

4. The side effects of anti-coagulants (blood thinners, such as warfarin), oral anti-diabetic agents, phenytoin, and methotrexate may be increased by the aspirin in this product.

5. Large doses of antacids increase the elimination of the aspirin portion of this medication from the body and decrease its effectiveness.

6. Aspirin may decrease the anti-gout effects of probenecid and sulfinpyrazone.

TELL YOUR DOCTOR if you are currently taking any of the medications listed above.

WARNINGS

• Tell your doctor about unusual or allergic reactions you have had to medications, especially to aspirin, methyl salicylate (oil of wintergreen), fenoprofen, ibuprofen, indomethacin, meclofenamate, mefenamic acid, naproxen, piroxicam, sulindac, tolmetin, and zomepirac; or to codeine or other narcotic analgesics (hydrocodone, hydromorphone, meperidine, methadone, morphine, oxycodone, or propoxyphene).

• Tell your doctor if you now have, or if you have ever had, abdominal disease, Addison's disease, blood disorders, brain disease, colitis, epilepsy, gallstones or gallbladder disease, head injuries, heart disease, hemophilia, kidney disease, liver disease, lung disease, peptic ulcer, porphyria, prostate disease, or thyroid disease.

• If this drug makes you dizzy or drowsy, do not take part in any activity that requires alertness, such as driving a car or operating potentially dangerous equipment.

- Before having any surgery or other medical or dental treatment, be sure to tell your doctor or dentist that you are taking this medication. Aspirin-containing medication should usually be discontinued five to seven days before surgery.
- Because this drug contains codeine, it has the potential for abuse, and must be used with caution. Usually, it should not be taken on a regular schedule for longer than ten days at a time. Tolerance develops quickly; do not increase the dosage or stop taking the drug abruptly unless you first consult your doctor. If you have been taking large amounts of this medication for long periods, you may experience a withdrawal reaction (muscle aches, diarrhea, gooseflesh, runny nose, nausea, vomiting, shivering, trembling, stomach cramps, sleep disorders, irritability, weakness, yawning, and sweating). Your doctor may therefore want to reduce the dosage gradually.
- Diabetic patients should be aware that large doses of aspirin (more than eight 325 mg tablets per day) may interfere with urine sugar testing. Diabetics should therefore check with their doctor before changing their insulin dose.
- Be sure to tell your doctor if you are pregnant. The effects of this medication during pregnancy have not yet been thoroughly studied in humans. Codeine, used regularly in large doses during pregnancy, may result in addiction of the fetus, leading to withdrawal symptoms (irritability, excessive crying, tremors, fever, vomiting, diarrhea, sneezing, and yawning) at birth. Large amounts of aspirin taken close to the end of pregnancy may prolong labor and cause heart problems in the newborn infant. Also, tell your doctor if you are breastfeeding an infant. Small amounts of this medication may pass into breast milk and cause excessive drowsiness in the nursing infant.

aspirin and meprobamate combination —see meprobamate and aspirin combination

aspirin and oxycodone combination

BRAND NAMES (Manufacturers)
Codóxy (Halsey)
oxycodone hydrochloride, oxycodone terephthalate, and
  aspirin (various manufacturers)
Percodan (Endo)
Percodan-Demi (Endo)
SK-Oxycodone with Aspirin (Smith Kline & French)

TYPE OF DRUG
Analgesic combination (pain reliever)

INGREDIENTS
aspirin and oxycodone as the hydrochloride and
  terephthalate salts

DOSAGE FORM
Tablets (325 mg aspirin with 4.5 mg oxycodone hydrochloride and 0.38 mg oxycodone terephthalate;
  325 mg aspirin with 2.25 mg oxycodone hydrochloride
  and 0.19 mg oxycodone terephthalate)

STORAGE
Aspirin and oxycodone tablets should be stored at room
temperature in a tightly closed container. Moisture causes
the aspirin in this product to decompose.

USES
This combination medication is used to relieve moderate
to severe pain. Oxycodone is a narcotic analgesic that
acts on the central nervous system to relieve pain.

TREATMENT
In order to avoid stomach upset, you can take this medication with food or milk.

This medication works most effectively if you take it at
the onset of pain, rather than waiting until the pain becomes intense.

If you are taking this medication on a regular schedule
and you miss a dose, take the missed dose as soon as
possible, unless it is close to the time for your next dose. In
that case, don't take the missed dose at all; just return to
your regular dosing schedule. Don't double the dose.

SIDE EFFECTS

Minor. Constipation; dizziness; drowsiness; dry mouth; false sense of well-being; flushing; indigestion; itching; light-headedness; loss of appetite; nausea; rash; sweating; and vomiting. These side effects should disappear in several days, as your body adjusts to the medication.

If you are constipated, increase the amount of fiber in your diet (raw vegetables, fruits, salads, bran, and whole-grain breads), drink more water, and exercise (unless your doctor directs you to do otherwise).

Chew sugarless gum, or suck on ice chips or a piece of hard candy, to reduce mouth dryness.

If you feel dizzy, light-headed, or nauseated, sit or lie down awhile; get up from a sitting or lying position slowly, and be careful on stairs.

Major. Tell your doctor about any side effects that are persistent or particularly bothersome. IT IS ESPECIALLY IMPORTANT TO TELL YOUR DOCTOR about bloody or black, tarry stools; chest tightness; difficulty breathing; difficult or painful urination; fatigue; palpitations; rash; ringing in the ears; severe abdominal pain; tremors; or yellowing of the eyes or skin.

INTERACTIONS

This medication interacts with several other drugs.
1. Concurrent use of this medication with other central nervous system depressants (drugs that slow the activity of the nervous system), such as antihistamines, barbiturates, benzodiazepine tranquilizers, muscle relaxants, phenothiazine tranquilizers, or alcohol, or with tricyclic anti-depressants can cause extreme drowsiness.
2. A monoamine oxidase (MAO) inhibitor, taken within 14 days of this medication, can lead to unpredictable and severe side effects.
3. Alcohol and anti-inflammation medication can increase the gastrointestinal side effects of this medication.
4. The side effects of anti-coagulants (blood thinners, such as warfarin), oral anti-diabetic agents, phenytoin, and methotrexate may be increased by the aspirin in this product.
5. Large doses of antacids increase the elimination of the aspirin portion of this medication from the body and de-

crease its effectiveness.

6. The aspirin portion of this medication may decrease the anti-gout effects of probenecid and sulfinpyrazone. TELL YOUR DOCTOR if you are currently taking any of the medications listed above.

WARNINGS

• Tell your doctor about unusual or allergic reactions you have had to medications, especially to aspirin, methyl salicylate (oil of wintergreen), fenoprofen, ibuprofen, indomethacin, meclofenamate, mefenamic acid, naproxen, piroxicam, sulindac, tolmetin, and zomepirac; or to oxycodone or other narcotic analgesics (codeine, hydrocodone, hydromorphone, meperidine, methadone, morphine, or propoxyphene).

• Tell your doctor if you now have, or if you have ever had, abdominal disease, Addison's disease, blood disorders, brain disease, colitis, epilepsy, gallstones or gallbladder disease, head injuries, heart disease, hemophilia, kidney disease, liver disease, lung disease, peptic ulcer, porphyria, prostate disease, or thyroid disease.

• If this drug makes you dizzy or drowsy, do not take part in any activity that requires alertness, such as driving a car or operating potentially dangerous equipment.

• Before having any surgery or other medical or dental treatment, be sure to tell your doctor or dentist that you are taking this medication. Aspirin-containing medications are usually stopped 5 to 7 days before surgery.

• Because this drug contains oxycodone, it has the potential for abuse, and must be used with caution. Usually, it should not be taken on a regular schedule for longer than ten days at a time. Tolerance develops quickly; do not increase the dosage or stop taking the drug abruptly, unless you first consult your doctor. If you have been taking large amounts of this medication for long periods, you may experience a withdrawal reaction (muscle aches, diarrhea, gooseflesh, runny nose, nausea, vomiting, shivering, trembling, stomach cramps, sleep disorders, irritability, weakness, yawning, and sweating). Your doctor may therefore want to reduce the dosage gradually.

• Diabetic patients should be aware that large doses of

aspirin (more than eight 325 mg tablets per day) may interfere with urine sugar testing. Diabetics should therefore check with their doctor before changing their insulin dose.

• Be sure to tell your doctor if you are pregnant. The effects of this medication during pregnancy have not yet been thoroughly studied in humans. Oxycodone, used regularly in large doses during pregnancy, may result in addiction of the fetus, leading to withdrawal symptoms (irritability, excessive crying, tremors, fever, vomiting, diarrhea, sneezing, and yawning) at birth. Large amounts of aspirin taken close to the end of pregnancy may prolong labor and cause heart problems in the newborn infant. Also, tell your doctor if you are breastfeeding an infant. Small amounts of this medication may pass into breast milk and cause excessive drowsiness in the nursing infant.

---

aspirin, caffeine, and butalbital combination

BRAND NAMES (Manufacturers)
Buff-A-Comp (Maynard)
Butal Compound (Cord)
butalbital with aspirin and caffeine
   (various manufacturers)
Fiorinal (Sandoz)
Isollyl (Rugby)
Lanorinal (Lannett)
Marnal (Vortech)
Protension (Dwyer)
Tenstan (Halsom)
TYPE OF DRUG
Analgesic combination (pain reliever) and sedative
INGREDIENTS
aspirin, caffeine, and butalbital
DOSAGE FORMS
Tablets (325 mg aspirin, 40 mg caffeine; and 50 mg butalbital)

Capsules (325 mg aspirin, 40 mg caffeine; and 50 mg
  butalbital)
STORAGE
Aspirin, caffeine, and butalbital tablets and capsules
should be stored at room temperature in tightly closed
containers. Moisture causes the aspirin in this product to
decompose.

USES
This combination medication is used to relieve tension
headaches and mild to moderate pain. Butalbital belongs
to a group of drugs known as barbiturates. The barbiturates act on the central nervous system (brain and spinal
cord) to produce relaxation. Caffeine is a central nervous
system stimulant. It constricts blood vessels in the head,
which may help to relieve headaches.

TREATMENT
In order to avoid stomach upset, you can take this medication with food or milk.
  This medication works most effectively if you take it at
the onset of pain, rather than waiting until the pain becomes intense
  If you are taking this medication on a regular schedule
and you miss a dose, take the missed dose as soon as
possible, unless it is close to the time for your next dose. In
that case, don't take the missed dose at all; just return to
your regular dosing schedule. Do not double the next
dose.

SIDE EFFECTS
Minor. Dizziness; drowsiness; gas; light-headedness;
loss of appetite; nausea; nervousness; sleeping disorders;
and vomiting. These side effects should disappear in several days, as your body adjusts to the medication.
  If you feel dizzy or light-headed, sit or lie down awhile;
get up from a sitting or lying position slowly, and be careful on stairs.
Major. Tell your doctor about any side effects that are
persistent or particularly bothersome. IT IS ESPECIALLY
IMPORTANT TO TELL YOUR DOCTOR about bloody or
black, tarry stools; chest tightness; confusion; difficult or

painful urination; loss of coordination; palpitations; rash; ringing in the ears; shortness of breath; severe abdominal pain; sore throat and fever; or yellowing of the eyes or skin.

INTERACTIONS

This medication interacts with several other types of drugs.

1. Concurrent use of this medication with other central nervous system depressants (drugs that slow the activity of the nervous system), such as antihistamines, barbiturates, benzodiazepine tranquilizers, muscle relaxants, phenothiazine tranquilizers, or alcohol, or with tricyclic anti-depressants can cause extreme drowsiness.

2. Alcohol and anti-inflammation medication can increase the gastrointestinal side effects of this medication.

3. The side effects of anti-coagulants (blood thinners, such as warfarin), oral anti-diabetic agents, phenytoin, and methotrexate may be increased by the aspirin in this product.

4. Large doses of antacids increase the elimination of the aspirin portion of this medication from the body and decrease its effectiveness.

5. Aspirin may decrease the anti-gout effects of probenecid and sulfinpyrazone.

6. Butalbital can increase the elimination from the body of oral contraceptives (birth control pills), carbamazepine, adrenocorticosteroids (cortisone-like drugs), digoxin, doxycycline, tricyclic anti-depressants, griseofulvin, theophylline, aminophylline, and quinidine, thereby decreasing the effectiveness of these medications.

7. The side effects of cyclophosphamide may be increased by butalbital.

TELL YOUR DOCTOR if you are currently taking any of the medications listed above.

WARNINGS

• Tell your doctor about unusual or allergic reactions you have had to medications, especially to aspirin, methyl salicylate (oil of wintergreen), fenoprofen, ibuprofen, indomethacin, meclofenamate, mefenamic acid, naproxen, piroxicam, sulindac, tolmetin, and zomepirac; to caffeine; or to butalbital or other barbiturates (phenobarbital, pentobarbital, or secobarbital).

• Tell your doctor if you now have, or if you have ever had, bleeding problems, blood disorders, diabetes mellitus (sugar diabetes), heart disease, hemophilia, hyperactivity, kidney disease, liver disease, mental depression, peptic ulcers, or thyroid disease.

• If this drug makes you dizzy or drowsy, do not take part in any activity that requires alertness, such as driving a car or operating potentially dangerous equipment.

• Before having any surgery or other medical or dental treatment, be sure to tell your doctor or dentist that you are taking this medication. Aspirin-containing medication should usually be discontinued five to seven days before surgery.

• Because this drug contains butalbital, it has the potential for abuse, and must be used with caution. Tolerance develops quickly; do not increase the dosage or stop taking the drug abruptly unless you first consult your doctor. If you have been taking large amounts of this medication for long periods, you may experience a withdrawal reaction (muscle aches, diarrhea, convulsions, sleep disorders, nervousness, irritability, and weakness). Your doctor may therefore want to reduce the dosage gradually.

• You should not take more than six tablets or capsules of this drug in one day, unless your doctor specifically directs you to do so.

• Diabetic patients should be aware that large doses of aspirin (more than eight 325 mg tablets or capsules per day) may interfere with urine sugar testing. Diabetics should therefore check with their doctor before changing their insulin dose.

• Be sure to tell your doctor if you are pregnant. The effects of this medication during pregnancy have not yet been thoroughly studied in humans. Butalbital, used regularly in large doses during pregnancy, may result in addiction of the fetus, leading to withdrawal symptoms (irritability, excessive crying, tremors, fever, vomiting, diarrhea, sneezing, and yawning) at birth. Large amounts of aspirin taken close to the end of pregnancy may prolong labor and cause heart problems in the newborn infant. Also, tell your doctor if you are breastfeeding an infant. Small amounts of this medication may pass into breast milk and cause excessive drowsiness in the nursing infant.

---

aspirin, caffeine, butalbital, and codeine combination

BRAND NAMES (Manufacturers)
Buff-A-Comp #3 (Mayrand)
Fiorinal with Codeine (Sandoz)
Isollyl with Codeine (Rugby)
TYPE OF DRUG
Analgesic combination (pain reliever) and sedative
INGREDIENTS
aspirin, caffeine, butalbital, and codeine
DOSAGE FORMS
Tablets (325 mg aspirin, 40 mg caffeine, 50 mg butalbital, and 7.5 mg, 15 mg, or 30 mg codeine)
Capsules (325 mg aspirin, 40 mg caffeine, 50 mg butalbital, and 7.5 mg, 15 mg, or 30 mg codeine)
   Note that on the label of the vial of tablets or capsules the name of this drug is followed by a number. This number refers to the amount of codeine present. Hence, #1 contains ⅛ grain or 7.5 mg codeine; #2 has ¼ grain (15 mg); and #3 contains ½ grain (30 mg) of codeine.
STORAGE
Aspirin, caffeine, butalbital, and codeine tablets and capsules should be stored at room temperature in tightly closed containers. Moisture causes the aspirin in this product to decompose.

USES

This combination medication is used to relieve tension headaches and mild to moderate pain. Codeine is a narcotic analgesic that acts on the central nervous system to relieve pain. Butalbital belongs to a group of drugs known as barbiturates. The barbiturates act on the central nervous system (brain and spinal cord) to produce relaxation. Caffeine is a central nervous system stimulant. It constricts blood vessels in the head, which may help to relieve headaches.

TREATMENT

In order to avoid stomach upset, you can take this medication with food or milk.

This medication works most effectively if you take it at the onset of pain, rather than waiting until the pain becomes intense.

If you are taking this medication on a regular schedule and you miss a dose, take the missed dose as soon as possible, unless it is close to the time for your next dose. In that case, don't take the missed dose at all; just return to your regular dosing schedule. Don't double the dose.

SIDE EFFECTS

Minor. Blurred vision; constipation; dizziness; drowsiness; flushing; headache; indigestion; sleep disorders; loss of appetite; nausea; nervousness; sweating; tiredness; and vomiting. These side effects should disappear in several days, as your body adjusts to the medication.

If you feel dizzy or light-headed, sit or lie down awhile; get up from a sitting or lying position slowly, and be careful on stairs.

If you are constipated, increase the amount of fiber in your diet (raw vegetables, fruits, salads, bran, and whole-grain breads), drink more water, and exercise (unless your doctor directs you to do otherwise).

Major. Tell your doctor about any side effects that are persistent or particularly bothersome. IT IS ESPECIALLY IMPORTANT TO TELL YOUR DOCTOR about bloody or black, tarry stools; chest tightness; confusion; difficult or painful urination; loss of coordination; palpitations; rash; ringing in the ears; shortness of breath; severe abdominal pain; sore throat and fever; or yellowing of the eyes or skin.

INTERACTIONS

This medication interacts with several other drugs.

1. Concurrent use of this medication with other central nervous system depressants (drugs that slow the activity of the nervous system), such as antihistamines, barbiturates, benzodiazepine tranquilizers, muscle relaxants, phenothiazine tranquilizers, or alcohol, or with tricyclic anti-depressants, can cause extreme drowsiness.

2. Alcohol and anti-inflammation medication can increase the gastrointestinal side effects of this medication.

3. The side effects of anti-coagulants (blood thinners, such as warfarin), oral anti-diabetic agents, phenytoin, and methotrexate may be increased by the aspirin in this product.

4. Large doses of antacids increase the elimination of the aspirin portion of this medication from the body and decrease its effectiveness.

5. Aspirin may decrease the anti-gout effects of probenecid and sulfinpyrazone.

6. Butalbital can increase the elimination from the body of oral contraceptives (birth control pills), carbamazepine, adrenocorticosteroids (cortisone-like drugs), digoxin, doxycycline, tricyclic anti-depressants, griseofulvin, theophylline, aminophylline, and quinidine, thereby decreasing the effectiveness of these medications.

7. The side effects of cyclophosphamide may be increased by butalbital.

TELL YOUR DOCTOR if you are currently taking any of the medications listed above.

WARNINGS

• Tell your doctor about unusual or allergic reactions you have had to medications, especially to aspirin, methyl salicylate (oil of wintergreen), fenoprofen, ibuprofen, indomethacin, meclofenamate, mefenamic acid, naproxen, piroxicam, sulindac, tolmetin, and zomepirac; to codeine or other narcotic analgesics (such as hydrocodone, hydromorphone, meperidine, methadone, morphine, oxycodone, or propoxyphene); to caffeine; or to butalbital or other barbiturates.

• Tell your doctor if you now have, or if you have ever

had, abdominal disease, Addison's disease, blood disorders, brain disease, colitis, epilepsy, gallstones or gallbladder disease, head injuries, heart disease, hemophilia, kidney disease, liver disease, lung disease, peptic ulcers, porphyria, prostate disease, or thyroid disease.

• If this drug makes you dizzy or drowsy, do not take part in any activity that requires alertness, such as driving a car or operating potentially dangerous equipment.

• Before having any surgery or other medical or dental treatment, be sure to tell your doctor or dentist that you are taking this medication. Aspirin-containing medication should usually be discontinued five to seven days before surgery.

• Because this drug contains codeine and butalbital, it has the potential for abuse, and must be used with caution. Usually, it should not be taken on a regular schedule for longer than ten days at a time. Tolerance develops quickly; do not increase the dosage or stop taking the drug abruptly, unless you first consult your doctor. If you have been taking large amounts of this medication for long periods, you may experience a withdrawal reaction (muscle aches, diarrhea, gooseflesh, runny nose, nausea, vomiting, shivering, trembling, stomach cramps, sleep disorders, irritability, weakness, yawning, and sweating). Your doctor may therefore want to reduce the dosage gradually.

• You should not take more than six tablets or capsules of this drug in one day, unless your doctor specifically directs you to do so.

• Diabetic patients should be aware that large doses of aspirin (more than eight 325 mg tablets or capsules per day) may interfere with urine sugar testing. Diabetics should therefore check with their doctor before changing their insulin dose.

• Be sure to tell your doctor if you are pregnant. The effects of this medication during pregnancy have not yet been thoroughly studied in humans. Codeine and butalbital, used regularly in large doses during pregnancy, may result in addiction of the fetus, leading to withdrawal symptoms (irritability, excessive crying, tremors, fever, vomiting, diarrhea, sneezing, and yawning) at birth.

Large amounts of aspirin taken close to the end of pregnancy may prolong labor and cause heart problems in the newborn infant. Also, tell your doctor if you are breastfeeding an infant. Small amounts of this medication may pass into breast milk and cause excessive drowsiness in the nursing infant.

---

aspirin, caffeine, dihydrocodeine, and promethazine combination

BRAND NAME (Manufacturer)
Synalgos-DC (Ives)
TYPE OF DRUG
Analgesic combination (pain reliever)
INGREDIENTS
aspirin, caffeine, dihydrocodeine as the bitartrate salt, and promethazine as the hydrochloride salt
DOSAGE FORM
Capsules (356.4 mg aspirin, 30 mg caffeine, 16 mg dihydrocodeine, and 6.25 mg promethazine)
STORAGE
Aspirin, caffeine, dihydrocodeine, and promethazine capsules should be stored at room temperature in a tightly closed container. Moisture causes the aspirin in this product to decompose.

USES
Aspirin, caffeine, dihydrocodeine, and promethazine combination is used to relieve mild to moderate pain. Dihydrocodeine is a narcotic analgesic that acts on the central nervous system (brain and spinal cord) to relieve pain. Caffeine is a central nervous system stimulant, which constricts the blood vessels in the head. This may help to relieve headaches. Promethazine is a phenothiazine tranquilizer that acts on the central nervous system to relieve tension.

TREATMENT

In order to avoid stomach upset, you can take this medication with food or milk.

This medication works most effectively if you take it at the onset of pain, rather than waiting until the pain becomes intense.

If you are taking this medication on a regular schedule and you miss a dose, take the missed dose as soon as possible, unless it is close to the time for your next dose. In that case, don't take the missed dose at all; just return to your regular dosing schedule. Do not double the next dose.

SIDE EFFECTS

Minor. Blurred vision; constipation; dizziness; drowsiness; dry mouth; false sense of well-being; headache; indigestion; itching; light-headedness; loss of appetite; nausea; nervousness; restlessness; sleep disorders; sweating; and vomiting. These side effects should disappear in several days, as your body adjusts to the medication.

If you are constipated, increase the amount of fiber in your diet (raw vegetables, fruits, salads, bran, and whole-grain breads), drink more water, and exercise (unless your doctor directs you to do otherwise).

Chew sugarless gum, or suck on ice chips or a piece of hard candy, to reduce mouth dryness.

If you feel dizzy or light-headed, sit or lie down awhile; get up from a sitting or lying position slowly, and be careful on stairs.

This medication can increase your sensitivity to sunlight. It is important, therefore, to avoid prolonged exposure to sunlight and sunlamps. Wear protective clothing and sunglasses, and use an effective sunscreen.

Major. Tell your doctor about any side effects that are persistent or particularly bothersome. IT IS ESPECIALLY IMPORTANT TO TELL YOUR DOCTOR about unusual bleeding or bruising; chest tightness; difficulty breathing; difficult or painful urination; fainting; sore throat and fever; loss of coordination; palpitations; ringing in the ears; skin rash; yellowing of the eyes or skin; severe abdominal pain; or black, tarry stools.

INTERACTIONS

This medication interacts with several other types of drugs.

1. Concurrent use of this medication with other central nervous system depressants (drugs that slow the activity of the nervous system), such as antihistamines, barbiturates, benzodiazepine tranquilizers, muscle relaxants, phenothiazine tranquilizers, or alcohol, or with tricyclic anti-depressants can cause extreme drowsiness.

2. A monoamine oxidase (MAO) inhibitor taken within 14 days of this medication can lead to unpredictable and severe side effects.

3. Alcohol and anti-inflammation medication can increase the gastrointestinal side effects of this medication.

4. The aspirin in this product may increase the side effects of anti-coagulants (blood thinners, such as warfarin), oral anti-diabetic agents, phenytoin, and methotrexate.

5. Large doses of antacids increase the elimination of the aspirin portion of this medication from the body and decrease its effectiveness.

6. This medication can decrease the effectiveness of amphetamines, guanethidine, anti-convulsants, and levodopa.

7. The side effects of epinephrine and tricyclic anti-depressants may be increased by the promethazine component of this drug.

8. The aspirin portion of this medication may decrease the anti-gout effects of probenecid and sulfinpyrazone.

TELL YOUR DOCTOR if you are currently taking any of the medications listed above.

WARNINGS

• Tell your doctor about unusual or allergic reactions you have had to medications, especially to aspirin, methyl salicylate (oil of wintergreen), fenoprofen, ibuprofen, indomethacin, meclofenamate, mefenamic acid, naproxen, piroxicam, sulindac, tolmetin, and zomepirac; to dihydrocodeine or other narcotic analgesics (such as codeine, hydrocodone, hydromorphone, meperidine, methadone, morphine, oxycodone, or propoxyphene); to caffeine; or to promethazine or any other phenothiazine tranquilizer (such as chlorpromazine, fluphenazine, mesoridazine, perphenazine, promazine, thioridazine, or trifluoperazine).

• Tell your doctor if you now have, or if you have ever had, abdominal disease, Addison's disease, blood disorders, brain disease, colitis, epilepsy, gallstones or gallbladder disease, glaucoma, head injuries, heart disease, hemophilia, high blood pressure, kidney disease, liver disease, lung disease, peptic ulcer, prostate disease, or thyroid disease.

• If this drug makes you dizzy or drowsy, do not take part in any activity that requires alertness, such as driving a car or operating potentially dangerous equipment.

• Before having any surgery or other medical or dental treatment, be sure to tell your doctor or dentist that you are taking this medication. Aspirin-containing medication should usually be discontinued five to seven days before surgery.

• Because this drug contains dihydrocodeine, it has the potential for abuse, and must be used with caution. Usually, it should not be taken on a regular schedule for longer than ten days at a time. Tolerance develops quickly; do not increase the dosage or stop taking the drug abruptly, unless you first consult your doctor. If you have been taking large amounts of this medication for long periods, you may experience a withdrawal reaction (muscle aches, diarrhea, gooseflesh, runny nose, nausea, vomiting, shivering, trembling, stomach cramps, sleep disorders, irritability, weakness, yawning, and sweating). Your doctor may therefore want to reduce the dosage gradually.

• Diabetic patients should be aware that large doses of aspirin (more than eight 325 mg tablets of aspirin per day) may interfere with urine sugar testing. Diabetics should therefore check with their doctor before changing their insulin dose.

• Be sure to tell your doctor if you are pregnant. The effects of this medication during pregnancy have not yet been thoroughly studied in humans. Dihydrocodeine, used regularly in large doses during pregnancy, may result in addiction of the fetus, leading to withdrawal symptoms (irritability, excessive crying, tremors, fever, vomiting, diarrhea, sneezing, and yawning) at birth. Large amounts of aspirin taken close to the end of pregnancy may prolong labor and cause heart problems in the newborn infant. Also, tell your doctor if you are breastfeeding an infant. Small amounts of this medication may pass into breast milk and cause excessive drowsiness in the nursing infant.

aspirin, caffeine, and propoxyphene combination

BRAND NAMES (Manufacturers)
Bexophene (Mallard)
Darvon Compound-65 (Lilly)
Dolene Compound-65 (Lederle)
Doxaphene Compound (Major)
propoxyphene hydrochloride compound
     (various manufacturers)
SK-65 Compound (Smith Kline & French)
TYPE OF DRUG
Analgesic combination (pain reliever)
INGREDIENTS
aspirin, caffeine, and propoxyphene as the
     hydrochloride salt
DOSAGE FORM
Capsules (389 mg aspirin, 32.4 mg caffeine, and 32 mg
     propoxyphene; 389 mg aspirin, 32.4 mg caffeine, and
     65 mg propoxyphene)
STORAGE
Aspirin, caffeine, and propoxyphene capsules should be stored at room temperature in a tightly closed container. Moisture causes the aspirin in this product to decompose.

USES
Aspirin, caffeine, and propoxyphene combination is used to relieve mild to moderate pain. Propoxyphene is a nar-

cotic analgesic that acts on the central nervous system (brain and spinal cord) to relieve pain. Caffeine is a central nervous system stimulant. It constricts blood vessels in the head, which may help to relieve headaches.

TREATMENT

In order to avoid stomach upset, you can take this medication with food or milk.

This medication works most effectively if you take it at the onset of pain, rather than waiting until the pain becomes intense.

If you are taking this medication on a regular schedule and you miss a dose, take the missed dose as soon as possible, unless it is close to the time for your next dose. In that case, don't take the missed dose at all; just return to your regular dosing schedule. Do not double the next dose.

SIDE EFFECTS

Minor. Constipation; dizziness; drowsiness; dry mouth; false sense of well-being; flushing; indigestion; itching; light-headedness; loss of appetite; nausea; sweating; and vomiting. These side effects should disappear in several days, as your body adjusts to the medication.

If you feel dizzy or light-headed, sit or lie down awhile; get up from a sitting or lying position slowly, and be careful on stairs.

If you are constipated, increase the amount of fiber in your diet (raw vegetables, fruits, salads, bran, and whole-grain breads), drink more water, and exercise (unless your doctor directs you to do otherwise).

Major. Tell your doctor about any side effects that are persistent or particularly bothersome. IT IS ESPECIALLY IMPORTANT TO TELL YOUR DOCTOR about severe abdominal pain; bloody or black, tarry stools, chest tightness; difficulty breathing; difficult or painful urination; fatigue; palpitations; rash; ringing in the ears; tremors; or yellowing of the eyes or skin.

INTERACTIONS

This medication interacts with several other drugs.

1. Concurrent use of this medication with other central nervous system depressants (drugs that slow the activity of the nervous system), such as antihistamines, barbiturates, benzodiazepine tranquilizers, muscle relaxants, phenothiazine tranquilizers, or alcohol, or with tricyclic anti-depressants can cause extreme drowsiness.

2. A monoamine oxidase (MAO) inhibitor taken within 14 days of this medication can lead to unpredictable and severe side effects.

3. Alcohol and anti-inflammation medication can increase the gastrointestinal side effects of this medication.

4. The aspirin in this product may increase the side effects of anti-coagulants (blood thinners, such as warfarin), oral anti-diabetic agents, phenytoin, and methotrexate.

5. Large doses of antacids increase the elimination of the aspirin portion of this medication from the body and decrease its effectiveness.

6. The aspirin portion of this medication may decrease the anti-gout effects of probenecid and sulfinpyrazone.

7. The propoxyphene portion of this medication can decrease the elimination of carbamazepine from the body, which can lead to an increase in side effects.

TELL YOUR DOCTOR if you are currently taking any of the medications listed above.

WARNINGS

• Tell your doctor about unusual or allergic reactions you have had to medications, especially to aspirin, methyl salicylate (oil of wintergreen), fenoprofen, ibuprofen, indomethacin, meclofenamate, mefenamic acid, naproxen, piroxicam, sulindac, tolmetin, and zomepirac; to propoxyphene or other narcotic analgesics (such as codeine, hydrocodone, hydromorphone, meperidine, methadone, morphine, or oxycodone); or to caffeine.

• Tell your doctor if you now have, or if you have ever had, abdominal disease, Addison's disease, blood disorders, brain disease, colitis, epilepsy, gallstones or gallbladder disease, head injuries, heart disease, hemophilia, kidney disease, liver disease, lung disease, peptic ulcer, prostate disease, or thyroid disease.

• If this drug makes you dizzy or drowsy, do not take part in any activity that requires alertness, such as driving a car or operating potentially dangerous equipment.

• Before having any surgery or other medical or dental treatment, be sure to tell your doctor or dentist that you are taking this medication. Aspirin-containing medication should usually be discontinued five to seven days before surgery.

• Because this drug contains propoxyphene, it has the potential for abuse, and must be used with caution. Usually, it should not be taken on a regular schedule for longer than ten days at a time. Tolerance develops quickly; do not increase the dosage or stop taking the drug abruptly, unless you first consult your doctor. If you have been taking large amounts of this medication for long periods, you may experience a withdrawal reaction (muscle aches, diarrhea, gooseflesh, runny nose, nausea, vomiting, shivering, trembling, stomach cramps, sleep disorders, irritability, weakness, yawning, and sweating). Your doctor may therefore want to reduce the dosage gradually.

• Diabetic patients should be aware that large doses of aspirin (more than eight 325 mg tablets of aspirin per day) may interfere with urine sugar testing. Diabetics should therefore check with their doctor before changing their insulin dose.

• Be sure to tell your doctor if you are pregnant. The effects of this medication during pregnancy have not yet been thoroughly studied in humans. Propoxyphene, used regularly in large doses during pregnancy, may result in addiction of the fetus, leading to withdrawal symptoms (irritability, excessive crying, tremors, fever, vomiting, diarrhea, sneezing, and yawning) at birth. Large amounts of aspirin taken close to the end of pregnancy may prolong labor and cause heart problems in the newborn infant. Also, tell your doctor if you are breastfeeding an infant. Small amounts of this medication may pass into breast milk and cause excessive drowsiness in the nursing infant.

Atarax — see hydroxyzine

atenolol

BRAND NAME (Manufacturer)
Tenormin (Stuart)
TYPE OF DRUG
Beta-adrenergic blocking agent
INGREDIENT
atenolol
DOSAGE FORM
Tablets (50 mg and 100 mg)
STORAGE
Atenolol should be stored at room temperature in a tightly closed, light-resistant container.

USES
Atenolol is used to treat high blood pressure. It belongs to a group of medicines known as beta-adrenergic blocking agents or, more commonly, beta-blockers. These drugs work by controlling nerve impulses along certain nerve pathways.

TREATMENT
Atenolol can be taken with a glass of water, with meals, immediately following meals, or on an empty stomach, depending on your doctor's instructions. Try to take the medication at the same time(s) each day.

Try not to miss any doses of this medication. If you do miss a dose, take the missed dose as soon as possible. However, if the next scheduled dose is within eight hours (if you are taking this medicine only once a day) or within four hours (if you are taking this medicine more than once a day), do not take the missed dose at all; just return to your regular dosing schedule. Do not double the next dose.

It is important to remember that atenolol does not cure high blood pressure, but it will help to control the condition, as long as you continue to take it.

SIDE EFFECTS
Minor. Diarrhea; drowsiness; dryness of the eyes, mouth and skin; nausea; numbness or tingling of the fingers or toes; cold hands or feet (due to decreased blood circula-

tion to skin, fingers, and toes); tiredness; weakness; anxiety; nervousness; constipation; decreased sexual ability; headache; stomach discomfort; and difficulty sleeping. These side effects should disappear as your body adjusts to the medicine.

If you are extra-sensitive to the cold, be sure to dress warmly during cold weather.

Plain, non-medicated eye drops (artificial tears) may help to relieve eye dryness.

Sucking on ice chips or chewing sugarless gum helps relieve mouth or throat dryness.

Major. Tell your doctor about any side effects that are persistent or particularly bothersome. IT IS ESPECIALLY IMPORTANT TO TELL YOUR DOCTOR about hallucinations; nightmares; dizziness; light-headedness; breathing difficulty or wheezing; confusion; mental depression; reduced alertness; swelling of the ankles, feet, or lower legs; fever and sore throat; skin rash; hair loss; or unusual bleeding or bruising.

INTERACTIONS

Atenolol interacts with a number of other medications.

1. Indomethacin has been shown to decrease the blood-pressure-lowering effects of the beta-blockers. This may also happen with aspirin or other salicylates.

2. Concurrent use of beta-blockers and calcium channel blockers (diltiazem, nifedipine, and verapamil) can possibly lead to heart failure or very low blood pressure.

3. Side effects may also be increased when beta-blockers are taken with clonidine, digoxin, epinephrine, phenylephrine, phenylpropanolamine, phenothiazine tranquilizers, reserpine, or monoamine oxidase (MAO) inhibitors. At least 14 days should separate the use of a beta-blocker and an MAO inhibitor.

4. Beta-blockers may antagonize (work against) the effects of theophylline, aminophylline, albuterol, metaproterenol, and terbutaline.

5. Beta-blockers can also interact with insulin or oral anti-diabetic agents—raising or lowering blood sugar levels or masking the symptoms of low blood sugar.

BE SURE TO TELL YOUR DOCTOR if you are currently taking any of the medications listed above.

WARNINGS

- Before starting to take this medication, it is important to tell your doctor if you have ever had unusual or allergic reactions to any beta-blocker (atenolol, metoprolol, nadolol, pindolol, propranolol, and timolol).
- Tell your doctor if you now have, or if you have ever had, allergies, asthma, hay fever, eczema, slow heartbeat, bronchitis, diabetes mellitus (sugar diabetes), emphysema, heart or blood vessel disease, kidney disease, liver disease, thyroid disease, or poor circulation in the fingers or toes.
- You may want to check your pulse while taking this medication. If your pulse is much slower than your usual rate (or if it is less than 50 beats per minute), check with your doctor. A pulse rate that is too slow may cause circulation problems.
- This medicine may affect your body's response to exercise. Make sure you discuss with your doctor a safe amount of exercise for your medical condition.
- It is important that you do not stop taking this medicine without first checking with your doctor. Some conditions may become worse when the medicine is stopped suddenly, and the danger of a heart attack is increased in some patients. Your doctor may want you to gradually reduce the amount of medicine you take before stopping completely. Make sure that you have enough medicine on hand to last through vacations, holidays, and weekends.
- Before having surgery or any other medical or dental treatment, tell the physician or dentist that you are taking this medicine. Often, this medication will be discontinued 48 hours prior to any major surgery.
- This medicine can cause dizziness, drowsiness, lightheadedness, or decreased alertness. Therefore, exercise caution while driving a car or using any machinery.
- While taking this medicine, do not use any over-the-counter (non-prescription) asthma, allergy, cough, cold, sinus, or diet preparations unless you first check with your pharmacist or doctor. Some of these medicines can cause high blood pressure and slow heartbeat when taken at the same time as a beta-blocker.

• Be sure to tell your doctor if you are pregnant. Animal studies have shown that some beta-blockers can cause problems in pregnancy when used at very high doses. Adequate studies have not been done in humans, but there has been some association between beta-blockers used during pregnancy and low birth rate, as well as breathing problems and slow heart rate in the newborn infants. However, other reports have shown no effects on newborn infants. Also, tell your doctor if you are breastfeeding an infant. Small amounts of atenolol may pass into breast milk.

Ativan — see lorazepam

Atozine — see hydroxyzine

Atromid-S — see clofibrate

---

atropine, scopolamine, hyoscyamine, and phenobarbital combination

BRAND NAMES (Manufacturers)
Barophen (various manufacturers)
Bay-Ase (Bay)
belladonna alkaloids with phenobarbital
  (various manufacturers)
Bellalphen (CMC)
Bellastal (Wharton)
Donnamor (H.L. Moore)
Donna-Sed (Vortech)
Donnatal (Robins)
Hyosophen (Rugby)
Malatal (Mallard)
Neoquess (O'Neal)
Palbar (Hauck)
Pylora (Hyrex)

Relaxadon (Geneva Generics)
Seds (Pasadena Research)
Spalix (Reid-Provident)
Spasaid (Century)
Spaslin (Blaine)
Spasmolin (various manufacturers)
Spasmophen (Lannett)
Spasquid (Geneva Generics)
Susano (Halsey)
Vanatal (Vangard)

TYPE OF DRUG

Anti-cholinergic and sedative

INGREDIENTS

atropine as the sulfate salt, scopolamine as the hydro-bromide salt, hyoscyamine as the sulfate salt, and phenobarbital

DOSAGE FORMS

Tablets (0.0194 mg atropine, 0.0065 mg scopolamine, 0.1037 mg hyoscyamine, and 16.2 or 32.4 mg phenobarbital)

Capsules (0.0194 mg atropine, 0.0065 mg scopolamine, 0.1037 mg hyoscyamine, and 16.2 mg phenobarbital)

Sustained-release tablets (0.0582 mg atropine, 0.0195 mg scopolamine, 0.3111 mg hyoscyamine, and 48.16 mg phenobarbital)

Oral elixir (0.0194 mg atropine, 0.0065 mg scopolamine, 0.1037 mg hyoscyamine, 16.2 mg phenobarbital, and 23% alcohol)

STORAGE

The tablets, capsules, and oral elixir should be stored at room temperature, in tightly closed, light-resistant containers. This medication should never be frozen.

USES

This medication is used to treat bed-wetting, lack of bladder control, motion sickness, premenstrual tension, and stomach and intestinal disorders.

Atropine, scopolamine, and hyoscyamine belong to a group of drugs known as belladonna alkaloids or anti-cholinergic agents. These drugs block certain nerve pathways, thereby slowing the gastrointestinal tract and decreasing urination. Phenobarbital is a sedative that acts directly on the brain to slow the activity of the nervous system.

TREATMENT

This medication should be taken 30 minutes to one hour before meals (unless your doctor directs you to do otherwise). In order to reduce stomach upset, you can take it with food or with a glass of water or milk.

At least one hour should separate doses of this drug and either antacids or anti-diarrhea medications—they may prevent gastrointestinal absorption of this drug.

Measure the liquid form of this medication carefully with a specially designed, 5 ml measuring spoon. An ordinary kitchen teaspoon is not accurate enough.

The sustained-release tablets should be swallowed whole. Chewing, crushing, or breaking them destroys their sustained-release activity, and possibly increases the side effects.

If you miss a dose of this medication, do not take the missed dose at all; just return to your regular dosing schedule. Do not double the next dose.

SIDE EFFECTS

Minor. Blurred vision; confusion; constipation; decreased sexual desire; dizziness; drowsiness; dry mouth, nose, and throat; headache; insomnia; loss of taste; muscle pain; nausea; nervousness; reduced sweating; sensitivity of eyes to sunlight; vomiting; and weakness. These side effects should disappear in several days, as your body adjusts to the medication.

If you are constipated, increase the amount of fiber in your diet (fresh fruits and vegetables, salads, bran, and whole-grain breads), exercise, and drink more water (unless your doctor directs you to do otherwise).

Chew sugarless gum, or suck on ice chips or a piece of hard candy, to reduce mouth dryness.

Wear sunglasses if your eyes become sensitive to light

To avoid dizziness or light-headedness when you stand, contract and relax the muscles of your legs for a few moments before rising. Do this by pushing one foot

against the floor while raising the other foot slightly, alternating feet so that you are "pumping" your legs in a pedaling motion.

Major. Tell your doctor about any side effects that are persistent or particularly bothersome. IT IS ESPECIALLY IMPORTANT TO TELL YOUR DOCTOR about difficulty breathing; difficulty urinating; hallucinations; hot and dry skin; palpitations; rash; slurred speech; sore throat; or yellowing of the eyes or skin.

INTERACTIONS
This medication interacts with several other drugs.

1. The belladonna alkaloids and phenobarbital can cause extreme drowsiness when combined with central nervous system depressants (drugs that slow the activity of the nervous system), such as antihistamines, barbiturates, benzodiazepine tranquilizers, muscle relaxants, narcotics, pain medications, or alcohol, or with tricyclic anti-depressants.

2. Amantadine, antihistamines, haloperidol, monoamine oxidase (MAO) inhibitors, phenothiazine tranquilizers, procainamide, quinidine, and tricyclic anti-depressants can increase the side effects of the belladonna alkaloids.

3. Phenobarbital can increase the elimination from the body, and decrease the effectiveness, of oral anticoagulants (blood thinners, such as warfarin), cortisone-like medications, digoxin, griseofulvin, doxycycline, phenytoin, and tricyclic anti-depressants.

Before starting to take this medication, BE SURE TO TELL YOUR DOCTOR if you are taking any of the medications listed above.

WARNINGS
• Tell your doctor about unusual or allergic reactions you have had to medications, especially to atropine, scopolamine, hyoscyamine, phenobarbital, or any other barbiturate (butalbital, primidone, pentobarbital, or secobarbital).

• Tell your doctor if you now have, or if you have ever had, glaucoma, heart disease, hiatal hernia, high blood pressure, internal bleeding, kidney disease, liver disease, lung disease, myasthenia gravis, porphyria, enlarged prostate gland, obstructed bladder, obstructed intestine, severe ulcerative colitis, or thyroid disease.

- If this medication makes you dizzy or drowsy, or blurs your vision, do not take part in any activity that requires alertness, such as driving a car or operating potentially dangerous equipment. Be careful on stairs, and avoid getting up from a lying or sitting position suddenly.
- This medication can decrease sweating and heat release from the body. Therefore, avoid getting overheated by strenuous exercise in hot weather, and avoid taking hot baths, showers, and saunas.
- Before having any surgery or other medical or dental treatment, be sure to tell the doctor or dentist that you are taking this medication.
- Be sure to tell your doctor if you are pregnant. This medication crosses the placenta. Phenobarbital given to the mother close to term can cause breathing problems and bleeding complications in a newborn infant. Also, tell your doctor if you are breastfeeding an infant. Small amounts of this medication pass into breast milk and may cause excessive drowsiness or irritability in the nursing infant.

Aventyl—see nortriptyline

azatadine

BRAND NAME (Manufacturer)
Optimine (Schering)
TYPE OF DRUG
Antihistamine
INGREDIENT
azatadine as the maleate salt
DOSAGE FORM
Tablets (1 mg)
STORAGE
Azatadine should be stored at room temperature in a tightly closed container.

USES

This medication belongs to a group of drugs known as antihistamines (antihistamines block the action of histamine, a chemical released by the body during an allergic reaction). It is therefore used to treat or prevent symptoms of allergy.

TREATMENT

To avoid stomach upset, you can take azatadine with food or with a full glass of milk or water (unless your doctor directs you to do otherwise).

If you miss a dose of this medication, take the missed dose as soon as possible, unless it is close to the time for your next dose. In that case, don't take the missed dose at all; just return to your regular dosing schedule. Do not double the next dose.

SIDE EFFECTS

Minor. Blurred vision; constipation; diarrhea; difficult or painful urination; dizziness; dry mouth, throat, or nose; headache; irritability; loss of appetite; confusion; nausea; restlessness; ringing or buzzing in the ears; rash; stomach upset; and unusual increase in sweating. These side effects should disappear in several days, as your body adjusts to the medication.

If you are constipated, increase the amount of fiber in your diet (raw vegetables, fruits, salads, bran, and whole-grain breads) and drink more water (unless your doctor tells you not to do so).

Chew sugarless gum, or suck on ice chips or a piece of hard candy, to reduce mouth dryness.

This medication can cause increased sensitivity to sunlight. It is therefore important to avoid prolonged exposure to sunlight and sunlamps. Wear protective clothing, and use an effective sunscreen.

If you feel dizzy or light-headed, sit or lie down awhile; get up from a sitting or lying position slowly, and be careful on stairs.

Major. Tell your doctor about any side effects that are persistent or particularly bothersome. IT IS ESPECIALLY IMPORTANT TO TELL YOUR DOCTOR about unusual bleeding or bruising; change in menstruation; clumsiness; feeling faint; flushing of the face; hallucinations; sleeping disorders; seizures; shortness of breath; sore throat and fever; palpitations; tightness in the chest; or unusual tiredness or weakness.

INTERACTIONS

Azatadine interacts with several other types of medication.

1. Concurrent use of this medication with other central nervous system depressants (drugs that slow the activity of the nervous system), such as barbiturates, benzodiazepine tranquilizers, muscle relaxants, narcotics, pain medication, phenothiazine tranquilizers, or alcohol, or with tricyclic anti-depressants can cause extreme drowsiness.

2. Monoamine oxidase (MAO) inhibitors (isocarboxazid, pargyline, phenelzine, tranylcypromine) can increase the side effects of this medication.

3. Azatadine can also decrease the activity of oral anticoagulants (blood thinners, such as warfarin).

TELL YOUR DOCTOR if you are currently taking any of the medications listed above.

WARNINGS

● Tell your doctor about unusual or allergic reactions you have had to medications, especially to azatadine or any other antihistamine (bromodiphenhydramine, brompheniramine, carbinoxamine, chlorpheniramine, clemastine, cyproheptadine, dexchlorpheniramine, dimenhydrinate, dimethindene, diphenhydramine, diphenylpyraline, doxylamine, hydroxyzine, promethazine, pyrilamine, trimeprazine, tripelennamine, or tripolidine).

● Tell your doctor if you now have, or if you have ever had, asthma, blood vessel disease, glaucoma, high blood pressure, kidney disease, peptic ulcers, enlarged prostate gland, or thyroid disease.

● Azatadine can cause drowsiness or dizziness. Your ability to perform tasks that require alertness, such as driving a car or operating potentially dangerous machinery, may be decreased. Appropriate caution should therefore be taken.

• Be sure to tell your doctor if you are pregnant. The effects of this medication during pregnancy have not yet been thoroughly studied in humans. Also, tell your doctor if you are breastfeeding an infant. Small amounts of azatadine pass into breast milk and may cause unusual excitement or irritability in nursing infants.

azathioprine

BRAND NAME (Manufacturer)
Imuran (Burroughs Wellcome)
TYPE OF DRUG
Immunosuppressant
INGREDIENT
azathioprine
DOSAGE FORM
Tablets (25 mg and 50 mg)
STORAGE
Azathioprine should be stored at room temperature, in a tightly closed, light-resistant container.

USES

This medication is used to prevent rejection of kidney transplants and to control the symptoms of severe rheumatoid arthritis. It is not clear exactly how azathioprine works, but it is known to act on the body's immune system.

TREATMENT

In order to prevent nausea and vomiting, you can take azathioprine with food or after a meal (unless your doctor directs you to do otherwise).

Try not to miss any doses of this medication. If you do miss a dose, take the missed dose as soon as possible, unless it is almost time for the next scheduled dose. In that case, do not take the missed dose at all; just return to your regular dosing schedule. Do not double the next dose. If you miss more than one dose, CHECK WITH YOUR DOCTOR.

SIDE EFFECTS

Minor. Diarrhea; nausea; and vomiting. These side effects should disappear in several weeks, as your body adjusts to the medication.

Major. Tell your doctor about any side effects that are persistent or particularly bothersome. IT IS ESPECIALLY IMPORTANT TO TELL YOUR DOCTOR about unusual bleeding or bruising; darkened urine; fever; hair loss; joint pains; mouth sores; muscle aches; skin rash; sore throat; or yellowing of the eyes or skin.

INTERACTIONS

BE SURE TO TELL YOUR DOCTOR if you are already taking allopurinol. It can increase the blood levels of azathioprine, which can lead to serious side effects.

WARNINGS

- Tell your doctor about unusual or allergic reactions you have had to any medications, especially to azathioprine.
- Before starting to take this medication, be sure to tell your doctor if you now have, or if you have ever had, gout, kidney disease, liver disease, pancreatitis, or recurrent infections.
- Azathioprine is potent medicine. Your doctor will want to carefully monitor your therapy with blood tests, so that you will obtain the maximum benefit with the least possible side effects.
- Do not stop taking this drug unless you first check with your doctor. Stopping this drug abruptly may lead to a worsening of your condition. Your doctor may want to start you on another drug before azathioprine is stopped.
- Azathioprine has been shown to produce cancers in animals. Organ transplant patients also appear to be at a higher risk for developing cancers while taking azathioprine.
- Azathioprine can increase your susceptibility to infections. It is therefore important to contact your doctor at the first sign of infection. Your dose of azathioprine may need to be adjusted.
- Be sure to tell your doctor if you are pregnant. Birth defects have been reported in animals whose mothers received large doses of azathioprine during pregnancy.

This drug also has the potential for producing birth defects in human offspring. Also, tell your doctor if you are breastfeeding an infant. It is not known whether or not azathioprine passes into breast milk.

Azodine—see phenazopyridine

Azo Gantanol—see sulfamethoxazole and phenazopyridine combination

Azo Gantrisin—see sulfisoxazole and phenazopyridine combination

Azolid—see phenylbutazone

Azo-Sulfisoxazole—see sulfisoxazole and phenazopyridine combination

Azo-Sulfizin—see sulfisoxazole and phenazopyridine combination

Azulfidine—see sulfasalazine

Azulfidine EN-tabs—see sulfasalazine

Bacarate—see phendimetrazine

---

baclofen

BRAND NAMES (Manufacturers)
Lioresal (Geigy)
Lioresal DS (Geigy)
TYPE OF DRUG
Muscle relaxant
INGREDIENT
baclofen
DOSAGE FORM
Tablets (10 mg and 20 mg)
STORAGE
Baclofen should be stored at room temperature in a tightly closed container.

USES

This medication is used to relieve muscle spasms. It is unclear exactly how baclofen works to relieve spasticity, but it is known that the drug acts on the brain and spinal cord.

TREATMENT

Baclofen can be taken either on an empty stomach or with food or a full glass of milk or water.

If you miss a dose of this medication and remember within an hour, take the missed dose immediately. If more than an hour has passed, do not take the missed dose at all; just return to your regular dosing schedule. Do not double the next dose.

SIDE EFFECTS

Minor. Abdominal pain; constipation; dizziness; diarrhea; drowsiness; dry mouth; fatigue; headache; insomnia; loss of appetite; nasal congestion; vomiting; and weight gain. These side effects should disappear in several days, as your body adjusts to the medication.

To relieve constipation, increase the amount of fiber in your diet (bran, salads, fresh fruits and vegetables, and whole-grain breads), and drink more water (unless your doctor directs you to do otherwise).

If you feel dizzy, sit or lie down awhile; get up slowly, and be careful on stairs.

To relieve mouth dryness, chew sugarless gum, or suck on ice chips or a piece of hard candy.

Major. Tell your doctor about any side effects that are persistent or particularly bothersome. IT IS ESPECIALLY IMPORTANT TO TELL YOUR DOCTOR about chest pain, confusion, convulsions, depression, false sense of well-being, fainting, hallucinations, muscle pain, palpitations, ringing in the ears, slurred speech, tremors, or visual disturbances.

INTERACTIONS

Baclofen interacts with several other types of medication.
1. Concurrent use of baclofen with other central nervous system depressants (drugs that slow the activity of the brain and spinal cord), such as alcohol, antihistamines,

barbiturates, benzodiazepine tranquilizers, muscle relaxants, narcotics, pain medications, phenothiazine tranquilizers, or sleeping medicines, or with tricyclic anti-depressants can lead to extreme drowsiness.

2. The dosage of oral anti-diabetic medications may need to be altered when baclofen is started.

BE SURE TO TELL YOUR DOCTOR if you are already taking any of the medications listed above.

WARNINGS

● Before starting to take baclofen, be sure to tell your doctor if you now have, or if you have ever had, diabetes mellitus (sugar diabetes), epilepsy, kidney disease, mental disorders, or stroke.

● If this drug makes you dizzy or drowsy, avoid taking part in any activity that requires alertness, such as driving a car or operating potentially dangerous equipment.

● Do not stop taking this medication unless you first check with your doctor. Stopping this drug abruptly can lead to hallucinations, nervousness, convulsions, and mood changes. Your doctor may therefore want to reduce your dosage gradually.

● Be sure to tell your doctor if you are pregnant. Although baclofen appears to be safe in humans, birth defects have been reported in animals whose mothers received large doses of this drug during pregnancy. Also, tell your doctor if you are breastfeeding an infant. It is not known whether or not baclofen passes into breast milk.

Bactocill—see oxacillin

Bactrim—see sulfamethoxazole and trimethoprim combination

Bactrim DS—see sulfamethoxazole and trimethoprim combination

Bancap HC—see acetaminophen and hydrocodone combination

Barbita—see phenobarbital

Barophen—see atropine, scopolamine, hyoscyamine, and phenobarbital combination

Bayapap with Codeine—see acetaminophen and codeine combination

Bay-Ase—see atropine, scopolamine, hyoscyamine, and phenobarbital combination

Bay-Ornade—see phenylpropanolamine and caramiphen combination

Beepen-VK—see penicillin VK

Belix—see diphenhydramine

belladonna alkaloids with phenobarbital—see atropine, scopolamine, hyoscyamine, and phenobarbital combination

Bellalphen—see atropine, scopolamine, hyoscyamine, and phenobarbital combination

Bellastal—see atropine, scopolamine, hyoscyamine, and phenobarbital combination

Benadryl—see diphenhydramine

Benaphen   see diphenhydramine

---

bendroflumethiazide

BRAND NAME (Manufacturer)
Naturetin (Squibb)
TYPE OF DRUG
Diuretic (water pill) and anti-hypertensive
INGREDIENT
bendroflumethiazide
DOSAGE FORM
Tablets (2.5 mg, 5 mg, and 10 mg)

STORAGE
This medication should be stored at room temperature in a tightly closed container.

USES
Bendroflumethiazide is prescribed to treat high blood pressure. It is also used to reduce fluid accumulation in the body caused by conditions such as heart failure, cirrhosis of the liver, kidney disease, and the long-term use of some medications. This medication reduces fluid accumulation by increasing the elimination of sodium and water through the kidneys.

TREATMENT
To decrease stomach irritation, you can take this medication with a glass of milk or with a meal (unless your doctor directs you to do otherwise). Try to take it at the same time every day. Avoid taking a dose after 6:00 P.M.—this will prevent you from having to get up during the night to urinate.

If you miss a dose of medication, take the missed dose as soon as possible, unless it is almost time for the next dose. In that case, do not take the missed dose at all; just wait until the next scheduled dose. Do not double the dose.

This medication does not cure high blood pressure, but it will help to control the condition, as long as you continue to take it.

SIDE EFFECTS
Minor. Constipation; cramps; diarrhea; dizziness; drowsiness; headache; heartburn; itching; loss of appetite; nausea; restlessness; upset stomach; vomiting. As your body adjusts to the medication, these side effects should disappear.

This medication can cause increased sensitivity to sunlight. It is therefore important to avoid prolonged exposure to sunlight and sunlamps. Wear protective clothing, and use an effective sunscreen.

To avoid dizziness or light-headedness when you stand, contract and relax the muscles of your legs for a few moments before rising. Do this by pushing one foot

against the floor while raising the other foot slightly, alternating the feet so that you are "pumping" your legs in a pedaling motion.

Major. Tell your doctor about any side effects that are persistent or particularly bothersome. IT IS ESPECIALLY IMPORTANT TO TELL YOUR DOCTOR about any unusual bleeding or bruising; blurred vision; confusion; difficulty breathing; dry mouth; fever; joint pain; mood changes; muscle spasms; palpitations; skin rash; excessive thirst; sore throat; tingling in the fingers or toes; excessive weakness; or yellowing of the eyes or skin.

INTERACTIONS

Bendroflumethiazide interacts with several other types of medication.

1. It may decrease the effectiveness of oral anti-coagulants, anti-gout medications, insulin, oral anti-diabetic medicines, and methenamine.

2. Fenfluramine can increase the blood-pressure-lowering effects of bendroflumethiazide (which can be dangerous).

3. Indomethacin can decrease the blood-pressure-lowering effects (thereby counteracting the desired effects) of bendroflumethiazide.

4. Cholestyramine and colestipol decrease the absorption of this medication from the gastrointestinal tract. Bendroflumethiazide should therefore be taken one hour before, or four hours after, a dose of cholestyramine or colestipol (if you have also been prescribed one of these medications).

5. The side effects of amphotericin B, calcium, cortisone-like steroids (such as cortisone, dexamethasone, hydrocortisone, prednisone, prednisolone), digoxin, digitalis, lithium, quinidine, sulfonamide antibiotics, and vitamin D may be increased when taken concurrently with bendroflumethiazide.

BE SURE TO TELL YOUR DOCTOR if you are already taking any of the medicines listed above.

WARNINGS

• Tell your doctor about unusual or allergic reactions you have had to any medications, especially to diuretics (water pills), oral anti-diabetic medications, or sulfonamide antibiotics.

• Before you start taking bendroflumethiazide, tell your doctor if you now have, or if you have ever had, kidney disease or problems with urination, diabetes mellitus (sugar diabetes), gout, liver disease, asthma, pancreas disease, or systemic lupus erythematosus (SLE).

• Bendroflumethiazide can cause potassium loss. Signs of potassium loss include dry mouth, thirst, weakness, muscle pain or cramps, nausea, and vomiting. If you experience any of these symptoms, call your doctor. To help avoid potassium loss, take this drug with a glass of fresh or frozen orange juice or cranberry juice, or eat a banana every day. The use of a salt substitute also helps to prevent potassium loss. Do not change your diet, however, before discussing it with your doctor. Too much potassium can also be dangerous. Your doctor may want you to have blood tests performed periodically, in order to monitor your potassium levels.

• Limit your intake of alcoholic beverages while taking this medication, in order to prevent dizziness and light-headedness.

• If you have high blood pressure, do not take any over-the-counter (non-prescription) medications for weight control or for allergy, asthma, cough, cold, or sinus problems, unless your doctor directs you to do so.

• To prevent dehydration (severe water loss) while taking this medication, check with your doctor if you have any illness that causes severe or continuous nausea, vomiting, or diarrhea.

• This medication can raise blood sugar in diabetic patients. Therefore, blood sugar levels should be carefully monitored by blood or urine tests when this medication is started.

• This product contains F.D. & C. Yellow Dye No. 5 (tartrazine), which can cause allergic-type reactions (difficulty breathing, rash, or fainting) in certain susceptible individuals.

• Be sure to tell your doctor if you are pregnant, because this drug is able to cross the placenta. Studies in humans have not been completed, but adverse effects have been observed on the fetuses of animals who were given large doses of this drug during pregnancy. Also, tell your doctor if you are breastfeeding an infant. Although problems in humans have not been reported, small amounts of this drug can pass into breast milk, so caution is warranted.

Bendylate—see diphenhydramine

Benemid—see probenecid

Bentyl—see dicyclomine

---

benzthiazide

BRAND NAMES (Manufacturers)
Aquatag (Reid-Provident)
benzthiazide (various manufacturers)
Exna (Robins)
Hydrex (Trimen)
Marazide (Vortech)
Proaqua (Reid-Provident)
TYPE OF DRUG
Diuretic (water pill) and anti-hypertensive
INGREDIENT
benzthiazide
DOSAGE FORM
Tablets (25 mg and 50 mg)
STORAGE
This medication should be stored at room temperature in a tightly closed container.

USES

Benzthiazide is prescribed to treat high blood pressure. It is also used to reduce fluid accumulation in the body caused by conditions such as heart failure, cirrhosis of the liver, kidney disease, and the long-term use of some medications. This medication reduces fluid accumulation by increasing the elimination of sodium and water through the kidneys.

TREATMENT

To decrease stomach irritation, you can take this medication with a glass of milk or with a meal (unless your doctor directs you to do otherwise). Try to take it at the same time every day. Avoid taking a dose after 6:00 P.M.—this will prevent you from having to get up during the night to urinate.

If you miss a dose of this medication, take the missed dose as soon as possible, unless it is almost time for the next dose. In that case, do not take the missed dose at all; just wait until the next scheduled dose. Do not double the dose.

This medication does not cure high blood pressure, but it will help to control the condition, as long as you continue to take it.

SIDE EFFECTS

Minor. Constipation; cramps; diarrhea; dizziness; drowsiness; headache; heartburn; itching; loss of appetite; nausea; restlessness; upset stomach; vomiting. As your body adjusts to this medication, these side effects should disappear.

This medication can cause increased sensitivity to sunlight. It is therefore important to avoid prolonged exposure to sunlight or sunlamps. Wear protective clothing, and use an effective sunscreen.

To avoid dizziness or light-headedness when you stand, contract and relax the muscles of your legs for a few moments before rising. Do this by pushing one foot against the floor while raising the other foot slightly, alternating the feet so that you are "pumping" your legs in a pedaling motion.

Major. Tell your doctor about any side effects that are persistent or particularly bothersome. IT IS ESPECIALLY IMPORTANT TO TELL YOUR DOCTOR about any unusual bleeding or bruising; blurred vision; confusion; difficulty breathing; dry mouth; fever; joint pain; mood changes; muscle spasms; palpitations; skin rash; excessive thirst; sore throat; tingling in the fingers or toes; excessive weakness; or yellowing of the eyes or skin.

INTERACTIONS

Benzthiazide interacts with several other types of medication.

1. It may decrease the effectiveness of oral anti-coagulants, anti-gout medications, insulin, oral anti-diabetic medicines, and methenamine.

2. Fenfluramine can increase the blood-pressure-lowering effects of benzthiazide (which can be dangerous).

3. Indomethacin can decrease the blood-pressure-lowering effects (thereby counteracting the desired effects) of benzthiazide.

4. Cholestyramine and colestipol decrease the absorption of this medication from the gastrointestinal tract. Benzthiazide should therefore be taken one hour before, or four hours after, a dose of cholestyramine or colestipol (if you have also been prescribed one of these medications).

5. The side effects of amphotericin B, calcium, cortisone-like steroids (such as cortisone, dexamethasone, hydrocortisone, prednisone, prednisolone), digoxin, digitalis, lithium, quinidine, sulfonamide antibiotics, and vitamin D may be increased when taken concurrently with benzthiazide.

BE SURE TO TELL YOUR DOCTOR if you are already taking any of the medicines listed above.

WARNINGS

- Tell your doctor about unusual or allergic reactions you have had to any medications, especially to diuretics (water pills), oral anti-diabetic medications, or sulfonamide antibiotics.

- Before you start taking benzthiazide, tell your doctor if you now have, or if you have ever had, kidney disease or problems with urination, diabetes mellitus (sugar diabetes), gout, liver disease, asthma, pancreas disease, or systemic lupus erythematosus (SLE).

- Benzthiazide can cause potassium loss. Signs of potassium loss include dry mouth, thirst, weakness, muscle pain or cramps, nausea, and vomiting. If you experience any of these symptoms, call your doctor. To help avoid potassium loss, take this drug with a glass of fresh or frozen orange juice or cranberry juice, or eat a banana every day. The use of a salt substitute also helps to prevent potassium loss. Do not change your diet, however, before discussing it with your doctor. Too much potassium can also be dangerous. Your doctor may want you to have blood tests performed periodically, in order to monitor your potassium levels.

- Limit your intake of alcoholic beverages while taking this medication, in order to prevent dizziness and light-headedness.
- If you have high blood pressure, do not take any over-the-counter (non-prescription) medications for weight control or for allergy, asthma, cough, cold, or sinus problems, unless your doctor directs you to do so.
- To prevent dehydration (severe water loss) while taking this medication, check with your doctor if you have any illness that causes severe or continuous nausea, vomiting, or diarrhea.
- This medication can raise blood sugar in diabetic patients. Therefore, blood sugar levels should be carefully monitored by blood or urine tests when this medication is started.
- Some of these products contain F.D. & C. Yellow Dye No. 5 (tartrazine), which can cause allergic-type reactions (difficulty breathing, wheezing, rash, or fainting) in certain susceptible individuals.
- Be sure to tell your doctor if you are pregnant, because this drug is able to cross the placenta. Studies in humans have not been completed, but adverse effects have been observed on the fetuses of animals who were given large doses of this drug during pregnancy. Also, tell your doctor if you are breastfeeding an infant. Although problems in humans have not been reported, small amounts of this drug can pass into breast milk, so caution is warranted.

---

benztropine

BRAND NAME (Manufacturer)
Cogentin (Merck Sharp & Dohme)
TYPE OF DRUG
Anti-parkinson
INGREDIENT
benztropine as the mesylate salt
DOSAGE FORM
Tablets (0.5 mg, 1 mg, and 2 mg)

STORAGE

Benztropine tablets should be stored at room temperature in a tightly closed container.

USES

Benztropine is used to treat the symptoms of Parkinson's disease or to control the side effects of phenothiazine tranquilizers. It is not clearly understood how this medication works, but it is thought to act by balancing certain chemicals in the brain.

TREATMENT

In order to reduce stomach irritation, you can take benztropine tablets with food, or just after a meal.

Antacids and diarrhea medicines prevent the absorption of this medication, so at least one hour should separate doses of benztropine and one of these medicines.

If you miss a dose of this medication, take the missed dose as soon as possible, unless it is within two hours of your next dose. In that case, don't take the missed dose at all; just return to your regular dosing schedule. Do not double the next dose.

SIDE EFFECTS

Minor. Bloating; blurred vision; constipation; dizziness; drowsiness; dry mouth, throat, and nose; false sense of well-being; headache; increased sensitivity of the eyes to light; muscle cramps; nausea; nervousness; reduced sweating; and weakness. These side effects should disappear in several days, as your body adjusts to the medication.

If you are constipated, increase the amount of fiber in your diet (fresh fruits and vegetables, salads, bran, and whole-grain breads), exercise, and drink more water (unless your doctor directs you to do otherwise).

Chew sugarless gum, or suck on ice chips or a piece of hard candy, to reduce mouth dryness.

Wear sunglasses if your eyes become sensitive to light.

To avoid dizziness and light-headedness when you stand, contract and relax the muscles of your legs for a few moments before rising. Do this by pushing one foot against the floor while raising the other foot slightly, alternating feet so that you are "pumping" your legs in a pedaling motion.

Major. Tell your doctor about any side effects that are persistent or particularly bothersome. IT IS ESPECIALLY IMPORTANT TO TELL YOUR DOCTOR about depression; difficulty urinating; hallucinations; involuntary muscle movements; numbness of the fingers; palpitations; or unusual excitement.

INTERACTIONS

Benztropine interacts with several other types of medication.

1. It can cause extreme drowsiness when combined with alcohol or other central nervous system depressants (drugs that slow the activity of the nervous system), such as antihistamines, barbiturates, benzodiazepine tranquilizers, muscle relaxants, narcotics, or pain medication, or with tricyclic anti-depressants.

2. Amantadine, antihistamines, haloperidol, monoamine oxidase (MAO) inhibitors, phenothiazine tranquilizers, procainamide, quinidine, and tricyclic anti-depressants can increase the side effects of benztropine.

Before starting to take this medication, BE SURE TO TELL YOUR DOCTOR if you are already taking any of the medications listed above.

WARNINGS

• Tell your doctor about unusual or allergic reactions you have had to any medications, especially to benztropine.

• Tell your doctor if you now have, or if you have ever had, achalasia, glaucoma, heart disease, high blood pressure, kidney disease, liver disease, myasthenia gravis, blockage of the intestinal tract or urinary tract, enlarged prostate gland, stomach ulcers, or thyroid disease.

• If this medication makes you dizzy or drowsy, do not take part in any activity that requires alertness, such as driving a car or operating potentially dangerous equipment. Be careful on stairs; and avoid getting up suddenly from a lying or sitting position.

• This medication can decrease sweating and heat release from the body. You should therefore avoid getting overheated by strenuous exercise in hot weather, and should avoid taking hot baths, showers, and saunas.

• Be sure to tell your doctor if you are pregnant. Although benztropine appears to be safe during pregnancy, extensive studies have not yet been completed. Also, tell your doctor if you are breastfeeding an infant. Small amounts of this medication may pass into breast milk.

Beta-2—see isoetharine

---

betamethasone (systemic)

BRAND NAME (Manufacturer)
Celestone (Schering)
TYPE OF DRUG
Adrenocorticosteroid hormone
INGREDIENT
betamethasone
DOSAGE FORMS
Tablets (0.6 mg)
Oral syrup (0.6 mg per 5 ml teaspoonful)
STORAGE
Betamethasone tablets and oral syrup should be stored at room temperature in a tightly closed container.

USES
Your adrenal glands naturally produce certain cortisone-like chemicals. These chemicals are involved in various regulatory processes in the body (such as maintenance of fluid balance, temperature, and reactions to inflammation). Betamethasone belongs to a group of drugs known as adrenocorticosteroids (or cortisone-like medications). It is used to treat a variety of disorders, including endocrine and rheumatic disorders; asthma; blood diseases; certain cancers; eye disorders; gastrointestinal disturbances such as ulcerative colitis; respiratory diseases; and inflammations such as arthritis, dermatitis, and poison ivy. How this drug acts to relieve these disorders is not completely understood.

TREATMENT

In order to prevent stomach irritation, you can take betamethasone with food or milk.

The oral syrup form of this medication should be measured carefully, with a specially designed, 5 ml measuring spoon. An ordinary kitchen teaspoon is not accurate enough.

If you are taking only one dose of this medication each day, try to take it before 9:00 A.M. This will mimic the body's normal production of this type of chemical.

It is important to try not to miss any doses of betamethasone. However, if you do miss a dose of this medication:

1. If you are taking it more than once a day, take the missed dose as soon as possible and return to your regular schedule. If it is already time for the next dose, double the dose.

2. If you are taking this medication once a day, take the dose you missed as soon as possible, unless you don't remember until the next day. In that case, do not take the missed dose at all; just follow your regular schedule. Do not double the next dose.

3. If you are taking this drug every other day, take it as soon as you remember. If you missed the scheduled time by a whole day, take it when you remember; then skip a day before you take the next dose. Do not double the dose.

If you miss more than one dose, CONTACT YOUR DOCTOR.

SIDE EFFECTS

Minor. Dizziness; false sense of well-being; increased appetite; increased susceptibility to infections; increased sweating; indigestion; menstrual irregularities; muscle weakness; nausea; reddening of the skin on the face; restlessness; sleep disorders; thinning of the skin; and weight gain. These side effects should disappear in several days, as your body adjusts to the medication.

To help avoid potassium loss while using this drug, take your dose with a glass of fresh or frozen orange juice, or eat a banana each day. The use of a salt substitute also helps prevent potassium loss. Discuss this with your doctor.

Major. Tell your doctor about any side effects that are persistent or particularly bothersome. IT IS ESPECIALLY IMPORTANT TO TELL YOUR DOCTOR about abdominal enlargement; acne or other skin problems; back or rib pain; bloody or black, tarry stools; blurred vision; unusual bruising or bleeding; convulsions; fever and sore throat; glaucoma; growth impairment (in children); headaches; impaired healing of wounds; increased thirst and urination; mental depression; mood changes; muscle wasting; nightmares; peptic ulcers; rapid weight gain (three to five pounds within a week); rash; shortness of breath; or unusual weakness.

INTERACTIONS

Betamethasone interacts with other medication.

1. Alcohol, aspirin, and anti-inflammation medications (diflunisal, ibuprofen, indomethacin, mefenamic acid, meclofenamate, naproxen, piroxicam, sulindac, tolmetin) aggravate the stomach problems that are common with use of this medication.

2. A change in the dosage requirements of oral anticoagulants (blood thinners, such as warfarin) and oral anti-diabetic drugs or insulin may be necessary when this medication is started or stopped.

3. The loss of potassium caused by betamethasone can lead to serious side effects in individuals taking digoxin. Thiazide diuretics (water pills) can increase the potassium loss caused by betamethasone.

4. Phenobarbital, phenytoin, rifampin, and ephedrine can increase the elimination of betamethasone from the body, thereby decreasing its effectiveness.

5. Oral contraceptives and estrogen-containing drugs may decrease the elimination of this drug from the body, which can lead to an increase in side effects.

6. Betamethasone can increase the elimination of aspirin and isoniazid, thereby decreasing the effectiveness of these two medications.

7. Cholestyramine and colestipol can chemically bind this medication in the stomach and gastrointestinal tract

and prevent its absorption.
TELL YOUR DOCTOR if you are currently taking any of
the medications listed above.

WARNINGS

• Tell your doctor about unusual or allergic reactions you
have had to any medications, especially to betamethasone or other adrenocorticosteroids (such as cortisone,
dexamethasone, fluprednisolone, hydrocortisone, methylprednisolone, paramethasone, prednisolone, prednisone, or triamcinolone).

• Be sure to tell your doctor if you now have, or if you
have ever had, bone disease; diabetes mellitus (sugar
diabetes); emotional instability; glaucoma; fungal infections; heart disease; high blood pressure; high
cholesterol levels; myasthenia gravis; peptic ulcers; osteoporosis; thyroid disease; tuberculosis; severe ulcerative colitis; kidney disease; or liver disease.

• If you are using this medication for longer than a week,
you may need to receive higher dosages if you are subjected to stress, such as serious infections, injury, or
surgery. Discuss this with your doctor.

• If you have been taking this drug for more than a week,
do not stop taking it suddenly. If it is stopped suddenly,
you may experience abdominal or back pain, dizziness,
fainting, fever, muscle or joint pain, nausea, vomiting,
shortness of breath, or extreme weakness. Your doctor
may therefore want to reduce the dosage gradually. Never
increase the dose or take the drug for longer than the
prescribed time, unless you first consult your doctor.

• While you are taking this drug, you should not be vaccinated or immunized. This medication decreases the effectiveness of vaccines and can lead to overwhelming
infection if a live virus is administered.

• Before having any surgery or other medical or dental
treatment, be sure your doctor or dentist knows that you
are taking betamethasone.

• Because this drug can cause glaucoma and cataracts
with long-term use, your doctor may want you to have
your eyes examined by an ophthalmologist periodically
during treatment.

• If you are taking this medication for prolonged periods,

you should wear or carry an identification card or notice stating that you are taking an adrenocorticosteroid.

• This medication can raise blood sugar levels in diabetic patients. Blood sugar should therefore be monitored carefully with blood or urine tests when this medication is started.

• Be sure to tell your doctor if you are pregnant. This type of drug crosses the placenta. Although studies in humans have not yet been completed, birth defects have been observed in animals whose mothers were given large doses of this drug during pregnancy. Also, tell your doctor if you are breastfeeding an infant. Small amounts of this type of drug pass into breast milk and may cause growth suppression or a decrease in natural adrenocorticosteroid production in the nursing infant.

---

betamethasone dipropionate (topical)

BRAND NAMES (Manufacturers)
Diprolene (Schering)
Diprosone (Schering)
TYPE OF DRUG
Adrenocorticosteroid hormone
INGREDIENT
betamethasone as the dipropionate salt
DOSAGE FORMS
Ointment (0.05%)
Cream (0.05%)
Lotion (0.05%)
Aerosol (0.1%)
STORAGE
Betamethasone dipropionate ointment, cream, and lotion should be stored at room temperature in tightly closed containers. This medication should never be frozen.

The aerosol form of this medication is packed under pressure. It should not be stored near heat or an open flame, or in direct sunlight; and the container should never be punctured.

USES

Your adrenal glands naturally produce certain cortisone-like chemicals. These chemicals are involved in various regulatory processes in the body (such as fluid balance, temperature, and reactions to inflammation). Betamethasone dipropionate belongs to a group of drugs known as adrenocorticosteroids (or cortisone-like medications). It is used to relieve the skin inflammation (redness, swelling, itching, and discomfort) associated with conditions such as dermatitis, eczema, and poison ivy. How this drug acts to relieve these disorders is not completely understood.

TREATMENT

Before applying this medication, wash your hands. Then, unless your doctor gives you different instructions, gently wash the area of the skin where the medication is to be applied. With a clean towel, pat the area almost dry; it should be slightly damp when you put the medicine on.

If you are using the lotion form of this medication, shake it well before pouring it out. The contents tend to settle on the bottom of the bottle, so it is necessary to shake the container to evenly distribute the ingredients and equalize the doses.

Apply a small amount of the medication to the affected area in a thin layer. Do not bandage the area unless your doctor tells you to do so. If you are to apply an occlusive dressing (like kitchen plastic wrap), be sure you understand the instructions.

If you are using the aerosol spray form of this medication, shake the can in order to disperse the medication evenly. Hold the can upright, six to eight inches from the area to be sprayed, and spray the area for one to three seconds. DO NOT SMOKE while you are using the aerosol spray; the contents are under pressure and may explode when exposed to heat or flames.

If you miss a dose of this medication, apply the dose as soon as possible, unless it is almost time for the next application. In that case, do not apply the missed dose;

just return to your regular schedule. Do not put twice as much medication on your skin at the next application.

SIDE EFFECTS

Minor. Acne; burning sensation; skin dryness; irritation of the affected area; itching; and rash.

If the affected area is extremely dry or scaling, the skin may be moistened before applying the medication by soaking in water or by applying water with a clean cloth. The ointment form is probably better for dry skin.

A mild, temporary stinging sensation may occur after this medication is applied. If this persists, contact your doctor.

Major. Tell your doctor about any side effects that are persistent or particularly bothersome. IT IS ESPECIALLY IMPORTANT TO TELL YOUR DOCTOR about blistering; increased hair growth; loss of skin color; secondary infection in the area being treated; or thinning of the skin with easy bruising.

INTERACTIONS

This medication does not interact with any other medications, as long as it is used according to directions.

WARNINGS

• Tell your doctor about unusual or allergic reactions you have had to medications, especially to betamethasone dipropionate or any other adrenocorticosteroid (such as amcinonide, clocortolone, cortisone, desonide, desoximetasone, dexamethasone, diflorasone, flumethasone, fluocinolone, fluocinonide, fluorometholone, flurandrenolide, halcinonide, hydrocortisone, methylprednisolone, prednisolone, prednisone, or triamcinolone).

• Tell your doctor if you now have, or if you have ever had, blood vessel disease, chicken pox, diabetes mellitus (sugar diabetes), fungal infection, peptic ulcer, shingles, tuberculosis, tuberculosis of the skin, vaccinia, or any other type of infection, especially at the site currently being treated.

- If irritation develops while using this drug, immediately discontinue its use and notify your doctor.
- This product is not for use in the eyes or on mucous membranes. Exposure of this medication to the eye may result in ocular (to the eye) side effects.
- Do not use this product with an occlusive wrap unless your doctor directs you to do so. Systemic absorption of this drug is increased if extensive areas of the body are treated, particularly if occlusive bandages are used. If it is necessary for you to use this drug under a wrap, follow your doctor's instructions exactly; do not leave the wrap in place longer than specified.
- If you are using this medication on a child's diaper area, do not put tight-fitting diapers or plastic pants on the child. This may lead to increased systemic absorption of the drug and a possible increase in side effects.
- In order to avoid freezing skin tissue when using the aerosol form of betamethasone dipropionate, make sure that you do not spray for more than three seconds; and hold the container at least six inches away.
- When using the aerosol form of this medication on the face, cover your eyes, and do not inhale the spray (in order to avoid side effects).
- Be sure to tell your doctor if you are pregnant. If large amounts of this drug are applied for prolonged periods, some of it will be absorbed and may cross the placenta. Although studies in humans have not yet been completed, birth defects have been observed in animals whose mothers were given large doses of this type of drug during pregnancy. Also, tell your doctor if you are breast-feeding an infant. If absorbed through the skin, small amounts of the drug pass into breast milk and may cause growth suppression or a decrease in natural adrenocorticosteroid production in the nursing infant.

---

betamethasone valerate (topical)

BRAND NAME (Manufacturer)
Valisone (Schering)
TYPE OF DRUG
Adrenocorticosteroid hormone

INGREDIENT
betamethasone as the valerate salt
DOSAGE FORMS
Cream (0.01% and 0.1%)
Ointment (0.1%)
Lotion (0.1%)
STORAGE
Betamethasone valerate ointment, cream, and lotion
should be stored at room temperature, in tightly closed
containers. This medication should never be frozen.

USES

Your adrenal glands naturally produce certain cortisone-
like chemicals. These chemicals are involved in various
regulatory processes in the body (such as fluid balance,
temperature, and reactions to inflammation). Betamethasone valerate belongs to a group of drugs known as
adrenocorticosteroids (or cortisone-like medications). It
is used to relieve the skin inflammation (redness, swelling, itching, and discomfort) associated with conditions
such as dermatitis, eczema, and poison ivy. How this
drug acts to relieve these disorders is not completely understood.

TREATMENT

Before applying this medication, wash your hands. Then,
unless your doctor gives you different instructions, gently
wash the area of the skin where the medication is to be
applied. With a clean towel, pat the area almost dry; it
should be slightly damp when you put the medicine on.
     If you are using the lotion form of this medication,
shake it well before pouring out the medicine. The contents tend to settle on the bottom of the bottle, so it is
necessary to shake the container to evenly distribute the
ingredients and equalize the doses.
     Apply a small amount of the medication to the affected
area in a thin layer. Do not bandage the area unless your
doctor tells you to do so. If you are to apply an occlusive
dressing (like kitchen plastic wrap), be sure you understand the instructions.
     If you miss a dose of this medication, apply the dose as
soon as possible, unless it is almost time for the next

application. In that case, do not apply the missed dose; just return to your regular schedule. Do not put twice as much of the medication on your skin at the next application.

SIDE EFFECTS

Minor. Acne; burning sensation; skin dryness; irritation of the affected area; itching; and rash.

If the affected area is extremely dry or scaling, the skin may be moistened before applying the medication by soaking in water or by applying water with a clean cloth. The ointment form is probably better for dry skin.

A mild, temporary stinging sensation may occur after this medication is applied. If this persists, contact your doctor.

Major. Tell your doctor about any side effects that are persistent or particularly bothersome. IT IS ESPECIALLY IMPORTANT TO TELL YOUR DOCTOR about blistering; increased hair growth; loss of skin color; secondary infection of the area being treated; and thinning of the skin with easy bruising.

INTERACTIONS

This medication does not interact with any other medications, as long as it is used according to directions.

WARNINGS

• Tell your doctor about unusual or allergic reactions you have had to any medications, especially to betamethasone valerate or other adrenocorticosteroids (such as amcinonide, clocortolone, cortisone, desonide, desoximetasone, dexamethasone, diflorasone, flumethasone, fluocinolone, fluocinonide, fluorometholone, flurandrenolide, halcinonide, hydrocortisone, methylprednisolone, prednisolone, prednisone, or triamcinolone).

• Tell your doctor if you now have, or if you have ever had, blood vessel disease, chicken pox, diabetes mellitus (sugar diabetes), fungal infection, peptic ulcers, shingles, tuberculosis, tuberculosis of the skin, vaccinia, or any other type of infection, especially at the site currently being treated.

- It irritation develops while using this drug, immediately discontinue its use and notify your doctor.
- This product is not for use in the eyes or mucous membranes. Exposure of this medication to the eye may result in ocular (to the eye) side effects.
- Do not use this product with an occlusive wrap unless your doctor directs you to do so. Systemic absorption of this drug is increased if extensive areas of the body are treated, particularly if occlusive bandages are used. If it is necessary for you to use this drug under a wrap, follow your doctor's instructions exactly; do not leave the wrap in place longer than specified.
- If you are using this medication on a child's diaper area, do not put tight-fitting diapers or plastic pants on the child. This may lead to increased systemic absorption of the drug and a possible increase in side effects.
- Be sure to tell your doctor if you are pregnant. If large amounts of this drug are applied for prolonged periods, some of it will be absorbed and may cross the placenta. Although studies in humans have not yet been completed, birth defects have been observed in animals whose mothers were given large doses of this type of drug during pregnancy. Also, tell your doctor if you are breastfeeding an infant. If absorbed through the skin, small amounts of this type of drug pass into breast milk, and may cause growth suppression or a decrease in natural adrenocorticosteroid production in the nursing infant.

Betapen-VK—see penicillin VK

---

bethanechol

BRAND NAMES (Manufacturers)
bethanechol chloride (various manufacturers)
Duvoid (Norwich-Eaton)
Myotonachol (Glenwood)
Urecholine (Merck Sharp & Dohme)
Vesicholine (Star)
TYPE OF DRUG
Cholinergic

INGREDIENT
bethanechol as the chloride salt
DOSAGE FORM
Tablets (5 mg, 10 mg, 25 mg, and 50 mg)
STORAGE
Bethanechol should be stored at room temperature, in a tightly closed container.

USES
Bethanechol is used to relieve retention of urine in the bladder. It acts on the nerves of the bladder to cause emptying.

TREATMENT
Bethanechol should be taken on an empty stomach one hour before or two hours after a meal. If it is taken soon after eating, nausea and vomiting may occur.

If you miss a dose of this medication and remember within an hour of the scheduled dose, take the missed dose immediately. If more than an hour has passed, do not take the missed dose at all; just return to your regular dosing schedule. Do not double the next dose.

SIDE EFFECTS
Minor. Abdominal cramps; belching; diarrhea; dizziness; flushing of the skin; headache; nausea; salivation; sweating; and vomiting. These side effects should disappear in several days, as your body adjusts to the medication.

If you feel dizzy, sit or lie down awhile; get up slowly, and be careful on stairs.

Major. Tell your doctor about any side effects that are persistent or particularly bothersome. IT IS ESPECIALLY IMPORTANT TO TELL YOUR DOCTOR about chest pain; feeling faint; or shortness of breath.

INTERACTIONS
Bethanechol interacts with several other types of medication.
1. Procainamide and quinidine decrease the therapeutic benefits of bethanechol.

2. Concurrent use of bethanechol and mecamylamine or trimethaphan can lead to a serious drop in blood pressure.

Before starting to take bethanechol, BE SURE TO TELL YOUR DOCTOR if you are already taking any of the medications listed above.

WARNINGS

• Tell your doctor about unusual or allergic reactions you have had to any medications, especially to bethanechol.

• Before starting to take bethanechol, be sure to tell your doctor if you now have, or if you have ever had, asthma, epilepsy, heart disease, high or low blood pressure, Parkinson's disease, stomach ulcers, thyroid disease, or an obstructed intestine or bladder.

• If this drug makes you dizzy, avoid taking part in any activity that requires alertness, such as driving a car or operating potentially dangerous equipment.

• Be sure to tell your doctor if you are pregnant. Although bethanechol appears to be safe during pregancy, extensive studies in humans have not yet been completed. Also, tell your doctor if you are breastfeeding an infant. Small amounts of bethanechol pass into breast milk.

bethanechol chloride—see bethanechol

Bethaprim SS—see sulfamethoxazole and trimethoprim combination

Bexophene—see aspirin, caffeine, and propoxyphene combination

Bleph-10—see sodium sulfacetamide (ophthalmic)

Blocadren—see timolol (systemic)

Bontril PDM—see phendimetrazine

Brethine—see terbutaline

Brevicon—see oral contraceptives

Brexin L.A.—see pseudoephedrine and chlorpheniramine combination

Bricanyl—see terbutaline

Bristamycin—see erythromycin

Bromanyl—see ammonium chloride, bromodiphenhydramine, diphenhydramine, codeine, and potassium guaiacolsulfonate combination

Brombay—see brompheniramine

---

bromocriptine

BRAND NAME (Manufacturer)
Parlodel (Sandoz)
TYPE OF DRUG
Dopamine agonist and anti-parkinson
INGREDIENT
bromocriptine as the mesylate salt
DOSAGE FORMS
Tablets (2.5 mg)
Capsules (5 mg)
STORAGE
Bromocriptine tablets and capsules should be stored at room temperature in tightly closed, light-resistant containers.

USES

This medication is used to treat the symptoms of Parkinson's disease, and to decrease milk production in women who choose not to breastfeed their infants. Bromocriptine relieves the symptoms of Parkinson's disease by replacing a chemical (dopamine) that is diminished in the brains of these patients. Bromocriptine prevents milk production by blocking the action of the responsible hormone (prolactin).

TREATMENT

In order to avoid stomach irritation, you can take bromocriptine with food or with a full glass of water or milk.

If you miss a dose of this medication and remember within four hours of the scheduled time, take the missed dose immediately. If more than four hours have passed, do not take the missed dose at all; just return to your regular dosing schedule. Do not double the next dose.

SIDE EFFECTS

Minor. Abdominal pain; constipation; diarrhea; dizziness; drowsiness; fatigue; headache; insomnia; lightheadedness; loss of appetite; nasal congestion; nausea; or vomiting. These side effects should disappear in several days, as your body adjusts to the medication.

Dizziness or fainting may occur, especially following the first dose. It is best, therefore, to take the first dose while lying down. If you feel dizzy or light-headed with later doses, sit or lie down awhile; get up slowly, and be careful on stairs.

To relieve constipation, increase the amount of fiber in your diet (bran, salads, fresh fruits and vegetables, and whole-grain breads), exercise, and drink more water (unless your doctor directs you to do otherwise).

Major. Tell your doctor about any side effects that are persistent or particularly bothersome. IT IS ESPECIALLY IMPORTANT TO TELL YOUR DOCTOR about abnormal, involuntary movements; anxiety; confusion; convulsions; depression; difficulty swallowing; fainting; fluid retention; hallucinations; nervousness; nightmares; skin rash; shortness of breath; tingling in the hands or feet; or visual disturbances.

INTERACTIONS

Bromocriptine interacts with several other types of medication.

1. Phenothiazine tranquilizers, methyldopa, haloperidol, metoclopramide, reserpine, and monoamine oxidase (MAO) inhibitors decrease the beneficial effects of bromocriptine.

2. Dosage of anti-hypertensive medications may require adjustment when bromocriptine is started.

Before starting to take bromocriptine, TELL YOUR DOCTOR if you are already taking any of these medications.

WARNINGS

- Tell your doctor about unusual or allergic reactions you have had to any medications, especially to bromocriptine or ergotamine.
- Before starting to take bromocriptine, be sure to tell your doctor if you now have, or if you have ever had, heart or blood vessel disease, kidney disease, liver disease, or mental disorders.
- If this drug makes you dizzy or drowsy, avoid tasks that require alertness, such as driving a car or operating potentially dangerous equipment.
- Do not stop taking bromocriptine unless you first check with your doctor. Stopping the drug abruptly may lead to a worsening of your condition.
- Be sure to tell your doctor if you are pregnant. It is generally recommended that bromocriptine not be used during pregnancy because there have been reports of birth defects in both animals and humans whose mothers received the drug during pregnancy. Also, tell your doctor if you are breastfeeding an infant. Bromocriptine blocks milk production.

Bromophen T.D. —see phenylpropanolamine, phenylephrine, and brompheniramine combination

Bromotuss with Codeine —see ammonium chloride, bromodiphenhydramine, diphenhydramine, codeine, and potassium guaiacolsulfonate combination

Bromphen —see phenylephrine, phenylpropanolamine, brompheniramine, and guaifenesin combination

Bromphen Compound T.D. —see phenylpropanolamine, phenylephrine, and brompheniramine combination

---

brompheniramine

BRAND NAMES (Manufacturers)
Brombay (Bay)
brompheniramine maleate (various manufacturers)

Diamine T.D. (Major)
Dimetane* (Robins)
Dimetane Extentabs* (Robins)
Veltane (Lannett)
*Brompheniramine is also available over-the-counter (non-prescription), under the brand name of Dimetane.

TYPE OF DRUG
Antihistamine

INGREDIENT
brompheniramine as the maleate salt

DOSAGE FORMS
Tablets (4 mg)
Sustained-release tablets (8 mg and 12 mg)
Oral elixir (2 mg per 5 ml teaspoonful)

STORAGE
Brompheniramine tablets and oral elixir should be stored at room temperature, in tightly closed containers.

USES
This medication belongs to a group of drugs known as antihistamines (antihistamines block the action of histamine, a chemical that is released by the body during an allergic reaction). Brompheniramine is used to treat or prevent symptoms of allergy.

TREATMENT
To avoid stomach upset, you can take brompheniramine with food or with a full glass of milk or water (unless your doctor directs you to do otherwise).

The oral elixir form of this medication should be measured carefully with a specially designed, 5 ml measuring spoon. An ordinary kitchen teaspoon is not accurate enough.

The sustained-release tablets should be swallowed whole. Breaking, chewing, or crushing these tablets destroys their sustained-release activity, and may increase the side effects.

If you miss a dose of this medication, take the missed dose as soon as possible, unless it is close to the time for your next dose. In that case, don't take the missed dose at all; just return to your regular dosing schedule. Do not double the next dose.

SIDE EFFECTS

Minor. Blurred vision; confusion; constipation; diarrhea; difficult or painful urination; dizziness; dry mouth, throat, or nose; headache; irritability; loss of appetite; nausea; restlessness; ringing or buzzing in the ears; rash; stomach upset; or unusual increase in sweating. These side effects should disappear in several days, as your body adjusts to the medication.

If you are constipated, increase the amount of fiber in your diet (raw vegetables, fruits, salads, bran, and whole-grain breads) and drink more water (unless your doctor tells you not to do so.)

Chew sugarless gum, or suck on ice chips or a piece of hard candy, to reduce mouth dryness.

This medication can cause increased sensitivity to sunlight. It is therefore important to avoid prolonged exposure to sunlight and sunlamps. Wear protective clothing, and use an effective sunscreen.

If you feel dizzy or light-headed, sit or lie down awhile; get up from a sitting or lying position slowly, and be careful on stairs.

Major. Tell your doctor about any side effects that are persistent or particularly bothersome. IT IS ESPECIALLY IMPORTANT TO TELL YOUR DOCTOR about unusual bleeding or bruising; change in menstruation; clumsiness; feeling faint; flushing of the face; hallucinations; seizures; shortness of breath; sleeping disorders; sore throat or fever; palpitations; tightness in the chest; or unusual tiredness or weakness.

INTERACTIONS

Brompheniramine interacts with several other types of medications.

1. Concurrent use of this medication with central nervous system depressants (drugs that slow the activity of the nervous system), such as barbiturates, benzodiazepine tranquilizers, muscle relaxants, narcotics, pain medication, phenothiazine tranquilizers, or alcohol, or with tricyclic anti-depressants can cause extreme drowsiness.

2. Monoamine oxidase (MAO) inhibitors (isocarboxazid, pargyline, phenelzine, tranylcypromine) can increase the side effects of this medication.

3. Brompheniramine can decrease the activity of oral anti-coagulants (blood thinners, such as warfarin).

TELL YOUR DOCTOR if you are currently taking any of the medications listed above.

WARNINGS

• Tell your doctor about unusual or allergic reactions you have had to medications, especially to brompheniramine or to any other antihistamine (bromodiphenhydramine, azatadine, carbinoxamine, chlorpheniramine, clemastine, cyproheptadine, dexchlorpheniramine, dimenhydrinate, dimethindene, diphenhydramine, diphenylpyraline, doxylamine, hydroxyzine, promethazine, pyrilamine, trimeprazine, tripelennamine, or tripolidine).

• Tell your doctor if you now have, or if you have ever had, asthma, blood vessel disease, glaucoma, high blood pressure, kidney disease, peptic ulcers, enlarged prostate gland, or thyroid disease.

• Brompheniramine can cause drowsiness or dizziness. Your ability to perform tasks that require alertness, such as driving a car or operating potentially dangerous machinery, may be decreased. Appropriate caution should therefore be taken.

• Be sure to tell your doctor if you are pregnant. The effects of this medication during pregnancy have not yet been thoroughly studied in humans. Also, tell your doctor if you are breastfeeding an infant. Small amounts of brompheniramine pass into breast milk and may cause unusual excitement or irritability in nursing infants.

brompheniramine maleate—see brompheniramine

Brompheniramine, Phenylephrine, and Phenylpropanolamine—see phenylpropanolamine, phenylephrine, and brompheniramine combination

Bronchial—see theophylline and guaifenesin combination

Bronkodyl—see theophylline

Bronkometer—see isoetharine

Bronkosol—see isoetharine

Buff-A-Comp—see aspirin, caffeine, and butalbital combination

Buff-A-Comp #3—see aspirin, caffeine, butalbital, and codeine combination

---

bumetanide

BRAND NAME (Manufacturer)
Bumex (Roche)
TYPE OF DRUG
Diuretic (water pill) and anti-hypertensive
INGREDIENT
bumetanide
DOSAGE FORM
Tablets (0.5 mg and 1 mg)
STORAGE
Bumetanide should be stored at room temperature in a tightly closed, light-resistant container.

USES
Bumetanide is prescribed to treat high blood pressure. It is also used to reduce fluid accumulation in the body caused by conditions such as heart failure, cirrhosis of the liver, kidney disease, and the long-term use of some medications. This medication reduces fluid accumulation by increasing the elimination of sodium and water through the kidneys.

TREATMENT
To decrease stomach irritation, you can take this medication with a glass of milk or with a meal (unless your doctor directs you to do otherwise). Try to take it at the same time every day. Avoid taking a dose after 6:00 P.M.—this will prevent you from having to get up during the night to urinate.

If you miss a dose of this medication, take the missed

dose as soon as possible, unless it is almost time for the next one. In that case, do not take the missed dose at all; just wait until the next scheduled dose. Do not double the dose.

This medication does not cure high blood pressure, but it will help to control the condition, as long as you continue to take it.

SIDE EFFECTS

Minor. Blurred vision; constipation; cramps; diarrhea; dizziness; headache; itching; loss of appetite; muscle spasms; nausea; sore mouth; stomach upset; vomiting; and weakness. As your body adjusts to the medication, these side effects should disappear.

This medication causes an increase in the amount of urine or frequency of urination when you first begin to take it. It may also cause you to have an unusual feeling of tiredness. These effects should lessen after several days.

This medication can cause increased sensitivity to sunlight. It is therefore important to avoid prolonged exposure to sunlight and sunlamps. Wear protective clothing, and use an effective sunscreen.

To avoid dizziness or light-headedness when you stand, contract and relax the muscles of your legs for a few moments before rising. Do this by pushing one foot against the floor while raising the other foot slightly, alternating feet so that you are "pumping" your legs in a pedaling motion.

Major. Tell your doctor about any side effects that are persistent or particularly bothersome. IT IS ESPECIALLY IMPORTANT TO TELL YOUR DOCTOR about abdominal pain; unusual bleeding or bruising; confusion; difficulty breathing; dry mouth; fainting; joint pains; loss of appetite; mood changes; muscle cramps; palpitations; rash; ringing in the ears; sore throat; increased thirst; tingling in the fingers and toes; or yellowing of the eyes or skin.

INTERACTIONS

Bumetanide interacts with several other types of medicines.

1. It can increase the side effects of alcohol, barbiturates, narcotics, cephalosporin antibiotics, chloral hydrate, cortisone-like steroids (such as cortisone, dexamethasone, hydrocortisone, prednisone, prednisolone), digoxin, digitalis, lithium, amphotericin B, cisplatin, mercaptopurine, and polymyxin B.

2. Probenecid and indomethacin may decrease the diuretic effectiveness of this medication.

Before taking bumetanide, BE SURE TO TELL YOUR DOCTOR if you are taking any of the medicines listed above.

WARNINGS

• Tell your doctor about unusual or allergic reactions you have had to any medications, especially to diuretics (water pills), oral anti-diabetic medicines, or sulfonamide antibiotics.

• Before you start taking this medication, tell your doctor if you now have, or if you have ever had, kidney disease or problems with urination, diabetes mellitus (sugar diabetes), gout, liver disease, or asthma.

• Bumetanide can cause potassium loss. Signs of potassium loss include dry mouth; thirst; weakness; muscle pain or cramps; nausea; and vomiting. If you experience any of these symptoms, call your doctor. Your doctor may want you to have blood tests performed periodically in order to monitor your potassium levels. To help avoid potassium loss, take this medication with a glass of fresh or frozen orange or cranberry juice, or eat a banana every day. The use of a salt substitute also helps prevent potassium loss. Do not change your diet, however, before discussing it with your doctor. Too much potassium may also be dangerous.

• Before having any surgery or other medical or dental treatment, be sure your doctor or dentist knows that you are taking bumetanide.

• In order to avoid dizziness or fainting while taking this medication, try not to stand for long periods of time; avoid drinking excessive amounts of alcohol; and avoid getting overheated (strenuous exercise in hot weather; hot baths, showers, and saunas).

• If you have high blood pressure, do not take any over-the-counter (non-prescription) medication for weight control, or for cough, cold, allergy, asthma, or sinus problems, unless you first check with your doctor.

• To prevent severe water loss (dehydration) while taking this medication, check with your doctor if you have any illness that causes severe or continuous nausea, vomiting, or diarrhea.

• This medication can raise blood sugar levels in diabetic patients. Therefore, blood sugar should be monitored carefully with blood or urine tests when this medication is started.

• Be sure to tell your doctor if you are pregnant. This drug crosses the placenta. Although studies in humans have not been completed, adverse effects have been reported on the fetuses of animals who were given large doses of this drug during pregnancy. Also, tell your doctor if you are breastfeeding an infant. Although problems in humans have not been reported, small amounts of this drug pass into breast milk.

Bumex — see bumetanide

---

busulfan

BRAND NAME (Manufacturer)
Myleran (Burroughs Wellcome)
TYPE OF DRUG
Anti-neoplastic (anti-cancer drug)
INGREDIENT
busulfan
DOSAGE FORM
Tablets (2 mg)
STORAGE
Busulfan should be stored at room temperature, in a tightly closed container.

USES
Busulfan belongs to a group of drugs known as alkylating agents. It is used to treat leukemia. This medication works by binding to the rapidly growing cancer cells, preventing their multiplication and growth.

TREATMENT

Busulfan can be taken either on an empty stomach or with food or milk (as directed by your doctor).

The timing of the doses of this medication is important. Be sure you completely understand your doctor's instructions on how this medication should be taken.

If you miss a dose of this medication, do not take the missed dose at all; just return to your regular dosing schedule. Do not double the next dose.

SIDE EFFECTS

Minor. Diarrhea; dizziness; itching; nausea; stomach upset; and vomiting. These side effects may disappear as your body adjusts to the medication. However, it is important to continue taking this medication despite any nausea and vomiting that may occur. Busulfan also causes hair loss, which is reversible when the medication is stopped.

If you feel dizzy, sit or lie down awhile; be careful on stairs, and get up from a sitting or lying position slowly.

Major. Tell your doctor about any side effects that are persistent or particularly bothersome. IT IS ESPECIALLY IMPORTANT TO TELL YOUR DOCTOR about unusual bleeding or bruising; blurred vision; breast enlargement (in both sexes); chills; confusion; cough; darkening of the skin; difficulty breathing; dry skin; fatigue; fever; joint pain; loss of appetite; menstrual irregularities; mouth sores; muscle weakness; skin rash; sore throat; weight loss; or yellowing of the eyes or skin.

INTERACTIONS

Busulfan can increase the blood levels of uric acid, which can block the effectiveness of anti-gout medications (allopurinol, probenecid, sulfinpyrazone).

Before starting to take busulfan, BE SURE TO TELL YOUR DOCTOR if you are already taking an anti-gout medication

WARNINGS

• Tell your doctor about unusual or allergic reactions you have had to any medications, especially to busulfan.
• Before starting to take this medication, be sure to tell

your doctor if you now have, or if you have ever had, blood disorders, chronic or recurrent infections, gout, or kidney stones.

• You should not receive any immunizations or vaccinations while taking this medication. Busulfan blocks the effectiveness of the vaccine, and may result in infection.

• It is important to drink plenty of fluid (up to two or three quarts each day) while taking this medication, in order to prevent uric acid kidney stones from developing.

• Busulfan can lower your platelet count, thereby decreasing your body's ability to form blood clots. You should therefore be especially careful while brushing your teeth, flossing, or using toothpicks, razors, or fingernail scissors. Try to avoid falls and other injuries.

• Before having any surgery or other medical or dental treatment, be sure your doctor or dentist knows that you are taking this medication.

• Busulfan can decrease fertility in both men and women.

• Be sure to tell your doctor if you are pregnant. Birth defects have been reported in both humans and animals whose mothers received busulfan during pregnancy. The risks should be discussed with your doctor. Also, tell your doctor if you are breastfeeding an infant. It is not known whether or not busulfan passes into breast milk.

butabarbital

BRAND NAMES (Manufacturers)
butabarbital sodium (various manufacturers)
Butalan (Lannett)
Butatran (Hauck)
Buticaps (Wallace)
Buticol (Wallace)
Sarisol (Halsey)
TYPE OF DRUG
Sedative/hypnotic
INGREDIENT
butabarbital as the sodium salt
DOSAGE FORMS
Tablets (15 mg, 30 mg, 50 mg, and 100 mg)

Capsules (15 mg and 30 mg)
Oral liquid (30 mg and 33.3 mg per 5 ml teaspoonful,
   with 7% alcohol)

STORAGE

Butabarbital tablets, capsules, and oral liquid should be
stored at room temperature in tightly closed containers.
This medication should never be frozen.

USES

This medication is used to relieve anxiety or tension, or as
a sleeping aid. It belongs to a group of drugs known as
barbiturates. The barbiturates are central nervous system
(brain and spinal cord) depressants (drugs that slow the
activity of the nervous system).

TREATMENT

In order to avoid stomach irritation, you can take butabarbital with food, milk, or water.

The oral liquid should be measured carefully, with a
specially designed, 5 ml measuring spoon. An ordinary
kitchen teaspoon is not accurate enough. The dose of the
liquid medication can be taken straight, or can be mixed
with water, milk, or fruit juice.

If butabarbital is being taken as a sleeping aid, take it 20
minutes to one hour before you want to go to sleep. The
use of this drug as a sleeping aid should be limited to two
weeks. After two weeks, butabarbital loses its ability to
produce or maintain sleep.

If you are taking this medication on a regular basis and
you miss a dose, take the missed dose as soon as possible
(if you remember within an hour or so). Then return to
your regular dosing schedule. If more than an hour has
passed, do not take the missed dose at all; just return to
your regular dosing schedule. Do not double the next
dose.

SIDE EFFECTS

Minor. Constipation; diarrhea; dizziness; drowsiness;
headache; a "hangover" feeling; muscle or joint pain;
nausea; stomach upset; and vomiting. These side effects
should disappear in several days, as your body adjusts to
the medication.

If you feel dizzy or light-headed, sit or lie down awhile; get up slowly, and be careful on stairs.

To relieve constipation, increase the amount of fiber in your diet (fresh fruits and vegetables, bran, salads, and whole-grain breads), exercise, and drink more water (unless your doctor directs you to do otherwise).

Major. Tell your doctor about any side effects that are persistent or particularly bothersome. IT IS ESPECIALLY IMPORTANT TO TELL YOUR DOCTOR about difficulty breathing; unusual bleeding or bruising; chest tightness; confusion; depression; excitation; feeling faint; hives or itching; loss of coordination; skin rash; slurred speech; sore throat; unusual weakness; or yellowing of the eyes or skin.

INTERACTIONS

Butabarbital interacts with several other types of medications.

1. Concurrent use of butabarbital with other central nervous system depressants, such as antihistamines, benzodiazepine tranquilizers, muscle relaxants, narcotics, pain medications, phenothiazine tranquilizers, sleeping medications, or alcohol, or with tricyclic anti-depressants can cause extreme drowsiness.

2. Valproic acid, chloramphenicol, and monoamine oxidase (MAO) inhibitors can prolong the effects of the barbiturates.

3. Butabarbital can increase the elimination from the body and thereby decrease the effectiveness of oral anticoagulants (blood thinners, such as warfarin), digoxin, tricyclic anti-depressants, cortisone-like medications, doxycycline, quinidine, estrogens, birth control pills, phenytoin, acetaminophen, and carbamazepine.

4. Butabarbital can decrease the absorption of griseofulvin from the gastrointestinal tract.

5. The combination of butabarbital and furosemide can cause low blood pressure and fainting.

6. Butabarbital can increase the side effects caused by large doses of acetaminophen or cyclophosphamide.

BE SURE TO TELL YOUR DOCTOR if you are already taking any of the medications listed above.

WARNINGS

- Tell your doctor about unusual or allergic reactions you have had to medications, especially to butabarbital or to any other barbiturate.

- Tell your doctor if you now have, or if you have ever had, acute or chronic (long-term) pain; Addison's disease (an underactive adrenal gland); diabetes mellitus (sugar diabetes); kidney disease; liver disease; lung disease; mental depression; porphyria; or thyroid disease.

- Before having surgery or other medical or dental treatment, be sure to tell your doctor or dentist that you are taking this medication.

- If this medication makes you dizzy or drowsy, do not take part in any activity that requires alertness, such as driving a car or operating potentially dangerous equipment.

- This drug has the potential for abuse and must be used with caution. Tolerance develops quickly; do not increase the dose or stop taking this drug unless you first consult your doctor. If you have been taking this drug for a long time or have been taking large doses, you may experience anxiety, muscle twitching, tremors, weakness, dizziness, nausea, vomiting, insomnia, or blurred vision, when you stop taking it. Your doctor may therefore want to reduce your dosage gradually to prevent this reaction.

- Some of these products contain F.D. & C. Yellow Dye No. 5 (tartrazine), which can cause allergic-type reactions (difficulty breathing, rash, hives, or fainting) in certain susceptible individuals.

- Be sure to tell your doctor if you are pregnant. Butabarbital crosses the placenta, and birth defects have been associated with the use of this medication during pregnancy. If butabarbital is used during the last three months of pregnancy, there is a chance that the infant will be born addicted to the medication and will experience a withdrawal reaction (seizures and irritability) at birth. The infant could also be born with bleeding problems. Also, tell your doctor if you are breastfeeding an infant. Small amounts of butabarbital pass into breast milk and may cause excessive drowsiness in the nursing infant.

butabarbital sodium—see butabarbital

Butalan—see butabarbital

butalbital with aspirin and caffeine—see aspirin, caffeine, and butalbital combination

Butal Compound—see aspirin, caffeine, and butalbital combination

Butatran—see butabarbital

Butazolidin—see phenylbutazone

Buticaps—see butabarbital

Butisol—see butabarbital

Cafergot—see ergotamine and caffeine combination

Cafertabs—see ergotamine and caffeine combination

Cafertrate—see ergotamine and caffeine combination

Calan—see verapamil

---

calcifediol

BRAND NAME (Manufacturer)
Calderol (Upjohn)
TYPE OF DRUG
Vitamin D analog
INGREDIENT
calcifediol (25-hydroxycholecalciferol)
DOSAGE FORM
Capsules (20 mcg and 50 mcg)
STORAGE
Calcifediol capsules should be stored at room temperature in a tightly closed, light-resistant container.

USES
Vitamin D is essential to many body systems, including

bone structure, regulation of blood calcium levels, and heart and muscle contraction. Since vitamin D is activated in the kidneys, patients with chronic (long-term) kidney failure are unable to produce enough active vitamin D on their own. Calcifediol is one of the active forms of vitamin D. This medication is used to treat bone disease and hypocalcemia (low blood calcium levels) in patients on dialysis.

TREATMENT

Calcifediol can be taken either on an empty stomach or with food or milk (as directed by your doctor).

If you miss a dose of this medication, take the missed dose as soon as possible, unless it is almost time for the next dose. In that case, do not take the missed dose at all; just return to your regular dosing schedule. Do not double the next dose.

SIDE EFFECTS

Minor. None, at the dosages normally prescribed.

Major. The side effects associated with calcifediol therapy are usually the result of too much medication (vitamin D toxicity). Tell your doctor about any side effects that are persistent or particularly bothersome. IT IS ESPECIALLY IMPORTANT TO TELL YOUR DOCTOR about blurred vision; bone pain; constipation; dry mouth; headache; irritability; loss of appetite; metallic taste in the mouth; mental disorders; muscle pain; nausea; palpitations; runny nose; increased thirst; increased urination; vomiting; weakness; or weight loss.

INTERACTIONS

Calcifediol interacts with a number of other drugs.

1. The dosage of calcifediol may need to be altered when anti-convulsion medication (such as phenytoin, phenobarbital, or primidone) is started.

2. Cholestyramine, colestipol, and mineral oil can decrease the absorption of calcifediol from the gastrointestinal tract.

BE SURE TO TELL YOUR DOCTOR if you are already taking any of these medications.

WARNINGS

- Tell your doctor about unusual or allergic reactions you have had to any medications, especially to calcifediol, calcitriol, dihydrotachysterol, ergocalciferol, or vitamin D.
- Before starting to take this medication, be sure to tell your doctor if you now have, or if you have ever had, heart or blood vessel disease, hypercalcemia (high levels of calcium in the bloodstream), hyperphosphatemia (high levels of phosphate in the bloodstream), vitamin D intoxication, or sarcoidosis.
- Before taking any over-the-counter (non-prescription) products that contain calcium, phosphates, magnesium, or vitamin D, check with your doctor. These ingredients can increase the side effects of calcifediol.
- Be sure to tell your doctor if you are pregnant. Although calcifediol (in normal doses) appears to be safe during pregnancy, extensive studies in humans have not yet been completed. Birth defects have been reported in the offspring of animals who received large doses of this medication during pregnancy. Also, tell your doctor if you are breastfeeding an infant. Small amounts of calcifediol pass into breast milk.

Calciferol—see ergocalciferol (vitamin D)

Calciparine—see heparin

---

calcitriol

BRAND NAME (Manufacturer)
Rocaltrol (Roche)
TYPE OF DRUG
Vitamin D analog
INGREDIENT
calcitriol (1, 25-dihydroxycholecalciferol)
DOSAGE FORM
Capsules (0.25 mcg and 0.5 mcg)
STORAGE
Calcitriol should be stored at room temperature in a tightly closed, light-resistant container.

USES

Vitamin D is essential to many body systems, including bone structure, regulation of blood calcium levels, and heart and muscle contraction. Since vitamin D is activated in the kidneys, patients with chronic (long-term) kidney failure are unable to produce enough active vitamin D on their own. Calcitriol is one of the active forms of vitamin D. This medication is used to treat bone disease and hypocalcemia (low blood calcium levels) in patients on dialysis.

TREATMENT

Calcitriol can be taken either on an empty stomach or with food or milk (as directed by your doctor).

If you miss a dose of this medication, take the missed dose as soon as possible, unless it is almost time for the next dose. In that case, do not take the missed dose at all; just return to your regular dosing schedule. Do not double the next dose.

SIDE EFFECTS

Minor. None, at the dosages normally prescribed.
Major. The side effects associated with calcitriol therapy are usually the result of too much medication (vitamin D toxicity). Tell your doctor about any side effects that are persistent or particularly bothersome. IT IS ESPECIALLY IMPORTANT TO TELL YOUR DOCTOR about blurred vision; bone pain; constipation; dry mouth; headache; irritability; loss of appetite; metallic taste in the mouth; mental disorders; muscle pain; nausea; palpitations; runny nose; increased thirst; increased urination; vomiting; weakness; or weight loss.

INTERACTIONS

Calcitriol interacts with a number of other drugs.
1. The dosage of calcitriol may need to be adjusted when anti-convulsion medication (phenytoin, phenobarbital, or primidone) is started.
2. Cholestyramine, colestipol, and mineral oil can decrease the absorption of calcitriol from the gastrointestinal tract.

BE SURE TO TELL YOUR DOCTOR if you are already taking any of these medications.

WARNINGS

- Tell your doctor about unusual or allergic reactions you have had to any medications, especially to calcitriol, calcifediol, dihydrotachysterol, ergocalciferol, or vitamin D.
- Before starting to take this medication, be sure to tell your doctor if you now have, or if you have ever had, heart or blood vessel disease, hypercalcemia (high levels of blood calcium), hyperphosphatemia (high levels of blood phosphate), vitamin D intoxication, or sarcoidosis.
- Before taking any over-the-counter (non-prescription) products that contain calcium, phosphates, magnesium, or vitamin D, check with your doctor. These ingredients can increase the side effects of calcitriol.
- Be sure to tell your doctor if you are pregnant. Although calcitriol appears to be safe during pregnancy in humans, birth defects have been reported in the offspring of animals who received large doses during pregnancy. Also, tell your doctor if you are breastfeeding an infant. Small amounts of calcitriol pass into breast milk.

Calderol—see calcifediol

Cam-ap-es—see hydralazine, hydrochlorothiazide, and reserpine combination

Candex see nystatin

Capital with Codeine—see acetaminophen and codeine combination

Capoten—see captopril

---

captopril

BRAND NAME (Manufacturer)
Capoten (Squibb)
TYPE OF DRUG
Anti-hypertensive

INGREDIENT
captopril
DOSAGE FORM
Tablets (25 mg, 50 mg, and 100 mg)
STORAGE
Captopril should be stored at room temperature in a tightly closed container.

USES
Captopril is used to treat high blood pressure and congestive heart failure. It is a vasodilator (it dilates the blood vessels) that acts by blocking the production of chemicals that may be responsible for constricting blood vessels.

TREATMENT
To obtain maximum benefit from captopril, you should take it on an empty stomach one hour before meals. In order to become accustomed to taking this medication, try to take it at the same time(s) every day.

It may be several weeks before you notice the full effects of this medication.

Captopril does not cure high blood pressure, but it will help to control the condition, as long as you continue to take it.

If you miss a dose of this medication, take the missed dose as soon as possible, unless it is almost time for the next dose. In that case, do not take the missed dose at all; just wait until the next scheduled dose. Do not double the dose.

SIDE EFFECTS
Minor. Abdominal pain; constipation; diarrhea; dizziness; dry mouth; fatigue; flushing; headache; insomnia; loss of taste; loss of appetite; nausea; and vomiting. These side effects should disappear in several days, as your body adjusts to the medication.

If you are constipated, increase the amount of fiber in your diet (raw vegetables, fruits, salads, bran, and whole-grain breads) and drink more water (unless your doctor directs you to do otherwise).

To relieve mouth dryness, suck on ice chips or a piece of hard candy, or chew sugarless gum.

To avoid dizziness or light-headedness when you stand, contract and relax the muscles of your legs for a few moments before rising. Do this by pushing one foot against the floor while raising the other foot slightly, alternating feet so that you are "pumping" your legs in a pedaling motion.

This medication can increase your sensitivity to sunlight. It is therefore important to avoid prolonged exposure to sunlight and sunlamps. Wear protective clothing and sunglasses, and use an effective sunscreen.

Major. Tell your doctor about any side effects that are persistent or particularly bothersome. IT IS ESPECIALLY IMPORTANT TO TELL YOUR DOCTOR about unusual bleeding or bruising; chest pain; chills; difficult or painful urination; fever; itching; mouth sores; palpitations; rash; sore throat; swelling of the face, hands, or feet; tingling in the fingers or toes; or yellowing of the eyes or skin.

INTERACTIONS

Captopril interacts with several other medications.

1. Diuretics (water pills) and other anti-hypertensive medications can cause an excessive drop in blood pressure when combined with captopril (especially with the first dose).

2. The combination of captopril with spironolactone, triamterene, amiloride, potassium supplements, or salt substitutes can lead to hyperkalemia (dangerously high levels of potassium in the bloodstream).

3. Anti neoplastic agents (anti-cancer drugs) or chloramphenicol can increase the bone marrow side effects of captopril.

BE SURE TO TELL YOUR DOCTOR if you are already taking any of the medications listed above.

WARNINGS

• Tell your doctor about any unusual or allergic reactions you have had to medications, especially to captopril.

• Tell your doctor if you now have, or if you have ever had, aortic stenosis, blood disorders, kidney disease, systemic lupus erythematosus (SLE), or a recent heart attack or stroke.

• Be careful—excessive perspiration, dehydration, or prolonged vomiting or diarrhea can lead to an excessive drop in blood pressure while you are taking this medication. Contact your doctor if you have any of these symptoms.

• Before having any surgery or other medical or dental treatment, be sure to tell your doctor or dentist that you are taking this medication.

• If you have high blood pressure, do not take any over-the-counter (non-prescription) medication for weight control, or for allergy, asthma, sinus, cough, or cold problems, unless you first check with your doctor.

• Do not stop taking this medication unless you first consult your doctor. Stopping this drug abruptly may lead to a rise in blood pressure.

• Be sure to tell your doctor if you are pregnant. Although this drug appears to be safe in animals, extensive studies in humans during pregnancy have not yet been completed. Also, tell your doctor if you are breastfeeding an infant. Small amounts of captopril pass into breast milk.

Caquin—see hydrocortisone and
   iodochlorhydroxyquin combination (topical)

Carafate—see sucralfate

**Caramiphen Edisylate and Phenylpropanolamine
   Hydrochloride**—see phenylpropanolamine and
   caramiphen combination

---

carbamazepine

BRAND NAME (Manufacturer)
Tegretol (Geigy)
TYPE OF DRUG
Anti-convulsant
INGREDIENT
carbamazepine
DOSAGE FORMS
Tablets (200 mg)
Chewable tablets (100 mg)

STORAGE
Carbamazepine tablets should be stored at room temperature in tightly closed containers.

USES
This medication is used for the treatment of seizure disorders and for relief of neuralgia (nerve pain). The mechanism of carbamazepine's anti-seizure activity is unknown, but it is not related to other anti-convulsants. Carbamazepine is not an ordinary pain reliever—it should not be used for minor aches or pains.

TREATMENT
Carbamazepine works best when the level of medicine in your bloodstream is kept constant. It is best therefore to take it at evenly spaced intervals, day and night. For example, if you are to take four doses a day, the doses should be spaced six hours apart.

Try not to miss any doses of this medication. If you do miss a dose, take the missed dose as soon as possible, unless it is almost time for the next dose. In that case, do not take the missed dose at all; just return to your regular dosing schedule. Do not double the next dose. If you are taking carbamazepine for a seizure disorder and you miss two or more doses, contact your doctor.

SIDE EFFECTS
Minor. Agitation; blurred vision; confusion; constipation; diarrhea; dizziness; drowsiness; dry mouth; headache; loss of appetite; muscle or joint pain; nausea; restlessness; sweating; vomiting; and weakness. These side effects should disappear in several weeks, as your body adjusts to the medication.

To relieve constipation, increase the amount of fiber in your diet (salads, bran, fresh fruits and vegetables, and whole-grain breads), exercise, and drink more water (unless your doctor directs you to do otherwise).

To relieve mouth dryness, suck on ice chips or a piece of hard candy, or chew sugarless gum.

If you feel dizzy or light-headed, sit or lie down awhile; get up slowly, and be careful on stairs.

This medication can increase your sensitivity to sunlight. It is therefore important to avoid prolonged exposure to sunlight and sunlamps. Wear protective clothing and sunglasses; and use an effective sunscreen.

Major. Tell your doctor about any side effects that are persistent or particularly bothersome. IT IS ESPECIALLY IMPORTANT TO TELL YOUR DOCTOR about abdominal pain; unusual bleeding or bruising; chills; depression; difficulty breathing; difficulty urinating; eye discomfort; fainting; fever; hair loss; hallucinations; impotence; loss of balance; mouth sores; nightmares; numbness or tingling; palpitations; ringing in the ears; skin rash; sore throat; swelling of the hands and feet; twitching; or yellowing of the eyes or skin.

INTERACTIONS

Carbamazepine interacts with several other types of medications.

1. Concurrent use of carbamazepine with central nervous system depressants (drugs that slow the activity of the nervous system), such as alcohol, antihistamines, barbiturates, benzodiazepine tranquilizers, muscle relaxants, narcotics, pain medications, or phenothiazine tranquilizers, or with tricyclic anti-depressants can cause extreme drowsiness.

2. Phenobarbital, phenytoin, and primidone can decrease blood levels of carbamazepine and decrease its effectiveness.

3. Isoniazid, propoxyphene, cimetidine, troleandomycin, and erythromycin can increase the blood levels of carbamazepine, which can lead to increased side effects.

4. The combination of lithium and carbamazepine can lead to central nervous system side effects.

5. Carbamazepine can decrease the effectiveness of phenytoin, oral anti-coagulants (blood thinners, such as warfarin), doxycycline, oral contraceptives (birth control pills), ethosuximide, and valproic acid.

6. The use of carbamazepine within 14 days of a monoamine oxidase (MAO) inhibitor can lead to serious side effects.

Before you start to take carbamazepine, BE SURE TO TELL YOUR DOCTOR if you are already taking any of the medications listed above.

WARNINGS

• Tell your doctor about unusual or allergic reactions you have had to medications, especially to carbamazepine, or to any tricyclic anti-depressants (amitriptyline, desipramine, doxepin, imipramine, protriptyline, or nortriptyline).

• Tell your doctor if you now have, or if you have ever had, bone marrow depression, blood disorders, glaucoma, heart disease, kidney disease, or liver disease.

• Before having any surgery or other medical or dental treatment, be sure to tell your doctor or dentist that you are taking this medication.

• If this medication makes you dizzy or drowsy, do not take part in any activity that requires alertness, such as driving a car or operating potentially dangerous equipment.

• If you are taking this medication to control a seizure disorder, do not stop taking it suddenly. If you stop abruptly, you may experience uncontrollable seizures.

• Be sure to tell your doctor if you are pregnant. Birth defects have been reported more often in infants whose mothers have seizure disorders. It is unclear if the increased risk of birth defects is associated with the disorder or with the anti-convulsion medications, such as carbamazepine, that are used to treat the condition. The risks and benefits of treatment should be discussed with your doctor. Also, tell your doctor if you are breastfeeding an infant. Small amounts of carbamazepine pass into breast milk.

---

carbenicillin

BRAND NAME (Manufacturer)
Geocillin (Roerig)
TYPE OF DRUG
Antibiotic (infection fighter)
INGREDIENT
carbenicillin indanyl sodium
DOSAGE FORM
Tablets (382 mg)

STORAGE
Carbenicillin tablets should be stored at room temperature in a tightly closed container.

USES
Carbenicillin is used to treat infections of the urinary tract and the prostate gland. It acts by severely injuring the cell walls of the infecting bacteria, thereby preventing them from growing and multiplying. Carbenicillin kills susceptible bacteria, but is not effective against viruses, parasites, or fungi.

TREATMENT
Carbenicillin should be taken on an empty stomach or with a glass of water one hour before, or two hours after, a meal.

It is important to continue to take this medication for the entire time prescribed by your doctor (usually seven to 14 days)—even if the symptoms of the infection disappear before the end of that period. If you stop taking the drug too soon, resistant bacteria are given the chance to continue growing, and the infection could recur.

Carbenicillin works best when the level of the medicine in your bloodstream is kept constant. Therefore, it is best to take the doses at evenly spaced intervals, day and night. For example, if you are taking four doses a day, the doses should be spaced six hours apart.

If you miss a dose of this medication, take the missed dose immediately. However, if you do not remember to take the missed dose until it is almost time for your next dose, take it; then space the next dose about halfway through the regular interval between doses. Then return to your regular schedule. Try not to skip any doses.

SIDE EFFECTS
Minor. Diarrhea; heartburn; nausea; and vomiting. These side effects should disappear in several days, as your body adjusts to the medication.
Major. Tell your doctor about any side effects that are persistent or particularly bothersome. IT IS ESPECIALLY IMPORTANT TO TELL YOUR DOCTOR about bloating; chills; cough; difficulty breathing; fever; irritation of the

mouth; muscle aches; rash; rectal or vaginal itching; severe diarrhea; sore throat; or darkened tongue. Also, if your symptoms of infection seem to be getting worse rather than improving, you should contact your doctor.

INTERACTIONS

Carbenicillin interacts with other types of medication.

1. Probenecid can increase the blood concentrations and side effects of this medication.

2. Carbenicillin may decrease the effectiveness of oral contraceptives (birth control pills), and pregnancy could result. You should therefore use another form of birth control while taking this medication. Discuss this with your doctor.

TELL YOUR DOCTOR if you are currently taking any of the medications listed above.

WARNINGS

• Tell your doctor about unusual or allergic reactions you have had to any medications, especially to carbenicillin or penicillins, or to cephalosporin antibiotics, penicillamine, or griseofulvin.

• Tell your doctor if you now have, or if you have ever had, kidney disease, asthma, or allergies.

• This medication has been prescribed for your current infection only. Another infection later on, or one that someone else has, may require a different medicine. You should not give your medicine to other people, or use it for other infections, unless your doctor specifically directs you to do so.

• Diabetics taking carbenicillin should know that this drug can cause a false-positive sugar reaction with a Clinitest urine glucose test. To avoid this problem, while taking carbenicillin you should switch to Clinistix or Tes-Tape to test your urine sugar.

• Be sure to tell your doctor if you are pregnant. Although carbenicillin appears to be safe during pregnancy, extensive studies in humans have not yet been completed. Also, tell your doctor if you are breastfeeding an infant. Small amounts of this medication pass into breast milk and may temporarily alter the bacteria in the intestinal tract of the nursing infant, resulting in diarrhea.

carbinoxamine

BRAND NAME (Manufacturer)
Clistin (McNeil)
TYPE OF DRUG
Antihistamine
INGREDIENT
carbinoxamine as the maleate salt
DOSAGE FORM
Tablets (4 mg)
STORAGE
Carbinoxamine should be stored at room temperature in a tightly closed container.

USES

This medication belongs to a group of drugs known as antihistamines (antihistamines block the action of histamine, a chemical that is released by the body during an allergic reaction). It is therefore used to treat or prevent symptoms of allergy.

TREATMENT

To avoid stomach upset, you can take carbinoxamine with food or with a full glass of milk or water (unless your doctor directs you to do otherwise).

If you miss a dose of this medication, take the missed dose as soon as possible, unless it is close to the time for your next dose. In that case, don't take the missed dose at all; just return to your regular dosing schedule. Do not double the next dose.

SIDE EFFECTS

Minor. Blurred vision; confusion; constipation; diarrhea; difficult or painful urination; dizziness; dry mouth, throat, or nose; headache; irritability; loss of appetite; nausea; rash; restlessness; ringing or buzzing in the ears; stomach upset; or unusual increase in sweating. These side effects should disappear in several days, as your body adjusts to the medication.

If you are constipated, increase the amount of fiber in your diet (raw vegetables, fruits, salads, bran, and whole-grain breads), and drink more water (unless your doctor tells you not to do so).

Chew sugarless gum, or suck on ice chips or a piece of hard candy, to reduce mouth dryness.

This medication can cause increased sensitivity to sunlight. It is therefore important to avoid prolonged exposure to sunlight and sunlamps. Wear protective clothing, and use an effective sunscreen.

If you feel dizzy or light-headed, sit or lie down awhile; get up from a sitting or lying position slowly, and be careful on stairs.

Major. Tell your doctor about any side effects that are persistent or particularly bothersome. IT IS ESPECIALLY IMPORTANT TO TELL YOUR DOCTOR about unusual bleeding or bruising; change in menstruation; clumsiness; feeling faint; flushing of the face; hallucinations; sleeping disorders; seizures; shortness of breath; sore throat or fever; palpitations; tightness in the chest; or unusual tiredness or weakness.

INTERACTIONS

Carbinoxamine interacts with several other types of medication.

1. Concurrent use of this medication with central nervous system depressants (drugs that slow the activity of the nervous system), such as barbiturates, benzodiazepine tranquilizers, muscle relaxants, narcotics, pain medications, phenothiazine tranquilizers, or alcohol, or with tricyclic anti-depressants can cause extreme drowsiness.

2. Monoamine oxidase (MAO) inhibitors (isocarboxazid, pargyline, phenelzine, tranylcypromine) can increase the side effects of this medication.

3. Carbinoxamine can decrease the activity of oral anticoagulants (blood thinners, such as warfarin).

TELL YOUR DOCTOR if you are currently taking any of the medications listed above.

WARNINGS

● Tell your doctor about unusual or allergic reactions you have had to medications, especially to carbinoxamine or to any other antihistamine (such as bromodiphenhydramine, brompheniramine, azatadine, chlorpheniramine,

clemastine, cyproheptadine, dexchlorpheniramine, dimenhydrinate, dimethindene, diphenhydramine, diphenylpyraline, doxylamine, hydroxyzine, promethazine, pyrilamine, trimeprazine, tripelennamine, or tripolidine).
• Tell your doctor if you now have, or if you have ever had, asthma, blood vessel disease, glaucoma, high blood pressure, kidney disease, peptic ulcers, enlarged prostate gland, or thyroid disease.
• Carbinoxamine can cause drowsiness or dizziness. Your ability to perform tasks that require alertness, such as driving a car or operating potentially dangerous machinery, may be decreased. Appropriate caution should therefore be taken.
• Be sure to tell your doctor if you are pregnant. The effects of this medication during pregnancy have not yet been thoroughly studied in humans. Also, tell your doctor if you are breastfeeding an infant. Small amounts of carbinoxamine pass into breast milk and may cause unusual excitement or irritability in nursing infants.

Cardioquin—see quinidine

Cardizem—see diltiazem

---

carisoprodol

BRAND NAMES (Manufacturers)
carisoprodol (various manufacturers)
Rela (Schering)
Soma (Wallace)
Soprodol (Henry Schein)
TYPE OF DRUG
Muscle relaxant
INGREDIENT
carisoprodol
DOSAGE FORM
Tablets (350 mg)
STORAGE
Carisoprodol should be stored at room temperature, in a tightly closed container.

USES

This medication is used to relieve painful muscle conditions. It should be used in conjunction with rest, physical therapy, and other measures to alleviate discomfort. It is not clear exactly how carisoprodol works, but it is thought to act as a central nervous system depressant (it slows the activity of the brain and spinal cord). It does NOT act directly on muscles.

TREATMENT

In order to avoid stomach irritation, you can take carisoprodol with food or with a full glass of water or milk (unless your doctor directs you to do otherwise).

If you miss a dose of this medication and remember within an hour of the scheduled dose, take the missed dose immediately. If more than an hour has passed, do not take the missed dose at all; just return to your regular dosing schedule. Do not double the next dose.

SIDE EFFECTS

Minor. Dizziness; drowsiness; headache; hiccups; insomnia; nausea; stomach pain; and vomiting. These side effects should disappear in several days, as your body adjusts to the medication.

If you feel dizzy, sit or lie down awhile; get up slowly, and be careful on stairs.

Major. Tell your doctor about any side effects that are persistent or particularly bothersome. IT IS ESPECIALLY IMPORTANT TO TELL YOUR DOCTOR about agitation; depression; irritability; loss of coordination; fainting; palpitations; and tremors.

INTERACTIONS

Carisoprodol interacts with several other types of medication. Concurrent use of it with other central nervous system depressants (such as alcohol, antihistamines, barbiturates, benzodiazepine tranquilizers, muscle relaxants, narcotics, pain medications, phenothiazine tranquilizers, or sleeping medications) or with tricyclic anti-depressants can lead to extreme drowsiness.

BE SURE TO TELL YOUR DOCTOR if you are already taking any of these medications.

WARNINGS

- Tell your doctor about unusual or allergic reactions you have had to any medications, especially to carisoprodol, meprobamate, or tybamate.
- Before starting to take carisoprodol, tell your doctor if you now have, or if you have ever had, kidney disease, liver disease, or porphyria.
- If this drug makes you dizzy or drowsy, avoid taking part in any activity that requires alertness, such as driving a car or operating potentially dangerous equipment.
- Some of these products contain F.D. & C. Yellow Dye No. 5 (tartrazine), which can cause allergic-type symptoms (rash, fainting, shortness of breath) in certain susceptible individuals.
- Carisoprodol has the potential for abuse, and should be used with caution. Do not increase the dose or stop taking the drug unless you first consult your doctor. If you have been taking carisoprodol for several months, and stop taking it abruptly, you could experience a withdrawal reaction. Your doctor may therefore want to decrease your dosage gradually to avoid this reaction.
- Be sure to tell your doctor if you are pregnant. Although carisoprodol appears to be safe during pregnancy, extensive studies have not yet been completed in humans. Also, tell your doctor if you are breastfeeding an infant. This medication passes into breast milk and can cause excessive drowsiness and stomach upset in nursing infants.

Catapres—see clonidine

Ceclor—see cefaclor

CeeNU—see lomustine

---

cefaclor

BRAND NAME (Manufacturer)
Ceclor (Dista)
TYPE OF DRUG
Cephalosporin antibiotic (infection fighter)

INGREDIENT
cefaclor
DOSAGE FORMS
Capsules (250 mg and 500 mg)
Oral suspension (125 mg and 250 mg per
   5 ml teaspoonful)
STORAGE
Cefaclor capsules should be stored at room temperature
in a tightly closed container. The oral suspension form of
this drug should be stored in the refrigerator in a tightly
closed container. Any unused portion of the oral suspension should be discarded after 14 days, because the drug
loses its potency after that time. This medication should
never be frozen.

USES

This medication is used to treat a wide variety of bacterial
infections, including those of the middle ear, upper and
lower respiratory tract, and urinary tract. This drug acts by
severely injuring the cell walls of the infecting bacteria,
thereby preventing them from growing and multiplying.
Cefaclor kills susceptible bacteria, but it is not effective
against viruses, parasites, or fungi.

TREATMENT

Cefaclor can be taken either on an empty stomach or with
food or milk (in order to avoid an upset stomach).
   The contents of the suspension form of cefaclor tend to
settle on the bottom of the bottle, so it is necessary to
shake the container well, to evenly distribute the ingredients and equalize the doses. Each dose should then be
measured carefully with a specially designed, 5 ml
measuring spoon or with the dropper provided. An ordinary kitchen spoon is not accurate enough.
   Cephalosporin antibiotics work best when the level of
medicine in your bloodstream is kept constant. It is therefore best to take the doses at evenly spaced intervals, day
and night. For example, if you are to take four doses a day,
the doses should be spaced six hours apart.
   If you miss a dose of this medication, take the missed
dose immediately. If you do not remember to take the
missed dose until it is almost time for your next dose, take

it; then space the next dose halfway through the regular interval between doses. Then return to your regular dosing schedule. Try not to skip any doses.

It is important to continue to take this medication for the entire time prescribed by your doctor (usually seven to 14 days)—even if the symptoms disappear before the end of that period. If you stop taking this drug too soon, resistant bacteria are given a chance to continue growing, and the infection could recur.

SIDE EFFECTS

Minor. Abdominal pain; diarrhea; dizziness; fatigue; headache; heartburn; itching; loss of appetite; nausea; and vomiting. These side effects should disappear in several days, as your body adjusts to the medication.

Major. Tell your doctor about any side effects that are persistent or particularly bothersome. IT IS ESPECIALLY IMPORTANT TO TELL YOUR DOCTOR about difficulty breathing; fever; joint pain; rash; rectal or vaginal itching; severe diarrhea (which can be watery, or contain pus or blood); sore mouth; stomach cramps; tingling in the hands or feet; darkened tongue; or unusual bleeding or bruising. Also, if your symptoms of infection seem to be getting worse rather than improving, you should contact your doctor.

INTERACTIONS

Cefaclor interacts with several other types of medication.
1. Probenecid can increase the blood concentrations and side effects of this medication.
2. The side effects, especially effects on the kidneys, of furosemide, bumetanide, ethacrynic acid, colistin, vancomycin, polymyxin B, and aminoglycoside antibiotics can be increased when used concurrently with cefaclor.
TELL YOUR DOCTOR if you are currently taking any of the medications listed above.

WARNINGS

• Tell your doctor about unusual or allergic reactions you have had to any medication, especially to cefaclor or other cephalosporin antibiotics (such as cefamandole, cephalexin, cephradine, cefadroxil, cefazolin, cefoperazone, cefotaxime, ceftizoxime, cephalothin, cephapirin, cefoxitin, cefuroxime, moxalactam), or to penicillin antibiotics.

• Tell your doctor if you now have, or if you have ever had, kidney disease.

• This medication has been prescribed for your current infection only. Another infection later on, or one that someone else has, may require a different medicine. You should not give your medication to other people, or use it for other infections, unless your doctor specifically directs you to do so.

• Diabetics taking cefaclor should know that this drug can cause a false-positive sugar reaction with a Clinitest urine glucose test. To avoid this problem, while taking cefaclor you should switch to Clinistix or Tes-Tape to test your urine sugar.

• Be sure to tell your doctor if you are pregnant. Although the cephalosprin antibiotics appear to be safe during pregnancy, extensive studies in humans have not yet been completed. Also, tell your doctor if you are breastfeeding an infant. Small amounts of this medication pass into breast milk and may temporarily alter the bacteria in the intestinal tract of the nursing infant, resulting in diarrhea.

---

cefadroxil

BRAND NAMES (Manufacturers)
Duricef (Mead Johnson)
Ultracef (Bristol)
TYPE OF DRUG
Cephalosporin antibiotic (infection fighter)
INGREDIENT
cefadroxil
DOSAGE FORMS
Tablets (1000 mg)
Capsules (250 mg and 500 mg)
Oral suspension (125 mg, 250 mg, and 500 mg per 5 ml teaspoonful)
STORAGE
Cefadroxil tablets and capsules should be stored at room temperature in tightly closed containers. The oral suspen-

sion form of this drug should be stored in the refrigerator in a tightly closed container. Any unused portion of the oral suspension should be discarded after 14 days, because the drug loses its potency after that time. This medication should never be frozen.

USES

This medication is used to treat a wide variety of bacterial infections, including those of the middle ear, upper and lower respiratory tract, and urinary tract. This drug acts by severely injuring the cell walls of the infecting bacteria, thereby preventing them from growing and multiplying. Cefadroxil kills susceptible bacteria, but it is not effective against viruses, parasites, or fungi.

TREATMENT

In order to avoid an upset stomach, you can take cefadroxil either on an empty stomach or with food or milk.

The contents of the suspension form of cefadroxil tend to settle on the bottom of the bottle, so it is necessary to shake the container well, to evenly distribute the ingredients and equalize the doses. Each dose should then be measured carefully with a specially designed, 5 ml measuring spoon or with the dropper provided. An ordinary kitchen spoon is not accurate enough.

Cephalosporin antibiotics work best when the level of medicine in your bloodstream is kept constant. It is therefore best to take the doses at evenly spaced intervals, day and night. For example, if you are to take four doses a day, the doses should be spaced six hours apart.

If you miss a dose of this medication, take the missed dose immediately. However, if you do not remember to take the missed dose until it is almost time for your next dose, take it; then space the next dose halfway through the regular interval between doses. Then return to your regular schedule. Try not to skip any doses.

It is important to continue to take this medication for the entire time prescribed by your doctor (usually seven to 14 days), even if the symptoms disappear before the end of that period. If you stop taking this drug too soon, resistant bacteria are given a chance to continue growing, and the infection could recur.

SIDE EFFECTS

Minor. Abdominal pain; diarrhea; dizziness; fatigue; headache; heartburn; itching; loss of appetite; nausea; and vomiting. These side effects should disappear in several days, as your body adjusts to the medication.

Major. Tell your doctor about any side effects that are persistent or particularly bothersome. IT IS ESPECIALLY IMPORTANT TO TELL YOUR DOCTOR about difficulty breathing; fever; joint pain; rash; rectal or vaginal itching; severe diarrhea (which can be watery, or contain pus or blood); sore mouth; stomach cramps; tingling in the hands or feet; darkened tongue; or unusual bleeding or bruising. Also, if your symptoms of infection seem to be getting worse rather than improving, you should contact your doctor.

INTERACTIONS

Cefadroxil interacts with other types of medication.

1. Probenecid can increase the blood concentrations and side effects of this medication.

2. The side effects, especially effects on the kidneys, of furosemide, bumetanide, ethacrynic acid, colistin, vancomycin, polymyxin B, and aminoglycoside antibiotics can be increased when used concurrently with cefadroxil.

TELL YOUR DOCTOR if you are currently taking any of the medications listed above.

WARNINGS

• Tell your doctor about unusual or allergic reactions you have had to any medication, especially to cefadroxil or other cephalosporin antibiotics, or to penicillin antibiotics.

• Tell your doctor if you now have, or if you have ever had, kidney disease.

• This medication has been prescribed for your current infection only. Another infection later on, or one that someone else has, may require a different medicine. You should not give your medication to other people, or use it for other infections, unless your doctor specifically directs you to do so.

• Diabetics taking cefadroxil should know that this drug

can cause a false-positive sugar reaction with a Clinitest urine glucose test. To avoid this problem, while taking cefadroxil you should switch to Clinistix or Tes-Tape to test your urine sugar.

• Be sure to tell your doctor if you are pregnant. Although the cephalosporin antibiotics appear to be safe during pregnancy, extensive studies in humans have not yet been completed. Also, tell your doctor if you are breastfeeding an infant. Small amounts of this medication pass into breast milk and may temporarily alter the bacteria in the intestinal tract of the nursing infant, resulting in diarrhea.

Celestone—see betamethasone (systemic)

Cena K—see potassium chloride

Centrax—see prazepam

---

cephalexin

BRAND NAME (Manufacturer)
Keflex (Dista)
TYPE OF DRUG
Cephalosporin antibiotic (infection fighter)
INGREDIENT
cephalexin
DOSAGE FORMS
Tablets (1,000 mg)
Capsules (250 mg and 500 mg)
Oral suspension (125 mg and 250 mg per 5 ml teaspoonful)
Pediatric oral suspension (100 mg per ml)
STORAGE
Cephalexin tablets and capsules should be stored at room temperature in tightly closed containers. The oral suspension forms of this drug should be stored in the refrigerator in tightly closed containers. Any unused portion of oral suspension should be discarded after 14 days, because the drug loses its potency after that time. This medication should never be frozen.

USES

This medication is used to treat a wide variety of bacterial infections, including those of the middle ear, upper and lower respiratory tract, and urinary tract. This drug acts by severely injuring the cell walls of the infecting bacteria, thereby preventing them from growing and multiplying. Cephalexin kills susceptible bacteria, but is not effective against viruses, parasites, or fungi.

TREATMENT

In order to avoid an upset stomach, you can take cephalexin either on an empty stomach or with food or milk.

The contents of the suspension form of cephalexin tend to settle on the bottom of the bottle, so it is necessary to shake the container well, to evenly distribute the ingredients and equalize the doses. Each dose should then be measured carefully with a specially designed, 5 ml measuring spoon or with the dropper provided. An ordinary kitchen spoon is not accurate enough.

Cephalosporin antibiotics work best when the level of medicine in your bloodstream is kept constant. It is therefore best to take the doses at evenly spaced intervals, day and night. For example, if you are to take four doses a day, the doses should be spaced six hours apart.

If you miss a dose of this medication, take the missed dose immediately. However, if you do not remember to take the missed dose until it is almost time for your next dose, take it; then space the next dose halfway through the regular interval between doses. Then return to your regular schedule. Try not to skip any doses.

It is important to continue to take this medication for the entire time prescribed by your doctor (usually seven to 14 days), even if the symptoms disappear before the end of that period. If you stop taking this drug too soon, resistant bacteria are given a chance to continue growing, and the infection could recur.

SIDE EFFECTS

Minor. Abdominal pain; diarrhea; dizziness; fatigue; headache; heartburn; itching; loss of appetite; nausea; and vomiting. These side effects should disappear in several days, as your body adjusts to the medication.

If you feel dizzy, sit or lie down awhile; get up slowly, and be careful on stairs.

Major. Tell your doctor about any side effects that are persistent or particularly bothersome. IT IS ESPECIALLY IMPORTANT TO TELL YOUR DOCTOR about difficulty breathing; fever; joint pain; rash; rectal or vaginal itching; severe diarrhea (which can be watery, or contain pus or blood); sore mouth; stomach cramps; tingling in the hands or feet; darkened tongue; or unusual bleeding or bruising. Also, if your symptoms of infection seem to be getting worse rather than improving, you should contact your doctor.

INTERACTIONS

Cephalexin interacts with several other types of medication.

1. Probenecid can increase the blood concentrations of this medication.

2. The side effects, especially effects on the kidneys, of furosemide, bumetanide, ethacrynic acid, colistin, vancomycin, polymyxin B, and aminoglycoside antibiotics can be increased when used concurrently with cephalexin.

TELL YOUR DOCTOR if you are currently taking any of the medications listed above

WARNINGS

• Tell your doctor about unusual or allergic reactions you have had to any medication, especially to cephalexin or other cephalosporin antibiotics (such as cefamandole, cephradine, cefaclor, cefadroxil, cefazolin, cefoperazone, cefotaxime, ceftizoxime, cephalothin, cephapirin, cefoxitin, cefuroxime, moxalactam), or to penicillin antibiotics.

• Tell your doctor if you now have, or if you have ever had, kidney disease.

• This medication has been prescribed for your current infection only. Another infection later on, or one that someone else has, may require a different medicine. You should not give your medication to other people, or use it for other infections, unless your doctor specifically directs you to do so.

- Diabetics taking cephalexin should know that this drug can cause a false-positive sugar reaction with a Clinitest urine glucose test. To avoid this problem, while taking cephalexin you should switch to Clinistix or Tes-Tape to test your urine sugar.
- Be sure to tell your doctor if you are pregnant. Although the cephalosporin antibiotics appear to be safe during pregnancy, extensive studies in humans have not yet been completed. Also, tell your doctor if you are breastfeeding an infant. Small amounts of this medication pass into breast milk and may temporarily alter the bacteria in the intestinal tract of the nursing infant, resulting in diarrhea.

cephradine

BRAND NAMES (Manufacturers)
Anspor (Smith Kline & French)
Velosef (Squibb)
TYPE OF DRUG
Cephalosporin antibiotic (infection fighter)
INGREDIENT
cephradine
DOSAGE FORMS
Tablets (1,000 mg)
Capsules (250 mg and 500 mg)
Oral suspension (125 mg and 250 mg per
   5 ml teaspoonful)
STORAGE
Cephradine tablets and capsules should be stored at room temperature in tightly closed containers. The oral suspension form of this drug should be stored in the refrigerator in a tightly closed container. Any unused portion of the oral suspension should be discarded after 14 days, because the drug loses its potency after that time. This medication should never be frozen.

USES

This medication is used to treat a wide variety of bacterial infections, including those of the middle ear, upper and lower respiratory tract, and urinary tract. This drug acts by severely injuring the cell walls of the infecting bacteria, thereby preventing them from growing and multiplying. Cephradine kills susceptible bacteria, but it is not effective against viruses, parasites, or fungi.

TREATMENT

In order to avoid an upset stomach, you can take cephradine either on an empty stomach or with food or milk.

The contents of the suspension form of cephradine tend to settle on the bottom of the bottle, so it is necessary to shake the container well, to evenly distribute the ingredients and equalize the doses. Each dose should then be measured carefully with a specially designed, 5 ml measuring spoon or with the dropper provided. An ordinary kitchen spoon is not accurate enough.

Cephalosporin antibiotics work best when the level of medicine in your bloodstream is kept constant. It is therefore best to take the doses at evenly spaced intervals, day and night. For example, if you are to take four doses a day, the doses should be spaced six hours apart.

If you miss a dose of this medication, take the missed dose immediately. However, if you do not remember to take the missed dose until it is almost time for your next dose, take it; then space the next dose halfway through the regular interval between doses. Then return to your regular schedule. Try not to skip any doses.

It is important to continue to take this medication for the entire time prescribed by your doctor (usually seven to 14 days), even if the symptoms disappear before the end of that period. If you stop taking this drug too soon, resistant bacteria are given a chance to continue growing, and the infection could recur.

SIDE EFFECTS

Minor. Abdominal pain; diarrhea; dizziness; fatigue; headache; heartburn; itching; loss of appetite; nausea; and vomiting. These side effects should disappear in several days, as your body adjusts to the medication.

If you feel dizzy, sit or lie down awhile; get up slowly, and be careful on stairs.

Major. Tell your doctor about any side effects that are persistent or particularly bothersome. IT IS ESPECIALLY

IMPORTANT TO TELL YOUR DOCTOR about difficulty breathing; fever; joint pain; rash; rectal or vaginal itching; severe diarrhea (which can be watery, or contain pus or blood); sore mouth; stomach cramps; tingling in the hands or feet; darkened tongue; or unusual bleeding or bruising. Also, if your symptoms of infection seem to be getting worse rather than improving, you should contact your doctor.

INTERACTIONS

Cephradine interacts with several other medications.

1. Probenecid can increase the blood concentrations and side effects of this medication.

2. The side effects, especially effects on the kidneys, of furosemide, bumetanide, ethacrynic acid, colistin, vancomycin, polymyxin B, and aminoglycoside antibiotics can be increased when used concurrently with cephradine.

TELL YOUR DOCTOR if you are currently taking any of the medications listed above.

WARNINGS

• Tell your doctor about unusual or allergic reactions you have had to any medication, especially to cephradine or other cephalosporin antibiotics (such as cefamandole, cephalexin, cefaclor, cefadroxil, cefazolin, cefoperazone, cefotaxime, ceftizoxime, cephalothin, cephapirin, cefoxitin, cefuroxime, moxalactam), or to penicillin antibiotics.

• Tell your doctor if you now have, or if you have ever had, kidney disease.

• This medication has been prescribed for your current infection only. Another infection later on, or one that someone else has, may require a different medicine. You should not give your medication to other people, or use it for other infections, unless your doctor specifically directs you to do so.

• Diabetics taking cephradine should know that this drug can cause a false-positive sugar reaction with a Clinitest urine glucose test. To avoid this problem, while taking cephradine you should switch to Clinistix or Tes-Tape to test your urine sugar.

• Be sure to tell your doctor if you are pregnant. Although the cephalosporin antibiotics appear to be safe during pregnancy, extensive studies in humans have not yet been completed. Also, tell your doctor if you are breastfeeding an infant. Small amounts of this medication pass into breast milk and may temporarily alter the bacteria in the intestinal tract of the nursing infant, resulting in diarrhea.

Cerespan—see papaverine

Cetacort—see hydrocortisone (topical)

Cetamide—see sodium sulfacetamide (ophthalmic)

Chenix—see chenodiol

---

chenodiol

BRAND NAME (Manufacturer)
Chenix (Rowell)
TYPE OF DRUG
Gallstone dissolver
INGREDIENT
chenodiol
DOSAGE FORM
Tablets (250 mg)
STORAGE
Chenodiol tablets should be stored at room temperature in a tightly closed container.

USES

This medication is used to dissolve gallstones in individuals who cannot tolerate surgery. Chenodiol is a naturally occurring bile acid that blocks the body's production of cholesterol. This action leads to gradual dissolution of cholesterol gallstones. It has no effect on calcified gallstones.

TREATMENT

In order to obtain the maximum benefit from this medication, you should take it with food or milk. It is important to continue taking this medication for the entire time prescribed by your doctor (usually six months to two years), even if your symptoms disappear. If you stop using this drug too soon, your symptoms could recur (the gallstones may not have completely dissolved).

If you miss a dose of this medication, take the missed dose as soon as possible, unless it is almost time for the next dose. In that case, do not take the missed dose at all; just return to your regular dosing schedule. Do not double the next dose.

SIDE EFFECTS

Minor. Constipation; diarrhea; gas; heartburn; loss of appetite; nausea; stomach cramps; and vomiting. These side effects should disappear in several weeks, as your body adjusts to the medication.

To relieve constipation, increase the amount of fiber in your diet (bran, salads, fresh fruits and vegetables, and whole-grain breads), exercise, and drink more water (unless your doctor directs you to do otherwise).

If diarrhea continues to be a problem, contact your doctor. Anti-diarrhea medications may be effective for short periods, or your doctor may want to decrease your dose of chenodiol.

Major. Tell your doctor about any side effects that are persistent or particularly bothersome. IT IS ESPECIALLY IMPORTANT TO TELL YOUR DOCTOR about yellowing of the eyes or skin.

INTERACTIONS

Chenodiol interacts with other types of medication.

1. Cholestyramine, colestipol, and aluminum-containing antacids can decrease the absorption of chenodiol from the gastrointestinal tract.

2. Estrogens, oral contraceptives (birth control pills), and clofibrate can counteract the effectiveness of chenodiol. Before you start to take this medication, BE SURE TO TELL YOUR DOCTOR if you are already taking any of the medications listed above.

WARNINGS

• Tell your doctor about any unusual or allergic reactions

you have had to medications, especially to chenodiol.
- Tell your doctor if you now have, or if you have ever had, biliary tract disease, blood vessel disease, colon cancer, inflammatory bowel disease, liver disease, or pancreatitis.
- Body weight and diet influence the formation and dissolution of gallstones. A high-fiber, low-fat diet and weight reduction are recommended to increase the effectiveness of chenodiol.
- Be sure to tell your doctor if you are pregnant. Extensive studies in humans during pregnancy have not yet been completed. However, this medication has caused birth defects in the offspring of animals that received large doses of it during pregnancy. Also, tell your doctor if you are breastfeeding an infant. It is not known whether or not chenodiol passes into breast milk.

Chlorafed Adult Timecelles—see pseudoephedrine and chlorpheniramine combination

Chlorafed (Half-Strength)—see pseudoephedrine and chlorpheniramine combination

---

chloral hydrate

BRAND NAMES (Manufacturers)
Aquachloral Supprettes (Webcon)
chloral hydrate (various manufacturers)
Noctec (Squibb)
Oradrate (Coast)
SK-Chloral Hydrate (Smith Kline & French)
TYPE OF DRUG
Sedative/hypnotic (sleeping aid)
INGREDIENT
chloral hydrate
DOSAGE FORMS
Capsules (250 mg and 500 mg)
Oral syrup (250 mg and 500 mg per 5 ml teaspoonful)
Oral elixir (500 mg per 5 ml teaspoonful)
Suppositories (325 mg, 500 mg, and 650 mg)

STORAGE

Chloral hydrate capsules, oral syrup, oral elixir, and suppositories should be stored at room temperature in tightly closed, light-resistant containers. This medication should never be frozen. The suppositories should be kept in the glass container in which they were dispensed.

USES

Chloral hydrate is used as a sleeping aid in the treatment of insomnia. Exactly how chloral hydrate works is not clearly understood, but it is known to be a central nervous system depressant (a drug that slows the activity of the brain and spinal cord).

TREATMENT

Chloral hydrate should be taken 15 to 30 minutes before bedtime.

In order to prevent stomach irritation, you should take chloral hydrate capsules with a full glass of water (unless your doctor directs you to do otherwise). The capsules should be swallowed whole to avoid their bad taste.

Each dose of the oral syrup or oral elixir should be measured carefully, with a specially designed, 5 ml measuring spoon. An ordinary kitchen spoon is not accurate enough. The syrup and elixir should then be mixed with at least ½ glass (4 ounces) of a non-alcoholic beverage (to avoid stomach irritation and to mask the unpleasant taste).

To insert the suppository form of this medication, first unwrap it and moisten it slightly with water (if the suppository is too soft, run cold water over it or refrigerate it for 30 minutes before you unwrap it). Lie down on your left side, with your right knee bent. Push the suppository well into the rectum with your finger. Try to avoid having a bowel movement for at least an hour.

The use of this drug as a sleeping aid should be limited to two weeks. After that period, chloral hydrate loses its ability to produce and maintain sleep.

SIDE EFFECTS

Minor. Diarrhea; dizziness; drowsiness during the day; gas; headache; nausea; stomach irritation; unpleasant taste in the mouth; and vomiting. These side effects should disappear in several days, as your body adjusts to the medication.

If you feel dizzy or light-headed, sit or lie down awhile; get up slowly, and be careful on stairs.

Major. Tell your doctor about any side effects that are persistent or particularly bothersome. IT IS ESPECIALLY IMPORTANT TO TELL YOUR DOCTOR about confusion; difficulty breathing; disorientation; excitation; fatigue; feeling faint; hallucinations; hives or itching; loss of coordination; nightmares; skin rash; or yellowing of the eyes or skin.

INTERACTIONS

Chloral hydrate interacts with a number of other medications.

1. Concurrent use of chloral hydrate with other central nervous system depressants (such as alcohol, barbiturates, benzodiazepine tranquilizers, muscle relaxants, narcotics, pain medications, phenothiazine tranquilizers, or other sleeping medications) or with tricyclic anti-depressants can lead to extreme drowsiness.

2. Chloral hydrate can increase the effects of oral anticoagulants (blood thinners, such as warfarin), which can lead to bleeding complications.

BE SURE TO TELL YOUR DOCTOR if you are currently taking any of these types of medication.

WARNINGS

• Tell your doctor about unusual or allergic reactions you have had to any medications, especially to chloral hydrate or to triclofos.

• Before starting to take this medication, be sure to tell your doctor if you now have, or if you have ever had, gastritis; heart disease; kidney disease; liver disease; or porphyria.

• If this drug makes you dizzy or drowsy, do not take part in any activity that requires alertness, such as driving a car or operating potentially dangerous equipment.

• This drug has the potential for abuse and must be used with caution. Tolerance develops quickly—do not increase the dose or stop taking this drug unless you first consult your doctor. If you have been taking chloral hydrate for a long time or have been taking large doses, you may experience anxiety, muscle twitching, tremors, weakness, dizziness, nausea, vomiting, insomnia, or blurred vision when you stop taking it. Your doctor may therefore want to reduce your dosage gradually.

• Be sure to tell your doctor if you are pregnant. Although extensive studies in animals and humans have not yet been completed, it is known that chloral hydrate crosses the placenta. If it is used for prolonged periods during the last three months of pregnancy, there is a chance that the infant will be born addicted to the medication and will experience a withdrawal reaction (convulsions and irritability) at birth. Also, tell your doctor if you are breastfeeding an infant. Small amounts of chloral hydrate pass into breast milk and may cause excessive drowsiness in the nursing infant.

chlorambucil

BRAND NAME (Manufacturer)
Leukeran (Burroughs Wellcome)
TYPE OF DRUG
Anti-neoplastic (anti-cancer drug)
INGREDIENT
chlorambucil
DOSAGE FORM
Tablets (2 mg)
STORAGE
Chlorambucil should be stored at room temperature in a tightly closed, light-resistant container.

USES

Chlorambucil belongs to a group of drugs known as alkylating agents. It is used to treat a variety of cancers. Chlorambucil works by binding to the rapidly growing cancer cells, preventing their multiplication and growth.

TREATMENT

Chlorambucil can be taken either on an empty stomach or with food or milk (as directed by your doctor).

The timing of the doses of this medication is important. Be sure you completely understand your doctor's instructions on how this medication should be taken.

If you miss a dose of this medication, take the missed dose as soon as possible, unless it is almost time for the next dose. In that case, do not take the missed dose at all; just return to your regular dosing schedule. Do not double the next dose.

SIDE EFFECTS

Minor. Itching; nausea; stomach upset; and vomiting. These side effects may disappear as your body adjusts to this medication. It is important, however, to continue taking this medication despite any nausea and vomiting that may occur.

Chlorambucil can also cause hair loss, which is reversible when the medication is stopped.

Major. Tell your doctor about any side effects that are persistent or particularly bothersome. IT IS ESPECIALLY IMPORTANT TO TELL YOUR DOCTOR about unusual bleeding or bruising; chills; convulsions; difficulty breathing; fever; joint pain; menstrual irregularities; mouth sores; skin rash; sore throat; or yellowing of the eyes or skin.

INTERACTIONS

Chlorambucil can increase the blood levels of uric acid, which can block the effectiveness of anti-gout medications (allopurinol, probenecid, sulfinpyrazone). BE SURE TO TELL YOUR DOCTOR if you are already taking any of these medications.

WARNINGS

• Tell your doctor about unusual or allergic reactions you have had to any medications, especially to chlorambucil or melphalan.

• Before starting to take this medication, be sure to tell your doctor if you now have, or if you have ever had, blood disorders, chronic or recurrent infections, gout, or kidney stones.

• You should not receive any immunizations or vaccinations while taking this medication. Chlorambucil blocks the effectiveness of the vaccine, and may lead to over-whelming infection if a live virus is administered.

• While you are taking this medication it is important that you drink plenty of fluids to prevent the formation of uric acid kidney stones.

• Chlorambucil can lower your platelet count, which can decrease your body's ability to form blood clots. You should therefore be especially careful while brushing your teeth; flossing; or using toothpicks, razors, or finger-nail scissors. Try to avoid falls and other injuries. Before having any surgery or other medical or dental treatment, be sure your doctor or dentist knows that you are taking this medication.

• Chlorambucil can decrease fertility in both men and women.

• Be sure to tell your doctor if you are pregnant. Birth defects have been reported in both humans and animals whose mothers received chlorambucil during pregnancy. The risks should be discussed with your doctor. Also, tell your doctor if you are breastfeeding an infant. It is not known whether or not chlorambucil passes into breast milk.

Chloramead—see chlorpromazine

---

chloramphenicol (systemic)

BRAND NAMES (Manufacturers)
chloramphenicol (various manufacturers)
Chloromycetin Kapseals (Parke-Davis)
Mychel (Rachelle)
TYPE OF DRUG
Antibiotic (infection fighter)
INGREDIENT
chloramphenicol
DOSAGE FORMS
Capsules (250 mg and 500 mg)
Oral suspension (150 mg per 5 ml teaspoonful)
STORAGE
Chloramphenicol capsules and oral suspension should

be stored at room temperature, in tightly closed light-resistant containers. This medication should never be frozen.

USES

This medication is an antibiotic that is used to treat a wide variety of bacterial infections. It attaches to the bacteria and blocks their production of protein, thereby preventing their growth and multiplication. Chloramphenicol kills susceptible bacteria, but is not effective against viruses, parasites, or fungi.

TREATMENT

Chloramphenicol is most effective if it is taken on an empty stomach one hour before or two hours after a meal.

The suspension form of this medication should be shaken well, just before measuring each dose. The contents tend to settle on the bottom of the bottle, so it is necessary to shake it in order to evenly distribute the ingredients and equalize the doses. Each dose should then be measured carefully with a specially designed, 5 ml measuring spoon. An ordinary kitchen teaspoon is not accurate enough.

Chloramphenicol works best when the level of medicine in your bloodstream is kept constant. It is best therefore to take the doses at evenly spaced intervals, day and night. For example, if you are to take four doses a day, the doses should be spaced six hours apart.

Try not to miss any doses of this medication. If you do miss a dose, take it as soon as you remember. Even if you do not remember to take the missed dose until it is almost time for your next dose, take the missed dose immediately. Space the following dose about halfway through the regular interval between doses. Then continue with your regular dosing schedule.

It is important to continue to take this medication for the entire time prescribed by your doctor (usually seven to 14 days), even if the symptoms disappear before the end of that period. If you stop taking the drug too soon, resistant bacteria are given a chance to continue growing and your infection could recur.

SIDE EFFECTS

Minor. Diarrhea; headache; and nausea or vomiting. These side effects should disappear in several days, as your body adjusts to the medication.

Major. Tell your doctor about any side effects that are persistent or particularly bothersome. IT IS ESPECIALLY IMPORTANT TO TELL YOUR DOCTOR about unusual bleeding or bruising; confusion; depression; fever; itching; mouth sores; skin rash; sore throat; sores on the tongue; tingling sensations; or unusual weakness. Also, if your symptoms of infection seem to be getting worse rather than improving, you should contact your doctor.

INTERACTIONS

Chloramphenicol interacts with several other types of medication.

1. It can increase the blood levels of dicumarol, phenytoin, phenobarbital, tolbutamide, and chlorpropamide, thereby leading to an increase in side effects.

2. Chloramphenicol can reduce the effectiveness of iron, vitamin B_{12}, and cyclophosphamide.

3. The blood levels and side effects of chloramphenicol may be increased by acetaminophen and penicillin.

4. Concurrent use of chloramphenicol and anti-neoplastic drugs (anti-cancer medicines), colchicine, gold, oxyphenbutazone, penicillamine, or phenylbutazone can lead to an increase in side effects, especially to the bone marrow.

Before starting to take chloramphenicol, BE SURE TO TELL YOUR DOCTOR if you are already taking any of the medications listed above.

WARNINGS

• Tell your doctor about unusual or allergic reactions you have had to any medications, especially to chloramphenicol.

• Before starting to take this medication, tell your doctor if you now have, or if you have ever had, kidney disease, liver disease, or porphyria.

• Diabetic patients should know that chloramphenicol can cause false-positive readings with the Clinitest urine glucose test. Temporarily switching to Clinistix or Tes-Tape to monitor urine glucose levels avoids this problem.

● Chloramphenicol has been prescribed for your current infection only. Another infection later on, or one that someone else has, may require a different medicine. You must not give your medication to other people, or use it for other infections, unless your doctor specifically directs you to do so.

● Be sure to tell your doctor if you are pregnant. Chloramphenicol crosses the placenta. Although it appears to be safe during the early stages of pregnancy, chloramphenicol can cause serious side effects in a newborn infant if it is given to the mother late in pregnancy. Also, tell your doctor if you are breastfeeding an infant. Small amounts of chloramphenicol pass into breast milk and can cause serious side effects in nursing infants.

Chlorate—see chlorpheniramine

Chlorazine—see prochlorperazine

---

chlordiazepoxide

BRAND NAMES (Manufacturers)
A-poxide (Abbott)
chlordiazepoxide hydrochloride (various manufacturers)
Libritabs (Roche)
Librium (Roche)
Lipoxide (Major)
Murcil (Reid-Provident)
Reposans-10 (Wesley)
Sereen (Foy)
SK-Lygen (Smith Kline & French)
TYPE OF DRUG
Sedative/hypnotic (anti-anxiety medication)
INGREDIENT
chlordiazepoxide as the hydrochloride salt
DOSAGE FORMS
Capsules (5 mg, 10 mg, and 25 mg)
Tablets (5 mg, 10 mg, and 25 mg)

STORAGE
This medication should be stored at room temperature in tightly closed, light-resistant containers.

USES
Chlordiazepoxide is prescribed to treat the symptoms of anxiety and alcohol withdrawal. It is not clear exactly how this medicine works, but it may relieve anxiety by acting as a depressant of the central nervous system. Chlordiazepoxide is currently used by many people to relieve nervousness. It is effective for this purpose for short periods, but it is important to try to remove the cause of the anxiety as well.

TREATMENT
This medication should be taken exactly as directed by your doctor. It can be taken with food or a full glass of water if stomach upset occurs. Do not take this medication with a dose of antacids, since they may retard its absorption.

If you are taking this medication regularly and you miss a dose, and remember within an hour of the scheduled time, take the missed dose immediately. If more than an hour has passed, however, skip the dose you missed and wait for the next scheduled dose. Do not double the dose.

SIDE EFFECTS
Minor. Bitter taste in mouth; constipation; depression; diarrhea; dizziness; drowsiness (after a night's sleep); dry mouth; fatigue; flushing; headache; heartburn; excess saliva; loss of appetite; nausea; nervousness; sweating; and vomiting. As your body adjusts to the medicine, these side effects should disappear.

Dry mouth can be relieved by chewing sugarless gum or by sucking on ice chips.

If you feel dizzy, sit or lie down awhile; get up slowly, and be careful on stairs.

Major. Tell your doctor about any side effects that are persistent or particularly bothersome. IT IS ESPECIALLY IMPORTANT TO TELL YOUR DOCTOR about blurred or double vision; chest pain; severe depression; difficulty urinating; fainting; falling; fever; joint pain; hallucinations; mouth sores; nightmares; palpitations; rash; shortness of breath; slurred speech; sore throat; uncoordinated movements; unusual excitement; unusual tiredness; or yellowing of the eyes or skin.

INTERACTIONS

Chlordiazepoxide interacts with a number of other medications.

1. To prevent over-sedation, this drug should not be taken with alcohol, other sedative drugs, central nervous system depressants, (such as antihistamines, barbiturates, muscle relaxants, pain medicines, narcotics, medicines for seizures, or phenothiazine tranquilizers), or with anti-depressants.

2. This medication may decrease the effectiveness of carbamazepine, levodopa, and oral anti-coagulants (blood thinners), and may increase the effects of phenytoin.

3. Disulfiram, isoniazid, and cimetidine can increase the blood levels of chlordiazepoxide, which can lead to toxic effects.

4. Concurrent use of rifampin may decrease the effectiveness of chlordiazepoxide.

If you are currently taking any of the medications listed above, CONSULT YOUR DOCTOR about their use.

WARNINGS

- Tell your doctor about unusual or allergic reactions you have had to any medications, especially to chlordiazepoxide or to other benzodiazepine tranquilizers (such as alprazolam, chlorazepate, diazepam, flurazepam, halazepam, lorazepam, oxazepam, prazepam, temazepam, or triazolam).
- Tell your doctor if you now have, or if you have ever had, liver disease, kidney disease, epilepsy, lung disease, myasthenia gravis, porphyria, mental depression, or mental illness.
- This medicine can cause drowsiness. Avoid tasks that require alertness, such as driving a car or operating poten-

tially dangerous machinery.

• This medication has the potential for abuse and must be used with caution. Tolerance may develop quickly; do not increase the dose of the drug without first consulting your doctor. It is also important not to stop this drug suddenly if you have been taking it in large amounts or if you have used it for several weeks. Your doctor may want to reduce your dosage gradually.

• This is a safe drug when used properly. When it is combined with other sedative drugs or alcohol, however, serious side effects may develop.

• Be sure to tell your doctor if you are pregnant. This medicine may increase the chance of birth defects if it is taken during the first three months of pregnancy. In addition, too much use of this medicine during the last six months of pregnancy may lead to addiction of the fetus, resulting in withdrawal side effects in the newborn. Also, use of this medicine during the last weeks of pregnancy may cause drowsiness, slowed heartbeat, and breathing difficulties in the infant. Tell your doctor if you are breastfeeding an infant. This medicine can pass into breast milk and cause drowsiness, slowed heartbeat, and breathing difficulties in the nursing infant.

---

chlordiazepoxide and amitriptyline combination

BRAND NAME (Manufacturer)
Limbitrol (Roche)
TYPE OF DRUG
Anti-anxiety and anti-depressant (mood elevator)
INGREDIENTS
chlordiazepoxide as the hydrochloride salt, and amitriptyline
DOSAGE FORM
Tablets (10 mg chlordiazepoxide and 25 mg amitriptyline; 5 mg chlordiazepoxide and 12.5 mg amitriptyline)

STORAGE
Chlordiazepoxide and amitriptyline tablets should be stored at room temperature in a tightly closed, light-resistant container.

USES
Chlordiazepoxide and amitriptyline is used for the treatment of depression associated with anxiety. Amitriptyline belongs to a group of drugs referred to as tricyclic antidepressants. These medicines are thought to relieve depression by increasing the concentration of certain chemicals necessary for nerve transmission in the brain. It is not clear exactly how chlordiazepoxide works, but it may relieve anxiety by acting as a depressant of the central nervous system (brain and spinal cord).

TREATMENT
This medication should be taken exactly as your doctor prescribes. In order to avoid stomach upset, it can be taken with food or with a full glass of milk or water (unless your doctor directs you to do otherwise). Do not take chlordiazepoxide and amitriptyline tablets with a dose of antacids— they retard absorption of this medication.

If you are taking this medication regularly and you miss a dose, take the missed dose as soon as possible, unless it is almost time for your next dose. In that case, do not take the missed dose at all; just return to your regular dosing schedule. Do not double the dose.

The benefits of therapy with this medication may not become apparent for two or three weeks.

SIDE EFFECTS
Minor. Agitation; anxiety; blurred vision; confusion; constipation; cramps; diarrhea; dizziness; drowsiness; dry mouth; fatigue; headache; heartburn; insomnia; loss of appetite; nausea; peculiar tastes in the mouth; restlessness; sweating; vomiting; weakness; and weight gain or loss. These side effects should disappear in several days, as your body adjusts to the medication.

Amitriptyline may cause the urine to turn blue-green in color—this is a harmless effect.

Dry mouth can be relieved by chewing sugarless gum or by sucking on ice chips or a piece of hard candy.

To relieve constipation, increase the amount of fiber in your diet (bran, fresh fruits and vegetables, salads, whole-grain breads), exercise, and drink more water (unless your doctor directs you to do otherwise).

To avoid dizziness or light-headedness when you stand, contract and relax the muscles of your legs for a few moments before rising. Do this by pushing one foot against the floor while raising the other foot slightly, alternating feet so that you are "pumping" your legs in a pedaling motion.

This medication may cause increased sensitivity to sunlight. Therefore, avoid prolonged exposure to the sun and sunlamps. Wear protective clothing and sunglasses; and use an effective sunscreen.

Major. Tell your doctor about any side effects that are persistent or particularly bothersome. IT IS ESPECIALLY IMPORTANT TO TELL YOUR DOCTOR about unusual bleeding or bruising; convulsions; difficult or painful urination; enlarged or painful breasts (in both sexes); fainting; fever; fluid retention; hair loss; hallucinations; chest tightness; impotence; mood changes; mouth sores; nervousness; nightmares; numbness in the fingers or toes; palpitations; ringing in the ears; skin rash; sore throat; tremors; uncoordinated movements, or balance problems; or yellowing of the eyes or skin.

INTERACTIONS

Chlordiazepoxide and amitriptyline interacts with several other types of medications.

1. Extreme drowsiness can occur when this medicine is taken with central nervous system depressants (drugs that slow the activity of the nervous system), including alcohol, antihistamines, barbiturates, benzodiazepine tranquilizers, muscle relaxants, narcotics, pain medications, phenothiazine tranquilizers, and sleeping medications.

2. Amitriptyline may decrease the effectiveness of antiseizure medications and block the blood-pressure-lowering effects of clonidine and guanethidine.

3. Estrogens and oral contraceptives can increase the

side effects and reduce the effectiveness of amitriptyline.
4. Amitriptyline may increase the side effects of thyroid medication and over-the-counter (non-prescription) cough, cold, allergy, asthma, sinus, and diet medications.
5. The concurrent use of amitriptyline and monoamine oxidase (MAO) inhibitors should be undertaken very carefully, because the combination may result in fever, convulsions, or high blood pressure.
6. Chlordiazepoxide may decrease the effectiveness of carbamazepine, levodopa, and oral anti-coagulants (blood thinners), and may increase the effects of phenytoin.
7. Disulfiram, isoniazid, and cimetidine can increase the blood levels of chlordiazepoxide, which could possibly lead to toxic effects.
8. Concurrent use of rifampin may decrease the effectiveness of chlordiazepoxide and amitriptyline.
Before starting to take this medication, BE SURE TO TELL YOUR DOCTOR if you are currently taking any of the medications listed above.

WARNINGS

• Tell your doctor about unusual or allergic reactions you have had to any medications, especially to chlordiazepoxide or other benzodiazepine tranquilizers (such as alprazolam, clorazepate, diazepam, flurazepam, halazepam, lorazepam, oxazepam, prazepam, temazepam, or triazolam); or to amitriptyline or other tricyclic antidepressants (such as desipramine, imipramine, nortriptyline, doxepin).
• Tell your doctor if you now have, or if you have ever had, asthma, high blood pressure, liver or kidney disease, lung disease, myasthenia gravis, heart disease, a recent heart attack, circulatory disease, stomach problems, intestinal problems, alcoholism, difficulty urinating, enlarged prostate gland, epilepsy, glaucoma, thyroid disease, mental illness, or electroshock therapy.
• If this drug makes you dizzy or drowsy, do not take part in any activity that requires alertness, such as driving a car or operating potentially dangerous equipment.
• Before having any surgery or other medical or dental

treatment, be sure to tell your doctor or dentist that you are taking this medication.

• The effects of this medication may last as long as seven days after you've stopped taking it, so continue to observe all precautions during this period.

• This medication has the potential for abuse, and must be used with caution. Tolerance develops quickly; do not increase the dosage of the drug unless you first consult your doctor. It is also important not to stop taking this drug suddenly, especially if it has been used in large amounts or has been used for longer than several weeks. Abruptly stopping this medication may cause nausea, headache, stomach upset, fatigue, or a worsening of your condition. Your doctor may therefore want to reduce the dosage gradually.

• Be sure to tell your doctor if you are pregnant. Chlordiazepoxide may increase the chance of birth defects if it is taken during the first three months of pregnancy. In addition, too much use of this medication during the last six months of pregnancy may lead to addiction of the fetus, resulting in withdrawal symptoms in the newborn. Use of this medication during the last weeks of pregnancy may cause drowsiness, slowed heartbeat, and breathing difficulties in the newborn infant. Also, tell your doctor if you are breastfeeding an infant. This medicine may pass into breast milk and cause drowsiness, slowed heartbeat, breathing difficulty, and irritability in the nursing infant.

---

chlordiazepoxide and clidinium combination

BRAND NAMES (Manufacturers)
Clindex (Rugby)
Clinoxide (Geneva Generics)
Clipoxide (Henry Schein)
Librax (Roche)
TYPE OF DRUG
Anti-anxiety and anti-cholinergic

INGREDIENTS
Chlordiazepoxide as the hydrochloride salt and clidinium as the bromide salt

DOSAGE FORM
Capsules (5 mg chlordiazepoxide and 2.5 mg clidinium)

STORAGE
Chlordiazepoxide and clindinium capsules should be stored at room temperature in a tightly closed, light-resistant container.

USES
Chlordiazepoxide and clidinium is used in conjunction with other drugs to treat peptic ulcer or irritable bowel syndrome. Clidinium is an anti-cholinergic agent that slows the activity of the gastrointestinal tract and reduces the production of stomach acid. Chlordiazepoxide belongs to a group of drugs known as benzodiazepine tranquilizers. It is not clear exactly how chlordiazepoxide works, but it may relieve anxiety by acting as a depressant of the central nervous system (brain and spinal cord).

TREATMENT
You should take chlordiazepoxide and clidinium 30 to 60 minutes before meals. It can be taken with water or milk. Do not take it with antacids, since they may interfere with its absorption.

If you miss a dose of this medication, take the missed dose as soon as possible, unless it is almost time for your next dose. In that case, do not take the missed dose at all; just return to your regular dosing schedule. Do not double the next dose.

SIDE EFFECTS
Minor. Blurred vision; change in your sense of taste; confusion; constipation; depression; diarrhea; dizziness; drowsiness; dry mouth; fatigue; headache; insomnia; nausea; reduced sweating; and vomiting. These side effects should disappear in several days, as your body adjusts to the medication.

Dry mouth can be relieved by chewing sugarless gum or by sucking on ice chips or a piece of hard candy.

To relieve constipation, increase the amount of fiber in your diet (bran, fresh fruit and vegetables, salads, and whole-grain breads), exercise, and drink more water (unless your doctor directs you to do otherwise).

To avoid dizziness or light-headedness when you stand, contract and relax the muscles of your legs for a few minutes before rising. Do this by pushing one foot against the floor while raising the other foot slightly, alternating feet so that you are "pumping" your legs in a pedaling motion.

This medication can cause increased sensitivity to sun light. You should therefore avoid prolonged exposure to the sun and sunlamps. Wear protective clothing and sunglasses, and use an effective sunscreen.

Major. Tell your doctor about any side effects that are persistent or particularly bothersome. IT IS ESPECIALLY IMPORTANT TO TELL YOUR DOCTOR about decreased sexual ability; difficulty breathing; difficult or painful urination; excitation; fluid retention; hallucinations; palpitations; rash; sore throat; uncoordinated movements; or yellowing of the eyes or skin.

INTERACTIONS

This medication interacts with several other types of medications.

1. Extreme drowsiness can occur when this medicine is taken with other central nervous system depressants (drugs that slow the activity of the nervous system), including alcohol, antihistamines, barbiturates, muscle relaxants, narcotics, pain medications, phenothiazine tranquilizers, and sleeping medications, or with tricyclic anti-depressants.

2. Chlordiazepoxide can decrease the effectiveness of carbamazepine, levodopa, and oral anti-coagulants (blood thinners), and may increase the effects of phenytoin.

3. Disulfiram, isoniazid, and cimetidine can increase the blood levels of chlordiazepoxide, which could possibly lead to toxic effects.

4. Concurrent use of rifampin may decrease the effectiveness of chlordiazepoxide and clidinium.

5. Amantadine, haloperidol, phenothiazine tranquilizers, procainamide, quinidine, and tricyclic antidepressants may increase the side effects of clidinium. Before starting to take this medication, BE SURE TO TELL YOUR DOCTOR if you are already taking any of the medications listed above.

WARNINGS

• Tell your doctor if you have ever had unusual or allergic reactions to any medications, especially to chlordiazepoxide or other benzodiazepine tranquilizers (such as alprazolam, clorazepate, diazepam, flurazepam, halazepam, lorazepam, oxazepam, prazepam, temazepam, or triazolam); or to clidinium.

• Tell your doctor if you now have, or if you have ever had, glaucoma, obstructed bladder or intestine, enlarged prostate gland, heart disease, lung disease, liver disease, kidney disease, ulcerative colitis, porphyria, high blood pressure, myasthenia gravis, epilepsy, thyroid disease, emotional instability, or hiatal hernia.

• This medication can decrease sweating and heat release from the body. You should therefore avoid getting overheated by strenuous exercise in hot weather, and should avoid taking hot baths, showers, and saunas.

• This medicine can cause drowsiness. Avoid tasks that require alertness, such as driving a car or using potentially dangerous machinery.

• This medication has the potential for abuse, and must be used with caution. Tolerance develops quickly; do not increase the dose unless you first consult your doctor. It is also important not to stop taking this drug suddenly if you have been using it in large amounts or for longer than several weeks. Your doctor may want to reduce the dosage gradually.

• This is a safe drug when used properly. When it is combined with other sedative drugs or alcohol, however, serious side effects may develop.

• Be sure to tell your doctor if you are pregnant. This medicine may increase the chance of birth defects if it is taken during the first three months of pregnancy. In addition, too much use of this medicine during the last six months of pregnancy may cause the baby to become dependent on it. This may result in withdrawal symptoms in the infant after birth. Use of this medicine during the last weeks of pregnancy may cause drowsiness, slowed heartbeat, and breathing difficulties in the newborn infant. Also, tell your doctor if you are breastfeeding an infant. This medicine may pass into breast milk and cause drowsiness, slowed heartbeat, and breathing difficulties in the nursing infant.

chlordiazepoxide hydrochloride—see
  chlordiazepoxide

Chlorofon-F—see chlorzoxazone and acetaminophen
  combination

Chloromycetin Kapseals—see chloramphenicol
  (systemic)

---

chlorothiazide

BRAND NAMES (Manufacturers)
chlorothiazide (various manufacturers)
Diachlor (Major)
Diuril (Merck Sharp & Dohme)
SK-Chlorothiazide (Smith Kline & French)
TYPE OF DRUG
Diuretic (water pill) and anti-hypertensive
INGREDIENT
chlorothiazide
DOSAGE FORMS
Tablets (250 mg and 500 mg)
Oral suspension (250 mg per 5 ml teaspoonful)
STORAGE
This medication should be stored at room temperature in a tightly closed container.

USES

Chlorothiazide is prescribed to treat high blood pressure. It is also used to reduce fluid accumulation in the body caused by conditions such as heart failure, cirrhosis of the liver, kidney disease, and the long-term use of some medications. This medication reduces fluid accumulation by increasing the elimination of sodium and water through the kidneys.

TREATMENT

This medication can be taken with a glass of milk or with a meal to decrease stomach irritation (unless your doctor directs you to do otherwise). Try to take it at the same time every day. Avoid taking a dose after 6:00 P.M.—this will prevent you from having to get up during the night to urinate.

If you miss a dose of this medication, take the missed dose as soon as possible, unless it is almost time for the next dose. In that case, do not take the missed dose at all, just wait until the next scheduled dose. Do not double the dose.

This medication does not cure high blood pressure, but it will help to control the condition, as long as you continue to take it.

SIDE EFFECTS

Minor. Constipation; cramps; diarrhea; dizziness; drowsiness; headache; heartburn; itching; loss of appetite; nausea; restlessness; upset stomach; vomiting. As your body adjusts to the medication, these side effects should disappear.

This medication can cause increased sensitivity to sunlight. It is therefore important to avoid prolonged exposure to sunlight or sunlamps. Wear protective clothing, and use an effective sunscreen.

To avoid dizziness or light-headedness when you stand, contract and relax the muscles of your legs for a few moments before rising. Do this by pushing one foot against the floor while raising the other foot slightly, alternating feet so that you are "pumping" your legs in a pedaling motion.

Major. Tell your doctor about any side effects that are persistent or particularly bothersome. IT IS ESPECIALLY IMPORTANT TO TELL YOUR DOCTOR about unusual bleeding or bruising; blurred vision; confusion; difficulty breathing; dry mouth; excessive thirst; fever; joint pain; mood changes; muscle spasms; palpitations; skin rash; sore throat; tingling in the fingers or toes; excessive weakness; or yellowing of the eyes or skin.

INTERACTIONS

Chlorothiazide interacts with other types of medication.

1. It may decrease the effectiveness of oral anti-coagulants, anti-gout medications, insulin, oral anti-diabetic medicines, and methenamine.

2. Fenfluramine can increase the blood-pressure-lowering effects of chlorothiazide, which can be dangerous.

3. Indomethacin can decrease the blood-pressure-lowering effects (thereby counteracting the desired effects) of chlorothiazide.

4. Cholestyramine and colestipol decrease the absorption of this medication from the gastrointestinal tract. Chlorothiazide should therefore be taken one hour before, or four hours after, a dose of cholestyramine or colestipol (if you have also been prescribed one of these medications).

5. The side effects of amphotericin B, calcium, cortisone-like steroids (such as cortisone, dexamethasone, hydrocortisone, prednisone, prednisolone), digoxin, digitalis, lithium, quinidine, sulfonamide antibiotics, and vitamin D may be increased when taken concurrently with chlorothiazide.

BE SURE TO TELL YOUR DOCTOR if you are already taking any of the medicines listed above.

WARNINGS

• Tell your doctor about unusual or allergic reactions you have had to any medications, especially to diuretics (water pills), oral anti-diabetic medications, or sulfonamide antibiotics.

• Before you start taking chlorothiazide, tell your doctor if you now have, or if you have ever had, kidney disease or problems with urination, diabetes mellitus (sugar diabetes), gout, liver disease, asthma, pancreas disease, or systemic lupus erythematosus (SLE).

• Chlorothiazide can cause potassium loss. Signs of potassium loss include dry mouth, thirst, weakness, muscle pain or cramps, nausea, and vomiting. If you experience any of these symptoms, call your doctor. To help avoid potassium loss, take this drug with a glass of fresh or frozen orange or cranberry juice, or eat a banana every day. The use of a salt substitute also helps to prevent potassium loss. Do not change your diet, however, before discussing it with your doctor. Too much potassium can also be dangerous. Your doctor may want you to have blood tests performed periodically, in order to monitor your potassium levels.

• Limit your intake of alcoholic beverages while taking this medication, in order to prevent dizziness and light-headedness.

• If you have high blood pressure, do not take any over-the-counter (non-prescription) medications for weight control or for cough, cold, allergy, asthma, or sinus problems, unless your doctor directs you to do so.

• To prevent dehydration (severe water loss) while taking this medication, check with your doctor if you have any illness that causes severe nausea, vomiting, or diarrhea.

• This medication can raise blood sugar levels in diabetic patients. Therefore, blood sugar should be carefully monitored by blood or urine tests when this medication is started.

• Be sure to tell your doctor if you are pregnant. Although studies in humans have not been completed, adverse effects have been observed on animals whose mothers were given large doses of this drug during pregnancy. Also, tell your doctor if you are breastfeeding an infant. Although problems in humans have not been reported, small amounts of this drug can pass into breast milk, so caution is warranted.

chlorpheniramine

BRAND NAMES (Manufacturers)
Alermine* (Reid-Provident)
Aller-Chlor* (Rugby)
Allerid-O.D. (Trimen)
Chlorate (Major)
Chlor-Niramine* (Whiteworth)

chlorpheniramine maleate (various manufacturers)
Chlorspan (Vortech)
Chlortab (Vortech)
Chlor-Trimeton* (Schering)
Hal-Chlor (Halsom)
Histrey* (Bowman)
Phenetron (Lannett)
T.D. Alermine (Reid-Provident)
Telachlor S.R. (Major)
Teldrin* (Menley & James)
Trymegen (Medco Supply)
*Chlorpheniramine is also available over-the-counter
   (non-prescription), under several brand names.

TYPE OF DRUG
Antihistamine
INGREDIENT
chlorpheniramine as the maleate salt
DOSAGE FORMS
Tablets (4 mg)
Sustained-release tablets (8 mg and 12 mg)
Oral syrup (2 mg per 5 ml teaspoonful)
STORAGE
Chlorpheniramine tablets, capsules, and oral syrup
should be stored at room temperature in tightly closed
containers.

USES

This medication belongs to a group of drugs known as
antihistamines (antihistamines block the action of histamine, a chemical that is released by the body during an
allergic reaction). It is therefore used to treat or prevent
symptoms of allergy.

TREATMENT

To avoid stomach upset, you can take chlorpheniramine
with food or with a full glass of milk or water (unless your
doctor directs you to do otherwise).

   The oral syrup form of chlorpheniramine should be
measured carefully, with a specially designed, 5 ml
measuring spoon. An ordinary kitchen teaspoon is not
accurate enough.

   The sustained-release tablets and capsules should be

swallowed whole. Breaking, chewing, or crushing these forms of the medication destroys the sustained-release activity, and may increase the side effects.

If you miss a dose of this medication, take the missed dose as soon as possible, unless it is close to the time for your next dose. In that case, don't take the missed dose at all; just return to your regular dosing schedule. Do not double the next dose.

SIDE EFFECTS

Minor. Blurred vision; confusion; constipation; diarrhea; difficult or painful urination; dizziness; dry mouth, throat, or nose; headache; irritability; loss of appetite; nausea; restlessness; ringing or buzzing in the ears; rash; stomach upset; and unusual increase in sweating. These side effects should disappear in several days, as your body adjusts to the medication.

If you are constipated, increase the amount of fiber in your diet (raw vegetables, fruits, salads, bran, and whole-grain breads), and drink more water (unless your doctor tells you not to do so).

Chew sugarless gum, or suck on ice chips or a piece of hard candy, to reduce mouth dryness.

This medication can cause increased sensitivity to sunlight. It is therefore important to avoid prolonged exposure to sunlight and sunlamps. Wear protective clothing, and use an effective sunscreen.

If you feel dizzy or light-headed, sit or lie down awhile; get up from a sitting or lying position slowly, and be careful on stairs.

Major. Tell your doctor about any side effects that are persistent or particularly bothersome. IT IS ESPECIALLY IMPORTANT TO TELL YOUR DOCTOR about unusual bleeding or bruising; change in menstruation; clumsiness; feeling faint; flushing of the face; hallucinations; seizures; shortness of breath; sleeping disorders; sore throat or fever; palpitations; tightness in the chest; or unusual tiredness or weakness.

INTERACTIONS

Chlorpheniramine interacts with several other types of medication.

1. Concurrent use of it with other central nervous system depressants (drugs that slow the activity of the nervous system), such as barbiturates, benzodiazepine tranquilizers, muscle relaxants, narcotics, pain medications, phenothiazine tranquilizers, or alcohol, or with tricyclic anti-depressants can cause extreme drowsiness.

2. Monoamine oxidase (MAO) inhibitors (isocarboxazid, pargyline, phenelzine, tranylcypromine) can increase the side effects of this medication.

3. Chlorpheniramine can also decrease the activity of oral anti-coagulants (blood thinners, such as warfarin).

TELL YOUR DOCTOR if you are currently taking any of the medications listed above.

WARNINGS

• Tell your doctor about unusual or allergic reactions you have had to medications, especially to chlorpheniramine or to any other antihistamines (such as bromodiphenhydramine, brompheniramine, carbinoxamine, azatadine, clemastine, cyproheptadine, dexchlorpheniramine, dimenhydrinate, dimethindene, diphenhydramine, diphenylpyraline, doxylamine, hydroxyzine, promethazine, or tripolidine).

• Tell your doctor if you now have, or if you have ever had, asthma, blood vessel disease, glaucoma, high blood pressure, kidney disease, peptic ulcers, enlarged prostate gland, or thyroid disease.

• Chlorpheniramine can cause drowsiness or dizziness. Your ability to perform tasks that require alertness, such as driving a car or operating potentially dangerous machinery, may be decreased. Appropriate caution should therefore be taken.

• Be sure to tell your doctor if you are pregnant. The effects of this medication during pregnancy have not yet been thoroughly studied in humans. Also, tell your doctor if you are breastfeeding an infant. Small amounts of chlorpheniramine pass into breast milk and may cause unusual excitement or irritability in nursing infants.

chlorpheniramine maleate—see chlorpheniramine

chlorpromazine

BRAND NAMES (Manufacturers)
Chloramead (Spencer-Mead)
chlorpromazine hydrochloride (various manufacturers)
Foypromazine (Foy)
Promapar (Parke-Davis)
Thorazine (Smith Kline & French)
Thorazine Spansules (Smith Kline & French)
Thor-Prom (Major)

TYPE OF DRUG
Phenothiazine tranquilizer

INGREDIENT
chlorpromazine as the hydrochloride salt

DOSAGE FORMS
Tablets (10 mg, 25 mg, 50 mg, 100 mg, and 200 mg)
Sustained-release capsules (30 mg, 75 mg, 150 mg, 200 mg, and 300 mg)
Oral concentrate (30 mg per ml and 100 mg per ml)
Oral syrup (10 mg per 5 ml teaspoonful)
Suppositories (25 mg and 100 mg)

STORAGE
The tablet and capsule forms of this medication should be stored at room temperature in tightly closed, light-resistant containers. The oral concentrate, oral syrup, and suppository forms of this medication should be stored in the refrigerator in tightly closed, light-resistant containers. If the oral concentrate or syrup turns to a slight yellow color, the medicine is still effective and can be used. However, if the oral concentrate or syrup change color markedly, or have particles floating in them, they should not be used, but discarded down the sink. Chlorpromazine should never be frozen.

USES
Chlorpromazine is prescribed to treat the symptoms of certain types of mental illness, such as emotional symptoms of psychosis, the manic phase of manic-depressive illness, and severe behavioral problems in children. This medication is thought to relieve the symptoms of mental illness by blocking certain chemicals involved with nerve transmission in the brain.

Chlorpromazine may also be used to treat tetanus, porphyria, uncontrollable hiccups, anxiety before surgery, and nausea and vomiting (this medication works at the vomiting center in the brain to relieve nausea and vomiting).

TREATMENT

In order to avoid stomach irritation, you can take the tablet or capsule forms of this medication with a meal or with a glass of water or milk (unless your doctor directs you to do otherwise).

The sustained-release capsules should be taken whole; do not crush, break, or open them prior to swallowing. Breaking the capsule would release the medication all at once—defeating the purpose of the extended-release capsules.

Measure the oral syrup carefully with a specially designed, 5 ml measuring spoon. An ordinary kitchen teaspoon is not accurate enough.

The oral concentrate form of this medication should be measured carefully with the dropper provided, then added to 4 ounces (½ cup) or more of water, milk, juice, or a carbonated beverage, or to applesauce or pudding, immediately prior to administration. To prevent possible loss of effectiveness, the medication should not be diluted in tea, coffee, or apple juice.

To use the suppository form of this medication, remove the foil wrapper and moisten the suppository with water (if the suppository is too soft to insert, refrigerate it for half an hour or run cold water over it before removing the wrapper). Lie on your left side with your right knee bent. Push the suppository into the rectum, pointed end first. Lie still for a few minutes. Try to avoid having a bowel movement for at least an hour.

If you miss a dose of this medication, take the missed dose as soon as possible, then return to your regular schedule. If it is almost time for the next dose, however, skip the one you missed and return to your regular schedule. Do not double the dose (unless your doctor directs you to do so).

Antacids and diarrhea medicine may decrease the absorption of this medication from the gastrointestinal tract.

Therefore, at least one hour should separate doses of one of these medicines and chlorpromazine.

The full effects of this medication for the control of emotional or mental symptoms may not become apparent for two weeks after starting it.

SIDE EFFECTS

Minor. Blurred vision; constipation; decreased sweating; diarrhea; discoloration of the urine to red, pink, or red-brown; dizziness; drooling; drowsiness; dry mouth; fatigue; jitteriness; menstrual irregularities; nasal congestion; restlessness; tremors; vomiting; and weight gain. As your body adjusts to the medication, these side effects should disappear.

If you are constipated, increase the amount of fiber in your diet (raw vegetables, fruits, salads, bran, and whole-grain breads) and drink more water (unless your doctor directs you to do otherwise).

Chew sugarless gum, or suck on ice chips or a piece of hard candy, to reduce mouth dryness.

This medication can cause increased sensitivity to sunlight. It is therefore important to avoid prolonged exposure to sunlight or sunlamps. Wear protective clothing, and use an effective sunscreen.

To avoid dizziness or light-headedness when you stand, contract and relax the muscles of your legs for a few moments before rising. Do this by pushing one foot against the floor while raising the other foot slightly, alternating feet so that you are "pumping" your legs in a pedaling motion.

Major. Tell your doctor about any side effects that are persistent or particularly bothersome. IT IS ESPECIALLY IMPORTANT TO TELL YOUR DOCTOR about unusual bleeding or bruising; breast enlargement (in both sexes); chest pain; convulsions; darkened skin; difficulty swallowing or breathing; fainting; fever; impotence; involuntary movements of the face, mouth, jaw, or tongue; palpitations; rash; sleep disorders; sore throat; uncoordinated movements; visual disturbances; or yellowing of the eyes or skin.

INTERACTIONS

Chlorpromazine interacts with several other types of medication.

1. It can cause extreme drowsiness when combined with alcohol or other central nervous system depressants (drugs that slow the activity of the nervous system), such as barbiturates, benzodiazepine tranquilizers, muscle relaxants, narcotics, or pain medication, or with tricyclic anti-depressants.

2. Chlorpromazine can decrease the effectiveness of amphetamines, guanethidine, anti-convulsants, and levodopa.

3. The side effects of epinephrine, monoamine oxidase (MAO) inhibitors, propranolol, phenytoin, and tricyclic anti-depressants may be increased when combined with this medication.

4. Lithium may increase the side effects and decrease the effectiveness of this medication.

Before starting to take chlorpromazine, BE SURE TO TELL YOUR DOCTOR if you are already taking any of the medications listed above.

WARNINGS

• Tell your doctor about unusual or allergic reactions you have had to medications, especially to chlorpromazine or any other phenothiazine tranquilizers (such as acetophenazine, carphenazine, fluphenazine, mesoridazine, perphenazine, piperacetazine, prochlorperazine, promazine, thioridazine, trifluoperazine, triflupromazine), or to loxapine.

• Tell your doctor if you now have, or if you have ever had, any blood disease, bone marrow disease, brain disease, breast cancer, blockage in the urinary or digestive tract, alcoholism, drug-induced depression, epilepsy, severe high or low blood pressure, diabetes mellitus (sugar diabetes), glaucoma, heart or circulatory disease, liver disease, lung disease, Parkinson's disease, peptic ulcer disease, or an enlarged prostate gland.

• Tell your doctor about any recent exposure to a pesticide or an insecticide. Chlorpromazine may increase the side effects from the exposure.

• To prevent over-sedation, avoid drinking alcoholic

beverages while taking this medication.

- If this medication makes you dizzy or drowsy, do not take part in any activity that requires alertness, such as driving a car or operating potentially dangerous equipment. Be careful on stairs, and avoid getting up suddenly from a lying or sitting position.
- Before having any surgery or other medical or dental treatment, be sure to tell your doctor or dentist that you are taking this medication.
- Some of the side effects caused by this drug can be prevented by taking an anti-parkinson drug. Discuss this with your doctor.
- Chlorpromazine has been reported to cause certain tumors in rats. This effect has not been shown to occur in humans.
- This medication can decrease sweating and heat release from the body. You should therefore avoid getting overheated by strenuous exercise in hot weather, and should avoid hot baths, showers, and saunas.
- Do not stop taking this medication suddenly. If the drug is stopped abruptly you may experience nausea, vomiting, stomach upset, headache, increased heart rate, insomnia, tremulousness, or a worsening of your condition. Your doctor may want to reduce the dosage gradually.
- If you are planning to have a myelogram, or any procedure in which dye will be injected into your spinal cord, tell your doctor that you are taking this medication.
- Avoid spilling the oral concentrate or oral syrup forms of this medication on your skin or clothing; they may cause redness and irritation of the skin.
- While taking this medication, do not take any over-the-counter (non-prescription) medication for weight control, or for cough, cold, allergy, asthma, or sinus problems, without first checking with your doctor. The combination of these medications with chlorpromazine may cause high blood pressure.
- Be sure to tell your doctor if you are pregnant. Small amounts of this medication cross the placenta. Although there are reports of safe use of this drug during pregnancy, there are also reports of liver disease and tremors in newborn infants whose mothers received this medication close to term. Also, tell your doctor if you are breastfeed-

ing an infant. Small amounts of this medication pass into breast milk and may cause unwanted effects in the nursing infant.

chlorpromazine hydrochloride—see chlorpromazine

---

chlorpropamide

BRAND NAMES (Manufacturers)
chlorpropamide (various manufacturers)
Diabinese (Pfizer)
TYPE OF DRUG
Oral anti-diabetic
INGREDIENT
chlorpropamide
DOSAGE FORM
Tablets (250 mg and 500 mg)
STORAGE
This medication should be stored at room temperature in a tightly closed container.

USES

Chlorpropamide is used for the treatment of diabetes mellitus (sugar diabetes) that appears in adulthood and cannot be managed by control of diet alone. This type of diabetes is known as noninsulin-dependent diabetes (sometimes called maturity-onset or Type II diabetes). Chlorpropamide lowers blood sugar by increasing the release of insulin from the pancreas.

TREATMENT

In order for this medication to work correctly, it must be taken as directed by your doctor. It is best to take this medicine at the same time each day, in order to maintain a constant blood sugar level. It is important therefore to try not to miss any doses of this medication. If you do miss a dose, take it as soon as possible, unless it is almost time for the next dose. In that case, do not take the missed dose at all; just return to your regular dosing schedule. Do not double the next dose. Tell your doctor if you feel any side effects from missing a dose of this drug.

Diabetics who are taking oral anti-diabetic medication may need to be switched to insulin if they develop diabetic coma, have a severe infection, are scheduled for major surgery, or become pregnant.

SIDE EFFECTS

Minor. Diarrhea; headache; heartburn; loss of appetite; nausea; vomiting; stomach pain; or stomach discomfort. These side effects usually disappear during treatment, as your body adjusts to the medication.

Major. If any side effects are persistent or particularly bothersome, it is important to notify your doctor. IT IS ESPECIALLY IMPORTANT TO TELL YOUR DOCTOR about dark urine; fatigue; itching of the skin; light-colored stools; sore throat and fever; unusual bleeding or bruising; or yellowing of the eyes or skin.

Chlorpropamide can also cause retention of body water, which in turn can lead to drowsiness; muscle cramps; seizures; swelling or puffiness of the face, hands, or ankles; and tiredness or weakness. IT IS IMPORTANT TO TELL YOUR DOCTOR if you notice any of these side effects.

INTERACTIONS

Chlorpropamide interacts with a number of other medications.

1. Chloramphenicol; guanethidine; insulin; monoamine oxidase (MAO) inhibitors; oxyphenbutazone; oxytetracycline; phenylbutazone; probenecid; aspirin or other salicylates; or sulfonamide antibiotics, when combined with chlorpropamide, can lower blood sugar levels —sometimes to dangerously low levels.

2. Thyroid hormones; dextrothyroxine; epinephrine; phenytoin; thiazide diuretics (water pills); or cortisone-like medications (such as dexamethasone, hydrocortisone, or prednisone), when combined with chlorpropamide, can actually increase blood sugar levels—just what you are trying to avoid.

3. Anti-diabetic medications can increase the effects of anti-coagulants (blood thinners, such as warfarin), which can lead to bleeding complications.

4. Beta-blocking medications (such as atenolol, metoprolol, nadolol, pindolol, propranolol, and timolol), combined with chlorpropamide, can result in either high or low blood sugar levels. Beta-blockers can also mask the symptoms of low blood sugar, which can be dangerous.

5. Avoid drinking alcoholic beverages while taking this medication (unless otherwise directed by your doctor). Some patients who take this medicine suffer nausea; vomiting; dizziness; stomach pain; pounding headache; sweating; and redness of the face and skin when they drink alcohol. Also, large amounts of alcohol can lower blood sugar to dangerously low levels.

BE SURE TO TELL YOUR DOCTOR if you are already taking any of the medications listed above.

WARNINGS

• It is important to tell your doctor if you have ever had unusual or allergic reactions to this medicine or to any sulfa medication [sulfonamide antibiotics, diuretics (water pills), or other oral anti-diabetics].

• Tell your doctor if you now have, or if you have ever had, kidney disease, liver disease, severe infection, or thyroid disease.

• It is important to follow the special diet that your doctor gave you. This is an essential part of controlling your blood sugar and is necessary in order for this medicine to work properly.

• Before having any kind of surgery or other medical or dental treatment, be sure to tell your doctor or dentist that you are taking this medicine.

• Test for sugar in your urine as directed by your doctor. It is a convenient way to determine whether or not your diabetes is being controlled by this medicine.

• Chlorpropamide may increase your sensitivity to sunlight. It is therefore important to use caution during exposure to the sun. You may want to wear protective clothing and sunglasses. Use an effective sunscreen, and avoid exposure to sunlamps.

• Eat or drink something containing sugar right away if you experience any symptoms of low blood sugar (such as anxiety; chills; cold sweats; cool or pale skin; drowsiness; excessive hunger; headache; nausea; nervousness;

rapid heartbeat; shakiness or unusual tiredness or weakness). It is important that your family and friends know the symptoms of low blood sugar and what to do if they observe any of these symptoms in you.

Check with your doctor as soon as possible—even if these symptoms are corrected by the sugar. The blood-sugar-lowering effects of this medicine can last for hours, and the symptoms may return during this period. Good sources of sugar are orange juice, corn syrup, honey, sugar cubes, and table sugar. You are at greatest risk of developing low blood sugar if you skip or delay meals, exercise more than usual, cannot eat because of nausea or vomiting, or drink large amounts of alcohol.

• Be sure to tell your doctor if you are pregnant. Studies in animals have shown that this medicine can cause birth defects. Studies have not yet been completed in humans. It is also important to tell your doctor if you are breastfeeding an infant. Although this medicine has not been shown to cause problems in breast-fed infants, small amounts may pass into breast milk.

---

chlorprothixene

BRAND NAME (Manufacturer)
Taractan (Roche)
TYPE OF DRUG
Anti-psychotic
INGREDIENT
chlorprothixene
DOSAGE FORMS
Tablets (10 mg, 25 mg, 50 mg, and 100 mg)
Oral suspension (100 mg per 5 ml teaspoonful)
STORAGE
Chlorprothixene tablets and oral suspension should be stored at room temperature in tightly closed, light-resistant containers. This medication should never be frozen.

USES

Chlorprothixene is prescribed to treat the symptoms of

certain types of mental illness, such as emotional symptoms of psychosis. This medication is thought to relieve the symptoms of mental illness by blocking certain chemicals involved with nerve transmission in the brain.

TREATMENT

To avoid stomach irritation, you can take the tablet form of this medication with a meal or with a glass of water or milk (unless your doctor directs you to do otherwise).

Measure the oral suspension carefully, with a specially designed, 5 ml measuring spoon. An ordinary kitchen spoon is not accurate enough.

If you miss a dose of this medication, take the missed dose as soon as possible and return to your regular schedule. If it is within two hours of your next dose, however, skip the dose you missed and return to your regular schedule. Do not double the dose (unless your doctor directs you to do so).

Antacids and diarrhea medicine may decrease the absorption of this medication from the gastrointestinal tract. Therefore, at least one hour should separate doses of chlorprothixene and one of these medicines.

The full effects of this medication for the control of emotional or mental symptoms may not become apparent for two weeks after starting to take it.

SIDE EFFECTS

Minor. Blurred vision; constipation; decreased sweating; diarrhea; discoloration of the urine to red, pink, or red brown; dizziness; drooling; drowsiness; dry mouth; fatigue; jitteriness; menstrual irregularities; nasal congestion; restlessness; tremors; vomiting; and weight gain. As your body adjusts to the medication, these side effects should disappear.

If you are constipated, increase the amount of fiber in your diet (raw vegetables, fruits, salads, bran, and whole-grain breads) and drink more water (unless your doctor directs you to do otherwise).

Chew sugarless gum, or suck on ice chips or a piece of hard candy, to reduce mouth dryness.

This medication can cause increased sensitivity to sunlight. It is therefore important to avoid prolonged exposure to sunlight and sunlamps. Wear protective clothing, and use an effective sunscreen.

To avoid dizziness or light-headedness when you stand, contract and relax the muscles of your legs for a few moments before rising. Do this by pushing one foot against the floor while raising the other foot slightly, alternating feet so that you are "pumping" your legs in a pedaling motion.

Major. Tell your doctor about any side effects that are persistent or particularly bothersome. IT IS ESPECIALLY IMPORTANT TO TELL YOUR DOCTOR about unusual bleeding or bruising; breast enlargement (in both sexes); chest pain; convulsions; darkened skin; difficulty swallowing or breathing; fainting; fever; impotence; involuntary movements of the face, mouth, jaw, or tongue; palpitations; rash; sleep disorders; sore throat; uncoordinated movements; visual disturbances; or yellowing of the eyes or skin.

INTERACTIONS

Chlorprothixene interacts with several other types of medication.

1. It can cause extreme drowsiness when combined with alcohol or other central nervous system depressants (drugs that slow the activity of the nervous system), such as barbiturates, benzodiazepine tranquilizers, muscle relaxants, narcotics, or pain medication, or with tricyclic anti-depressants.

2. This medication can decrease the effectiveness of amphetamines, guanethidine, anti-convulsants, and levodopa.

3. The side effects of epinephrine, monoamine oxidase (MAO) inhibitors, and tricyclic anti-depressants may be increased when combined with this medication.

4. Lithium may increase the side effects and decrease the effectiveness of this medication.

Before starting to take chlorprothixene, BE SURE TO TELL YOUR DOCTOR if you are taking any of the medications listed above.

WARNINGS

• Tell your doctor about unusual or allergic reactions you

have had to medications, especially to chlorprothixene, thiothixene, or any phenothiazine tranquilizer.

• Tell your doctor if you now have, or if you have ever had, blood disease; bone marrow disease; brain disease; breast cancer; blockage in the urinary or digestive tract; alcoholism; drug-induced depression; epilepsy; severe high or low blood pressure; diabetes mellitus (sugar diabetes); glaucoma; heart or circulatory disease; liver disease; lung disease; Parkinson's disease; peptic ulcers; or an enlarged prostate gland.

• Avoid drinking alcoholic beverages while taking this medication, in order to prevent over-sedation.

• If this medication makes you dizzy or drowsy, do not take part in any activity that requires alertness, such as driving a car or operating potentially dangerous equipment. Be careful on stairs, and avoid getting up suddenly from a lying or sitting position.

• Prior to having surgery or other medical or dental treatment, be sure your doctor or dentist knows that you are taking this medication.

• Some of the side effects caused by this drug can be prevented by taking an anti parkinson drug. Discuss this with your doctor.

• This drug has been reported to cause certain tumors in rats. This effect has not been shown to occur in humans.

• Chlorprothixene can decrease sweating and heat release from the body. You should therefore avoid getting overheated by strenuous exercise in hot weather, and should avoid taking hot baths, showers, and saunas.

• Do not stop taking this medication suddenly. If the drug is stopped abruptly you may experience nausea; vomiting; stomach upset; headache; increased heart rate; insomnia; tremulousness; or a worsening of your condition. Your doctor may want to reduce the dosage gradually.

• If you are planning to have a myelogram, or any procedure in which dye will be injected into your spinal cord, tell your doctor that you are taking this medication.

• Avoid spilling the oral suspension form of this medication on your skin or clothing; it can cause redness and irritation of the skin.

• While taking this medication, do not take any over-the-counter (non-prescription) medication for weight control, or for cough, cold, allergy, asthma, or sinus problems, without first checking with your doctor. The combination of these medications with chlorprothixene may cause high blood pressure.

• Be sure to tell your doctor if you are pregnant. Small amounts of this medication can cross the placenta. Although there are reports of safe use of this drug during pregnancy, there are also reports of liver disease and tremors in newborn infants whose mothers received this type of medication close to term. Also, tell your doctor if you are breastfeeding an infant. Small amounts of this medication pass into breast milk and may cause unwanted effects in the nursing infant.

Chlorspan—see chlorpheniramine

Chlortab—see chlorpheniramine

---

chlorthalidone

BRAND NAMES (Manufacturers)
chlorthalidone (various manufacturers)
Hygroton (USV)
Hylidone (Major)
Thalitone (Boehringer Ingelheim)
TYPE OF DRUG
Diuretic (water pill) and anti-hypertensive
INGREDIENT
chlorthalidone
DOSAGE FORM
Tablets (25 mg, 50 mg, and 100 mg)
STORAGE
This medication should be stored at room temperature in a tightly closed container.

USES

Chlorthalidone is prescribed to treat high blood pressure. It is also used to reduce fluid accumulation in the body caused by conditions such as heart failure, cirrhosis of the liver, kidney disease, and the long-term use of some medications. This medication reduces fluid accumulation by increasing the elimination of sodium and water through the kidneys.

TREATMENT

To decrease stomach irritation, you can take this medication with a glass of milk or with a meal (unless your doctor directs you to do otherwise). Try to take it at the same time every day. Avoid taking a dose after 6:00 P.M.—this will prevent you from having to get up during the night to urinate.

If you miss a dose of this medication, take the missed dose as soon as possible, unless it is almost time for the next dose. In that case, do not take the missed dose at all, just wait until the next scheduled dose. Do not double the dose.

This medication does not cure high blood pressure, but it will help to control the condition, as long as you continue to take it.

SIDE EFFECTS

Minor. Constipation; cramps; diarrhea; dizziness; drowsiness; headache; heartburn; itching; loss of appetite; nausea; restlessness; upset stomach; vomiting. As your body adjusts to the medication, these side effects should disappear.

This medication can cause increased sensitivity to sunlight. It is therefore important to avoid prolonged exposure to sunlight or sunlamps. Wear protective clothing, and use an effective sunscreen.

To avoid dizziness or light-headedness when you stand, contract and relax the muscles of your legs for a few moments before rising. Do this by pushing one foot against the floor while raising the other foot slightly, alternating the feet so that you are "pumping" your legs in a pedaling motion.

Major. Tell your doctor about any side effects that are persistent or particularly bothersome. IT IS ESPECIALLY IMPORTANT TO TELL YOUR DOCTOR about any unusual bleeding or bruising; blurred vision; confusion; difficulty breathing; dry mouth; fever; joint pain; mood changes; muscle spasms; palpitations; skin rash; excessive thirst; sore throat; tingling in the fingers or toes; excessive weakness; or yellowing of the eyes or skin.

INTERACTIONS

Chlorthalidone interacts with several other types of medication.

1. It may decrease the effectiveness of oral anticoagulants, anti-gout medications, insulin, oral anti-diabetic medicines, and methenamine.

2. Fenfluramine can increase the blood-pressure-lowering effects of chlorthalidone (which can be dangerous).

3. Indomethacin can decrease the blood-pressure-lowering effects (thereby counteracting the desired effects) of chlorthalidone.

4. Cholestyramine and colestipol decrease the absorption of this medication from the gastrointestinal tract. Chlorthalidone should therefore be taken one hour before, or four hours after, a dose of cholestyramine or colestipol (if you have also been prescribed one of these medications).

5. The side effects of amphotericin B, calcium, cortisone-like steroids (such as cortisone, dexamethasone, hydrocortisone, prednisone, prednisolone), digoxin, digitalis, lithium, quinidine, sulfonamide antibiotics, and vitamin D may be increased when taken concurrently with chlorthalidone.

BE SURE TO TELL YOUR DOCTOR if you are already taking any of the medicines listed above.

WARNINGS

• Tell your doctor about unusual or allergic reactions you have had to any medications, especially to diuretics (water pills), oral anti-diabetic medications, or sulfonamide antibiotics.

• Before you start taking chlorthalidone, tell your doctor if you now have, or if you have ever had, kidney disease or problems with urination, diabetes mellitus (sugar diabetes), gout, liver disease, asthma, pancreas disease, or systemic lupus erythematosus (SLE).

• Chlorthalidone can cause potassium loss. Signs of potassium loss include dry mouth, thirst, weakness, muscle pain or cramps, nausea, and vomiting. If you experience any of these symptoms, call your doctor. To help avoid potassium loss, take this drug with a glass of fresh or frozen orange or cranberry juice, or eat a banana every day. The use of a salt substitute also helps to prevent potassium loss. Do not change your diet, however, before discussing it with your doctor. Too much potassium can also be dangerous. Your doctor may want you to have blood tests performed periodically, in order to monitor your potassium levels.

• Limit your intake of alcoholic beverages while taking this medication, in order to prevent dizziness and light-headedness.

• If you have high blood pressure, do not take any over-the-counter (non-prescription) medications for weight control or for cough, cold, allergy, asthma, or sinus problems, unless your doctor directs you to do so.

• To prevent dehydration (severe water loss) while taking this medication, check with your doctor if you have any illness that causes severe or continuous nausea, vomiting, or diarrhea.

• This medication can raise blood sugar levels in diabetic patients. Therefore, blood sugar should be carefully monitored by blood or urine tests when this medication is started.

• Be sure to tell your doctor if you are pregnant. Although studies in humans have not been completed, adverse effects have been observed on animals whose mothers were given large doses of this drug during pregnancy. Also, tell your doctor if you are breastfeeding an infant. Although problems in humans have not been reported, small amounts of this drug can pass into breast milk, so caution is warranted.

Chlorzide—see hydrochlorothiazide

Chlorzone Forte—see chlorzoxazone and acetaminophen combination

chlorzoxazone and acetaminophen combination

BRAND NAMES (Manufacturers)
Chlorofon-F (Rugby)
Chlorzone Forte (Schein)
chlorzoxazone and acetaminophen
  (various manufacturers)
Paracet Forte (Major)
Parafon Forte (McNeil)
Polyflex (Holloway)
Tuzon (Tutag)
Zoxaphen (Mallard)
TYPE OF DRUG
Muscle relaxant and analgesic (pain reliever)
INGREDIENTS
chlorzoxazone and acetaminophen
DOSAGE FORM
Tablets (250 mg chlorzoxazone and
  300 mg acetaminophen)
STORAGE
Chlorzoxazone and acetaminophen tablets should be stored at room temperature in a tightly closed container.

USES

Chlorzoxazone and acetaminophen is used to relax muscles and to relieve the pain of sprains, strains, and other muscle injuries. Chlorzoxazone acts as a central nervous system (brain and spinal cord) depressant, which blocks reflexes involved in producing and maintaining muscle spasms. It does not act directly on tense muscles.

TREATMENT

These tablets should be taken with a full glass of water. In order to avoid stomach irritation, you can also take this medication with food or milk (unless your doctor directs you to do otherwise).

If you miss a dose of this medication, take the missed dose as soon as possible, unless it is within three hours of your next scheduled dose. In that case, don't take the missed dose at all; just return to your regular dosing schedule. Do not double the next dose.

SIDE EFFECTS

Minor. Constipation; diarrhea; dizziness; drowsiness; fatigue; headache; heartburn; light-headedness; nausea; nervousness; overstimulation; stomach cramps; and vomiting. These side effects should disappear in several days, as your body adjusts to the medication.

If you are constipated, increase the amount of fiber in your diet (fresh fruits and vegetables, salads, bran, and whole-grain breads), and drink more water (unless your doctor directs you to do otherwise).

If you feel dizzy or light-headed, sit or lie down awhile; get up slowly, and be careful on stairs.

Chlorzoxazone can cause your urine to become orange or reddish-purple in color. This is a harmless effect that will disappear when you stop taking the drug.

Major. Tell your doctor about any side effects that are persistent or particularly bothersome. IT IS ESPECIALLY IMPORTANT TO TELL YOUR DOCTOR about bloody or black, tarry stools; unusual bleeding or bruising; difficulty urinating; fever; rash; sore throat; severe abdominal pain; unusual weakness; or yellowing of the eyes or skin.

INTERACTIONS

Chlorzoxazone and acetaminophen interacts with several other types of medications.

1. Concurrent use of chlorzoxazone with other central nervous system depressants (drugs that slow the activity of the nervous system), such as alcohol, antihistamines, barbiturates, benzodiazepine tranquilizers, pain medications, narcotics, phenothiazine tranquilizers, and sleeping medications, or with tricyclic anti-depressants can cause extreme drowsiness.

2. Alcohol, barbiturates, and anti-convulsants can increase the liver toxicity of large doses of acetaminophen.

3. Long-term use of large doses of acetaminophen can increase the effects of oral anti-coagulants (blood thinners, such as warfarin), which can lead to bleeding complications.

Before starting to take this medication, BE SURE TO TELL YOUR DOCTOR if you are already taking any of the medications listed above.

WARNINGS

- Tell your doctor about unusual or allergic reactions you have had to any medications, especially to chlorzoxazone or to acetaminophen.
- Tell your doctor if you now have, or if you have ever had, blood disorders, or heart, kidney, liver, or lung disease.
- If this medication makes you dizzy or drowsy, or blurs your vision, do not take part in any activity that requires alertness, such as driving a car or operating potentially dangerous equipment.
- This medication should not be taken as a substitute for rest, physical therapy, or other measures recommended by your doctor to treat your condition.
- Because this product contains acetaminophen, additional medications that contain acetaminophen should not be taken without your doctor's approval. Check the labels on over-the-counter (non-prescription) pain, sinus, allergy, asthma, diet, cough, and cold products to see if they contain acetaminophen.
- Be sure to tell your doctor if you are pregnant. Although this drug appears to be safe during pregnancy, extensive studies have not yet been completed. Also, tell your doctor if you are breastfeeding an infant. Small amounts of acetaminophen pass into breast milk. It is not known whether or not chlorzoxazone passes into the milk.

Choledyl—see oxtriphylline

Choledyl SA—see oxtriphylline

---

cholestyramine

BRAND NAME (Manufacturer)
Questran (Mead Johnson)

TYPE OF DRUG
Anti-hyperlipidemic (lipid-lowering drug)
INGREDIENT
cholestyramine
DOSAGE FORM
Oral powder (4 grams of cholestyramine per 9 grams of
    powder)
STORAGE
Cholestyramine should be stored at room temperature in
a tightly closed container.

USES

This medication is used to lower blood cholesterol and
to treat itching associated with liver disease. Cholestyramine chemically binds to bile salts in the gastrointestinal
tract and prevents the body from producing cholesterol.

TREATMENT

Cholestyramine is usually taken before meals. Each dose
should be measured carefully, then placed on the surface
of 2 to 6 ounces of a beverage (water, milk, fruit juice, or
other non-carbonated beverage). The powder should be
allowed to sit for one to two minutes without stirring (to
prevent lumpiness). The mixture should then be stirred
and completely mixed (the powder does not completely
dissolve). After the solution is drunk, the glass should be
refilled with the same beverage and this solution swallowed as well (this assures that the whole dose is taken).
The powder can also be mixed with soup, applesauce, or
crushed pineapple. You should never take cholestyramine dry; you might accidentally inhale the powder
which could irritate your throat and lungs.

Cholestyramine does not cure hypercholesterolemia
(high blood cholesterol levels), but it will help to control
the condition, as long as you continue to take it.

If you miss a dose of this medication, take the missed
dose as soon as possible, unless it is almost time for the
next dose. In that case, do not take the missed dose at all;
just return to your regular dosing schedule. Do not double
the next dose.

SIDE EFFECTS

Minor. Anxiety; belching; constipation; diarrhea; dizziness; drowsiness; fatigue; gas; headache; hiccups; loss of appetite; nausea; stomach pain; vomiting; weight loss or gain. These side effects should disappear in several weeks, as your body adjusts to the medication.

To relieve constipation, increase the amount of fiber in your diet (bran, salads, fresh fruits and vegetables, and whole-grain breads), exercise, and drink more water (unless your doctor directs you to do otherwise).

If you feel dizzy, sit or lie down awhile; get up slowly, and be careful on stairs.

Major. Tell your doctor about any side effects that are persistent or particularly bothersome. IT IS ESPECIALLY IMPORTANT TO TELL YOUR DOCTOR about unusual bleeding or bruising; bloody or black, tarry stools; backaches; difficult or painful urination; fluid retention; muscle or joint pains; rash or irritation of the skin, tongue, or rectal area; ringing in the ears; swollen glands; tingling sensations; or unusual weakness.

INTERACTIONS

Cholestyramine interferes with the absorption of a number of other drugs, including phenylbutazone, warfarin, thiazide diuretics (water pills), digoxin, penicillins, tetracycline, phenobarbital, folic acid, iron, thyroid hormones, cephalexin, clindamycin, trimethoprim, and fat-soluble vitamins (A, D, E, and K). The effectiveness of these medications will be decreased by cholestyramine. To avoid this interaction, take the other medications one hour before, or four to six hours after, a dose of cholestyramine.

BE SURE TO TELL YOUR DOCTOR if you are already taking any of these medications.

WARNINGS

• Tell your doctor about unusual or allergic reactions you have had to any medications, especially to cholestyramine.

• Tell your doctor if you now have, or if you have ever had, bleeding disorders; biliary obstruction; heart disease; hemorrhoids; gallstones or gallbladder disease;

kidney disease; malabsorption; stomach ulcers; or an obstructed intestine.

• Cholestyramine should be used only in conjunction with diet, weight reduction, or correction of other conditions that could be causing high blood cholesterol levels.

• This product contains F.D. & C. Yellow Dye No. 5 (tartrazine), which can cause allergic-type symptoms (fainting, rash, shortness of breath) in certain susceptible individuals

• The color of cholestyramine powder may vary from batch to batch. This does not affect the effectiveness of the medication.

• Be sure to tell your doctor if you are pregnant. Although cholestyramine appears to be safe (because very little is absorbed into the bloodstream), extensive studies in humans during pregnancy have not yet been completed. Also, tell your doctor if you are breastfeeding an infant. It is not known whether or not cholestyramine passes into breast milk.

Cibalith-S—see lithium

---

cimetidine

BRAND NAME (Manufacturer)
Tagamet (Smith Kline & French)
TYPE OF DRUG
Gastric acid secretion inhibitor (decreases stomach acid)
INGREDIENT
cimetidine
DOSAGE FORMS
Tablets (200 mg, 300 mg, and 400 mg)
Oral liquid (300 mg per 5 ml teaspoonful)
STORAGE
Cimetidine tablets and oral liquid should be stored at room temperature in tightly closed, light-resistant containers. This medication should never be frozen.

USES
Cimetidine is used to treat duodenal and gastric ulcers. It is also used in the long-term treatment of excessive

stomach acid secretion, and in the prevention of recurrent ulcers. Cimetidine works by blocking the effects of histamine in the stomach, which reduces stomach acid secretion.

TREATMENT

In order to obtain the maximum effect, cimetidine should be taken with, or shortly after, meals, and again at bedtime.

The tablets should not be crushed or chewed, because cimetidine has a bitter taste and an unpleasant odor.

The oral liquid should be measured carefully, with a specially designed, 5 ml measuring spoon. An ordinary kitchen teaspoon is not accurate enough.

Antacids can block the absorption of cimetidine. If you are taking antacids as well as cimetidine, at least one hour should separate doses of the two medications.

If you miss a dose of cimetidine, take the missed dose as soon as possible, unless it is almost time for the next dose. In that case, do not take the missed dose at all; just return to your regular dosing schedule. Do not double the next dose.

SIDE EFFECTS

Minor. Diarrhea; drowsiness; dizziness; headache; and muscle pain. These side effects should disappear in several days, as your body adjusts to the medication.

If you feel dizzy, sit or lie down awhile; get up slowly, and be careful on stairs.

Major. Tell your doctor about any side effects that are persistent or particularly bothersome. IT IS ESPECIALLY IMPORTANT TO TELL YOUR DOCTOR about unusual bleeding or bruising; confusion; fever; hair loss; enlarged or painful breasts (in both sexes); hallucinations; impotence; palpitations; rash; sore throat; weakness; or yellowing of the eyes or skin.

INTERACTIONS

Cimetidine interacts with several other types of medication.

1. It can decrease the elimination from the body, and increase the side effects, of theophylline; aminophylline; oxtriphylline; phenytoin; carbamazepine; beta-blockers; benzodiazepine tranquilizers (such as clorazepate, chlordiazepoxide, diazepam, flurazepam, halazepam, and prazepam); oral anti-coagulants (blood thinners, such as warfarin); lidocaine; and morphine.

2. The combination of cimetidine and anti-neoplastic agents (anti-cancer drugs) may increase the risk of blood disorders.

3. The absorption of ketoconazole is decreased by cimetidine; at least two hours should separate doses of these two medications.

4. Cimetidine may decrease the blood levels and effectiveness of digoxin.

Before starting to take this medication, BE SURE TO TELL YOUR DOCTOR if you are already taking any of the medications listed above.

WARNINGS

● Tell your doctor about any unusual or allergic reactions you have had to medications, especially to cimetidine.

● Tell your doctor if you now have, or if you have ever had, arthritis, kidney disease, liver disease, or organic brain syndrome.

● Cimetidine should be taken continuously for as long as your doctor prescribes. Stopping therapy early may be a cause of ineffective treatment.

● Cigarette smoking may block the beneficial effects of cimetidine.

● If this drug makes you dizzy or drowsy, do not take part in any activity that requires alertness, such as driving a car or operating potentially dangerous equipment.

● Be sure to tell your doctor if you are pregnant. Cimetidine appears to be safe during pregnancy; however, extensive testing has not yet been completed. Also, tell your doctor if you are breastfeeding an infant. Small amounts of cimetidine pass into breast milk.

Cinobac—see cinoxacin

cinoxacin

BRAND NAME (Manufacturer)
Cinobac (Dista)
TYPE OF DRUG
Antibiotic (infection fighter)
INGREDIENT
cinoxacin
DOSAGE FORM
Capsules (250 mg and 500 mg)
STORAGE
Cinoxacin capsules should be stored at room temperature, in a tightly closed container.

USES

Cinoxacin is an antibiotic that is used to treat bacterial urinary tract infections. It chemically attaches to the bacteria, preventing their growth and multiplication. It kills susceptible bacteria, but is not effective against viruses, parasites, or fungi.

TREATMENT

In order to prevent stomach irritation, you can take cinoxacin with food or with a full glass of water or milk (unless your doctor directs you to do otherwise).

Cinoxacin works best when the level of the medicine in your urine is kept constant. It is best therefore to take the doses at evenly spaced intervals, day and night. For example, if you are to take four doses a day, the doses should be spaced six hours apart.

Try not to miss any doses of this medication. If you do miss a dose, take it as soon as you remember. However, if you do not remember to take the missed dose until it is almost time for your next dose, take the missed dose immediately. Space the following dose about halfway through the regular interval between doses; then continue with your regular dosing schedule.

It is important to continue to take this medication for the entire time prescribed by your doctor (usually seven to 14 days), even if the symptoms disappear before the end of that period. If you stop taking the drug too soon, resistant bacteria are given a chance to continue growing, and your infection could recur.

SIDE EFFECTS

Minor. Abdominal cramps; diarrhea; dizziness; headache; insomnia; loss of appetite; nausea; nervousness; rectal itching; and increased sensitivity of the eyes to light. These side effects should disappear in several days, as your body adjusts to the medication.

To relieve the increased sensitivity of your eyes to light, avoid prolonged exposure to sunlight and bright lights; and wear sunglasses.

Major. Tell your doctor about any side effects that are persistent or particularly bothersome. IT IS ESPECIALLY IMPORTANT TO TELL YOUR DOCTOR about confusion; itching; rapid weight gain (three to five pounds within a week); ringing in the ears; skin rash; tingling sensations; visual disturbances; or yellowing of the eyes or skin.

INTERACTIONS

Probenecid blocks the excretion of cinoxacin into the urinary tract, decreasing its effectiveness. BE SURE TO TELL YOUR DOCTOR if you are already taking probenecid.

WARNINGS

• Tell your doctor about unusual or allergic reactions you have had to any medications, especially to cinoxacin or nalidixic acid.

• Tell your doctor if you now have, or if you have ever had, kidney disease or liver disease.

• If this drug makes you dizzy, do not take part in activities that require alertness, such as driving a car or operating potentially dangerous equipment.

• Be sure to tell your doctor if you are pregnant. Although cinoxacin appears to be safe during pregnancy, extensive studies in humans have not yet been completed. Also, tell your doctor if you are breastfeeding an infant. It is not known whether or not cinoxacin passes into breast milk.

Cin-Quin—see quinidine

Circanol—see ergoloid mesylates

---

clemastine

BRAND NAMES (Manufacturers)
Tavist (Sandoz)
Tavist-1 (Sandoz)
TYPE OF DRUG
Antihistamine
INGREDIENT
clemastine as the fumarate salt
DOSAGE FORM
Tablets (1 mg and 2 mg)
STORAGE
Clemastine should be stored at room temperature in a tightly closed container.

USES

This medication belongs to a group of drugs known as antihistamines (antihistamines block the action of histamine, a chemical that is released by the body during an allergic reaction). It is therefore used to treat or prevent symptoms of allergy.

TREATMENT

To avoid stomach upset, you can take clemastine with food or with a full glass of milk or water (unless your doctor directs you to do otherwise).

If you miss a dose of this medication, take the missed dose as soon as possible, unless it is close to the time for your next dose. In that case, don't take the missed dose at all; just return to your regular dosing schedule. Do not double the next dose.

SIDE EFFECTS

Minor. Blurred vision; confusion; constipation; diarrhea; difficult or painful urination; dizziness; dry mouth, throat, or nose; headache; irritability; loss of appetite; nausea; restlessness; ringing or buzzing in the ears; rash; stomach upset; and unusual increase in sweating. These side effects should disappear in several days, as your body adjusts to the medication.

If you are constipated, increase the amount of fiber in your diet (raw vegetables, fruits, salads, bran, and whole-grain breads), and drink more water (unless your doctor tells you not to do so).

Chew sugarless gum, or suck on ice chips or a piece of hard candy, to reduce mouth dryness.

This medication can cause increased sensitivity to sunlight. It is therefore important to avoid prolonged exposure to sunlight and sunlamps. Wear protective clothing, and use an effective sunscreen.

If you feel dizzy or light-headed, sit or lie down awhile; get up from a sitting or lying position slowly, and be careful on stairs.

Major. Tell your doctor about any side effects that are persistent or particularly bothersome. IT IS ESPECIALLY IMPORTANT TO TELL YOUR DOCTOR about unusual bleeding or bruising; change in menstruation; clumsiness; feeling faint; flushing of the face; hallucinations; seizures; shortness of breath; sleeping disorders; sore throat or fever; palpitations; tightness in the chest; or unusual tiredness or weakness.

INTERACTIONS

Clemastine interacts with several other types of medication.

1. Concurrent use of it with central nervous system depressants (drugs that slow the activity of the nervous system), such as barbiturates, benzodiazepine tranquilizers, muscle relaxants, narcotics, pain medications, phenothiazine tranquilizers, and alcohol, or with tricyclic antidepressants can cause extreme drowsiness.

2. Monoamine oxidase (MAO) inhibitors (isocarboxazid, pargyline, phenelzine, tranylcypromine) can increase the side effects of this medication.

3. Clemastine can also decrease the activity of oral anticoagulants (blood thinners, such as warfarin).

TELL YOUR DOCTOR if you are already taking any of the medications listed above.

WARNINGS

• Tell your doctor about unusual or allergic reactions you

have had to medications, especially to clemastine or to any other antihistamines (such as bromodiphenhydramine, brompheniramine, carbinoxamine, chlorpheniramine, azatadine, cyproheptadine, dexchlorpheniramine, dimenhydrinate, dimethindene, diphenhydramine, diphenylpyraline, doxylamine, hydroxyzine, promethazine, pyrilamine, trimeprazine, tripelennamine, or tripolidine).

• Tell your doctor if you now have, or if you have ever had, asthma, blood vessel disease, glaucoma, high blood pressure, kidney disease, peptic ulcers, enlarged prostate gland, or thyroid disease.

• Clemastine can cause drowsiness or dizziness. Your ability to perform tasks that require alertness, such as driving a car or operating potentially dangerous machinery, may be decreased. Appropriate caution should therefore be taken.

• Be sure to tell your doctor if you are pregnant. The effects of this medication during pregnancy have not yet been thoroughly studied in humans. Also, tell your doctor if you are breastfeeding an infant. Small amounts of clemastine pass into breast milk and may cause unusual excitement or irritability in nursing infants.

Cleocin — see clindamycin (systemic)

Cleocin Pediatric — see clindamycin (systemic)

Cleocin T — see clindamycin (topical)

---

clindamycin (systemic)

BRAND NAMES (Manufacturers)
Cleocin (Upjohn)
Cleocin Pediatric (Upjohn)
TYPE OF DRUG
Antibiotic (infection fighter)
INGREDIENT
clindamycin as the hydrochloride salt
DOSAGE FORMS
Capsules (75 mg and 150 mg)

Oral liquid (75 mg per 5 ml teaspoonful)
STORAGE
Clindamycin capsules and oral liquid should be stored at room temperature, in tightly closed containers. The oral liquid should not be refrigerated or frozen; when chilled it thickens and becomes difficult to pour. The liquid form of this medication should be discarded after 14 days because it loses potency after that time.

USES
Clindamycin is an antibiotic that is used to treat a wide variety of bacterial infections. It chemically attaches to the bacteria and prevents their growth and multiplication. Clindamycin kills susceptible bacteria, but is not effective against viruses, parasites, or fungi.

TREATMENT
In order to prevent irritation to your esophagus (swallowing tube) or stomach, you should take clindamycin with food or a full glass of water or milk (unless your doctor directs you to do otherwise).

The liquid form of this medication should be shaken well, just before measuring each dose. The contents tend to settle on the bottom of the bottle, so it is necessary to shake the container to evenly distribute the ingredients and equalize the doses. Each dose should then be measured carefully, with a specially designed, 5 ml measuring spoon. An ordinary kitchen teaspoon is not accurate enough.

Clindamycin works best when the level of medicine in your bloodstream is kept constant. It is best therefore to take the doses at evenly spaced intervals, day and night. For example, if you are to take four doses a day, the doses should be spaced six hours apart.

Try not to miss any doses of this medication. If you do miss a dose, take it as soon as you remember. However, if you do not remember to take the missed dose until it is almost time for your next dose, take the missed dose immediately; space the following dose about halfway through the regular interval between doses. Then continue with your regular dosing schedule.

It is important to continue to take this medication for

the entire time prescribed by your doctor (usually seven to 14 days), even if your symptoms of infection disappear before the end of that period. If you stop taking the drug too soon, resistant bacteria are given a chance to continue growing, and your infection could recur.

SIDE EFFECTS

Minor. Diarrhea; loss of appetite; nausea; stomach or throat irritation; and vomiting. These side effects should disappear in several days, as your body adjusts to the medication. If the diarrhea becomes prolonged, CONTACT YOUR DOCTOR. Do not take diarrhea medicine.

Major. Tell your doctor about any side effects that are persistent or particularly bothersome. IT IS ESPECIALLY IMPORTANT TO TELL YOUR DOCTOR about unusual bleeding or bruising; bloody or pus-containing diarrhea; hives; itching; muscle or joint pain; skin rash; or yellowing of the eyes or skin. Also, if the symptoms of your infection do not improve in several days, contact your doctor. This medication may not be effective for your particular infection.

INTERACTIONS

Clindamycin should not interact with other medications, if it is used according to directions.

WARNINGS

• Tell your doctor about unusual or allergic reactions you have had to any medications, especially to clindamycin or lincomycin.

• Before starting to take this medication, be sure to tell your doctor if you now have, or if you have ever had, colitis; kidney disease; or liver disease.

• Before having any surgery or other medical or dental treatment, be sure your doctor or dentist knows that you are taking clindamycin.

• The capsule form of this medication contains F.D. & C. Yellow Dye No. 5 (tartrazine), which can cause allergic-type symptoms (fainting, shortness of breath, rash) in certain susceptible individuals.

• Clindamycin has been prescribed for your current infection only. Another infection later on, or one that someone else has, may require a different medicine. You should not give your medicine to other people, or use it for other infections, unless your doctor specifically directs you to do so.

• Be sure to tell your doctor if you are pregnant. Although clindamycin appears to be safe during pregnancy, extensive studies in humans have not yet been completed. Also, tell your doctor if you are breastfeeding an infant. Small amounts of clindamycin pass into breast milk.

---

clindamycin (topical)

BRAND NAME (Manufacturer)
Cleocin T (Upjohn)
TYPE OF DRUG
Antibiotic (infection fighter)
INGREDIENT
clindamycin as the phosphate salt
DOSAGE FORM
Topical solution (10 mg per ml)
STORAGE
Clindamycin topical solution should be stored at room temperature, in a tightly closed container. It should be kept away from flames and heat, because the solution is flammable (it contains alcohol).

USES

Clindamycin topical solution is used to treat acne vulgaris. It is an antibiotic that is thought to act by suppressing the growth of the bacteria *Propionibacterium acnes*. This bacteria is probably responsible for the formation of the acne sores.

TREATMENT

Before applying topical clindamycin, wash the affected area thoroughly with a mild soap and warm water. Then rinse well and pat dry. To avoid skin irritation from the alcohol, wait at least 30 minutes after washing or shaving before applying this medication.

Clindamycin is packaged in a bottle with an applicator tip that can be used to apply the solution directly to the skin. Press the applicator tip firmly against your skin. The pressure applied determines the amount of medicine released. Use the applicator with a dabbing motion rather than a rolling motion. A thin film of medication should be applied to the entire area of skin affected by acne.

Topical clindamycin does not cure acne, but it helps to control the condition, as long as you continue to use it.

It is important to continue to apply this medication for the entire time prescribed by your doctor (which may be several months), even if your symptoms disappear in several days. If you stop applying the medication too soon, the bacteria are given a chance to continue growing, and your infection could recur.

If you miss a dose of this medication, apply it as soon as possible, unless it is almost time for the next dose. In that case, do not apply the missed dose at all; just return to your regular dosing schedule.

If there is no improvement in your condition after six weeks of using this medication, check with your doctor. However, it may take up to 12 weeks before improvement in your acne is readily apparent.

SIDE EFFECTS

Minor. Diarrhea; dry skin; fatigue; headache; nausea; oily skin; and stomach irritation. These side effects should disappear in several weeks, as your body adjusts to the medication.

If diarrhea becomes severe or prolonged, contact your doctor. Do not take any diarrhea medicine.

Major. Tell your doctor about any side effects that are persistent or particularly bothersome. IT IS ESPECIALLY IMPORTANT TO TELL YOUR DOCTOR about bloody or pus-containing diarrhea; itching; sore throat; swelling of the face; or increased urination.

INTERACTIONS

If you are using another topical medication as well as clindamycin, it is best to apply them at different times, to increase their effectiveness and to reduce the chance of skin irritation.

Use of abrasive or medicated cleansers, medicated cosmetics, or any topical, alcohol-containing preparations (such as after-shave lotions or perfume) along with topical clindamycin can result in excessive skin dryness and irritation.

WARNINGS
- Tell your doctor about unusual or allergic reactions you have had to any medications, especially to clindamycin or lincomycin.
- Tell your doctor if you now have, or if you have ever had, colitis.
- Because this medication contains alcohol, it can cause skin irritation to sensitive areas. You should therefore avoid getting this medication in your eyes, nose, or mouth, or in the areas surrounding scratches or burns.
- You may continue to use cosmetics while applying this medication (unless otherwise directed by your doctor), but it is best to use only "water-based" cosmetics rather than ones with an oil base.
- Be sure to tell your doctor if you are pregnant. Although topical clindamycin appears to be safe during pregnancy, extensive studies in humans have not yet been completed. Also, tell your doctor if you are breastfeeding an infant. It is not known whether or not topical clindamycin passes into breast milk.

Clindex—see chlordiazepoxide and clidinium combination

Clinoril—see sulindac

Clinoxide—see chlordiazepoxide and clidinium combination

Clipoxide—see chlordiazepoxide and clidinium combination

Clistin—see carbinoxamine

clofibrate
BRAND NAME (Manufacturer)
Atromid-S (Ayerst)

TYPE OF DRUG
Anti-hyperlipidemic
INGREDIENT
clofibrate
DOSAGE FORM
Capsules (500 mg)
STORAGE
Clofibrate should be stored at room temperature in a tightly closed, light-resistant container.

USES
Clofibrate is used to reduce fat (lipid) or cholesterol in the blood in patients with atherosclerosis (hardening of the arteries) and in patients having certain kinds of skin lesions caused by excessive fat levels in the blood. It is not clearly understood how clofibrate works, but it appears to decrease the body's production of cholesterol and fats.

Attempts are usually made to control serum fat levels with diet, exercise, weight loss, or control of diabetes before therapy with this drug is initiated.

TREATMENT
Clofibrate should be taken with food or immediately after a meal (unless your doctor directs you to do otherwise).

If you miss a dose of this medication, take the missed dose as soon as possible, unless it is almost time for the next dose. In that case, do not take the missed dose at all; just return to your regular dosing schedule. Do not double the next dose.

SIDE EFFECTS
Minor. Abdominal cramps; bloating; blurred vision; decreased sexual desire; diarrhea; dizziness; drowsiness; dry and brittle hair; dry skin; fatigue; gas; headache; increased sweating; itching; muscle cramps; nausea; rash; sore mouth; vomiting; weakness; and weight gain. These side effects should disappear in several weeks, as your body adjusts to the medication.

If you feel dizzy, sit or lie down awhile; get up slowly, and be careful on stairs.

Major. Tell your doctor about any side effects that are persistent or particularly bothersome. IT IS ESPECIALLY

IMPORTANT TO TELL YOUR DOCTOR about unusual bleeding or bruising; bloody or black, tarry stools; chest pain; difficult or painful urination; impotence; loss of hair; palpitations; sore joints; or tremors.

INTERACTIONS

Clofibrate interacts with other types of medication.

1. It can increase the side effects of oral anti-coagulants (blood thinners, such as warfarin) and oral anti-diabetic agents.

2. Rifampin can decrease the effectiveness of clofibrate.

3. Probenecid and furosemide can increase the side effects of clofibrate.

Before starting to take clofibrate, BE SURE TO TELL YOUR DOCTOR if you are already taking any of the medicines listed above.

WARNINGS

● Tell your doctor about unusual or allergic reactions you have had to any medications, especially to clofibrate.

● Before starting to take this medication, be sure to tell your doctor if you now have, or if you have ever had, diabetes mellitus (sugar diabetes); gallstones; heart disease; kidney disease; liver disease; stomach ulcers; or thyroid disease.

● Do not stop taking this medication without first checking with your doctor. Stopping this medication abruptly may lead to an increase in your blood fat levels. Your doctor may want you to follow a special diet to prevent this from happening.

● Clofibrate has been shown to cause tumors when administered to animals in large doses. This effect has not been observed in humans.

● Be sure to tell your doctor if you are pregnant. Clofibrate crosses the placenta and can build up in the body of the developing fetus. Because clofibrate has long-term effects on the body, you should not become pregnant for at least two months after you stop taking this drug. Also, tell your doctor if you are breastfeeding an infant. It is not known whether or not clofibrate passes into breast milk.

Clomid—see clomiphene

clomiphene

BRAND NAMES (Manufacturers)
Clomid (Merrell Dow)
Serophene (Serono)
TYPE OF DRUG
Fertility drug
INGREDIENT
clomiphene as the citrate salt
DOSAGE FORM
Tablets (50 mg)
STORAGE
Clomiphene should be stored at room temperature in a tightly closed, light-resistant container.

USES

Clomiphene is used to treat infertility in women. It reverses some types of infertility by stimulating ovulation.

TREATMENT

Clomiphene can be taken either on an empty stomach or with food or milk, as directed by your doctor.

It is very important to follow your dosing schedule carefully. If you have any questions about how to take this medication, BE SURE TO CHECK WITH YOUR DOCTOR.

If you miss a dose of this medication, take the missed dose as soon as possible. If you don't remember until it is time for the next dose, double the dose, then return to your regular dosing schedule. If you miss more than one dose, CHECK WITH YOUR DOCTOR.

SIDE EFFECTS

Minor. Abdominal discomfort; bloating; dizziness; hair loss; headache; insomnia; nausea; nervousness; and vomiting. As your body adjusts to the medicine, these side effects should disappear.

If you feel dizzy, sit or lie down awhile; get up slowly, and be careful on stairs.

Major. Tell your doctor about any side effects that are persistent or particularly bothersome. IT IS ESPECIALLY

IMPORTANT TO TELL YOUR DOCTOR about breast tenderness; depression; fatigue; hot flashes; skin rash; or visual disturbances.

INTERACTIONS

Clomiphene should not interact with other medications, if it is used according to directions.

WARNINGS

• Tell your doctor about unusual or allergic reactions you have had to any medications, especially to clomiphene.
• Before starting to take clomiphene, tell your doctor if you now have, or if you have ever had, abnormal vaginal bleeding, clotting problems, tumors or cysts of the uterus or ovary, liver disease, or mental depression.
• If this drug makes you dizzy, do not take part in any activity that requires alertness, such as driving a car or operating potentially dangerous equipment.
• While taking this medication, it is important to carefully follow your doctor's directions for recording your body temperature and the timing of sexual intercourse.
• The risk of a multiple pregnancy is increased when clomiphene is used. This medication should not be taken if you are already pregnant. It has been reported to cause birth defects in animals whose mothers received large doses of clomiphene during pregnancy. Also, tell your doctor if you are breastfeeding an infant. It is not known whether or not clomiphene passes into breast milk.

---

clonazepam

BRAND NAME (Manufacturer)
Clonopin (Roche)
TYPE OF DRUG
Anti-convulsant
INGREDIENT
clonazepam
DOSAGE FORM
Tablets (0.5 mg, 1 mg, and 2 mg)

STORAGE

Clonazepam should be stored at room temperature in a tightly closed, light-resistant container.

USES

This medication is used to treat certain seizure disorders. It is unclear exactly how clonazepam works to treat convulsions, but it appears to prevent the spread of seizures to all parts of the brain.

TREATMENT

This medication can be taken either on an empty stomach or with food or milk (as directed by your doctor).

Clonazepam works best when the level of medicine in your bloodstream is kept constant. It is best therefore to take the doses at evenly spaced intervals, day and night. For example, if you are to take three doses a day, the doses should be spaced eight hours apart.

Try not to miss any doses of this medication. If you do miss a dose, and remember within an hour of the scheduled time, take the dose immediately. If more than an hour has passed, do not take the missed dose at all; just return to your regular dosing schedule. Do not double the next dose. If you miss two or more doses, CONTACT YOUR DOCTOR.

SIDE EFFECTS

Minor. Increased appetite; constipation; diarrhea; drowsiness; dry mouth; headache; insomnia; loss of appetite; nausea; runny nose; or weight loss or gain. These side effects should disappear in several weeks, as your body adjusts to the medication.

In order to relieve constipation, increase the amount of fiber in your diet (bran, salads, fresh fruits and vegetables, and whole-grain breads), exercise, and drink more water (unless your doctor directs you to do otherwise).

To relieve mouth dryness, suck on ice chips or a piece of hard candy.

Major. Tell your doctor about any side effects that are persistent or particularly bothersome. IT IS ESPECIALLY IMPORTANT TO TELL YOUR DOCTOR about behavioral problems; unusual bleeding or bruising; confu-

sion; depression; fever; fluid retention; hair loss; hallu-
.inations; hysteria; increased or decreased urination;
muscle weakness; palpitations; skin rash; slurred speech;
sore gums; tremors; unusual body movements; or yellowing of the eyes or skin.

Clonazepam can also produce an increase in salivation, so it should be used cautiously by people who have
swallowing difficulties. Contact your doctor if salivation
becomes a problem.

INTERACTIONS

Clonazepam interacts with several other types of medica-
tioi.
1. Concurrent use of clonazepam with other central
nervous system depressants (drugs that slow the activity
of the brain and spinal cord), such as alcohol, antihistamines, barbiturates, benzodiazepine tranquilizers,
muscle relaxants, narcotics, pain medications, phenothiazine tranquilizers, or sleeping medications, or with
tricyclic anti-depressants can cause extreme drowsiness.
2. Phenobarbital and phenytoin can decrease the blood
levels and effectiveness of clonazepam.
3. Concurrent use of clonazepam and valproic acid can
lead to increased seizure activity.
Before starting to take this medication, BE SURE TO TELL
YOUR DOCTOR if you are already taking any of the
medications listed above.

WARNINGS

• Tell your doctor about unusual or allergic reactions you
have had to any medications, especially to clonazepam
or to other benzodiazepine tranquilizers (such as alprazolam, chlordiazepoxide, clorazepate, diazepam, flurazepam, halazepam, lorazepam, oxazepam, prazepam, temazepam, or triazolam).
• Tell your doctor if you now have, or if you have ever
had, glaucoma, kidney disease, liver disease, or lung disease.
• If this drug makes you dizzy or drowsy, do not take part
in any activity that requires alertness, such as driving a car
or operating potentially dangerous equipment. Children
should be careful while playing or while climbing trees.

- Do not stop taking this medication unless you first check with your doctor. If you have been taking this medication for several months or longer, stopping the drug abruptly could lead to a withdrawal reaction and a worsening of your condition. Your doctor may therefore want to reduce your dosage gradually.
- Be sure to tell your doctor if you are pregnant. Although no harmful effects have been reported during pregnancy, extensive studies have not yet been completed. The risks and benefits of clonazepam therapy during pregnancy should be discussed with your doctor. Also, tell your doctor if you are breastfeeding an infant. Small amounts of clonazepam pass into breast milk and may cause excessive drowsiness in nursing infants.

---

clonidine

BRAND NAME (Manufacturer)
Catapres (Boehringer Ingelheim)
TYPE OF DRUG
Anti-hypertensive
INGREDIENT
clonidine as the hydrochloride salt
DOSAGE FORM
Tablets (0.1 mg, 0.2 mg, and 0.3 mg)
STORAGE
Clonidine should be stored at room temperature in a tightly closed container.

USES

This medication is used to treat high blood pressure. It works on the central nervous system (brain and spinal cord) to prevent the release of chemicals responsible for maintaining high blood pressure.

TREATMENT

To avoid stomach irritation, you can take clonidine with food or with a full glass of milk or water. In order to become accustomed to taking this medication, try to take it at the same time(s) every day.

Clonidine does not cure high blood pressure, but it will

help to control the condition, as long as you continue to take it.

If you miss a dose of this medication, take the missed dose as soon as possible, unless it is almost time for your next dose. In that case, do not take the missed dose at all; just return to your regular dosing schedule. Do not double the next dose. If you miss more than two doses of this medication, contact your doctor.

SIDE EFFECTS

Minor. Anxiety; constipation; decreased sexual desire; dizziness; drowsiness; dry eyes; dry mouth; fatigue; headache; insomnia; jaw pain; loss of appetite; nasal congestion; nausea; nervousness; and vomiting. These side effects should disappear in several days, as your body adjusts to the medication.

To relieve constipation, increase the amount of fiber in your diet (salads, bran, fresh fruits and vegetables, and whole-grain breads), exercise, and drink more water (unless your doctor directs you to do otherwise).

To relieve mouth dryness, suck on ice chips or a piece of hard candy, or chew sugarless gum.

Artificial tears eye drops may help relieve eye dryness

To avoid dizziness or light-headedness when you stand, contract and relax the muscles of your legs for a few moments before rising. Do this by pushing one foot against the floor while raising the other foot slightly, alternating feet so that you are "pumping" your legs in a pedaling motion.

Major. Tell your doctor about any side effects that are persistent or particularly bothersome. IT IS ESPECIALLY IMPORTANT TO TELL YOUR DOCTOR about chest pain; cold fingertips or toes; depression; difficulty breathing; difficulty urinating; enlarged, painful breasts (in both sexes); hair loss; hives; itching; impotence; nightmares; rash; swelling of the hands or feet; weight gain; or yellowing of the eyes or skin.

INTERACTIONS

Clonidine interacts with other types of medication.
1. Concurrent use of clonidine with other central nervous system depressants (drugs that slow the activity of

the nervous system), such as alcohol, antihistamines, barbiturates, benzodiazepine tranquilizers, muscle relaxants, narcotics, pain medications, phenothiazine tranquilizers, and sleeping medications, or with tricyclic anti-depressants can cause extreme drowsiness.

2. Tolazoline and tricyclic anti-depressants may block the blood-pressure-lowering effects of clonidine.

Before you start to take this medication, BE SURE TO TELL YOUR DOCTOR if you are already taking any of the medications listed above.

WARNINGS

• Tell your doctor about any unusual or allergic reactions you have had to medications, especially to clonidine.

• Tell your doctor if you now have, or if you have ever had, heart disease, kidney disease, depression, Raynaud's disease, or a recent heart attack or stroke.

• Before having any kind of surgery or other medical or dental treatment, be sure to tell your doctor or dentist that you are taking this medication.

• If you have high blood pressure, do not take any over-the-counter (non-prescription) medication for weight control, or for allergy, asthma, sinus, cough, or cold problems, unless you first check with your doctor.

• If this drug makes you dizzy or drowsy, do not take part in any activity that requires alertness, such as driving a car or operating potentially dangerous equipment.

• Tolerance to this medication develops occasionally; consult your doctor if you feel that the drug is becoming less effective.

• Do not stop taking this medication without first consulting your doctor. If this drug is stopped abruptly, you may experience nervousness, agitation, headache, and a *rise in blood pressure*. Your doctor may therefore want to reduce your dosage gradually or start you on another medication.

• Make sure you have enough medication on hand to last through weekends, vacations, and holidays.

• Drinking alcoholic beverages, standing for prolonged periods, exercising, and hot weather can each increase the blood-pressure-lowering effects of clonidine, and can cause fainting or dizziness.

- Be sure to tell your doctor if you are pregnant. Although clonidine appears to be safe in animals, extensive studies in humans during pregnancy have not yet been completed. Also, tell your doctor if you are breastfeeding an infant. It is not known whether or not clonidine passes into breast milk.

Clonopin—see clonazepam

---

clorazepate

BRAND NAMES (Manufacturers)
Tranxene (Abbott)
Tranxene SD (Abbott)
TYPE OF DRUG
Sedative/hypnotic (anti-anxiety medication)
INGREDIENT
clorazepate as the dipotassium salt
DOSAGE FORMS
Capsules (3.75 mg, 7.5 mg, and 15 mg)
Tablets (3.75 mg, 7.5 mg, 11.25 mg, 15 mg, and 22.5 mg)
STORAGE
This medication should be stored at room temperature in tightly closed, light-resistant containers.

USES

Clorazepate is prescribed to treat the symptoms of anxiety, and sometimes to treat seizures and alcohol withdrawal. It is not clear exactly how this medicine works, but it may relieve anxiety by acting as a depressant of the central nervous system. Clorazepate is currently used by many people to relieve nervousness. It is effective for this purpose for short periods, but it is important to try to remove the cause of the anxiety as well.

TREATMENT

This medication should be taken exactly as directed by your doctor. It can be taken with food or a full glass of water if stomach upset occurs. Do not take this medication with a dose of antacids, since they may retard its absorption.

If you are taking this medication regularly and you miss a dose, take the missed dose immediately, if you remember within an hour of the scheduled time. If more than an hour has passed, skip the dose you missed and wait for the next scheduled dose. Do not double the dose.

SIDE EFFECTS

Minor. Bitter taste in mouth; constipation; depression; diarrhea; dizziness; drowsiness (after a night's sleep); dry mouth; fatigue; flushing; headache; heartburn; excess saliva; loss of appetite; nausea; nervousness; sweating; and vomiting. As your body adjusts to the medicine, these side effects should disappear.

Dry mouth can be relieved by chewing sugarless gum or by sucking on ice chips.

If you feel dizzy, sit or lie down awhile; get up slowly, and be careful on stairs.

Major. Tell your doctor about any side effects that are persistent or particularly bothersome. IT IS ESPECIALLY IMPORTANT TO TELL YOUR DOCTOR about blurred vision; chest pain; severe depression; difficulty urinating; double vision; fainting; falling; fever; joint pain; hallucinations; mouth sores; nightmares; palpitations; rash; shortness of breath; slurred speech; sore throat; uncoordinated movements; unusual excitement; unusual tiredness; or yellowing of the eyes or skin.

INTERACTIONS

Clorazepate interacts with several other medications.

1. To prevent over-sedation, this drug should not be taken with alcohol; other sedative drugs; central nervous system depressants, such as antihistamines, barbiturates, muscle relaxants, pain medicines, narcotics, medicines for seizures, and phenothiazine tranquilizers, or with anti-depressants.

2. This medication may decrease the effectiveness of carbamazepine, levodopa, and oral anti-coagulants (blood thinners), and may increase the effects of phenytoin.

3. Disulfiram, isoniazid, and cimetidine can increase the blood levels of clorazepate, which can lead to toxic effects.

4. Concurrent use of rifampin may decrease the effectiveness of clorazepate.

If you are currently taking any of the medications listed above, CONSULT YOUR DOCTOR about their use.

WARNINGS

• Tell your doctor about any unusual or allergic reactions you have had to medications, especially to clorazepate or any other benzodiazepine tranquilizers (such as alprazolam, chlordiazepoxide, diazepam, flurazepam, halazepam, lorazepam, oxazepam, prazepam, temazepam, or triazolam).

• Tell your doctor if you now have, or if you have ever had, liver disease, kidney disease, epilepsy, lung disease, myasthenia gravis, porphyria, depression, or mental illness.

• This medicine can cause drowsiness. Avoid tasks that require alertness, such as driving a car or using potentially dangerous machinery.

• This medication has the potential for abuse and must be used with caution. Tolerance may develop quickly; do not increase the dose of the drug without first consulting your doctor. It is also important not to stop this drug suddenly if you have been taking it in large amounts, or if you have used it for several weeks. Your doctor may want to reduce the dosage gradually.

• This is a safe drug when used properly. When it is combined with other sedative drugs or alcohol, however, serious side effects may develop.

• Be sure to tell your doctor if you are pregnant. This medicine may increase the chance of birth defects if it is taken during the first three months of pregnancy. In addition, too much use of this medicine during the last six months of pregnancy may cause the baby to become dependent on it. This may result in withdrawal side effects in the newborn. Also, use of this medicine during the last weeks of pregnancy may cause drowsiness, slowed heartbeat, and breathing difficulties in the infant. Tell your doctor if you are breastfeeding an infant. This medicine can pass into the breast milk and cause drowsiness, slowed heartbeat, and breathing difficulties in the nursing infant.

clotrimazole (topical)

BRAND NAMES (Manufacturers)
Lotrimin (Schering)
Mycelex (Miles)
TYPE OF DRUG
Anti-fungal
INGREDIENT
clotrimazole
DOSAGE FORMS
Topical cream (1%)
Topical solution (1%)
Topical lotion (1%)
STORAGE
Clotrimazole cream, solution, or lotion should be stored at room temperature in tightly closed containers. This medication should never be frozen.

USES

This medication is used to treat superficial fungal infections of the skin. Clotrimazole is an anti-fungal agent that is active against a broad range of fungi and yeast. It acts by preventing the growth and multiplication of the organisms.

TREATMENT

Before applying clotrimazole you should wash your hands. Then, unless your doctor tells you to do otherwise, cleanse the affected area with soap and water. Pat the skin with a clean towel until it is almost dry. Gently massage a small amount of the cream, solution, or lotion over the entire area that is affected and the skin immediately surrounding this area. Don't bandage or cover the infection after applying the medication, unless your doctor instructs you to do so.

Improvement in your condition may not become apparent for as much as a week after you begin treatment with this drug. However, you should be sure to complete the full course of therapy. If you stop using this drug too soon, resistant fungi are given a chance to continue growing, and the infection could recur. If your condition has not improved after four weeks, however, CONTACT

YOUR DOCTOR. Clotrimazole may not be effective against the organism causing your infection.

If you miss a dose of this medication, apply the missed dose as soon as possible. If you do not remember until it is almost time for the next dose, however, do not apply the missed dose at all; just return to your regular dosing schedule. Do not use a double dose of the medication at the next application.

SIDE EFFECTS

Minor. You may experience some burning, itching, stinging, or redness when this drug is applied to the skin. This sensation should disappear in several days, as your body adjusts to the medication.

Major. Tell your doctor about any side effects that are persistent or particularly bothersome. IT IS ESPECIALLY IMPORTANT TO TELL YOUR DOCTOR about blistering, irritation, peeling of the skin, or swelling.

INTERACTIONS

Clotrimazole does not interact with other medications, as long as it is used according to directions.

WARNINGS

• Tell your doctor about any unusual or allergic reactions you have had to medications, especially to clotrimazole.
• This medication has been prescribed for your current infection only. Another infection later on, or one that someone else has, may require a different medication. Therefore, you should not give your medicine to other people or use it for other infections, unless your doctor specifically directs you to do so.
• Clotrimazole should not be used in or around the eyes.
• In order to avoid reinfection, keep the affected area clean and dry, wear freshly laundered clothing, and try to avoid wearing tight-fitting clothing.
• Be sure to tell your doctor if you are pregnant. Small amounts of clotrimazole may be absorbed through the skin. It should therefore be used cautiously, especially during the first three months of pregnancy. Also, tell your doctor if you are breastfeeding an infant. It is not known whether or not clotrimazole passes into breast milk.

clotrimazole (vaginal)

BRAND NAMES (Manufacturers)
Gyne-Lotrimin (Schering)
Mycelex-G (Miles)
TYPE OF DRUG
Anti-fungal
INGREDIENT
clotrimazole
DOSAGE FORMS
Vaginal cream (1%)
Vaginal tablets (100 mg)
STORAGE
Clotrimazole vaginal cream or tablets should be stored at room temperature, in tightly closed containers.

USES
This medication is used to treat fungal infections of the vagina. Clotrimazole is an anti-fungal agent that prevents the growth and multiplication of a wide range of fungi and yeast, including Candida.

TREATMENT
Clotrimazole vaginal cream and tablets are packaged with detailed directions for use. Follow these instructions carefully. An applicator will probably be provided for inserting the cream into the vagina.

You should wash the area carefully prior to inserting the cream or tablet into the vagina.

If you begin to menstruate while you are being treated with clotrimazole, continue with your regular dosing schedule.

It is important to continue to insert this medication for the entire time prescribed by your doctor—even if the symptoms disappear before the end of that period. If you stop using the drug too soon, resistant fungus is given a chance to continue growing, and your infection could recur.

If you miss a dose of this medication, insert the missed dose as soon as possible. However, if you do not remember until the following day, do not insert the missed dose at all; just return to your regular dosing schedule. Do not use a double dose of the medication at the next application.

SIDE EFFECTS

Minor. You may experience vaginal burning, itching, or irritation when this drug is inserted. This sensation should disappear in several days, as your body adjusts to the medication.

Do not treat any side effects that occur in the area of the infection, unless you first consult your doctor.

Your sexual partner may also experience some burning or irritation.

Major. Tell your doctor about any side effects that are persistent or particularly bothersome. IT IS ESPECIALLY IMPORTANT TO TELL YOUR DOCTOR about abdominal cramps; blistering; bloating; irritation; painful urination; or peeling of the skin.

INTERACTIONS

Clotrimazole does not interact with other medications, if it is used according to directions.

WARNINGS

• Tell your doctor about unusual or allergic reactions you have had to any medications, especially to clotrimazole.

• Tell your doctor if you have had other vaginal infections, especially if they have been resistant to treatment.

• In order to prevent reinfection, avoid sexual intercourse, or ask your partner to use a condom, until treatment is completed.

• There may be some vaginal drainage while using this medication; therefore, you may want to use a sanitary napkin or panty liner to prevent the staining of clothing.

• Wear cotton panties rather than those made of nylon or other non-porous materials while being treated for a vaginal fungus infection. Also, in order to prevent reinfection, always wear freshly laundered underclothes.

• If there is no improvement in your condition, or if irritation in the area continues after several days of treatment,

CONTACT YOUR DOCTOR. This medication may be causing an allergic reaction, or it may not be effective against the organism causing your infection.

• This medication has been prescribed for your current infection only. Another infection later on, or one that someone else has, may require a different medication. Therefore, you should not give your medication to other women or use it for other infections, unless your doctor specifically directs you to do so.

• Be sure to tell your doctor if you are pregnant. Clotrimazole appears to be safe during pregnancy. However, extensive studies have not yet been completed. In addition, your doctor may want to change the instructions on how you are to use this medication if you are pregnant. Also, tell your doctor if you are breastfeeding an infant. It is not known whether or not this medication passes into breast milk.

---

cloxacillin

BRAND NAMES (Manufacturers)
cloxacillin sodium (various manufacturers)
Cloxapen (Beecham)
Tegopen (Bristol)
TYPE OF DRUG
Antibiotic (infection fighter)
INGREDIENT
cloxacillin as the sodium salt
DOSAGE FORMS
Capsules (250 mg and 500 mg)
Oral solution (125 mg per 5 ml teaspoonful)
STORAGE
Cloxacillin capsules should be stored at room temperature in a tightly closed container. The oral solution should be stored in the refrigerator in a tightly closed container. Any unused portion of the solution should be discarded after 14 days, because the drug loses its potency after that time. This medication should never be frozen.

USES

Cloxacillin is used to treat a wide variety of bacterial

infections, usually involving the *Staphylococcus* bacteria. It acts by severely injuring the cell walls of the infecting bacteria, thereby preventing them from growing and multiplying. Cloxacillin kills susceptible bacteria, but is not effective against viruses, parasites, or fungi.

TREATMENT

Cloxacillin should be taken on an empty stomach or with a glass of water, one hour before or two hours after a meal. This medication should never be taken with fruit juices or carbonated beverages, because the acidity of these drinks destroys the drug in the stomach.

The oral solution should be measured carefully, with a specially designed, 5 ml measuring spoon. An ordinary kitchen teaspoon is not accurate enough.

Cloxacillin works best when the level of the medicine in your bloodstream is kept constant. Therefore, it is best to take the doses at evenly spaced intervals, day and night. For example, if you are taking four doses a day, the doses should be spaced six hours apart.

If you miss a dose of this medication, take the missed dose immediately. However, if you do not remember to take the missed dose until it is almost time for your next dose, take it; then space the next dose about halfway through the regular interval between doses. Then return to your regular schedule. Try not to skip any doses.

It is important to continue to take this medication for the entire time prescribed by your doctor (usually seven to 14 days), even if the symptoms of the infection disappear before the end of that period. If you stop taking the drug too soon, resistant bacteria are given the chance to continue growing, and the infection could recur.

SIDE EFFECTS

Minor. Diarrhea; heartburn; nausea; and vomiting. These side effects should disappear in several days, as your body adjusts to the medication.

Major. Tell your doctor about any side effects that are persistent or particularly bothersome. IT IS ESPECIALLY IMPORTANT TO TELL YOUR DOCTOR about bloating; chills; cough; difficulty breathing; fever; irritation of the mouth; muscle aches; rash; rectal or vaginal itching;

severe diarrhea; sore throat; or darkened tongue. Also, if your symptoms of infection seem to be getting worse rather than improving, you should contact your doctor.

INTERACTIONS

Cloxacillin interacts with other types of medication.

1. Probenecid can increase the blood concentrations and side effects of this medication.

2. Cloxacillin may decrease the effectiveness of oral contraceptives (birth control pills), and pregnancy could result. You should therefore use another form of birth control while taking this medication. Discuss this with your doctor.

TELL YOUR DOCTOR if you are already taking either of the medications listed above.

WARNINGS

• Tell your doctor about unusual or allergic reactions you have had to any medications, especially to cloxacillin or penicillins, or to cephalosporin antibiotics, penicillamine, or griseofulvin.

• Tell your doctor if you now have, or if you have ever had, kidney disease, asthma, or allergies.

• This medication has been prescribed for your current infection only. Another infection later on, or one that someone else has, may require a different medicine. You should not give your medicine to other people or use it for other infections, unless your doctor specifically directs you to do so.

• Diabetics taking cloxacillin should know that this drug can cause a false-positive sugar reaction with a Clinitest urine glucose test. To avoid this problem, while taking cloxacillin you should switch to Clinistix or Tes-Tape to test your urine sugar.

• Be sure to tell your doctor if you are pregnant. Although cloxacillin appears to be safe during pregnancy, extensive studies in humans have not yet been completed. Also, tell your doctor if you are breastfeeding an infant. Small amounts of this medication pass into breast milk and may temporarily alter the bacteria in the intestinal tract of the nursing infant and result in diarrhea.

cloxacillin sodium — see cloxacillin

Cloxapen — see cloxacillin

Codap — see acetaminophen and codeine combination

---

codeine

BRAND NAMES (Manufacturers)
codeine phosphate (various manufacturers)
codeine sulfate (various manufacturers)
TYPE OF DRUG
Analgesic (pain reliever) and cough suppressant
INGREDIENT
codeine as the phosphate or sulfate salt
DOSAGE FORM
Tablets (15 mg, 30 mg, and 60 mg)
STORAGE
Codeine tablets should be stored at room temperature in a tightly closed, light-resistant container.

USES
Codeine is a narcotic analgesic that acts directly on the central nervous system (brain and spinal cord). It is used to relieve mild to moderate pain or to suppress coughing.

TREATMENT
In order to avoid stomach upset, you can take codeine with food or milk.

This medication works most effectively if you take it at the onset of pain, rather than waiting until the pain becomes intense.

If you are taking this medication on a regular schedule and you miss a dose, take the missed dose as soon as possible, unless it is close to the time for your next dose. In that case, don't take the missed dose at all; just return to your regular dosing schedule. Do not double the next dose.

SIDE EFFECTS

Minor. Constipation; dizziness; drowsiness; dry mouth; false sense of well-being; flushing; light-headedness; loss of appetite; nausea; rash; sweating; and painful or difficult urination. These side effects should disappear in several days, as your body adjusts to the medication.

If you are constipated, increase the amount of fiber in your diet (raw vegetables, fruits, salads, bran, and whole-grain breads) and drink more water (unless your doctor directs you to do otherwise).

Chew sugarless gum, or suck on ice chips or a piece of hard candy, to reduce mouth dryness.

If you feel dizzy, light-headed, or nauseated, sit or lie down awhile; get up from a sitting or lying position slowly, and be careful on stairs.

Major. Tell your doctor about any side effects that are persistent or particularly bothersome. IT IS ESPECIALLY IMPORTANT TO TELL YOUR DOCTOR about anxiety; breathing difficulties; excitation; fatigue; palpitations; restlessness; sore throat and fever; tremors; or weakness.

INTERACTIONS

This medication interacts with several other types of drugs.

1. Concurrent use of this medication with other central nervous system depressants (drugs that slow the activity of the nervous system), such as antihistamines, barbiturates, benzodiazepine tranquilizers, muscle relaxants, phenothiazine tranquilizers, and alcohol, or with tricyclic anti-depressants can cause extreme drowsiness.

2. A monoamine oxidase (MAO) inhibitor taken within 14 days of this medication can lead to unpredictable and severe side effects.

3. Cimetidine, combined with this medication, can cause confusion, disorientation, seizures, and shortness of breath.

TELL YOUR DOCTOR if you are currently taking any of the medications listed above.

WARNINGS

• Tell your doctor about unusual or allergic reactions you have had to medications, especially to codeine or to any other narcotic analgesics (such as hydrocodone, hydromorphone, meperidine, methadone, morphine, oxycodone, or propoxyphene).

• Tell your doctor if you now have, or if you have ever had, acute abdominal conditions, asthma, brain disease, colitis, epilepsy, gallstones or gallbladder disease, head injuries, heart disease, kidney disease, liver disease, lung disease, mental illness, emotional disorders, prostate disease, thyroid disease, or urethral stricture.

• If this drug makes you dizzy or drowsy, do not take part in any activity that requires alertness, such as driving a car or operating potentially dangerous equipment.

• Before having any surgery or other medical or dental treatment, be sure to tell your doctor or dentist that you are taking this medication.

• Because this product contains codeine, it has the potential for abuse, and must be used with caution. Usually, it should not be taken on a regular schedule for longer than ten days (unless your doctor directs you to do so). Tolerance develops quickly; do not increase the dosage or stop taking the drug abruptly, unless you first consult your doctor. If you have been taking large amounts of this medication for long periods, you may experience a withdrawal reaction (muscle aches, diarrhea, gooseflesh, runny nose, nausea, vomiting, shivering, trembling, stomach cramps, sleep disorders, irritability, weakness, yawning, and sweating). Your doctor may therefore want to reduce the dosage gradually.

• Be sure to tell your doctor if you are pregnant. The effects of this medication during the early stages of pregnancy have not yet been thoroughly studied in humans. Codeine, used regularly in large doses during the later stages of pregnancy, can result in addiction of the fetus, leading to withdrawal symptoms (irritability, excessive crying, tremors, fever, vomiting, diarrhea, sneezing, and yawning) at birth. Also, tell your doctor if you are breast-feeding an infant. Small amounts of this medication may pass into breast milk and cause excessive drowsiness in the nursing infant.

codeine phosphate—see codeine

codeine sulfate—see codeine

Codimal-L.A. Cenules—see pseudoephedrine and chlorpheniramine combination

Codoxy—see aspirin and oxycodone combination

Cogentin—see benztropine

Co-Gesic—see acetaminophen and hydrocodone combination

---

colchicine

BRAND NAME (Manufacturer)
colchicine (various manufacturers)
TYPE OF DRUG
Anti-gout
INGREDIENT
colchicine
DOSAGE FORM
Tablets (0.5 mg and 0.6 mg)
STORAGE
Colchicine should be stored at room temperature, in a tightly closed, light-resistant container.

USES

Colchicine is used to relieve the symptoms of a gout attack and to prevent further attacks. Colchicine prevents the movement of uric acid crystals, which is responsible for the pain in the joints.

TREATMENT

Colchicine can be taken either on an empty stomach or with food or a full glass of water or milk (as directed by your doctor).

If you are taking colchicine to control a gout attack, it is important that you understand how to take it and when it should be stopped. CHECK WITH YOUR DOCTOR if you have any questions.

If you miss a dose of this medication, take the missed

dose as soon as possible, unless it is almost time for the next dose. In that case, do not take the missed dose at all; just return to your regular dosing schedule. Do not double the next dose.

SIDE EFFECTS

Minor. Abdominal pain; diarrhea; nausea; and vomiting. These side effects should disappear in several days, as your body adjusts to the medication.

Major. Tell your doctor about any side effects that are persistent or particularly bothersome. IT IS ESPECIALLY IMPORTANT TO TELL YOUR DOCTOR about unusual bleeding or bruising; difficult or painful urination; fever; loss of hair; muscle pain; skin rash; sore throat; or tingling in the hands or feet.

INTERACTIONS

Colchicine interacts with several other medications.

1. It can decrease absorption of vitamin B_{12}.

2. The action of colchicine can be blocked by vitamin C and can be enhanced by sodium bicarbonate or ammonium chloride.

3. Colchicine can increase the drowsiness caused by central nervous system depressants (drugs that slow the activity of the brain and spinal cord).

BE SURE TO TELL YOUR DOCTOR if you are already taking any of these medications.

WARNINGS

• Tell your doctor about unusual or allergic reactions you have had to any medications, especially to colchicine.

• Tell your doctor if you now have, or if you have ever had, blood disorders, gastrointestinal disorders, heart disease, kidney disease, or liver disease.

• Large amounts of alcohol can increase the blood levels of uric acid, which can decrease the effectiveness of colchicine. Alcohol ingestion should therefore be limited while you are taking this medication.

• Colchicine is not an analgesic (pain reliever) and does not relieve pain other than that of gout.

• Be sure to tell your doctor if you are pregnant. Colchicine is not recommended for use during pregnancy because it has been reported to cause birth defects in both animals and humans. Also, tell your doctor if you are breastfeeding an infant. It is not known whether or not colchicine passes into breast milk.

Colestid — see colestipol

---

colestipol

BRAND NAME (Manufacturer)
Colestid (Upjohn)
TYPE OF DRUG
Anti-hyperlipidemic (lipid-lowering drug)
INGREDIENT
colestipol as the hydrochloride salt
DOSAGE FORM
Oral granules (5 g per level teaspoon)
STORAGE
Colestipol should be stored at room temperature in a tightly closed container.

USES

This medication is used to lower blood cholesterol levels. It chemically binds to bile salts in the gastrointestinal tract and prevents the body from producing cholesterol.

TREATMENT

Colestipol is usually taken before meals. Each dose should be measured carefully, with a specially designed, 5 ml measuring spoon. An ordinary kitchen teaspoon is not accurate enough. The dose should then be added to at least 3 ounces of fluid (water, milk, fruit juice, or other carbonated or non-carbonated beverage). The mixture should be stirred and completely mixed (the granules do not completely dissolve). After the solution is drunk, the glass should be refilled with the same beverage, and this solution swallowed as well. This assures that the whole dose is taken. The granules can also be mixed with soup, applesauce, or crushed pineapple. You should never take colestipol dry; you might accidentally inhale the granules, which could irritate your throat and lungs.

Colestipol does not cure hypercholesterolemia (high blood cholesterol levels), but it will help to control the condition, as long as you continue to take it.

If you miss a dose of this medication, take the missed dose as soon as possible, unless it is almost time for the next dose. In that case, do not take the missed dose at all; just return to your regular dosing schedule. Do not double the next dose.

SIDE EFFECTS

Minor. Anxiety; belching; constipation; diarrhea; dizziness; drowsiness; fatigue; gas; headache; hiccups; loss of appetite; nausea; stomach pain; vomiting; or weight loss or gain. These side effects should disappear in several weeks, as your body adjusts to the medication.

To relieve constipation, increase the amount of fiber in your diet (bran, salads, fresh fruits and vegetables, and whole-grain breads), exercise, and drink more water (unless your doctor directs you to do otherwise). A stool softener may also be helpful; ask your pharmacist to recommend one.

Major. Tell your doctor about any side effects that are persistent or particularly bothersome. IT IS ESPECIALLY IMPORTANT TO TELL YOUR DOCTOR about any unusual bleeding or bruising; bloody or black, tarry stools; backache; difficult or painful urination; fluid retention; muscle or joint pains; rash or irritation of the skin, tongue, or rectal area; ringing in the ears; swollen glands; tingling sensations; or unusual weakness.

INTERACTIONS

Colestipol interferes with the absorption of a number of other drugs, including phenylbutazone, warfarin, thiazide diuretics (water pills), digoxin, penicillins, tetracycline, phenobarbital, folic acid, iron, thyroid hormones, cephalexin, clindamycin, trimethoprim, and the fat-soluble vitamins (vitamins A, D, E, and K). The effectiveness of these medications will be decreased by colestipol. To avoid this interaction, take the other medications 1 hour before or 4 to 6 hours after a dose of colestipol. BE SURE TO TELL YOUR DOCTOR if you are already taking any of these medications.

WARNINGS

- Tell your doctor about unusual or allergic reactions you have had to any medications, especially to colestipol.
- Before starting to take this medication, be sure to tell your doctor if you now have, or if you have ever had, bleeding disorders; biliary obstruction; heart disease; hemorrhoids; gallstones or gallbladder disease; kidney disease; malabsorption; stomach ulcers; or an obstructed intestine.
- Colestipol should be used only in conjunction with diet, weight reduction, or correction of other conditions that could be causing high blood cholesterol levels.
- Be sure to tell your doctor if you are pregnant. Although colestipol appears to be safe (because very little is absorbed into the bloodstream), extensive studies in humans during pregnancy have not yet been completed. Also, tell your doctor if you are breastfeeding an infant. It is not known whether or not colestipol passes into breast milk.

Combid—see prochlorperazine and isopropamide combination

Compazine—see prochlorperazine

Condecal—see phenylpropanolamine, phenylephrine, chlorpheniramine, and phenyltoloxamine combination

Condrin-LA—see phenylpropanolamine and chlorpheniramine combination

conjugated estrogens—see estrogens, conjugated

Constant-T—see theophylline

Control-D—see pseudoephedrine and chlorpheniramine combination

Cophed-C—see pseudoephedrine, tripolidine, guaifenesin, and codeine combination

Cordamine-PA—see phenylpropanolamine, phenylephrine, and brompheniramine combination

Cordilate—see dipyridamole

Cordran—see flurandrenolide (topical)

Corgard—see nadolol

Corque—see hydrocortisone and iodochlorhydroxyquin combination (topical)

Cortalone—see prednisolone (systemic)

Cortan—see prednisolone (systemic)

Cort-Dome—see hydrocortisone (topical)

Cortef—see hydrocortisone (systemic)

Cortef Acetate—see hydrocortisone (topical)

Cortef Fluid—see hydrocortisone (systemic)

Cortin—see hydrocortisone and iodochlorhydroxyquin combination (topical)

_____

cortisone (systemic)

BRAND NAMES (Manufacturers)
cortisone acetate (various manufacturers)
Cortone Acetate (Merck Sharp & Dohme)
TYPE OF DRUG
Adrenocorticosteroid hormone
INGREDIENT
cortisone as the acetate salt
DOSAGE FORM
Tablets (5 mg, 10 mg, and 25 mg)

STORAGE
Cortisone tablets should be stored at room temperature in a tightly closed container.

USES
Your adrenal glands naturally produce certain cortisone-like chemicals. These chemicals are involved in various regulatory processes in the body (such as maintenance of fluid balance, temperature, and reactions to inflammation). Cortisone belongs to a group of drugs known as adrenocorticosteroids (or cortisone-like medications). It is used to treat a variety of disorders, including endocrine and rheumatic disorders; asthma; blood diseases; certain cancers; eye disorders; gastrointestinal disturbances such as ulcerative colitis; respiratory diseases; and inflammations such as arthritis, dermatitis, and poison ivy. How this drug acts to relieve these disorders is not completely understood.

TREATMENT
In order to prevent stomach irritation, you can take cortisone with food or with milk.

If you are taking only one dose of this medication each day, try to take it before 9:00 A.M. This will mimic the body's normal production of this type of chemical.

It is important to try not to miss any doses of cortisone. However, if you do miss a dose of this medication:

1. If you are taking it more than once a day, take the missed dose as soon as possible and return to your regular schedule. If it is already time for the next dose, double the dose.

2. If you are taking this medication once a day, take the dose you missed as soon as possible, unless you don't remember until the next day. In that case do not take the missed dose at all; just follow your regular schedule. Do not double the next dose.

3. If you are taking this drug every other day, take it as soon as you remember. If you missed the scheduled time by a whole day, take it when you remember, then skip a day before you take the next dose. Do not double the dose.

If you miss more than one dose, CONTACT YOUR DOCTOR.

SIDE EFFECTS

Minor. Dizziness; false sense of well-being; fatigue; increased appetite; increased sweating; indigestion; menstrual irregularities; muscle weakness; nausea; reddening of the skin on the face; restlessness; sleep disorders; thinning of the skin; and weight gain. These side effects should disappear in several days, as your body adjusts to the medication.

To help avoid potassium loss while using this drug, take your dose with a glass of fresh or frozen orange juice, or eat a banana each day. The use of a salt substitute also helps prevent potassium loss. Check with your doctor.

Major. Tell your doctor about any side effects that are persistent or particularly bothersome. IT IS ESPECIALLY IMPORTANT TO TELL YOUR DOCTOR about abdominal enlargement; acne or other skin problems; back or rib pain; blurred vision; unusual bruising or bleeding; convulsions; eye pain; fever and sore throat; glaucoma; growth impairment (in children); headaches; impaired healing of wounds; increased thirst and urination; depression; mood changes; muscle wasting; nightmares; rapid weight gain (three to five pounds within a week); rash; severe abdominal pain; shortness of breath; unusual weakness; or bloody or black, tarry stools.

INTERACTIONS

Cortisone interacts with other types of medication.

1. Alcohol, aspirin, and anti-inflammation medications (such as diflunisal, ibuprofen, indomethacin, mefenamic acid, meclofenamate, naproxen, piroxicam, sulindac, tolmetin) aggravate the stomach problems that are common with use of this medication.

2. A change in the dosage requirements of oral anticoagulants (blood thinners, such as warfarin) and oral anti-diabetic drugs or insulin may be necessary when this medication is started or stopped.

3. The loss of potassium caused by cortisone can lead to serious side effects in individuals taking digoxin. Thiazide diuretics (water pills) can increase the potassium loss caused by cortisone.

4. Phenobarbital, phenytoin, rifampin, and ephedrine can increase the elimination of cortisone from the body, thereby decreasing its effectiveness.

5. Oral contraceptives and estrogen-containing drugs may decrease the elimination of this drug from the body, which can lead to an increase in side effects.

6. Cortisone can increase the elimination of aspirin and isoniazid from the body, thereby decreasing the effectiveness of these two medications.

7. Cholestyramine and colestipol can chemically bind this medication in the stomach and gastrointestinal tract, preventing its absorption.

TELL YOUR DOCTOR if you are currently taking any of the medications listed above.

WARNINGS

• Tell your doctor about unusual or allergic reactions you have had to any medications, especially to cortisone or other adrenocorticosteroids.

• Tell your doctor if you now have, or if you have ever had, bone disease; diabetes mellitus (sugar diabetes); emotional instability; glaucoma; fungal infections; heart disease; high blood pressure; high cholesterol levels; myasthenia gravis; peptic ulcers; osteoporosis; thyroid disease; tuberculosis; severe ulcerative colitis; kidney disease; or liver disease.

• If you are using this medication for longer than a week, you may need to receive higher dosages if you are subjected to stress, such as serious infections, injury, or surgery. Discuss this with your doctor.

• If you have been taking this drug for more than a week, do not stop taking it suddenly. If it is stopped suddenly, you may experience abdominal or back pain, dizziness, fainting, fever, muscle or joint pain, nausea, vomiting, shortness of breath, or extreme weakness. Your doctor may therefore want to reduce the dosage gradually. Never increase the dose or take the drug for longer than the prescribed time, unless you first consult your doctor.

• While you are taking this drug, you should not be vac-

cinated or immunized. This medication decreases the effectiveness of vaccines and can lead to overwhelming infection if a live virus is administered.
• Before having any surgery or other medical or dental treatment, be sure your doctor or dentist knows that you are taking this medication.
• If you are taking this medication for prolonged periods, you should wear or carry an identification card or notice stating that you are taking an adrenocorticosteroid.
• Because this drug can cause glaucoma and cataracts with long-term use, your doctor may want you to have your eyes examined by an ophthalmologist periodically during treatment.
• This medication can raise blood sugar levels in diabetic patients, so blood sugar should be monitored carefully with blood or urine tests when this medication is started.
• Be sure to tell your doctor if you are pregnant. This drug crosses the placenta. Although studies in humans have not yet been completed, birth defects have been observed in the fetuses of animals who were given large doses of this type of drug during pregnancy. Also, tell your doctor if you are breastfeeding an infant. Small amounts of this drug pass into breast milk and may cause growth suppression or a decrease in natural adrenocorticosteroid production in the nursing infant.

cortisone acetate—see cortisone (systemic)

Cortisporin Ophthalmic—see hydrocortisone, polymyxin B, neomycin, and bacitracin combination (ophthalmic)

Cortisporin Otic—see hydrocortisone, polymyxin B, and neomycin combination (otic)

Cortone Acetate—see cortisone (systemic)

Cortril—see hydrocortisone (topical)

Cotazym—see pancrelipase

Cotazym-S—see pancrelipase

Cotrim—see sulfamethoxazole and trimethoprim combination

Coufarin—see warfarin

Coumadin—see warfarin

---

cromolyn sodium (inhalation)

BRAND NAME (Manufacturer)
Intal (Fisons)
TYPE OF DRUG
Anti-allergic (anti-asthmatic)
INGREDIENT
cromolyn as the sodium salt (disodium cromoglycate)
DOSAGE FORMS
Capsules (20 mg): for inhalation only
Solution (20 mg per 2 ml vial): for inhalation only
STORAGE
Cromolyn sodium should be stored at room temperature in tightly closed, light-resistant containers.

USES
This medication is used to prevent asthma attacks. It is not effective in relieving asthma symptoms once an attack begins. Cromolyn sodium works by preventing the release of the body chemicals responsible for the asthma attack.

TREATMENT
Cromolyn sodium capsules are for inhalation only—they should NOT be swallowed. The medication is not effective if swallowed. This medication comes packaged with instructions for use of the capsules with the Spinhaler device. It is very important that you completely understand how to use this device.

The Spinhaler should be cleaned at least once a week. Take the Spinhaler apart and rinse it in clear, warm water. Do not use soap. Allow the inhaler to air-dry before you use it again. If properly cared for, the inhaler should last about six months.

The solution form of this medication should be used only with a power-operated nebulizer, equipped with a face mask. It should never be used with a hand-held nebulizer.

Cromolyn sodium is most effective when therapy is started before contact with allergens (the suspected offending agents causing your allergy), so if you expect to be exposed to something to which you know you are allergic, it is a good idea to start taking your medication first.

This medication works best when the level of medicine in your bloodstream is kept constant. It is best therefore to take the doses at evenly spaced intervals, day and night. For example, if you are to take four doses a day, the doses should be spaced six hours apart.

If you are using another inhaler to open up the lungs (a bronchodilator), it should be used 20 to 30 minutes before using cromolyn sodium. This allows the cromolyn sodium to penetrate deeper into the lungs.

The full benefits of this medication may not become apparent for up to four weeks after starting to take it.

If you miss a dose of this medication and remember within an hour or so of the scheduled time, take the missed dose immediately. If more than an hour has passed, do not take the missed dose at all; just return to your regular dosing schedule. Do not double the next dose.

SIDE EFFECTS

Minor. Cough; dizziness; drowsiness; headache; nasal congestion; nasal itching; nausea; sneezing; stomach irritation; tearing; and increased urination. These side effects should disappear in several weeks, as your body adjusts to the medication.

If you feel dizzy, sit or lie down awhile, get up slowly, and be careful on stairs.

This medication can cause mouth dryness, throat irritation, and hoarseness. Gargling and rinsing your mouth after each dose helps to prevent these effects.

Major. Tell your doctor about any side effects that are persistent or particularly bothersome. IT IS ESPECIALLY IMPORTANT TO TELL YOUR DOCTOR about itching;

joint swelling or pain; nosebleeds; nose burning; rash; swelling of the face or eyes; swollen glands; painful or increased urination; or wheezing.

INTERACTIONS

Cromolyn sodium does not interact with other medications, if it is used according to directions.

WARNINGS

• Tell your doctor about unusual or allergic reactions you have had to any medications, especially to cromolyn sodium.

• Patients who are allergic to lactose, milk, or milk products may also be allergic to the capsule form of this medication.

• Before starting to take this medication, be sure to tell your doctor if you now have, or if you have ever had, kidney or liver disease.

• Do not stop taking this medication unless you first check with your doctor. Stopping the drug abruptly may lead to a worsening of your condition.

• Be sure to tell your doctor if you are pregnant. Although cromolyn sodium appears to be safe during pregnancy, extensive studies in humans have not yet been completed. Also, tell your doctor if you are breastfeeding an infant. It is not known whether or not cromolyn sodium passes into breast milk.

---

cromolyn sodium (nasal)

BRAND NAME (Manufacturer)
Nasalcrom (Fisons)
TYPE OF DRUG
Anti-allergic
INGREDIENT
cromolyn as the sodium salt (disodium cromoglycate)
DOSAGE FORM
Nasal solution (each spray delivers 5.2 mg)
STORAGE
Cromolyn sodium should be stored at room temperature in its original container.

USES

Cromolyn sodium nasal solution is used to prevent and treat allergic rhinitis (inflammation of the nasal passages resulting from allergies). Cromolyn sodium works by preventing the release of the body chemicals responsible for the inflammation and swelling.

TREATMENT

This medication is for use within the nose only. The nasal passages should be cleared before using the spray. Inhale through the nose as you spray the solution.

This medication is most effective when therapy is started before contact with allergens (the suspected offending agents causing your allergy), so if you expect to be exposed to something to which you know you are allergic, it is a good idea to take your medication first.

This medication works best when the level of medicine in your bloodstream is kept constant. It is best therefore to take the doses at evenly spaced intervals, day and night. For example, if you are to take four doses a day, the doses should be spaced six hours apart.

Maximum benefits of this medication may not become apparent for up to four weeks after starting therapy.

If you miss a dose of this medication, take the missed dose as soon as possible, unless it is almost time for the next dose. In that case, do not take the missed dose at all; just return to your regular dosing schedule. Do not double the next dose.

SIDE EFFECTS

Minor. Bad taste in the mouth; headaches; nasal burning; irritation or stinging; post-nasal drip; and sneezing. These side effects should disappear as your body adjusts to the medication.

Major. Tell your doctor about any side effects that are persistent or particularly bothersome. IT IS ESPECIALLY IMPORTANT TO TELL YOUR DOCTOR about nosebleeds or skin rash.

INTERACTIONS

Cromolyn sodium does not interact with other medications, if it is used according to directions.

WARNINGS
• Tell your doctor about unusual or allergic reactions you have had to any medication, especially to cromolyn sodium.
• Before starting to take this medication, be sure to tell your doctor if you now have, or if you have ever had, kidney or liver disease.
• Do not stop taking this medication unless you first check with your doctor, even if the symptoms of your disorder disappear. Stopping the drug abruptly can lead to a worsening of your condition. Cromolyn sodium should be continued as long as you have contact with the substance causing your allergic symptoms.
• Be sure to tell your doctor if you are pregnant. Although the medication appears to be safe during pregnancy, extensive studies in humans have not yet been completed. Also, tell your doctor if you are breastfeeding an infant. It is not known whether or not cromolyn sodium passes into breast milk.

Crystodigin—see digitoxin

Cuprimine—see penicillamine

Curretab—see medroxyprogesterone

---

cyclacillin

BRAND NAME (Manufacturer)
Cyclapen-W (Wyeth)
TYPE OF DRUG
Antibiotic (infection fighter)
INGREDIENT
cyclacillin
DOSAGE FORMS
Tablets (250 mg and 500 mg)
Oral suspension (125 mg and 250 mg per
  5 ml teaspoonful)
STORAGE
Cyclacillin tablets should be stored at room temperature in a tightly closed container. The oral suspension form of

this drug should be stored in the refrigerator in a tightly closed container. Any unused portion of the suspension should be discarded after 14 days, because the drug loses its potency after that time. This medication should never be frozen.

USES

Cyclacillin is used to treat a wide variety of bacterial infections, including infections in the middle ear, upper and lower respiratory tracts, and the urinary tract. It acts by severely injuring the cell walls of the infecting bacteria, thereby preventing them from growing and multiplying.

Cyclacillin kills susceptible bacteria, but is not effective against viruses, parasites, or fungi.

TREATMENT

Cyclacillin should be taken on an empty stomach or with a glass of water, one hour before or two hours after a meal. This medication should never be taken with fruit juices or carbonated beverages, because the acidity of these drinks destroys the drug in the stomach.

The suspension form of this medication should be shaken well, just before measuring each dose. The contents tend to settle on the bottom of the bottle, so it is necessary to shake the container to evenly distribute the ingredients and equalize the doses. Each dose should then be measured carefully with a specially designed, 5 ml measuring spoon. An ordinary kitchen teaspoon is not accurate enough.

Cyclacillin works best when the level of medicine in your bloodstream is kept constant. It is best therefore to take the doses at evenly spaced intervals, day and night. For example, if you are to take four doses a day, the doses should be spaced six hours apart.

If you miss a dose of this medication, take the missed dose immediately. However, if you do not remember to take the missed dose until it is almost time for your next dose, take it; space the next dose halfway through the regular interval between doses. Then return to your regular dosing schedule. Try not to skip any doses.

It is important to continue to take this medication for

the entire time prescribed by your doctor (usually seven to 14 days), even if the symptoms of the infection disappear before the end of that period. If you stop taking the drug too soon, resistant bacteria are given the chance to continue growing, and the infection could recur.

SIDE EFFECTS

Minor. Diarrhea; heartburn; nausea; and vomiting. These side effects should disappear in several days, as your body adjusts to the medication.

Major. Tell your doctor about any side effects that are persistent or particularly bothersome. IT IS ESPECIALLY IMPORTANT TO TELL YOUR DOCTOR about bloating; chills; cough; difficulty breathing; fever; irritation of the mouth; muscle aches; rash; rectal or vaginal itching; severe diarrhea; sore throat; or darkened tongue. Also, if your symptoms of infection seem to be getting worse rather than improving, you should contact your doctor.

INTERACTIONS

Cyclacillin interacts with other types of medication.

1. Probenecid can increase the blood concentrations of this medication.

2. Cyclacillin may decrease the effectiveness of oral contraceptives (birth control pills), and pregnancy could result. You should therefore use another form of birth control while taking this medication. Discuss this with your doctor.

TELL YOUR DOCTOR if you are already taking either of the medications listed above.

WARNINGS

• Tell your doctor about unusual or allergic reactions you have had to any medications, especially to cyclacillin or penicillins, or to cephalosporin antibiotics, penicillamine, or griseofulvin.

• Tell your doctor if you now have, or if you have ever had, kidney disease, asthma, or allergies.

• This medication has been prescribed for your current infection only. Another infection later on, or one that someone else has, may require a different medicine. You should not give your medication to other people, or use it for other infections, unless your doctor specifically directs you to do so.

• Diabetics taking cyclacillin should know that this drug can cause a false-positive sugar reaction with a Clinitest urine glucose test. To avoid this problem, while taking cyclacillin you should switch to Clinistix or Tes-Tape to test your urine sugar.

• Be sure to tell your doctor if you are pregnant. Although cyclacillin appears to be safe during pregnancy, extensive studies in humans have not yet been completed. Also, tell your doctor if you are breastfeeding an infant. Small amounts of this medication pass into breast milk and may temporarily alter the bacteria in the intestinal tract of the nursing infant, resulting in diarrhea.

Cyclan—see cyclandelate

---

cyclandelate

BRAND NAMES (Manufacturers)
Cyclan (Major)
cyclandelate (various manufacturers)
Cyclospasmol (Ives)
Cydel (Hauck)
TYPE OF DRUG
Vasodilator
INGREDIENT
cyclandelate
DOSAGE FORMS
Tablets (100 mg)
Capsules (200 mg and 400 mg)
STORAGE
Cyclandelate should be stored at room temperature in tightly closed containers.

USES
Cyclandelate is used to treat vascular (blood vessel) disease in the legs or brain. It acts directly on the muscle of the blood vessels to increase the blood supply to various parts of the body.

TREATMENT

You can take cyclandelate on an empty stomach (unless your doctor gives you different instructions). However, if the drug causes stomach irritation, ask your doctor if you may take it with food, milk, or antacids.

If you miss a dose of this medication, take the missed dose as soon as possible, unless it is almost time for the next dose. In that case, do not take the missed dose at all; just return to your regular dosing schedule. Do not double the next dose.

SIDE EFFECTS

Minor. Dizziness; drowsiness; flushing; headache; heartburn; stomach distress; and sweating. These side effects should disappear in several days, as your body adjusts to the medication.

If you feel dizzy, sit or lie down awhile; get up slowly, and be careful on stairs.

Major. Tell your doctor about any side effects that are persistent or particularly bothersome. IT IS ESPECIALLY IMPORTANT TO TELL YOUR DOCTOR about palpitations; skin rash; tingling in the hands or feet; or weakness.

INTERACTIONS

Cyclandelate does not interact with other medications, if it is used according to directions.

WARNINGS

• Tell your doctor about unusual or allergic reactions you have had to any medications, especially to cyclandelate.

• Before starting to take this medication, tell your doctor if you now have, or if you have ever had, angina, bleeding disorders, glaucoma, or a recent heart attack.

• A government panel has recently reviewed the effectiveness of this medication in the treatment of leg cramps or hardening of the arteries, and in the prevention of stroke. This drug may not be as effective as once thought. Discuss this with your doctor.

• Before taking any over-the-counter (non-prescription) cough, cold, allergy, asthma, sinus, or diet medication, check with your doctor or pharmacist. Some of these products can decrease the effectiveness of cyclandelate.

• If this drug makes you dizzy or drowsy, do not take part in any activity that requires alertness, such as driving a car or operating potentially dangerous equipment.

• The beneficial effects of this medication may be decreased by the nicotine in cigarettes. Try to stop smoking.

• To prevent dizziness and fainting while taking this medication, avoid getting overheated (strenuous exercise in hot weather; hot baths, showers, and saunas).

• Be sure to tell your doctor if you are pregnant. Although cyclandelate appears to be safe during pregnancy, extensive studies in humans have not yet been completed. Also, tell your doctor if you are breastfeeding an infant. It is not known whether or not cyclandelate passes into breast milk.

Cyclapen-W — see cyclacillin

Cycline-250 — see tetracycline

cyclobenzaprine

BRAND NAME (Manufacturer)
Flexeril (Merck Sharp & Dohme)
TYPE OF DRUG
Muscle relaxant
INGREDIENT
cyclobenzaprine as the hydrochloride salt
DOSAGE FORM
Tablets (10 mg)
STORAGE
Cyclobenzaprine tablets should be stored at room temperature in a tightly closed container.

USES

Cyclobenzaprine is prescribed to relieve muscle pain and stiffness caused by injuries such as sprains or strains. It is not clear how this drug works, but it is thought to act as a central nervous system (brain and spinal cord) depressant that blocks reflexes involved in producing and maintaining muscle spasms. It does not act directly on tense muscles.

TREATMENT

In order to avoid stomach irritation, you can take cyclo-benzaprine with food or with a full glass of water or milk.

If you miss a dose of this medication and remember within an hour, take the missed dose; then return to your regular dosing schedule. If it has been longer than an hour, don't take the missed dose at all; just return to your dosing schedule. Do not double the next dose.

SIDE EFFECTS

Minor. Abdominal pain; black tongue; blurred vision; constipation; dizziness; drowsiness; dry mouth; fatigue; indigestion; insomnia; muscle pain; nausea; nervous-ness; sweating; unpleasant taste in the mouth; and weak-ness. These side effects should disappear in several days, as your body adjusts to the medication.

If you are constipated, increase the amount of fiber in your diet (fresh fruits and vegetables, salads, bran, and whole-grain breads), and drink more water (unless your doctor directs you to do otherwise).

If you feel dizzy or light-headed, sit or lie down awhile; get up slowly, and be careful on stairs.

To relieve mouth dryness, suck on ice chips or a piece of hard candy, or chew sugarless gum.

Major. Tell your doctor about any side effects that are persistent or particularly bothersome. IT IS ESPECIALLY IMPORTANT TO TELL YOUR DOCTOR about confu-sion; depression; difficulty urinating; disorientation; hal-lucinations; headache; itching; numbness in the fingers or toes; palpitations; rash; swelling of the face or tongue; or tremors.

INTERACTIONS

Cyclobenzaprine interacts with several other types of medication.

1. Concurrent use of cyclobenzaprine with other central nervous system depressants (drugs that slow the activity of the nervous system), such as alcohol, antihistamines, barbiturates, benzodiazepine tranquilizers, narcotics, pain medications, phenothiazine tranquilizers, and sleeping medications, or with tricyclic anti-depressants can cause extreme drowsiness.

2. Cyclobenzaprine can block the blood-pressure-lowering effects of clonidine and guanethidine.

3. Use of this drug within 14 days of a monoamine oxidase (MAO) inhibitor can lead to severe reactions and high blood pressure.

Before starting to take this medication, BE SURE TO TELL YOUR DOCTOR if you are already taking any of the medications listed above.

WARNINGS

• Tell your doctor about unusual or allergic reactions you have had to medications, especially to cyclobenzaprine or to tricyclic anti-depressants (such as amitriptyline, imipramine, desipramine, or nortriptyline).

• Tell your doctor if you now have, or if you have ever had, blood clots, epilepsy, heart disease, a recent heart attack, narrow-angle glaucoma, thyroid disease, or urinary retention.

• Use of cyclobenzaprine for periods longer than two to three weeks is not recommended, because there is no evidence of benefit with prolonged use, and because muscle spasm due to sprain or strain is generally of short duration.

• This medication should not be taken as a substitute for rest, physical therapy, or other measures recommended by your doctor to treat your condition.

• If this medication makes you dizzy or drowsy, or blurs your vision, do not take part in any activity that requires alertness, such as driving a car or operating potentially dangerous equipment.

• If you have been taking large doses of this medication for prolonged periods, you may experience nausea, headache, or fatigue when you stop taking it, as your body adjusts to the drug being removed.

• Be sure to tell your doctor if you are pregnant. Although cyclobenzaprine appears to be safe during pregnancy, extensive studies in humans have not yet been completed. Also, tell your doctor if you are breastfeeding an infant. It is not known whether or not cyclobenzaprine passes into breast milk.

Cyclopar—see tetracycline

cyclophosphamide

BRAND NAME (Manufacturer)
Cytoxan (Mead Johnson)
TYPE OF DRUG
Anti-neoplastic (anti-cancer drug)
INGREDIENT
cyclophosphamide
DOSAGE FORM
Tablets (25 mg and 50 mg)
STORAGE
Cyclophosphamide should be stored at room temperature, in a tightly closed container.

USES

Cyclophosphamide belongs to a group of drugs known as alkylating agents or nitrogen mustards. It is used to treat a variety of cancers. Cyclophosphamide works by binding to the rapidly growing cancer cells, preventing their multiplication and growth. This drug has also been used as an immunosuppressant, to treat severe rheumatoid arthritis.

TREATMENT

In order to obtain maximum benefit, you should take cyclophosphamide on an empty stomach. However, if stomach upset occurs, you can take it with food or milk (unless your doctor directs you to do otherwise).

The timing of the doses of this anti-cancer medication is important. Be sure you completely understand your doctor's instructions on how and when this medication should be taken. Try not to miss any doses.

If you miss a dose of this medication, do not take the missed dose at all; just return to your regular dosing schedule. Do not double the next dose.

SIDE EFFECTS

Minor. Diarrhea; loss of appetite; nausea; and vomiting. These side effects may disappear as your body adjusts to the medication. However, it is important to continue taking this medication despite the nausea and vomiting that may occur. Cyclophosphamide also causes hair loss, which is reversible when the medication is stopped.

Major. Tell your doctor about any side effects that are persistent or particularly bothersome. IT IS ESPECIALLY IMPORTANT TO TELL YOUR DOCTOR about unusual bleeding or bruising; chills; cough; darkening of the skin or fingernails; difficult or painful urination; fever; menstrual irregularities; mouth sores; sore throat; blood in the urine; or yellowing of the eyes or skin.

INTERACTIONS

Cyclophosphamide interacts with several other types of medication.

1. It can decrease the absorption of digoxin from the gastrointestinal tract.

2. Phenobarbital can increase the side effects of cyclophosphamide.

3. Concurrent use of allopurinol, chloramphenicol, or thiazide diuretics (water pills) with cyclophosphamide can lead to bone marrow toxicity.

Before starting to take this medication, BE SURE TO TELL YOUR DOCTOR if you are already taking any of the medications listed above.

WARNINGS

• Tell your doctor about unusual or allergic reactions you have had to any medication, especially to cyclophosphamide.

• Before starting to take this medication, be sure to tell your doctor if you now have, or if you have ever had, blood disorders, chronic or recurrent infections, gout, kidney disease, or liver disease.

• Before having any surgery or other medical or dental treatment, be sure your doctor or dentist knows that you are taking this medication.

• Cyclophosphamide tablets contain F.D. & C. Yellow Dye No. 5 (tartrazine), which can cause allergic-type symptoms (fainting, shortness of breath, rash) in certain susceptible individuals.

• You should not receive any immunizations or vaccinations while taking this medication. Cyclophosphamide decreases the effectiveness of the vaccine, and may result in an infection.

• It is important to drink plenty of fluids (3 quarts each

day) while taking this medication. If the drug is allowed to concentrate in the bladder, it could cause hemorrhaging and bloody urine.

• This medication can lower your platelet count, which can decrease your body's ability to form blood clots. You should therefore be especially careful while brushing your teeth, flossing, or using toothpicks, razors, or fingernail scissors. Try to avoid falls and other injuries.

• Cyclophosphamide can decrease fertility in both men and women.

• Be sure to tell your doctor if you are pregnant. Birth defects have been reported in both humans and animals whose mothers received cyclophosphamide during pregnancy. The risks should be discussed with your doctor. Also, tell your doctor if you are breastfeeding an infant. Small amounts of cycloposphamide pass into breast milk.

Cyclospasmol—see cyclandelate

---

cyclosporine

BRAND NAME (Manufacturer)
Sandimmune (Sandoz)
TYPE OF DRUG
Immunosuppressant
INGREDIENT
cyclosporine
DOSAGE FORM
Oral solution (100 mg per ml)
STORAGE
Cyclosporine oral solution should be stored in the original container at room temperature. This medication should never be refrigerated or frozen. Once the container has been opened, the contents should be used within two months.

USES

Cyclosporine is used to prevent organ rejection after kidney, liver, and heart transplants. It is not clearly understood how cyclosporine works, but it appears to prevent the body's rejection of foreign tissue.

TREATMENT

To make cyclosporine more palatable, the oral solution should be diluted with milk, chocolate milk, or orange juice (preferably at room temperature). The dose should be taken from the container with the dropper provided and placed in a glass container of one of the fluids listed above. Stir well and drink at once—do not allow the medication mixture to stand before drinking. After the solution is drunk, the glass should be refilled with the same beverage, and this solution swallowed as well. This assures that the whole dose is taken. It is best to use a glass container (cyclosporine chemically binds to the surfaces of a plastic cup).

It is important not to miss any doses of this medication. If you do miss a dose, take the missed dose as soon as possible, unless it is almost time for the next dose. In that case, do not take the missed dose at all; just return to your regular dosing schedule. Do not double the next dose.

SIDE EFFECTS

Minor. Abdominal discomfort; diarrhea; flushing; headache; hiccups; loss of appetite; nausea; and vomiting. These side effects should disappear in several days, as your body adjusts to the medication.

Major. Tell your doctor about any side effects that are persistent or particularly bothersome. IT IS ESPECIALLY IMPORTANT TO TELL YOUR DOCTOR about acne; unusual bleeding or bruising; convulsions; difficult or painful urination; enlarged and painful breasts (in both sexes); enlarged gums; fever; hair growth; hearing loss; muscle pain; rapid weight gain (three to five pounds within a week); tremors; tingling of the hands or feet; or yellowing of the eyes or skin.

INTERACTIONS

Cyclosporine interacts with several other medications.
1. Rifampin, phenytoin, phenobarbital, and co-trimoxazole can decrease the blood levels of cyclosporine, decreasing its effectiveness.
2. Cimetidine, ketoconazole, and amphotericin B can

increase the blood levels of cyclosporine, which can lead
to an increase in side effects.
BE SURE TO TELL YOUR DOCTOR if you are already
taking any of the medications listed above

WARNINGS
- Tell your doctor about unusual or allergic reactions you
have had to any medications, especially to cyclosporine.
- Before starting to take this medication, be sure to tell
your doctor if you now have, or if you have ever had,
hypertension (high blood pressure) or gastrointestinal
disorders.
- Repeated laboratory tests are necessary while you are
taking cyclosporine, to assure that you are receiving the
correct dose, and to avoid liver and kidney damage.
- Certain cancers have occurred in patients receiving
cyclosporine and other immunosuppressant drugs after
transplantation. No causal effect has been established,
however.
- Do not stop taking this medication without first consulting your doctor. If the drug is stopped abruptly, organ
rejection may occur. Your doctor may therefore want to
reduce your dosage gradually or start you on another
drug if treatment with this drug is to be discontinued.
- Be sure to tell your doctor if you are pregnant. Although
cyclosporine appears to be safe during pregnancy, extensive studies in humans have not yet been completed.
Also, tell your doctor if you are breastfeeding an infant.
Cyclosporine passes into breast milk.

---

cyclothiazide

BRAND NAMES (Manufacturers)
Anhydron (Lilly)
Fluidil (Adria)
TYPE OF DRUG
Diuretic (water pill) and anti-hypertensive
INGREDIENT
cyclothiazide
DOSAGE FORM
Tablets (2 mg)

STORAGE

This medication should be stored at room temperature in a tightly closed container..

USES

Cyclothiazide is prescribed to treat high blood pressure. It is also used to reduce fluid accumulation in the body caused by conditions such as heart failure, cirrhosis of the liver, kidney disease, and the long-term use of some medications. This medication reduces fluid accumulation by increasing the elimination of sodium and water through the kidneys.

TREATMENT

To decrease stomach irritation, you can take cyclothiazide with a glass of milk or with a meal (unless your doctor directs you to do otherwise). Try to take it at the same time every day. Avoid taking a dose after 6:00 P.M.—this will prevent you from having to get up during the night to urinate.

If you miss a dose of this medication, take the missed dose as soon as possible, unless it is almost time for the next dose. In that case, do not take the missed dose at all; just wait until the next scheduled dose. Do not double the dose.

This medication does not cure high blood pressure, but it will help to control the condition, as long as you continue to take it.

SIDE EFFECTS

Minor. Constipation; cramps; diarrhea; dizziness; drowsiness; headache; heartburn; itching; loss of appetite; nausea; restlessness; upset stomach; vomiting. As your body adjusts to the medication, these side effects should disappear

This medication can cause increased sensitivity to sunlight. It is therefore important to avoid prolonged exposure to sunlight or sunlamps. Wear protective clothing, and use an effective sunscreen.

To avoid dizziness or light-headedness when you stand, contract and relax the muscles of your legs for a few moments before rising. Do this by pushing one foot

against the floor while raising the other foot slightly, alternating the feet so that you are "pumping" your legs in a pedaling motion.

Major. Tell your doctor about any side effects that are persistent or particularly bothersome. IT IS ESPECIALLY IMPORTANT TO TELL YOUR DOCTOR about unusual bleeding or bruising; blurred vision; confusion; difficulty breathing; dry mouth; fever; joint pain; mood changes; muscle spasms; palpitations; skin rash; excessive thirst; sore throat; tingling in the fingers or toes; excessive weakness; or yellowing of the eyes or skin.

INTERACTIONS

Cyclothiazide interacts with several other types of medication.

1. It may decrease the effectiveness of oral anticoagulants, anti-gout medications, insulin, oral antidiabetic medicines, and methenamine.

2. Fenfluramine can increase the blood-pressure-lowering effects of cyclothiazide (which can be dangerous).

3. Indomethacin can decrease the blood-pressure-lowering effects (thereby counteracting the desired effects) of cyclothiazide.

4. Cholestyramine and colestipol decrease the absorption of this medication from the gastrointestinal tract. Cyclothiazide should therefore be taken one hour before, or four hours after, a dose of cholestyramine or colestipol (if you have also been prescribed one of these medications).

5. The side effects of amphotericin B, calcium, cortisone-like steroids (such as cortisone, dexamethasone, hydrocortisone, prednisone, prednisolone), digoxin, digitalis, lithium, quinidine, sulfonamide antibiotics, and vitamin D may be increased when taken concurrently with cyclothiazide.

Before taking cyclothiazide, BE SURE TO TELL YOUR DOCTOR if you are taking any of the medicines listed above.

WARNINGS

• Tell your doctor about unusual or allergic reactions you have had to any medications, especially to diuretics (water pills), oral anti-diabetic medications, or sulfonamide antibiotics.

• Before you start taking cyclothiazide, tell your doctor if you now have, or if you have ever had, kidney disease or problems with urination, diabetes mellitus (sugar diabetes), gout, liver disease, asthma, pancreas disease, or systemic lupus erythematosus (SLE).

• Cyclothiazide can cause potassium loss. Signs of potassium loss include dry mouth, thirst, weakness, muscle pain or cramps, nausea, and vomiting. If you experience any of these symptoms, call your doctor. To help avoid potassium loss, take this drug with a glass of fresh or frozen orange or cranberry juice, or eat a banana every day. The use of a salt substitute also helps to prevent potassium loss. Do not change your diet, however, before discussing it with your doctor. Too much potassium can also be dangerous. Your doctor may want to have blood tests performed periodically, in order to monitor your potassium levels.

• Limit your intake of alcoholic beverages while taking this medication, in order to prevent dizziness and lightheadedness.

• If you have high blood pressure, do not take any over-the-counter (non-prescription) medications for weight control or for cough, cold, allergy, asthma, or sinus problems, unless your doctor directs you to do so.

• To prevent dehydration (severe water loss) while taking this medication, check with your doctor if you have any illness that causes severe or continuous nausea, vomiting, or diarrhea.

• This medication can raise blood sugar in diabetic patients. Therefore, blood sugar levels should be carefully monitored by blood or urine tests when this medication is started.

• Be sure to tell your doctor if you are pregnant. Although studies in humans have not yet been completed, adverse effects have been observed on the fetuses of animals who were given large doses of this drug during pregnancy. Also, tell your doctor if you are breastfeeding an infant. Although problems in humans have not been reported, small amounts of this drug can pass into breast milk, so caution is warranted.

Cydel—see cyclandelate

Cylert—see pemoline

---

cyproheptadine

BRAND NAMES (Manufacturers)
cyproheptadine hydrochloride (various manufacturers)
Periactin (Merck Sharp & Dohme)
TYPE OF DRUG
Antihistamine
INGREDIENT
cyproheptadine as the hydrochloride salt
DOSAGE FORMS
Tablets (4 mg)
Oral syrup (2 mg per 5 ml teaspoonful)
STORAGE
Cyproheptadine tablets and oral syrup should be stored at
room temperature in tightly closed containers.

USES

This medication belongs to a group of drugs known as
antihistamines (antihistamines block the action of histamine, a chemical that is released by the body during an
allergic reaction). It is therefore used to treat or prevent
symptoms of allergy.

TREATMENT

To avoid stomach upset, you can take cyproheptadine
with food or with a full glass of milk or water (unless your
doctor directs you to do otherwise).

The oral syrup form of this medication should be measured carefully, with a specially designed, 5 ml measuring
spoon. An ordinary kitchen teaspoon is not accurate
enough.

If you miss a dose of this medication, take the missed
dose as soon as possible, unless it is almost time for your
next dose. In that case, don't take the missed dose at all;
just return to your regular dosing schedule. Do not double
the next dose.

SIDE EFFECTS

Minor. Blurred vision; confusion; constipation; diarrhea; difficult or painful urination; dizziness; dry mouth, throat, or nose; headache; irritability; loss of appetite; nausea; restlessness; ringing or buzzing in the ears; rash; stomach upset; and unusual increase in sweating. These side effects should disappear in several days, as your body adjusts to the medication.

If you are constipated, increase the amount of fiber in your diet (raw vegetables, fruits, salads, bran, and whole-grain breads), and drink more water (unless your doctor directs you not to do so).

Chew sugarless gum, or suck on ice chips or a piece of hard candy, to reduce mouth dryness.

This medication can cause increased sensitivity to sunlight. It is therefore important to avoid prolonged exposure to sunlight and sunlamps. Wear protective clothing, and use an effective sunscreen.

If you feel dizzy or light-headed, sit or lie down awhile; get up from a sitting or lying position slowly, and be careful on stairs.

Major. Tell your doctor about any side effects that are persistent or particularly bothersome. IT IS ESPECIALLY IMPORTANT TO TELL YOUR DOCTOR about unusual bleeding or bruising; change in menstruation; clumsiness; feeling faint; flushing of the face; hallucinations; seizures; shortness of breath; sleeping disorders; sore throat or fever; palpitations; tightness in the chest; or unusual tiredness or weakness.

INTERACTIONS

Cyproheptadine interacts with several other types of medication.

1. Concurrent use of this medication with other central nervous system depressants (drugs that slow the activity of the nervous system), such as barbiturates, benzodiazepine tranquilizers, muscle relaxants, narcotics, pain medications, phenothiazine tranquilizers, and alcohol, or with tricyclic anti-depressants can cause extreme drowsiness.

2. Monoamine oxidase (MAO) inhibitors (such as isocarboxazid, pargyline, phenelzine, tranylcypromine) can increase the side effects of this medication.

3. Cyproheptadine can also decrease the activity of oral anti-coagulants (blood thinners, such as warfarin).

TELL YOUR DOCTOR if you are already taking any of the medications listed above.

WARNINGS

• Tell your doctor about unusual or allergic reactions you have had to any medications, especially to cyproheptadine or to other antihistamines (such as bromodiphenhydramine, brompheniramine, carbinoxamine, chlorpheniramine, clemastine, azatadine, dexchlorpheniramine, dimenhydrinate, dimethindene, diphenhydramine, diphenylpyraline, doxylamine, hydroxyzine, promethazine, pyrilamine, trimeprazine, tripelennamine, or tripolidine).

• Tell your doctor if you now have, or if you have ever had, asthma, blood vessel disease, glaucoma, high blood pressure, kidney disease, peptic ulcers, enlarged prostate gland, or thyroid disease.

• Cyproheptadine can cause drowsiness or dizziness. Your ability to perform tasks that require alertness, such as driving a car or operating potentially dangerous machinery, may be decreased. Appropriate caution should therefore be taken.

• Be sure to tell your doctor if you are pregnant. The effects of this medication during pregnancy have not yet been thoroughly studied in humans. Also, tell your doctor if you are breastfeeding an infant. Small amounts of cyproheptadine pass into breast milk and may cause unusual excitement or irritability in nursing infants.

cyproheptadine hydrochloride—see cyproheptadine

Cytomel—see liothyronine

Cytoxan—see cyclophosphamide

Dalmane—see flurazepam

Dantrium—see dantrolene

dantrolene

BRAND NAME (Manufacturer)
Dantrium (Norwich-Eaton)
TYPE OF DRUG
Muscle relaxant
INGREDIENT
dantrolene as the sodium salt
DOSAGE FORM
Capsules (25 mg, 50 mg, and 100 mg)
STORAGE
Dantrolene should be stored at room temperature in a tightly closed container.

USES

This medication is used to relieve the spasticity caused by spinal cord injury, stroke, cerebral palsy, or multiple sclerosis. It works directly on muscles to prevent contraction. Dantrolene is also used prior to anesthesia to prevent malignant hyperthermia in patients known or suspected to be at risk for developing this complication.

TREATMENT

You can take dantrolene either on an empty stomach or with food or milk (as directed by your doctor). If you are unable to swallow the capsule, you can open it and mix the contents with fruit juice or other non-alcoholic beverage. You should then take the dose immediately.

If you miss a dose of this medication and remember within an hour of the scheduled time, take the missed dose immediately. If more than an hour has passed, do not take the missed dose at all; just return to your regular dosing schedule. Do not double the next dose.

SIDE EFFECTS

Minor. Abnormal hair growth; alteration of taste; constipation; diarrhea; dizziness; drowsiness; fatigue; headache; insomnia; loss of appetite; stomach upset; and excessive tearing. These side effects should disappear in several weeks, as your body adjusts to the medication.

To relieve constipation, increase the amount of fiber in your diet (bran, salads, fresh fruits and vegetables, and whole-grain breads), and drink more water (unless your doctor directs you to do otherwise).

If you feel dizzy, sit or lie down awhile; get up slowly, and be careful on stairs.

This medication can increase your sensitivity to sunlight. You should therefore try to avoid prolonged exposure to sunlight and sunlamps. Wear protective clothing and sunglasses, and use an effective sunscreen.

Major. Tell your doctor about any side effects that are persistent or particularly bothersome. IT IS ESPECIALLY IMPORTANT TO TELL YOUR DOCTOR about backaches; bloody or black, tarry stools; blurred vision; chills; confusion; convulsions; depression; difficult or painful urination; difficulty breathing; difficulty swallowing; feeling of suffocation; fever; increased urination; muscle pain; nervousness; palpitations; skin rash; speech disturbances; unusual weakness; or yellowing of the eyes or skin.

INTERACTIONS

Dantrolene interacts with a number of other medications.

1. Concurrent use of dantrolene with central nervous system depressants (drugs that slow the activity of the brain and spinal cord), such as alcohol, antihistamines, barbiturates, benzodiazepine tranquilizers, muscle relaxants, narcotics, pain medications, phenothiazine tranquilizers, and sleeping medications, or with tricyclic anti-depressants can lead to extreme drowsiness.

2. The use of dantrolene in combination with estrogen by women over 35 years of age can increase their risk of liver damage.

BE SURE TO TELL YOUR DOCTOR if you are already taking any of these medications.

WARNINGS

• Tell your doctor about unusual or allergic reactions you have had to any medications, especially to dantrolene.

• Before starting to take this medication, be sure to tell your doctor if you now have, or if you have ever had, heart disease, liver disease, or lung disease.

• If this drug makes you dizzy or drowsy, or blurs your

vision, do not take part in any activities that require alertness, such as driving a car or operating potentially dangerous equipment.

• An increased risk of benign and malignant cancers has been observed in some experimental animals who received large doses of dantrolene. This increase has not yet been observed in humans, but the risks should be discussed with your doctor.

• Be sure to tell your doctor if you are pregnant. Although dantrolene appears to be safe during pregnancy, extensive studies in humans have not yet been completed. Also, tell your doctor if you are breastfeeding an infant. It is not known whether or not dantrolene passes into breast milk.

Darvocet-N—see acetaminophen and propoxyphene combination

Darvon—see propoxyphene

Darvon Compound-65—see aspirin, caffeine, and propoxyphene combination

Darvon-N—see propoxyphene

Deapril-ST—see ergoloid mesylates

Decadron—see dexamethasone (systemic)

Deconade—see phenylpropanolamine and chlorpheniramine combination

Deconamine—see pseudoephedrine and chlorpheniramine combination

Deconamine SR—see pseudoephedrine and chlorpheniramine combination

Decongestabs—see phenylpropanolamine, phenylephrine, chlorpheniramine, and phenyltoloxamine combination

Delapav — see papaverine

Delaxin — see methocarbamol

Delta-Cortef — see prednisolone (systemic)

Delta-E — see erythromycin

Deltalin Gelseals — see ergocalciferol (vitamin D)

Deltamycin — see tetracycline

Deltapen-VK — see penicillin VK

Deltasone — see prednisone (systemic)

Demerol — see meperidine

Demulen — see oral contraceptives

Depakene — see valproic acid

Depakote — see valproic acid

Depen Titratabs — see penicillamine

Depletite-25 — see diethylpropion

Dermacort — see hydrocortisone (topical)

Dermtex HC — see hydrocortisone (topical)

DES — see diethylstilbestrol

---

desipramine

BRAND NAMES (Manufacturers)
Norpramin (Merrell Dow)
Pertofrane (USV)
TYPE OF DRUG
Tricyclic anti-depressant (mood elevator)

INGREDIENT
desipramine as the hydrochloride salt
DOSAGE FORM
Capsules (10 mg, 25 mg, 50 mg, 75 mg, 100 mg, and
150 mg)
STORAGE
This medication should be stored at room temperature in
a tightly closed container.

USES

Desipramine is used to relieve the symptoms of mental
depression. This medication belongs to a group of drugs
referred to as the tricyclic anti-depressants. These
medicines are thought to relieve depression by increasing
the concentration of certain chemicals necessary for
nerve transmission in the brain.

TREATMENT

This medication should be taken exactly as your doctor
prescribes. You can take it with water or with food to
lessen the chance of stomach irritation, unless your doctor tells you to do otherwise.

If you miss a dose of this medication, take the missed
dose as soon as possible, then return to your regular dosing schedule. If, however, the dose you missed was a
once-a-day bedtime dose, do not take that dose in the
morning; check with your doctor instead. If the dose is
taken in the morning, it may cause some unwanted side
effects. Never double the dose.

The effects of therapy with this medication may not
become apparent for two or three weeks.

SIDE EFFECTS

Minor. Agitation; anxiety; blurred vision; confusion;
constipation; cramps; diarrhea; dizziness; drowsiness;
dry mouth; fatigue; heartburn; insomnia; loss of appetite;
nausea; peculiar tastes in the mouth; restlessness; sweating; vomiting; weakness; or weight gain or loss. As your
body adjusts to the medication, these side effects should
disappear.

Dry mouth can be relieved by chewing sugarless gum
or by sucking on ice chips or a piece of hard candy.

To relieve constipation, increase the amount of fiber (bran, salads, whole-grain breads, fresh fruits and vegetables) in your diet, and drink more water (unless your doctor directs you to do otherwise).

To avoid dizziness or light-headedness when you stand, contract and relax the muscles of your legs for a few moments before rising. Do this by pushing one foot against the floor while raising the other foot slightly, alternating feet so that you are "pumping" your legs in a pedaling motion.

This medication may cause increased sensitivity to sunlight. You should therefore avoid prolonged exposure to sunlight and sunlamps. Wear protective clothing, and use an effective sunscreen.

Major. Tell your doctor about any side effects that are persistent or particularly bothersome. IT IS ESPECIALLY IMPORTANT TO TELL YOUR DOCTOR about unusual bleeding or bruising; chest pain; convulsions; difficulty urinating; enlarged or painful breasts (in both sexes); fainting; fever; fluid retention; hair loss; hallucinations; headaches; impotence; mood changes; mouth sores; nervousness; nightmares; nosebleeds; numbness in the fingers or toes; palpitations; ringing in the ears; seizures; skin rash; sleep disorders; sore throat; tremors; uncoordinated movements or balance problems; or yellowing of the eyes or skin.

INTERACTIONS

Desipramine interacts with a number of other types of medication.

1. Extreme drowsiness can occur when this medicine is taken with central nervous system depressants (medicines that slow the activity of the nervous system), including alcohol, antihistamines, barbiturates, benzodiazepine tranquilizers, muscle relaxants, narcotics, pain medications, phenothiazine tranquilizers, and sleeping medications.

2. Desipramine may decrease the effectiveness of anti-seizure medications.

3. It may block the blood-pressure-lowering effects of clonidine and guanethidine.

4. Oral contraceptives (estrogens) can increase the side effects and reduce the effectiveness of the tricyclic anti-depressants (including desipramine).

5. Tricyclic anti-depressants may increase the side effects of thyroid medication and of over-the-counter (non-prescription) cough, cold, allergy, asthma, sinus, and diet medications.

6. The concurrent use of tricyclic anti-depressants and monoamine oxidase (MAO) inhibitors should be undertaken very carefully, because the combination may result in fever, convulsions, or high blood pressure.

Before starting to take desipramine, BE SURE TO TELL YOUR DOCTOR if you are already taking any of the medications listed above.

WARNINGS

• Tell your doctor if you have had unusual or allergic reactions to medications, especially to desipramine or any of the other tricyclic anti-depressants (such as amitriptyline, imipramine, doxepin, trimipramine, amoxapine, protriptyline, maprotiline, or nortriptyline).

• Tell your doctor if you now have, or if you have ever had, asthma, high blood pressure, liver or kidney disease, heart disease, a recent heart attack, circulatory disease, stomach problems, intestinal problems, alcoholism, difficulty urinating, enlarged prostate gland, epilepsy, glaucoma, thyroid disease, mental illness, or electroshock therapy.

• If this drug makes you dizzy or drowsy, do not take part in any activity that requires alertness, such as driving a car or operating potentially dangerous equipment.

• Before having any surgery or other medical or dental treatment, be sure to tell your doctor or dentist that you are taking this medication.

• Do not stop taking this drug suddenly. Abruptly stopping it can cause nausea, headache, stomach upset, fatigue, or a worsening of your condition. Your doctor may want to reduce the dosage gradually.

• The effects of this medication may last as long as seven days after you have stopped taking it, so continue to observe all precautions during that period.

• Be sure to tell your doctor if you are pregnant. Problems in humans have not been reported; however, studies in animals have shown that this medication can cause side effects to the fetus when given to the mother in large doses during pregnancy. Also, tell your doctor if you are breastfeeding an infant. Small amounts of this drug can pass into the breast milk, which may cause unwanted effects, such as irritability or sleeping problems, in the nursing infant.

Desoxyn — see methamphetamine

Desoxyn Gradumets — see methamphetamine

Desyrel — see trazodone

Dexameth — see dexamethasone (systemic)

---

dexamethasone (systemic)

BRAND NAMES (Manufacturers)
Decadron (Merck Sharp & Dohme)
Dexameth (Major)
dexamethasone (various manufacturers)
Dexone (Rowell)
Hexadrol (Organon)
SK-Dexamethasone (Smith Kline & French)
TYPE OF DRUG
Adrenocorticosteroid hormone
INGREDIENT
dexamethasone
DOSAGE FORMS
Tablets (0.25 mg, 0.5 mg, 0.75 mg, 1.5 mg, 2 mg, 4 mg, and 6 mg)
Oral elixir (0.5 mg per 5 ml teaspoonful with 5% alcohol)
STORAGE
Dexamethasone tablets and oral elixir should be stored at room temperature in tightly closed containers.

USES
Your adrenal glands naturally produce certain cortisone-like chemicals. These chemicals are involved in various regulatory processes in the body (such as maintenance of

fluid balance, temperature, and reactions to inflammation). Dexamethasone belongs to a group of drugs known as adrenocorticosteroids (or cortisone-like medications). It is used to treat a variety of disorders, including endocrine and rheumatic disorders; asthma; blood diseases; certain cancers; eye disorders; gastrointestinal disturbances such as ulcerative colitis; respiratory diseases; and inflammations such as arthritis, dermatitis, and poison ivy. How this drug acts to relieve these disorders is not completely understood.

TREATMENT

In order to prevent stomach irritation, you can take dexamethasone with food or milk.

If you are taking only one dose of this medication each day, try to take it before 9 A.M. This will mimic the body's normal production of this type of chemical.

The oral elixir form of this medication should be measured carefully, with a specially designed, 5 ml measuring spoon. A kitchen teaspoon is not accurate enough.

It is important to try not to miss any doses of dexamethasone. However, if you do miss a dose of this medication:

1. If you are taking it more than once a day, take the missed dose as soon as possible and return to your regular schedule. If it is already time for the next dose, double the dose.

2. If you are taking this medication once a day, take the dose you missed as soon as possible, unless you don't remember until the next day. In that case do not take the missed dose at all, just follow your regular dosing schedule. Do not double the next dose.

3. If you are taking this drug every other day, take it as soon as you remember. If you missed the scheduled dose by a whole day, take it when you remember, then skip a day before you take the next dose. Do not double the dose.

If you miss more than one dose, CONTACT YOUR DOCTOR.

SIDE EFFECTS

Minor. Dizziness; false sense of well-being; increased appetite; fatigue; increased sweating; indigestion; leg cramps; menstrual irregularities; muscle weakness; nausea; reddening of the skin on the face; restlessness; sleep disorders; thinning of the skin; and weight gain These side effects should disappear in several days, as your body adjusts to the medication.

To help avoid potassium loss while using this drug, take your dose with a glass of fresh or frozen orange juice, or eat a banana each day. The use of a salt substitute also helps prevent potassium loss. Check with your doctor.

Major. Tell your doctor about any side effects that are persistent or particularly bothersome. IT IS ESPECIALLY IMPORTANT TO TELL YOUR DOCTOR about abdominal enlargement or pain; acne or other skin problems; back or rib pain; bloody or black, tarry stools; blurred vision; unusual bruising or bleeding; convulsions; eye pain; fever and sore throat; growth impairment (in children); headaches; impaired healing of wounds; increased thirst and urination; mental depression; mood changes; muscle wasting; nightmares; peptic ulcers; rapid weight gain (three to five pounds within a week); rash; shortness of breath; or unusual weakness.

INTERACTIONS

Dexamethasone interacts with other medication.

1. Alcohol, aspirin, and anti-inflammation medications (such as diflunisal, ibuprofen, indomethacin, mefenamic acid, meclofenamate, naproxen, piroxicam, sulindac, tolmetin) aggravate the stomach problems that are common with use of this medication.

2. A change in the dosage requirements of oral anticoagulants (blood thinners, such as warfarin), oral antidiabetic drugs, or insulin may be necessary when this medication is started or stopped.

3. The loss of potassium caused by this medication can lead to serious side effects in individuals taking digoxin.

4. Thiazide diuretics (water pills) can increase the potassium loss caused by dexamethasone.

5. Phenobarbital, phenytoin, rifampin, and ephedrine can increase the elimination of dexamethasone from the body, thereby decreasing its effectiveness.

6. Oral contraceptives and estrogen-containing drugs may decrease the elimination of this drug from the body, which can lead to an increase in side effects.

7. Dexamethasone can increase the elimination of aspirin and isoniazid from the body, thereby decreasing the effectiveness of these two medications.

8. Cholestyramine and colestipol can chemically bind this medication in the stomach and gastrointestinal tract, preventing its absorption.

TELL YOUR DOCTOR if you are already taking any of the medications listed above.

WARNINGS

• Tell your doctor about unusual or allergic reactions you have had to any medications, especially to dexamethasone or other adrenocorticosteroids (amcinonide, betamethasone, clocortolone, cortisone, desonide, desoximetasone, diflorasone, flumethasone, fluocinolone, fluocinonide, fluorometholone, fluprednisolone, flurandrenolide, halcinonide, hydrocortisone, methylprednisolone, paramethasone, prednisolone, prednisone, or triamcinolone).

• Tell your doctor if you now have, or if you have ever had, bone disease; diabetes mellitus (sugar diabetes); emotional instability; glaucoma; fungal infections; heart disease; high blood pressure; high cholesterol levels; myasthenia gravis; peptic ulcers; osteoporosis; thyroid disease; tuberculosis; severe ulcerative colitis; kidney disease; or liver disease.

• If you are using this medication for longer than a week, you may need to receive higher doses if you are subjected to stress, such as serious infections, injury, or surgery. Discuss this with your doctor.

• If you have been taking this drug for more than a week, do not stop taking it suddenly. If it is stopped abruptly, you may experience abdominal or back pain, dizziness, extreme weakness, fainting, fever, muscle or joint pain, nausea, vomiting, or shortness of breath. Your doctor may therefore want to reduce the dosage gradually. Never increase the dose or take the drug for longer than the prescribed time, unless you first consult your doctor.

• While you are taking this drug, you should not be vaccinated or immunized. This medication decreases the effectiveness of vaccines and can lead to overwhelming

infection if a live virus is administered.
• Before having any surgery or other medical or dental treatment, be sure your doctor or dentist knows that you are taking this medication.
• Because this drug can cause glaucoma and cataracts with long-term use, your doctor may want you to have your eyes examined by an ophthalmologist periodically during treatment.
• If you are taking this medication for prolonged periods, you should wear or carry an identification card or notice stating that you are taking an adrenocorticosteroid.
• This medication can raise blood sugar levels in diabetic patients. Blood sugar should therefore be monitored carefully with blood or urine tests when this medication is started.
• Be sure to tell your doctor if you are pregnant. This drug crosses the placenta. Although studies in humans have not yet been completed, birth defects have been observed in the fetuses of animals who were given large doses of this type of drug during pregnancy. Also, tell your doctor if you are breastfeeding an infant. Small amounts of this drug pass into breast milk and may cause growth suppression or a decrease in natural adrenocorticosteroid production in the nursing infant.

Dexampex—see dextroamphetamine

Dexbrompheniramine and Pseudoephedrine—see pseudoephedrine and dexbrompheniramine combination

Dexchlor—see dexchlorpheniramine

---

dexchlorpheniramine

BRAND NAMES (Manufacturers)
Dexchlor (Henry Schein)
Poladex T.D. (Major)
Polaramine (Schering)
TYPE OF DRUG
Antihistamine

INGREDIENT
dexchlorpheniramine as the maleate salt
DOSAGE FORMS
Tablets (2 mg)
Repeat-action tablets (4 mg and 6 mg)
Oral syrup (2 mg per 5 ml teaspoonful)
STORAGE
Dexchlorpheniramine tablets and oral syrup should be stored at room temperature in tightly closed containers.

USES

This medication belongs to a group of drugs known as antihistamines (antihistamines block the action of histamine, a chemical that is released by the body during an allergic reaction). It is therefore used to treat or prevent symptoms of allergy.

TREATMENT

To avoid stomach upset, you can take dexchlorpheniramine with food or with a full glass of milk or water (unless your doctor directs you to do otherwise).

The syrup form of this medication should be measured carefully, with a specially designed, 5 ml measuring spoon. An ordinary kitchen teaspoon is not accurate enough.

The repeat-action tablets should be swallowed whole. Breaking, chewing, or crushing these tablets destroys their sustained-release activity, and may increase the side effects.

If you miss a dose of this medication, take the missed dose as soon as possible, unless it is almost time for your next dose. In that case, don't take the missed dose at all; just return to your regular dosing schedule. Do not double the next dose.

SIDE EFFECTS

Minor. Blurred vision; confusion; constipation; diarrhea; difficult or painful urination; dizziness; dry mouth, throat, or nose; headache; irritability; loss of appetite; nausea; restlessness; ringing or buzzing in the ears; rash; stomach upset; and unusual increase in sweating. These side effects should disappear in several days, as your body adjusts to the medication.

If you are constipated, increase the amount of fiber in your diet (raw vegetables, fruits, salads, bran, and whole-grain breads), and drink more water (unless your doctor tells you not to do so).

Chew sugarless gum, or suck on ice chips or a piece of hard candy, to reduce mouth dryness.

This medication can cause increased sensitivity to sunlight. It is therefore important to avoid prolonged exposure to sunlight and sunlamps. Wear protective clothing, and use an effective sunscreen.

If you feel dizzy or light-headed, sit or lie down awhile; get up from a sitting or lying position slowly, and be careful on stairs.

Major. Tell your doctor about any side effects that are persistent or particularly bothersome. IT IS ESPECIALLY IMPORTANT TO TELL YOUR DOCTOR about changes in menstruation; clumsiness; feeling faint; flushing of the face; hallucinations; seizures; shortness of breath; sleeping disorders; sore throat or fever; palpitations; tightness in the chest; unusual bleeding or bruising; or unusual tiredness or weakness.

INTERACTIONS

Dexchlorpheniramine interacts with several other types of medication.

1. Concurrent use of it with central nervous system depressants (drugs that slow the activity of the nervous system), such as barbiturates, benzodiazepine tranquilizers, muscle relaxants, narcotics, pain medications, phenothiazine tranquilizers, and alcohol, or with tricyclic antidepressants can cause extreme drowsiness.

2. Monoamine oxidase (MAO) inhibitors (such as isocarboxazid, pargyline, phenelzine, tranylcypromine) can increase the side effects of this medication.

3. Dexchlorpheniramine can also decrease the activity of oral anti-coagulants (blood thinners, such as warfarin). TELL YOUR DOCTOR if you are already taking any of the medications listed above.

WARNINGS

• Tell your doctor about unusual or allergic reactions you

have had to any medications, especially to dexchlorpheniramine or other antihistamines (such as bromodiphenhydramine, brompheniramine, carbinoxamine,
chlorpheniramine, clemastine, cyproheptadine, azatadine, dimenhydrinate, dimethindene, diphenhydramine,
diphenylpyraline, doxylamine, hydroxyzine, promethazine, pyrilamine, trimeprazine, or tripolidine).

● Tell your doctor if you now have, or if you have ever
had, asthma, blood vessel disease, glaucoma, high blood
pressure, kidney disease, peptic ulcers, enlarged prostate
gland, or thyroid disease.

● Dexchlorpheniramine can cause drowsiness or dizziness. Your ability to perform tasks that require alertness,
such as driving a car or operating potentially dangerous
machinery, may be decreased. Appropriate caution
should therefore be taken.

● Be sure to tell your doctor if you are pregnant. The
effects of this medication during pregnancy have not yet
been thoroughly studied in humans. Also, tell your doctor
if you are breastfeeding an infant. Small amounts of dexchlorpheniramine pass into breast milk and may cause
unusual excitement or irritability in nursing infants.

Dexedrine—see dextroamphetamine

Dexedrine Spansules—see dextroamphetamine

Dexone—see dexamethasone (systemic)

---

dextroamphetamine

BRAND NAMES (Manufacturers)
Dexampex (Lemmon)
Dexedrine (Smith Kline & French)
Dexedrine Spansules (Smith Kline & French)
dextroamphetamine sulfate (various manufacturers)
Ferndex (Ferndale)
Oxydess II (Vortech)
Spancap No. 1 (Vortech)
TYPE OF DRUG
Amphetamine (central nervous system stimulant)

INGREDIENT
dextroamphetamine as the sulfate salt
DOSAGE FORMS
Tablets (5 mg and 10 mg)
Capsules (15 mg)
Sustained-release capsules (5 mg, 10 mg, and 15 mg)
Oral elixir (5 mg per 5 ml teaspoonful with 10% alcohol)
STORAGE
Dextroamphetamine tablets, capsules, and oral elixir should be stored at room temperature in tightly closed containers

USES
This medication is a central nervous system stimulant that increases mental alertness and decreases fatigue. It is used to treat narcolepsy (problems in staying awake) and abnormal behavioral syndrome in children (hyperkinetic syndrome or attention deficit disorder). The way this medication acts to control abnormal behavioral syndrome in children is not clearly understood.

Dextroamphetamine is also used as an appetite suppressant during the first few weeks of dieting (while you are trying to establish new eating habits). It is thought to relieve hunger by altering nerve impulses to the appetite control center in the brain. Its effectiveness as an appetite suppressant lasts only for short periods (three to 12 weeks), however.

TREATMENT
In order to avoid stomach upset, you can take dextroamphetamine with food or with a full glass of milk or water (unless your doctor directs you to do otherwise).

If this medication is being used to treat narcolepsy or abnormal behavioral syndrome in children, the first dose each day should be taken soon after awakening. Subsequent doses should be spaced at 4- to 6-hour intervals.

If this medication has been prescribed as a diet aid, it should be taken one hour before each meal.

The oral elixir form of this medication should be measured carefully, with a specially designed, 5 ml measuring spoon. An ordinary kitchen teaspoon is not accurate enough.

The sustained-release form of this medication should be swallowed whole. Breaking, chewing, or crushing these capsules destroys their sustained-release activity, and may increase the side effects.

In order to avoid difficulty falling asleep, the last dose of this medication each day should be taken four to six hours before bedtime (tablets and capsules) or ten to 14 hours before bedtime (sustained-release capsules).

If you miss a dose of this medication, take the missed dose as soon as possible, unless it is almost time for your next dose. In that case, don't take the missed dose at all; just return to your regular dosing schedule. Do not double the next dose.

SIDE EFFECTS

Minor. Abdominal cramps; constipation; diarrhea; dry mouth; false sense of well-being; dizziness; insomnia; loss of appetite; irritability; nausea; overstimulation; restlessness; unpleasant taste in the mouth; and vomiting. These side effects should disappear in several days, as your body adjusts to the medication.

To prevent constipation, increase the amount of fiber in your diet (fresh fruits and vegetables, bran, salads, whole-grain cereals and breads), drink more water, and increase your exercise (unless your doctor directs you to do otherwise).

Dry mouth can be relieved by sucking on ice chips or a piece of hard candy, or by chewing sugarless gum.

If you feel dizzy, sit or lie down awhile; get up from a sitting or lying position slowly, and be careful on stairs.

Major. Tell your doctor about any side effects that are persistent or particularly bothersome. IT IS ESPECIALLY IMPORTANT TO TELL YOUR DOCTOR about blurred vision; confusion; fatigue; headaches; impotence; mental depression; nosebleeds; palpitations; rash; sweating; tightness in the chest; tremors; or uncoordinated movements.

INTERACTIONS

Dextroamphetamine interacts with several other types of medication.

1. Use of it within 14 days of a monoamine oxidase

(MAO) inhibitor (such as isocarboxazid, pargyline, phen-elzine, tranylcypromine) can result in high blood pressure and other side effects.

2. Barbiturate medications, phenothiazine tranquilizers (especially chlorpromazine), and tricyclic anti-depressants can antagonize (act against) this medication, decreasing its effectiveness

3. Amphetamines can decrease the blood-pressure-lowering effects of anti-hypertensive medications (especially guanethidine), and may alter insulin and oral anti-diabetic medication dosage requirements in diabetic patients.

4. The side effects of other central nervous system stimulants, such as caffeine, over-the-counter (non-prescription) appetite suppressants, and cough, sinus, allergy, asthma, or cold preparations, may be increased by dextroamphetamine.

5. Acetazolamide and sodium bicarbonate can decrease the elimination of the amphetamines from the body, thereby prolonging their duration of action.

BE SURE TO TELL YOUR DOCTOR if you are already taking any of the medications listed above.

WARNINGS

• Tell your doctor about unusual or allergic reactions you have had to any medications, especially to dextroamphetamine or other central nervous system stimulants (such as albuterol, amphetamine, ephedrine, epinephrine, isoproterenol, metaproterenol, norepinephrine, phenylephrine, phenylpropanolamine, pseudoephedrine, or terbutaline).

• Tell your doctor if you have a history of drug abuse or if you have ever had problems with agitation, diabetes mellitus (sugar diabetes), glaucoma, heart or blood vessel disease, high blood pressure, or thyroid disease.

• Dextroamphetamine can mask the symptoms of extreme fatigue and can cause dizziness. Your ability to perform tasks that require alertness, such as driving a car or operating potentially dangerous machinery, may be decreased. Appropriate caution should therefore be taken.

• Before having any surgery or other medical or dental

treatment, be sure to tell your doctor or dentist that you are taking this medication.

• Dextroamphetamine is related to amphetamine and may be habit-forming when taken for long periods of time (both physical and psychological dependence can occur). Therefore, you should not increase the dose of this medication or take it for longer than 12 weeks, unless you first consult your doctor. It is also important that you not stop taking this medication abruptly—fatigue; sleep disorders; mental depression; or nausea, vomiting, stomach cramps, or pain could occur. Your doctor may therefore want to decrease the dosage gradually, in order to prevent these side effects.

• Some of these products contain F.D. & C. Yellow Dye No. 5 (tartrazine), which can cause allergic-type reactions (difficulty breathing, fainting, rash, or wheezing) in certain susceptible individuals.

• Be sure to tell your doctor if you are pregnant. Although side effects in humans have not yet been thoroughly studied, some of the amphetamines have caused heart, brain, and biliary tract abnormalities in the fetuses of animals who received large doses of these drugs during pregnancy. Also, tell your doctor if you are breastfeeding an infant. Small amounts of this drug pass into breast milk.

dextroamphetamine sulfate—see
  dextroamphetamine

Dey-Dose Isoetharine—see isoetharine

Dey-Lute Isoetharine—see isoetharine

Diabeta—see glyburide

Diabinese—see chlorpropamide

Diachlor—see chlorothiazide

Diahist—see diphenhydramine

Diamine T.D.—see brompheniramine

Di-Ap-Trol—see phendimetrazine

Diaqua—see hydrochlorothiazide

---

diazepam

BRAND NAMES (Manufacturers)
Valium (Roche)
Valrelease (Roche)
TYPE OF DRUG
Sedative/hypnotic (anti-anxiety medication)
INGREDIENT
diazepam
DOSAGE FORMS
Tablets (2 mg, 5 mg, and 10 mg)
Sustained-release capsules (15 mg)
STORAGE
This medication should be stored at room temperature in a tightly closed, light-resistant container.

USES

Diazepam is prescribed to treat symptoms of anxiety, and sometimes to treat muscle spasms, convulsions, seizures, or alcohol withdrawal. It is not clear exactly how this medicine works, but it may relieve anxiety by acting as a depressant of the central nervous system. Diazepam is currently used by many people to relieve nervousness. It is effective for this purpose for short periods, but it is important to try to remove the cause of the anxiety as well.

TREATMENT

This medication should be taken exactly as directed by your doctor. It can be taken with food or a full glass of water if stomach upset occurs. Do not take this medication with a dose of antacids, since they may retard its absorption.

If you are taking this medication regularly and you miss a dose, then remember within an hour of the scheduled time, take the missed dose immediately. If more than an hour has passed, skip the dose you missed and wait for the next scheduled dose. Do not double the dose.

SIDE EFFECTS

Minor. Bitter taste in the mouth; constipation; depression; diarrhea; dizziness; drowsiness (after a night's sleep); dry mouth; fatigue; flushing; headache; heartburn; excess saliva; loss of appetite; nausea; nervousness; sweating; and vomiting. These side effects should disappear, as your body adjusts to the medication.

Dry mouth can be relieved by chewing sugarless gum or by sucking on ice chips.

If you feel dizzy, sit or lie down awhile; get up slowly, and be careful on stairs.

Major. Tell your doctor about any side effects that are persistent or particularly bothersome. IT IS ESPECIALLY IMPORTANT TO TELL YOUR DOCTOR about blurred or double vision; chest pain; difficulty urinating; fainting; falling; fever; joint pain; hallucinations; mouth sores; nightmares; palpitations; rash; severe depression; shortness of breath; slurred speech; sore throat; uncoordinated movements; unusual excitement; unusual tiredness; or yellowing of the eyes or skin

INTERACTIONS

Diazepam interacts with a number of other medications.
1. To prevent over-sedation, this drug should not be taken with alcohol, other sedative drugs, or central nervous system depressants (such as antihistamines, barbiturates, muscle relaxants, pain medicines, narcotics, medicines for seizures, phenothiazine tranquilizers), or with anti-depressants.
2. This medication may decrease the effectiveness of carbamazepine, levodopa, and oral anti-coagulants (blood thinners); and may increase the effects of phenytoin.
3. Disulfiram, isoniazid, and cimetidine can increase the blood levels of diazepam, which can lead to toxic effects.
4. Concurrent use of rifampin may decrease the effectiveness of diazepam.
If you are already taking any of the medications listed above, CONSULT YOUR DOCTOR about their use.

WARNINGS

• Tell your doctor about unusual or allergic reactions you have had to any medications, especially to diazepam or other benzodiazepine tranquilizers (such as alprazolam, chlordiazepoxide, clorazepate, flurazepam, halazepam, lorazepam, oxazepam, prazepam, temazepam, or triazolam).

• Tell your doctor if you now have, or if you have ever had, liver disease; kidney disease; epilepsy; lung disease; myasthenia gravis; porphyria; mental depression; or mental illness.

• This medicine can cause drowsiness. Avoid tasks that require alertness, such as driving a car or using potentially dangerous machinery.

• This medication has the potential for abuse and must be used with caution. Tolerance may develop quickly; do not increase your dosage of the drug without first consulting your doctor. It is also important not to stop taking this drug suddenly if you have been taking it in large amounts or if you have used it for several weeks. Your doctor may want to reduce your dosage gradually.

• This is a safe drug when used properly. When it is combined with other sedative drugs or alcohol, however, serious side effects can develop.

• Be sure to tell your doctor if you are pregnant. This medicine may increase the chance of birth defects if it is taken during the first three months of pregnancy. In addition, too much use of this medicine during the last six months of pregnancy may cause the baby to become dependent on it, resulting in withdrawal side effects in the newborn. Also, use of this medicine during the last weeks of pregnancy may cause drowsiness, slowed heartbeat, and breathing difficulties in the infant. Tell your doctor if you are breastfeeding an infant. This medicine can pass into breast milk and cause drowsiness, slowed heartbeat, and breathing difficulties in nursing infants.

Dibent —see dicyclomine

dicloxacillin

BRAND NAMES (Manufacturers)
dicloxacillin sodium (various manufacturers)
Dycill (Beecham)
Dynapen (Bristol)
Pathocil (Wyeth)
Veracillin (Ayerst)

TYPE OF DRUG
Antibiotic (infection fighter)

INGREDIENT
dicloxacillin as the sodium salt

DOSAGE FORMS
Capsules (125 mg, 250 mg, and 500 mg)
Oral suspension (62.5 mg per 5 ml teaspoonful)

STORAGE
Dicloxacillin capsules should be stored at room temperature in a tightly closed container. The oral suspension should be stored in the refrigerator in a tightly closed container. Any unused portion of the suspension should be discarded after 14 days, because the drug loses its potency after that time. This medication should never be frozen.

USES
Dicloxacillin is used to treat a wide variety of bacterial infections, usually involving the *Staphylococcus* bacteria. It acts by severely injuring the cell walls of the infecting bacteria, thereby preventing them from growing and multiplying. Dicloxacillin kills susceptible bacteria, but is not effective against viruses, parasites, or fungi.

TREATMENT
Dicloxacillin should be taken on an empty stomach or with a glass of water, one hour before or two hours after a meal. This medication should never be taken with fruit juices or carbonated beverages, because the acidity of these drinks destroys the drug in the stomach.

The suspension form of this medication should be shaken well, just before measuring each dose. The contents tend to settle on the bottom of the bottle, so it is necessary to shake the container to evenly distribute the ingredients and equalize the doses. Each dose should then be measured carefully, with a specially designed, 5 ml measuring spoon. An ordinary kitchen teaspoon is not accurate enough.

Dicloxacillin works best when the level of the medicine in your bloodstream is kept constant. It is therefore best to take the doses at evenly spaced times, day and night. For example, if you are taking four doses a day, the doses should be spaced six hours apart.

If you miss a dose of this medication, take the missed dose immediately. However, if you do not remember to take the missed dose until it is almost time for your next dose, take it; then space the next dose about halfway through the regular interval between doses. Then return to your regular schedule. Try not to skip any doses.

It is important to continue to take this medication for the entire time prescribed by your doctor (usually seven to 14 days), even if the symptoms of the infection disappear before the end of that period. If you stop taking the drug too soon, resistant bacteria are given the chance to continue growing, and the infection could recur.

SIDE EFFECTS

Minor. Diarrhea; heartburn; nausea; and vomiting. These side effects should disappear in several days, as your body adjusts to the medication.

Major. Tell your doctor about any side effects that are persistent or particularly bothersome. IT IS ESPECIALLY IMPORTANT TO TELL YOUR DOCTOR about bloating; chills; cough; darkened tongue; difficulty breathing; fever; irritation of the mouth; muscle aches; rash; rectal or vaginal itching; severe diarrhea; or sore throat. Also, if your symptoms of infection seem to be getting worse rather than improving, you should contact your doctor.

INTERACTIONS

Dicloxacillin interacts with other types of medication.
1. Probenecid can increase the blood concentrations and side effects of this medication.
2. Dicloxacillin may decrease the effectiveness of oral contraceptives (birth control pills), and pregnancy could result. You should therefore use another form of birth

control while taking this medication. Ask your doctor.
TELL YOUR DOCTOR if you are currently taking either of
the medications listed above.

WARNINGS

• Tell your doctor about unusual or allergic reactions you
have had to any medications, especially to dicloxacillin
or penicillins, or to cephalosporin antibiotics, penicillamine, or griseofulvin.
• Tell your doctor if you now have, or if you have ever
had, kidney disease, asthma, or allergies.
• This medication has been prescribed for your current
infection only. Another infection later on, or one that
someone else has, may require a different medicine. You
should not give your medicine to other people or use it for
other infections, unless your doctor specifically directs
you to do so.
• Diabetics taking dicloxacillin should know that this
drug can cause a false-positive sugar reaction with a
Clinitest urine glucose test. To avoid this problem, while
taking dicloxacillin you should switch to Clinistix or Tes-
Tape to test your urine sugar.
• Be sure to tell your doctor if you are pregnant. Although
dicloxacillin appears to be safe during pregnancy, extensive studies in humans have not yet been completed.
Also, tell your doctor if you are breastfeeding an infant.
Small amounts of this medication pass into breast milk
and may temporarily alter the bacteria in the intestinal
tract of the nursing infant, resulting in diarrhea.

dicloxacillin sodium — see dicloxacillin

---

dicyclomine

BRAND NAMES (Manufacturers)
Bentyl (Merrell Dow)
Dibent (Hauck)
dicyclomine hydrochloride (various manufacturers)
Di-Spaz (Vortech)
TYPE OF DRUG
Anti-spasmodic

INGREDIENT
dicyclomine as the hydrochloride salt
DOSAGE FORMS
Tablets (20 mg)
Capsules (10 mg and 20 mg)
Oral liquid (10 mg per 5 ml teaspoonful)
STORAGE
Dicyclomine tablets, capsules, and oral liquid should be stored at room temperature, in tightly closed containers. This medication should never be frozen.

USES
Dicyclomine is used to treat gastrointestinal tract disorders, including peptic ulcers, irritable colon, mucous colitis, acute enterocolitis, and neurogenic colon. Dicyclomine acts directly on the muscles of the gastrointestinal tract to decrease tone and slow their activity.

TREATMENT
Dicyclomine should be taken 30 to 60 minutes before meals (unless your doctor directs you to do otherwise). In order to reduce stomach upset, you can take this medication with food or with a glass of water or milk.

Antacids and anti-diarrhea medicines may prevent gastrointestinal absorption of this drug; therefore, at least one hour should separate doses of dicyclomine and one of these medications.

Measure the liquid form of dicyclomine carefully, with a specially designed, 5 ml measuring spoon. An ordinary kitchen teaspoon is not accurate enough. You can then dilute the oral liquid in other liquids to mask its unpleasant taste.

If you miss a dose of this medication, do not take the missed dose at all; just return to your regular dosing schedule. Do not double the next dose.

SIDE EFFECTS
Minor. Bloating; blurred vision; confusion; constipation; dizziness; drowsiness; dry mouth, throat, and nose; increased sensitivity to light; headache; insomnia; loss of taste; nausea; nervousness; reduced sweating; vomiting;

and weakness. These side effects should disappear in several days, as your body adjusts to the medication.

If you are constipated, increase the amount of fiber in your diet (fresh fruits and vegetables, salads, bran, and whole-grain breads), exercise, and drink more water (unless your doctor directs you to do otherwise).

Chew sugarless gum, or suck on ice chips or a piece of hard candy, to reduce mouth dryness.

Wear sunglasses if your eyes become sensitive to light.

To avoid dizziness or light-headedness when you stand, contract and relax the muscles of your legs for a few moments before rising. Do this by pushing one foot against the floor while raising the other foot slightly, alternating feet so that you are "pumping" your legs in a pedaling motion.

Major. Tell your doctor about any side effects that are persistent or particularly bothersome. IT IS ESPECIALLY IMPORTANT TO TELL YOUR DOCTOR about difficulty urinating, fever, impotence, palpitations, rash, or sore throat.

INTERACTIONS

Dicyclomine interacts with several other types of drugs.

1. It can cause extreme drowsiness when combined with alcohol or central nervous system depressants (drugs that slow the activity of the nervous system), such as antihistamines, barbiturates, benzodiazepine tranquilizers, muscle relaxants, narcotics, pain medications, and phenothiazine tranquilizers, or with tricyclic anti-depressants.

2. Amantadine, antihistamines, haloperidol, monoamine oxidase (MAO) inhibitors, phenothiazine tranquilizers, procainamide, quinidine, and tricyclic antidepressants can increase the side effects of dicyclomine Before starting to take this medication, BE SURE TO TELL YOUR DOCTOR if you are already taking any of the medications listed above.

WARNINGS

• Tell your doctor about unusual or allergic reactions you have had to any medications, especially to dicyclomine.

• Tell your doctor if you now have, or if you have ever

had, glaucoma, heart disease, hiatal hernia, high blood pressure, kidney disease, liver disease, myasthenia gravis, obstructed bladder, obstructed intestine, enlarged prostate gland, thyroid disease, severe ulcerative colitis, or internal bleeding.

• If this medication makes you dizzy or drowsy, or blurs your vision, do not take part in any activity that requires alertness, such as driving a car or operating potentially dangerous equipment. Be careful on stairs; and avoid getting up from a lying or sitting position suddenly.

• This medication can decrease sweating and heat release from the body. You should therefore avoid getting overheated by strenuous exercise in hot weather, and should avoid taking hot baths, showers, and saunas.

• Before having any surgery or other medical or dental treatment, be sure to tell your doctor or dentist that you are taking this medication.

• Be sure to tell your doctor if you are pregnant. Although this drug appears to be safe during pregnancy, extensive studies in humans have not yet been completed. Also, tell your doctor if you are breastfeeding an infant. Small amounts of dicyclomine pass into breast milk.

dicyclomine hydrochloride—see dicyclomine

---

diethylpropion

BRAND NAMES (Manufacturers)
Depletite-25 (Reid-Provident)
diethylpropion hydrochloride (various manufacturers)
Tenuate (Merrell Dow)
Tenuate Dospan (Merrell Dow)
Tepanil (Riker)
Tepanil Ten-Tab (Riker)
TYPE OF DRUG
Anorectic (appetite suppressant)
INGREDIENT
diethylpropion as the hydrochloride salt
DOSAGE FORMS
Tablets (25 mg)
Sustained-release tablets (75 mg)

STORAGE

Diethylpropion should be stored at room temperature in tightly closed, light-resistant containers.

USES

Diethylpropion is used as an appetite suppressant during the first few weeks of dieting, to help establish new eating habits. This medication is thought to relieve hunger by altering nerve impulses to the appetite control center in the brain. Its effectiveness lasts only for short periods (three to 12 weeks), however.

TREATMENT

You can take diethylpropion with a full glass of water one hour before meals (unless your doctor directs you to do otherwise).

If you miss a dose of this medication, take the missed dose as soon as possible, unless it is almost time for your next dose. In this case, don't take the missed dose at all; just return to your regular dosing schedule. Do not double the next dose.

In order to avoid difficulty falling asleep, the last dose of this medication each day should be taken four to six hours before bedtime (regular tablets) or ten to 14 hours before bedtime (sustained-release tablets).

The sustained-release form of this medication should be swallowed whole. Breaking, chewing, or crushing these tablets destroys their sustained-release activity, and may increase the side effects.

SIDE EFFECTS

Minor. Blurred vision; constipation; diarrhea; dizziness; dry mouth; euphoria; fatigue; insomnia; irritability; nausea; nervousness; restlessness; stomach pain; sweating; tremors; unpleasant taste in the mouth; and vomiting. These side effects should disappear in several days, as your body adjusts to the medication.

Dry mouth can be relieved by sucking on ice chips or a piece of hard candy, or by chewing sugarless gum.

In order to prevent constipation, increase the amount of fiber in your diet (raw vegetables, fruits, salads, bran, and whole-grain breads), and drink more water (unless your

doctor directs you to do otherwise).
Major. Tell your doctor about any side effects that are persistent or particularly bothersome. IT IS ESPECIALLY IMPORTANT TO TELL YOUR DOCTOR about changes in sexual desire; chest pain; difficulty urinating; enlarged breasts (in both sexes); fever; hair loss; headaches; impotence; menstrual irregularities; mental depression; mood changes; mouth sores; muscle pains; nosebleeds; palpitations; rash; or sore throat.

INTERACTIONS

Diethylpropion interacts with other medications.
1. Use of it within 14 days of a monoamine oxidase (MAO) inhibitor (such as isocarboxazid, pargyline, phenelzine, tranylcypromine) can result in high blood pressure and other side effects.
2. Barbiturate medications and phenothiazine tranquilizers (especially chlorpromazine) can antagonize (act against) the appetite suppressant activity of this medication, decreasing its effectiveness.
3. Diethylpropion can decrease the blood-pressure-lowering effects of anti-hypertensive medications (especially guanethidine) and may alter insulin and oral anti-diabetic medication dosage requirements in diabetic patients.
4. The side effects of other central nervous system stimulants, such as caffeine, over-the-counter (non-prescription) appetite suppressants, or cough, allergy, asthma, sinus, or cold preparations, may be increased by this medication.
TELL YOUR DOCTOR if you are already taking any of the medications listed above.

WARNINGS

● Tell your doctor about unusual or allergic reactions you have had to any medications, especially to diethylpropion or other appetite suppressants (including benzphetamine, phendimetrazine, phenmetrazine, fenfluramine, mazindol, or phentermine), or to epinephrine, norepinephrine, ephedrine, amphetamines, dextroamphetamine, phenylephrine, phenylpropanolamine, pseudoephedrine, albuterol, metaproterenol, or terbutaline.

- Tell your doctor if you have a history of drug abuse, or if you have ever had angina (chest pain); diabetes mellitus (sugar diabetes); emotional disturbances; glaucoma; heart or cardiovascular disease; high blood pressure; thyroid disease; or epilepsy.
- Diethylpropion can mask the symptoms of extreme fatigue, and can cause dizziness or light-headedness. Your ability to perform tasks that require alertness, such as driving a car or operating potentially dangerous machinery, may be decreased. Appropriate caution should therefore be taken.
- Before having any surgery or other medical or dental treatment, be sure to tell your doctor or dentist that you are taking this medication.
- Diethylpropion is related to amphetamine and may be habit-forming when taken for long periods of time (both physical and psychological dependence can occur). Therefore, you should not increase the dose of this medication or take it for longer than 12 weeks, unless you first consult your doctor. It is also important that you not stop taking this medication abruptly. Fatigue, sleep disorders, mental depression, nausea or vomiting, or stomach cramps or pain could occur. Your doctor may therefore want to decrease your dosage gradually.
- Be sure to tell your doctor if you are pregnant. Although side effects in humans have not yet been thoroughly studied, some of the appetite suppressants have been shown to cause side effects in the fetuses of animals who received large doses during pregnancy. Also, tell your doctor if you are breastfeeding an infant. It is not known whether or not this medication passes into breast milk.

diethylpropion hydrochloride—see diethylpropion

---

diethylstilbestrol

BRAND NAMES (Manufacturers)
DES (Lilly)
diethylstilbestrol (various manufacturers)
TYPE OF DRUG
Estrogen (female hormone)

INGREDIENT
diethylstilbestrol
DOSAGE FORMS
Tablets (0.1 mg, 0.25 mg, 0.5 mg, 1 mg, and 5 mg)
Enteric-coated tablets (0.25 mg, 0.5 mg, 1 mg, and 5 mg)
Vaginal suppositories (0.1 mg and 0.5 mg)
STORAGE
Diethylstilbestrol tablets and suppositories should be stored at room temperature, in tightly closed containers.

USES
This medication is a synthetic estrogen that is used to treat atrophic vaginitis, menopausal symptoms, breast cancer, and prostate cancer. As an emergency treatment following rape, diethylstilbestrol is also used as a post-coital contraceptive (a "morning after" pill).

TREATMENT
In order to avoid stomach irritation, you can take diethylstilbestrol with food or with a full glass of water or milk (unless your doctor directs you to do otherwise).

The enteric-coated tablets should be swallowed whole. Breaking, crushing, or chewing these tablets increases the risk of gastrointestinal side effects.

Detailed instructions for inserting the vaginal suppositories are provided on the package insert. If you are taking a single daily dose of this medication, it is best to insert the suppository at bedtime, to maximize its effectiveness.

If you miss a dose of this medication, take the missed dose as soon as possible, unless it is almost time for the next dose. In that case, do not take the missed dose at all; just return to your regular dosing schedule. Do not double the next dose.

SIDE EFFECTS
Minor. Abdominal cramping; abnormal vaginal bleeding; bloating; breast tenderness; diarrhea; dizziness; fluid retention; frequent and painful urination; hair loss; headache; itching; nausea; nervousness; skin rash; darkening of the skin; vomiting; or weight gain. These side effects should disappear in several days, as your body

adjusts to the medication.

If you feel dizzy, sit or lie down awhile; get up slowly, and be careful on stairs.

Eating a full breakfast or having a midmorning snack may relieve nausea and vomiting.

This medication can increase your sensitivity to sunlight. You should therefore avoid prolonged exposure to sunlight and sunlamps. Wear protective clothing and sunglasses, and use an effective sunscreen.

Major. Tell your doctor about any side effects that are persistent or particularly bothersome. IT IS ESPECIALLY IMPORTANT TO TELL YOUR DOCTOR about blurred vision; chest pain; convulsions; depression; pain or inflammation of the calves or thighs; shortness of breath; or yellowing of the eyes or skin.

INTERACTIONS

Diethylstilbestrol interacts with other medications.

1. It can decrease the effectiveness of oral anti-coagulants (blood thinners, such as warfarin).

2. Carbamazepine, phenobarbital, phenytoin, primidone, and rifampin can reduce the effectiveness of diethylstilbestrol.

3. Diethylstilbestrol can increase the side effects and decrease the effectiveness of tricyclic anti-depressants. BE SURE TO TELL YOUR DOCTOR if you are already taking any of the medications listed above.

WARNINGS

• Tell your doctor about unusual or allergic reactions you have had to medications, especially to diethylstilbestrol or to any other estrogens or oral contraceptives.

• Before starting to take this medication, be sure to tell your doctor if you now have, or if you have ever had, asthma, blood clots, breast disease, depression, diabetes, epilepsy, endometriosis, gallstones or gallbladder disease, heart disease, high blood pressure, kidney disease, liver disease, migraine headaches, porphyria, or uterine tumors.

• Estrogens can alter the blood's clotting ability, so be especially careful to avoid injuries.

• Before having any surgery or other medical or dental

treatment, be sure your doctor or dentist knows that you
are taking this medication.
• A package insert entitled "Information for the Patient"
should be dispensed with your prescription. Read it carefully—it is important that you understand the possible
risks and benefits of taking this medication. If you have
any questions, check with your doctor or pharmacist.
• Cigarette smoking can increase your risk of developing
heart or blood vessel disorders while taking this medication. The risks increase with the amount of smoking and
the age of the smoker.
• Be sure to tell your doctor if you are pregnant. It has
been found that daughters of women who took diethylstilbestrol during pregnancy have a greater risk of developing cancer of the vagina and/or uterine cervix and
other abnormalities of the reproductive tract. Also, tell
your doctor if you are breastfeeding an infant. Diethylstilbestrol passes into breast milk. It may also decrease milk
production.

diflunisal

BRAND NAME (Manufacturer)
Dolobid (Merck Sharp & Dohme)
TYPE OF DRUG
Non-steroidal anti-inflammatory analgesic (pain reliever)
INGREDIENT
diflunisal
DOSAGE FORM
Tablets (250 mg and 500 mg)
STORAGE
This medication should be stored in a closed container at
room temperature, away from heat and direct sunlight.

USES
Diflunisal is used to treat the inflammation (pain, swelling, and stiffness) of osteoarthritis and muscle or skeletal
injury.

TREATMENT
You should take this drug immediately after meals or with

food, in order to reduce stomach irritation. Do not break, crush, or chew the tablets before swallowing—they should be swallowed whole, to lessen side effects and to maintain their benefits for a full 12 hours. Ask your doctor if you can take diflunisal with an antacid.

If you are taking diflunisal to relieve osteoarthritis you must take it regularly, as directed by your doctor. It may take up to eight days before you feel the full benefits of this medication. Diflunisal does not cure osteoarthritis, but it will help to control the condition, as long as you continue to take it.

It is important to take diflunisal on schedule and not to miss any doses. If you do miss a dose of this medication, take the missed dose as soon as possible, unless more than six hours have passed. In that case, don't take the missed dose at all; just return to your regular dosing schedule. Do not double the next dose.

SIDE EFFECTS

Minor. Bloating; constipation; diarrhea; difficulty sleeping; dizziness; drowsiness; headache; heartburn; indigestion; light-headedness; loss of appetite; nausea; nervousness; unusual sweating; and vomiting. As your body adjusts to the drug, these side effects should disappear.

If you become dizzy, sit or lie down awhile; get up slowly, and be careful on stairs.

Acetaminophen may be helpful in relieving any headaches.

Major. If any side effects are persistent or particularly bothersome, you should report them to your doctor. IT IS ESPECIALLY IMPORTANT TO TELL YOUR DOCTOR about bloody or black, tarry stools; blurred vision; confusion; depression; difficult or painful urination; difficulty breathing, or wheezing; palpitations; ringing or buzzing in the ears or difficulty hearing; skin rash, hives, or itching; stomach pain; swelling of the feet; tightness in the chest; unexplained sore throat and fever; unusual bleeding or bruising; unusual fatigue or weakness; unusual weight gain; or yellowing of the eyes or skin.

INTERACTIONS

Diflunisal interacts with several types of medications.

1. Anti-coagulants (blood thinners, such as warfarin), in combination with diflunisal, can lead to an increase in bleeding complications.
2. Aspirin, salicylates, or other anti-inflammation medication may cause increased stomach irritation.
3. Antacids can lower blood diflunisal concentrations, decreasing its effectiveness.
4. Diflunisal can increase the blood concentrations and side effects of acetaminophen and of hydrochlorothiazide.
BE SURE TO TELL YOUR DOCTOR if you are already taking any of these medications.

WARNINGS

• Before you take this medication, it is important to tell your doctor if you have ever had unusual or allergic reactions to diflunisal or any chemically related drug (including aspirin or other salicylates, indomethacin, fenoprofen, ibuprofen, meclofenamate, mefenamic acid, naproxen, oxyphenbutazone, phenylbutazone, piroxicam, sulindac, tolmetin, and zomepirac).
• Tell your doctor if you now have, or if you have ever had, bleeding problems; colitis, stomach ulcers, or other stomach problems; epilepsy; heart disease; high blood pressure; asthma; kidney disease; liver disease; mental illness; or Parkinson's disease.
• If this drug makes you dizzy or drowsy, do not take part in any activity that requires alertness, such as driving a car or operating potentially dangerous equipment.
• Because this drug can prolong your bleeding time, it is important to tell your doctor or dentist that you are taking this drug, before having any surgery or other medical or dental treatment.
• Stomach problems are more likely to occur if you take aspirin regularly or drink alcohol while being treated with this medication. These should therefore be avoided (unless your doctor directs you to do otherwise).
• Be sure to tell your doctor if you are pregnant. Although studies in humans have not yet been completed, unwanted side effects (defects in the spine and ribs) have been reported in the offspring of animals who received diflunisal during pregnancy. If taken late in pregnancy, it

can also prolong labor. Also tell your doctor if you are breastfeeding an infant. Small amounts of diflunisal can pass into breast milk.

---

digitoxin

BRAND NAMES (Manufacturers)
Crystodigin (Lilly)
digitoxin (various manufacturers)
Purodigin (Wyeth)
TYPE OF DRUG
Cardiac glycoside (heart medication)
INGREDIENT
digitoxin
DOSAGE FORM
Tablets (0.05 mg, 0.1 mg, 0.15 mg, and 0.2 mg)
STORAGE
Digitoxin should be stored at room temperature, in a tightly closed container.

USES

Digitoxin belongs to a group of drugs known as digitalis glycosides. It is used to treat heart arrhythmias and congestive heart failure. Digitoxin improves the strength and efficiency of the heart, and controls the heart rhythm.

TREATMENT

In order to avoid stomach irritation, you can take digitoxin with food or with a full glass of water or milk (unless your doctor directs you to do otherwise).

In order to become accustomed to taking this medication, try to take it at the same time each day.

If you miss a dose of this medication, take the missed dose as soon as possible, unless it is almost time for the next dose. In that case, do not take the missed dose at all; just return to your regular dosing schedule. Do not double the next dose. If you miss two or more doses, check with your doctor.

Digitoxin does not cure heart failure, but it will help to control the condition, as long as you continue to take it.

SIDE EFFECTS

Minor. Drowsiness; headache; loss of appetite; nausea; stomach upset; and vomiting. These side effects should disappear in several weeks, as your body adjusts to the medication.

Major. Tell your doctor about any side effects that are persistent or particularly bothersome. IT IS ESPECIALLY IMPORTANT TO TELL YOUR DOCTOR about bad dreams; blurred vision; breast enlargement (in both sexes); confusion; depression; disorientation; hallucinations; muscle weakness; palpitations; or tingling sensations.

INTERACTIONS

Digitoxin interacts with other types of medication.

1. Barbiturates, phenytoin, oral anti-diabetic medications, phenylbutazone, and rifampin can decrease the blood levels and effectiveness of digitoxin.

2. The absorption of digitoxin from the gastrointestinal tract is reduced when it is taken with colestipol, cholestyramine, antacids, neomycin, or sulfasalazine.

3. Spironolactone can unpredictably increase or decrease the side effects of digitoxin.

4. Concurrent use of quinidine, procainamide, calcium, reserpine, ephedrine, or beta-blockers (atenolol, metoprolol, nadolol, pindolol, propranolol, timolol) with digitoxin can lead to additive effects on the heart.

5. The dosage of digitoxin may require adjustment when thyroid hormones, methimazole, or propylthiouracil is started.

6. Quinidine, diltiazem, nifedipine, and verapamil can increase the blood levels and side effects of digitoxin. Before starting to take digitoxin, BE SURE TO TELL YOUR DOCTOR if you are already taking any of the medications listed above.

WARNINGS

• Tell your doctor about unusual or allergic reactions you have had to medications, especially to digitoxin or any other digitalis glycoside (digitalis, digoxin, gitalin, or ouabain).

• Before starting to take this medication, be sure to tell

your doctor if you now have, or if you have ever had, blood electrolyte disorders (too much or too little calcium, magnesium, or potassium), heart disease, kidney disease, lung disease, liver disease, or thyroid disease.

• Before having any kind of surgery or other medical or dental treatment, be sure to tell your doctor or dentist that you are taking this medication.

• Check with your doctor or pharmacist before taking any over-the-counter (non-prescription) allergy, asthma, cough, cold, diet, or sinus product. Some of these products can increase the side effects of digitoxin.

• Do not stop taking this medication unless you first check with your doctor. Stopping abruptly may lead to a worsening of your condition.

• Some of these products contain F.D. & C. Yellow Dye No. 5 (tartrazine), which can cause allergic-type symptoms (fainting, shortness of breath, rash) in certain susceptible individuals.

• While you are taking digitoxin, your doctor may want you to check your pulse every day. If your pulse is slower than your doctor has told you it should be, or if the rhythm is irregular, CONTACT YOUR DOCTOR IMMEDIATELY.

• Be sure to tell your doctor if you are pregnant. Although digitoxin appears to be safe during pregnancy, extensive studies in humans have not yet been completed. In addition, the dosage of digitoxin required to control your disorder may change during pregnancy. Also, tell your doctor if you are breastfeeding an infant. Small amounts of digitoxin pass into breast milk.

---

digoxin

BRAND NAMES (Manufacturers)
digoxin (various manufacturers)
Lanoxicaps (Burroughs Wellcome)
Lanoxin (Burroughs Wellcome)
SK-Digoxin (Smith Kline & French)
TYPE OF DRUG
Cardiac glycoside (heart medication)
INGREDIENTS
digoxin

DOSAGE FORMS
Tablets (0.125 mg, 0.25 mg, and 0.5 mg)
Capsules (0.05 mg, 0.1 mg, and 0.2 mg)
Pediatric elixir (0.05 mg per ml with 10% alcohol)

STORAGE
Digoxin tablets, capsules, and pediatric elixir should be stored at room temperature in tightly closed, light-resistant containers. This medication should never be frozen.

USES
Digoxin is used to strengthen the heartbeat and improve heart rhythm. It works directly on the muscle of the heart to improve contraction.

TREATMENT
In order to avoid stomach irritation, you can take digoxin with a full glass of water or with food. Try to take it at the same time every day.

Measure the dose of the pediatric elixir carefully, with the dropper provided. An ordinary kitchen spoon is not accurate enough.

Antacids decrease the absorption of digoxin from the gastrointestinal tract. Therefore, if you are taking both of these types of medication, the dose of digoxin should be taken one hour before or two hours after a dose of antacids.

Try not to miss any doses of this medication. If you do miss a dose, take the missed dose as soon as possible, unless it is almost time for the next dose. In that case do not take the missed dose at all; just return to your regular dosing schedule. Do not double the next dose. If you miss more than two doses of digoxin, contact your doctor.

Digoxin does not cure congestive heart failure, but it will help to control the condition, as long as you continue to take it.

SIDE EFFECTS
Minor. Apathy; diarrhea; drowsiness; headache; muscle weakness; and tiredness. These side effects should disappear in several weeks, as your body adjusts to the medication.

Major. Tell your doctor about any side effects that are persistent or particularly bothersome. IT IS ESPECIALLY IMPORTANT TO TELL YOUR DOCTOR about disorientation; enlarged and painful breasts (in both sexes); hallucinations; loss of appetite; mental depression; nausea; palpitations; severe abdominal pain; slowed heart rate; visual disturbances (such as blurred or yellow vision); or vomiting.

INTERACTIONS

Digoxin interacts with several other types of medication.
1. Penicillamine can decrease the blood levels and effectiveness of digoxin.
2. Erythromycin, tetracycline, hydroxychloroquine, verapamil, nifedipine, quinidine, quinine, and spironolactone can increase the blood levels of digoxin, which can lead to an increase in side effects.
3. Thyroid hormone, propylthiouracil, and methimazole can change the dosage requirements of digoxin.
4. Antacids, kaolin-pectin, sulfasalazine, aminosalicylic acid, metoclopramide, anti-neoplastic agents (anticancer drugs), neomycin, colestipol, and cholestyramine can decrease the absorption of digoxin from the gastrointestinal tract, decreasing its effectiveness.
5. Calcium and reserpine can increase the side effects of digoxin.
6. Diuretics (water pills) and adrenocorticosteroids (cortisone-like medications) can cause hypokalemia (low potassium blood levels), which can increase the side effects of digoxin.
Before starting to take digoxin, BE SURE TO TELL YOUR DOCTOR if you are already taking any of the medications listed above.

WARNINGS

• Tell your doctor about unusual or allergic reactions you have had to any medications, especially to digoxin, digitoxin, gitalin, or ouabain.
• Tell your doctor if you now have, or if you have ever had, kidney disease, lung disease, thyroid disease, hypokalemia (low blood potassium levels), or hypercalcemia (high blood calcium levels).

• The pharmacological activity of the different brands of this drug varies widely—the tablets dissolve in the stomach and bowel at different rates and to varying degrees. Because of this variability, it is important not to change brands of the drug without consulting your doctor.

• Meals high in bran fiber may reduce the absorption of digoxin from the gastrointestinal tract. Avoid these types of meals when taking your dose of medication

• Your doctor may want you to take your pulse daily while you are using digoxin. Contact your doctor if your pulse becomes slower than normal, or if it drops below 50 beats per minute

• Before having any surgery or other medical or dental treatment, be sure to tell your doctor or dentist that you are taking this medication.

• Before taking any over-the-counter (non-prescription) asthma, allergy, cough, cold, sinus, or diet product, be sure to check with your doctor or pharmacist. Some of these drugs can increase the side effects of digoxin.

• Be sure to tell your doctor if you are pregnant. Although this drug appears to be safe during pregnancy, extensive studies in humans have not yet been completed. In addition, the dose of digoxin required to control your symptoms may change during pregnancy. Also, tell your doctor if you are breastfeeding an infant. Small amounts of digoxin pass into breast milk.

---

dihydrotachysterol

BRAND NAMES (Manufacturers)
dihydrotachysterol (Roxane)
Hytakerol (Winthrop)
TYPE OF DRUG
Vitamin D analog
INGREDIENT
dihydrotachysterol
DOSAGE FORMS
Tablets (0.125 mg, 0.2 mg, and 0.4 mg)
Capsules (0.125 mg)
Oral solution (0.25 mg per ml)

STORAGE
Dihydrotachysterol tablets, capsules, and oral solution should be stored at room temperature in tightly closed, light-resistant containers. This medication should never be frozen.

USES
Vitamin D is essential to many body systems (including muscle and heart function). Dihydrotachysterol is a vitamin D analog—it raises blood calcium levels. This medication is used to treat tetany and hypoparathyroidism, conditions characterized by low blood calcium levels.

TREATMENT
You can take dihydrotachysterol either on an empty stomach or with food or milk (as directed by your doctor).

Each dose of the oral solution form of this medication should be measured carefully, with the dropper provided. The solution can then be swallowed directly or mixed with fruit juice, cereal, or other foods.

If you miss a dose of this medication, take the missed dose as soon as possible, unless it is almost time for the next dose. In that case, do not take the missed dose at all; just return to your regular dosing schedule. Do not double the next dose.

SIDE EFFECTS
Minor. None, at the dosages normally prescribed.
Major. The side effects associated with dihydrotachysterol therapy are usually the result of too much medication (vitamin D intoxication). Tell your doctor about any side effects that are persistent or particularly bothersome. IT IS ESPECIALLY IMPORTANT TO TELL YOUR DOCTOR about blurred vision; bone pain; constipation; dry mouth; headache; irritability; loss of appetite; mental disorders; metallic taste in the mouth; muscle pain; nausea; palpitations; runny nose; increased thirst; increased urination; vomiting; weakness; or weight loss.

INTERACTIONS
If you are being treated for hypoparathyroidism, concurrent use of dihydrotachysterol and thiazide diuretics

(water pills) can lead to hypercalcemia (high blood calcium levels). BE SURE TO TELL YOUR DOCTOR if you are already taking this type of diuretic.

WARNINGS

• Tell your doctor about unusual or allergic reactions you have had to any medications, especially to dihydrotachysterol, calcitriol, calcifediol, ergocalciferol, or vitamin D.

• Before starting to take this medication, be sure to tell your doctor if you now have, or if you have ever had, heart or blood vessel disease, hypercalcemia, hyperphosphatemia, vitamin D intoxication, or sarcoidosis.

• Before taking any over-the-counter (non-prescription) products that contain calcium, phosphates, magnesium, or vitamin D, check with your doctor. These ingredients can increase the side effects of dihydrotachysterol.

• Dihydrotachysterol is more expensive than vitamin D products, but it is often prescribed instead of vitamin D because it is faster-acting and does not persist in the body once therapy is stopped.

• Be sure to tell your doctor if you are pregnant. Although dihydrotachysterol appears to be safe during pregnancy in humans, birth defects have been reported in the offspring of animals who received large doses of this medication during pregnancy. Also, tell your doctor if you are breastfeeding an infant. Small amounts of dihydrotachysterol may pass into breast milk.

Dilantin—see phenytoin

Dilantin Infatab—see phenytoin

Dilart—see papaverine

Dilatrate-SR — see isosorbide dinitrate

Dilaudid—see hydromorphone

diltiazem

BRAND NAME (Manufacturer)
Cardizem (Marion)
TYPE OF DRUG
Anti-anginal (calcium channel blocker)
INGREDIENT
diltiazem as the hydrochloride salt
DOSAGE FORM
Tablets (30 mg and 60 mg)
STORAGE
Diltiazem should be stored at room temperature in a tightly closed container.

USES
This medication is used to prevent the symptoms of angina (chest pain). It belongs to a group of drugs known as calcium channel blockers. It is unclear exactly how it does so, but diltiazem dilates the blood vessels of the heart and increases the amount of oxygen that reaches the heart muscle.

TREATMENT
To obtain maximum benefit, you should take diltiazem on an empty stomach, one hour before or two hours after a meal. If this drug upsets your stomach, however, check with your doctor to see if you can take it with food or milk.

In order to become accustomed to taking this medication, try to take it at the same times each day.

Diltiazem does not relieve chest pain once it has begun; this medication is used to prevent angina attacks from occurring.

This medication does not cure angina, but it will help to control the condition, as long as you continue to take it.

If you miss a dose of this medication, take the missed dose as soon as possible, unless it is within four hours of the next scheduled dose. In that case, do not take the missed dose at all; just return to your regular dosing schedule. Do not double the next dose.

SIDE EFFECTS
Minor. Constipation; diarrhea; dizziness; drowsiness;

headache; insomnia; light-headedness; nausea; nervousness; stomach upset; and vomiting. These side effects should disappear in several days, as your body adjusts to the medication.

If you feel dizzy or light-headed, sit or lie down awhile; get up slowly, and be careful on stairs.

To relieve constipation, increase the amount of fiber in your diet (bran, salads, fresh fruits and vegetables, and whole-grain breads), and drink more water (unless your doctor directs you to do otherwise).

This medication can increase your sensitivity to sunlight. You should therefore avoid prolonged exposure to sunlight and sunlamps. Wear protective clothing and sunglasses, and use an effective sunscreen.

Major. Tell your doctor about any side effects that are persistent or particularly bothersome. IT IS ESPECIALLY IMPORTANT TO TELL YOUR DOCTOR about confusion; depression; fainting; fatigue; flushing; fluid retention; hallucinations; palpitations; skin rash; tingling in the fingers or toes; unusual weakness; or yellowing of the eyes or skin.

INTERACTIONS

Diltiazem should be used cautiously with beta-blockers (atenolol, metoprolol, nadolol, propranolol, pindolol, timolol); digitoxin; digoxin; or disopyramide. Side effects on the heart may be increased by the concurrent use of these medications.

BE SURE TO TELL YOUR DOCTOR if you are already taking one of these medications.

WARNINGS

• Tell your doctor about unusual or allergic reactions you have had to any medications, especially to diltiazem.

• Before starting to take this medication, be sure to tell your doctor if you now have, or if you have ever had, bradycardia (slow heartbeat), heart block, heart failure, kidney disease, liver disease, low blood pressure, or sick sinus syndrome.

• If this drug makes you dizzy or drowsy, avoid taking part in any activities that require alertness, such as driving a car or operating potentially dangerous equipment.

- In order to prevent fainting while taking this medication, avoid drinking large amounts of alcohol. You should also avoid prolonged standing and strenuous exercise in hot weather.
- Your doctor may want you to check your heart rate regularly while taking this medication. If your heart rate drops below 50 beats per minute, CHECK WITH YOUR DOCTOR.
- Be sure to tell your doctor if you are pregnant. Extensive studies in pregnant women have not yet been completed, but birth defects have been reported in animals whose mothers received large doses of diltiazem during pregnancy. Also, tell your doctor if you are breastfeeding an infant. It is not known whether or not diltiazem passes into breast milk.

Dimetane Expectorant—see phenylephrine, phenylpropanolamine, brompheniramine, and guaifenesin combination

Dimetapp Extentabs—see phenylpropanolamine, phenylephrine, and brompheniramine combination

Diphen—see diphenydramine

Diphenatol—see diphenoxylate and atropine

---

diphenhydramine

BRAND NAMES (Manufacturers)
Belix (Halsey)
Benadryl (Parke-Davis)
Benaphen (Major)
Bendylate (Reid-Provident)
Benylin Cough Syrup* (Parke-Davis)
Compoz* (Jeffrey Martin)
Diahist (Century)
Diphen (Bay)
diphenhydramine hydrochloride (various manufacturers)
Fenylhist (Mallard)
Fynex (Mallard)

Hydril (Blaine)
Noradryl (Vortech)
Nordryl (Vortech)
Nytol with DPH* (Block)
Phen-Amin (Scrip)
Sleep-Eze 3* (Whitehall)
Sominex Formula 2* (Beecham)
Tusstat (Century)
Twilite* (Pfeiffer)
Valdrene (Vale)
*Diphenhydramine is also available over-the-counter
  (non-prescription), under several brand names.
TYPE OF DRUG
Antihistamine and sedative/hypnotic (sleeping aid)
INGREDIENTS
diphenhydramine as the hydrochloride salt
DOSAGE FORMS
Tablets (25 mg and 50 mg)
Capsules (25 mg and 50 mg)
Elixir (12.5 mg per 5 ml teaspoonful)
Oral syrup (12.5 mg and 13.3 mg per 5 ml teaspoonful)
STORAGE
Diphenhydramine tablets, capsules, elixir, and oral syrup
should be stored at room temperature, in tightly closed
containers.

USES

This medication has multiple uses. It belongs to a group of
drugs known as antihistamines (antihistamines block the
action of histamine, a chemical that is released by the
body during an allergic reaction). It is therefore used to
treat or prevent symptoms of allergy.

   Diphenhydramine is also used to treat motion sickness
and Parkinson's disease; and it is used as a night time
sleeping aid and non-narcotic cough suppressant.

TREATMENT

To avoid stomach upset, you can take diphenhydramine
with food or with a full glass of milk or water (unless your
doctor directs you to do otherwise).

   The elixir and oral syrup forms of this medication
should be measured carefully, with a specially designed,

5 ml measuring spoon. An ordinary kitchen spoon is not accurate enough.

If you miss a dose of this medication, take the missed dose as soon as possible, unless it is almost time for your next dose. In that case, don't take the missed dose at all; just return to your regular dosing schedule. Do not double the next dose.

SIDE EFFECTS

Minor. Blurred vision; confusion; constipation; diarrhea; difficult or painful urination; dizziness; dry mouth, throat, or nose; headache; irritability; loss of appetite; nausea; restlessness; ringing or buzzing in the ears; rash; stomach upset; and unusual increase in sweating. These side effects should disappear in several days, as your body adjusts to this medication.

If you are constipated, increase the amount of fiber in your diet (raw vegetables, fruits, salads, bran, and whole-grain breads), and drink more water (unless your doctor tells you not to do so).

Chew sugarless gum, or suck on ice chips or a piece of hard candy, to reduce mouth dryness.

This medication can cause increased sensitivity to sunlight. It is therefore important to avoid prolonged exposure to sunlight and sunlamps. Wear protective clothing, and use an effective sunscreen.

If you feel dizzy or light-headed, sit or lie down awhile; get up from a sitting or lying position slowly, and be careful on stairs.

Major. Tell your doctor about any side effects that are persistent or particularly bothersome. IT IS ESPECIALLY IMPORTANT TO TELL YOUR DOCTOR about change in menstruation; clumsiness; feeling faint; flushing of the face; hallucinations; seizures; shortness of breath; sleeping disorders; sore throat or fever; palpitations; tightness in the chest; unusual bleeding or bruising; or unusual tiredness or weakness.

INTERACTIONS

Diphenhydramine interacts with several other types of medication.

1. Concurrent use of this medication with other central

nervous system depressants (drugs that slow the activity of the nervous system), such as barbiturates, benzodiazepine tranquilizers, muscle relaxants, narcotics, pain medications, phenothiazine tranquilizers, and alcohol, or with tricyclic anti-depressants can cause extreme drowsiness.

2. Monoamine oxidase (MAO) inhibitors (isocarboxazid, pargyline, phenelzine, tranylcypromine) can increase the side effects of this medication.

3. Diphenhydramine can also decrease the activity of oral anti-coagulants (blood thinners, such as warfarin). TELL YOUR DOCTOR if you are currently taking any of the medications listed above.

WARNINGS

• Tell your doctor about unusual or allergic reactions you have had to medications, especially to diphenhydramine or to any other antihistamine (bromodiphenhydramine, brompheniramine, carbinoxamine, chlorpheniramine, clemastine, cyproheptadine, dexchlorpheniramine, dimenhydrinate, dimethindene, azatadine, diphenylpyraline, doxylamine, hydroxyzine, promethazine, pyrilamine, trimeprazine, tripelennamine, or tripolidine).

• Tell your doctor if you now have, or if you have ever had, asthma, blood vessel disease, glaucoma, high blood pressure, kidney disease, peptic ulcers, enlarged prostate gland, or thyroid disease.

• Diphenhydramine can cause drowsiness or dizziness. Your ability to perform tasks that require alertness, such as driving a car or operating potentially dangerous machinery, may be decreased. Appropriate caution should therefore be taken.

• Be sure to tell your doctor if you are pregnant. The effects of this medication during pregnancy have not yet been thoroughly studied in humans. Also, tell your doctor if you are breastfeeding an infant. Small amounts of diphenhydramine pass into breast milk and may cause unusual excitement or irritability in nursing infants.

diphenhydramine hydrochloride—see
diphenhydramine

diphenoxylate and atropine

BRAND NAMES (Manufacturers)
Diphenatol (Rugby)
diphenoxylate hydrochloride with atropine sulfate
(various manufacturers)
Elmotil (Elder)
Enoxa (Tutag)
Lofene (Lannett)
Lomotil (Searle)
Lonox (Geneva Generics)
Lo-Trol (Vangard)
Low-Quel (Halsey)
Nor-Mil (Vortech)
SK-Diphenoxylate (Smith Kline & French)

TYPE OF DRUG
Anti-diarrheal (anti-spasmodic and anti-cholinergic)

INGREDIENTS
diphenoxylate as the hydrochloride salt and atropine as
the sulfate salt

DOSAGE FORMS
Tablets (2.5 mg diphenoxylate and 0.025 mg atropine)
Oral liquid (2.5 mg diphenoxylate and 0.025 mg atropine
per 5 ml teaspoonful)

STORAGE
Diphenoxylate and atropine tablets and oral liquid
should be stored at room temperature in tightly closed,
light-resistant containers. This medication should never
be frozen.

USES
Diphenoxylate and atropine is used to treat severe diarrhea. Diphenoxylate is related to the narcotic analgesics
and acts by slowing the movement of the gastrointestinal
tract. Small amounts of atropine are added to this medication to prevent abuse of the narcotic, diphenoxylate.

TREATMENT
In order to avoid stomach upset, you can take this medication with food or with a full glass of water or milk.

The oral liquid form of this medication should be
measured carefully, using a specially designed, 5 ml

measuring spoon. An ordinary kitchen teaspoon is not accurate enough.

If you miss a dose of this medication, do not take the missed dose at all; just return to your regular dosing schedule. Do not double the next dose.

SIDE EFFECTS

Minor. Blurred vision; constipation; dizziness; drowsiness; dry mouth; flushing; headache; itching; loss of appetite; nervousness; sweating; and swollen gums. These side effects should disappear in several days, as your body adjusts to the medication.

If you become constipated, increase the amount of fiber in your diet (raw vegetables, fruits, salads, bran, and whole-grain breads), and drink more water (unless your doctor directs you to do otherwise).

Chew sugarless gum, or suck on ice chips or a piece of hard candy, to reduce mouth dryness.

If you feel dizzy or light-headed, sit or lie down awhile; get up from a sitting or lying position slowly, and be careful on stairs.

Major. Tell your doctor about any side effects that are persistent or particularly bothersome. IT IS ESPECIALLY IMPORTANT TO TELL YOUR DOCTOR about abdominal pain; bloating; breathing difficulties; depression; difficult or painful urination; false sense of well-being; fever; hives; numbness in the fingers or toes; palpitations; rash; severe nausea; vomiting; or weakness.

INTERACTIONS

This medication interacts with several other types of drugs.

1. Concurrent use of this medication with central nervous system depressants (drugs that slow the activity of the nervous system), such as antihistamines, barbiturates, benzodiazepine tranquilizers, muscle relaxants, narcotics, pain medications, phenothiazine tranquilizers, and alcohol, or with tricyclic anti-depressants can cause extreme drowsiness.

2. A monoamine oxidase (MAO) inhibitor taken within 14 days of this medication can lead to unpredictable and severe side effects.

3. The side effects of the atropine component of this medication may be increased by amantadine, haloperidol, phenothiazine tranquilizers, procainamide, and quinidine.

TELL YOUR DOCTOR if you are currently taking any of the medications listed above.

WARNINGS

• Tell your doctor about unusual or allergic reactions you have had, especially to diphenoxylate or to atropine.

• Tell your doctor if you now have, or if you have ever had, drug-induced diarrhea, gallstones or gallbladder disease, glaucoma, heart disease, hiatal hernia, high blood pressure, kidney disease, liver disease, lung disease, myasthenia gravis, enlarged prostate gland, thyroid disease, or ulcerative colitis.

• If this drug makes you dizzy or drowsy, do not take part in any activity that requires alertness, such as driving a car or operating potentially dangerous equipment.

• Before having any surgery or other medical or dental treatment, be sure to tell your doctor or dentist that you are taking this medication.

• Because this product contains diphenoxylate, it has the potential for abuse, and must be used with caution. Tolerance develops quickly; do not increase the dosage or stop taking the drug unless you first consult your doctor. If you have been taking large amounts of this medication for long periods, and then stop abruptly, you may experience a withdrawal reaction (muscle aches, diarrhea, gooseflesh, runny nose, nausea, vomiting, shivering, trembling, stomach cramps, sleep disorders, irritability, weakness, yawning, and sweating). Your doctor may therefore want to reduce the dosage gradually.

• Check with your doctor if your diarrhea does not subside within two to three days. Unless your doctor prescribes otherwise, do not take this drug for more than five days.

• While taking this medication, drink lots of fluids, to replace those lost with the diarrhea.

• Be sure to tell your doctor if you are pregnant. Although this medication has been shown to be safe in animals, its effects in humans during pregnancy have not yet been thoroughly studied. Also, tell your doctor if you are breastfeeding an infant. Small amounts of this medication pass into breast milk and may cause excessive drowsiness in nursing infants.

diphenoxylate hydrochloride with atropine sulfate
—see diphenoxylate and atropine

Diphenylan—see phenytoin

Diprolene—see betamethasone dipropionate (topical)

Diprosone—see betamethasone dipropionate (topical)

---

dipyridamole

BRAND NAMES (Manufacturers)
Cordilate (Foy)
dipyridamole (various manufacturers)
Persantine (Boehringer Ingelheim)
Pyridamole (Major)
TYPE OF DRUG
Anti-anginal
INGREDIENT
dipyridamole
DOSAGE FORM
Tablets (25 mg, 50 mg, and 75 mg)
STORAGE
Dipyridamole should be stored at room temperature in a tightly closed container.

USES
Dipyridamole is used to prevent chronic chest pain (angina) due to heart disease. It relieves chest pain by dilating the blood vessels of the heart and providing more oxygen to the heart muscle. Dipyridamole is also used to prevent blood clot formation.

TREATMENT
You should take this medication on an empty stomach

with a full glass of water, one hour before or two hours after a meal. If this drug upsets your stomach, check with your doctor to see if you can take it with food.

The full benefits of this medication may not become apparent for up to two months.

If you miss a dose of this medication, take the missed dose as soon as possible, unless it is within four hours of your next scheduled dose. In that case, do not take the missed dose at all; just return to your regular dosing schedule. Do not double the next dose.

SIDE EFFECTS

Minor. Dizziness; fatigue; flushing; headache; nausea; stomach cramps; and weakness. These side effects should disappear in several weeks, as your body adjusts to the medication.

To avoid dizziness or light-headedness when you stand, contract and relax the muscles of your legs for a few moments before rising. Do this by pushing one foot against the floor while raising the other foot slightly, alternating feet so that you are "pumping" your legs in a pedaling motion:

Major. Tell your doctor about any side effects that are persistent or particularly bothersome. IT IS ESPECIALLY IMPORTANT TO TELL YOUR DOCTOR about skin rash; fainting; or a worsening of your chest pain.

INTERACTIONS

Dipyridamole does not interact with other medications, if it is used according to directions.

WARNINGS

• Tell your doctor about unusual or allergic reactions you have had to any medications, especially to dipyridamole.
• Tell your doctor if you now have, or if you have ever had, low blood pressure.
• The effectiveness of dipyridamole in controlling chronic angina is controversial. This drug is more frequently prescribed to prevent blood clot formation, although use of dipyridamole for this purpose has not yet been approved by the Food and Drug Administration.

- This drug does not stop chest pain from angina that has already begun. It is used only to prevent such pain from occurring.
- If this drug makes you dizzy, do not take part in any activity that requires alertness, such as driving a car or operating potentially dangerous equipment.
- Before having any surgery or other medical or dental treatment, be sure to tell your doctor or dentist that you are taking this medication.
- Some of these products contain F.D. & C. Yellow Dye No. 5 (tartrazine), which can cause allergic-type symptoms (difficulty breathing, rash, or fainting) in certain susceptible individuals.
- Be sure to tell your doctor if you are pregnant. Although this drug appears to be safe in humans, extensive studies have not yet been completed. Also, tell your doctor if you are breastfeeding an infant. It is not known whether or not dipyridamole passes into breast milk.

Disophrol Chronotabs—see pseudoephedrine and dexbrompheniramine combination

---

disopyramide

BRAND NAMES (Manufacturers)
Norpace (Searle)
Norpace CR (Searle)
TYPE OF DRUG
Anti-arrhythmic
INGREDIENT
disopyramide as the phosphate salt
DOSAGE FORMS
Capsules (100 mg and 150 mg)
Sustained-release capsules (100 mg and 150 mg)
STORAGE
Disopyramide capsules should be stored at room temperature in tightly closed containers.

USES
Disopyramide is used for the treatment of heart arrhythmias. It corrects irregular heartbeats and helps to

achieve a more normal rhythm.

TREATMENT

Disopyramide should be taken with a full glass of water on an empty stomach, one hour before or two hours after a meal. If this medication upsets your stomach, however, check with your doctor to see if you can take it with food.

Try to take disopyramide at the same times(s) each day. This medication works best if the amount of drug in your bloodstream is kept at a constant level. It should therefore be taken at evenly spaced intervals, day and night. For example, if you are to take it three times per day, the doses should be spaced eight hours apart.

Try not to miss any doses of this medication. If you do miss a dose and you remember within two hours, take the missed dose as soon as possible. If more than two hours have passed, do not take the missed dose; just wait for your next scheduled dose. Do not double the next dose.

SIDE EFFECTS

Minor. Abdominal pain; aches and pain; blurred vision, constipation; diarrhea; dizziness; dry mouth, eyes, and throat; fatigue; gas; headache; impotence; loss of appetite; muscle pain; muscle weakness; nausea; nervousness; rash; and vomiting. These side effects should disappear in several weeks, as your body adjusts to the medication.

To relieve constipation, increase the amount of fiber in your diet (bran, salads, fresh fruits and vegetables, and whole-grain breads), and drink more water (unless your doctor directs you to do otherwise).

If you feel dizzy or light-headed, sit or lie down awhile; get up slowly, and be careful on stairs.

To relieve mouth dryness, suck on ice chips or a piece of hard candy, or chew sugarless gum.

Artificial tears eye drops may help to relieve eye dryness.

This medication may increase your sensitivity to sunlight. It is therefore important to avoid prolonged exposure to sunlight and sunlamps. Wear protective clothing and sunglasses, and use an effective sunscreen.

Major. Tell your doctor about any side effects that are

persistent or particularly bothersome. IT IS ESPECIALLY IMPORTANT TO TELL YOUR DOCTOR about chest pain; depression; difficulty urinating; enlarged, painful breasts (in both sexes); fainting; fever; numbness or tingling sensations; palpitations; shortness of breath; sore throat; swelling of the feet or ankles; weight gain; or yellowing of the eyes or skin.

INTERACTIONS

Disopyramide interacts with several other types of drugs.
1. Phenytoin, rifampin, barbiturates, and glutethimide can decrease its effectiveness.
2. The combination of alcohol and disopyramide can lead to dizziness and hypoglycemia (low blood sugar levels). You should therefore avoid drinking alcoholic beverages while you are taking this medication.
Before starting to take disopyramide, BE SURE TO TELL YOUR DOCTOR if you are already taking any of the medications listed above.

WARNINGS

• Tell your doctor about unusual or allergic reactions you have had to any medications, especially to disopyramide.
• Tell your doctor if you now have, or if you have ever had, glaucoma, hypoglycemia, hypokalemia (low blood potassium levels), kidney disease, liver disease, myasthenia gravis, urinary retention, or an enlarged prostate gland.
• If this drug makes you dizzy or drowsy, or blurs your vision, do not take part in any activities that require alertness, such as driving a car or operating potentially dangerous equipment.
• This medication can decrease sweating and heat release from the body. You should therefore avoid getting overheated by strenuous exercise in hot weather, and should avoid taking hot baths, showers, and saunas.
• Before having any surgery or other medical or dental treatment, be sure to tell your doctor or dentist that you are taking this medication.
• Disopyramide can cause hypoglycemia. Signs of hypoglycemia include anxiety, chills, pale skin, headache,

hunger, nausea, nervousness, shakiness, sweating, and weakness. If you experience this reaction, eat or drink food containing sugar, and CONTACT YOUR DOCTOR.
• Be sure to tell your doctor if you are pregnant. Although this drug appears to be safe, extensive studies in humans during pregnancy have not yet been completed. Also, tell your doctor if you are breastfeeding an infant. Small amounts of disopyramide pass into breast milk.

Di-Spaz—see dicyclomine

Dispos-a-Med—see isoetharine

disulfiram

BRAND NAMES (Manufacturers)
Antabuse (Ayerst)
disulfiram (various manufacturers)
TYPE OF DRUG
Anti-alcoholic
INGREDIENT
disulfiram
DOSAGE FORM
Tablets (250 mg and 500 mg)
STORAGE
Disulfiram should be stored at room temperature in a tightly closed, light-resistant container.

USES
Disulfiram is used as an aid to treat strongly motivated alcoholics who want to remain sober. Disulfiram blocks the breakdown of alcohol by the body, leading to an accumulation of the chemical acetaldehyde in the bloodstream. Buildup of acetaldehyde in the body can lead to a severe and very unpleasant reaction. Alcohol must therefore be avoided to prevent this reaction.

TREATMENT
Disulfiram can be taken either on an empty stomach or with food or milk (as directed by your doctor). The tablets

can also be crushed and mixed with beverages (non-alcoholic).

If you miss a dose of this medication, take the missed dose as soon as possible, unless it is almost time for the next dose. In that case do not take the missed dose at all; just return to your regular dosing schedule. Do not double the next dose.

SIDE EFFECTS

Minor. Drowsiness; fatigue; headache; metallic or garlic-like aftertaste; and restlessness. These side effects should disappear in several days, as your body adjusts to the medication.

Major. Tell your doctor about any side effects that are persistent or particularly bothersome. IT IS ESPECIALLY IMPORTANT TO TELL YOUR DOCTOR about blurred vision; impotence; joint pain; mental disorders; skin rash; tingling sensations; or yellowing of the eyes or skin.

INTERACTIONS

Disulfiram interacts with other types of medication.

1. It can increase the blood levels and side effects of diazepam, chlordiazepoxide, phenytoin, and oral anticoagulants (blood thinners, such as warfarin).

2. Concurrent use of disulfiram with isoniazid, metronidazole, paraldehyde, or marijuana can lead to severe reactions.

BE SURE TO TELL YOUR DOCTOR if you are currently taking any of these types of medication.

WARNINGS

• Tell your doctor about unusual or allergic reactions you have had to any medications, especially to disulfiram.

• Before starting to take this medication, be sure to tell your doctor if you now have, or if you have ever had, brain damage, dermatitis, diabetes mellitus (sugar diabetes), epilepsy, heart disease, kidney disease, liver disease, mental disorders, or thyroid disease.

• It is important to not drink or use any alcohol-containing preparations or medications (including beer, wine, liquor, vinegar, sauces, aftershave lotions, liniments, or colognes) while taking this medication. Be sure to check the labels on any over-the-counter (non-prescription) products for their alcohol content.

• It is important that you understand the serious nature of the disulfiram-alcohol reaction. If you take disulfiram within 12 hours after ingesting alcohol, or drink alcohol for up to two weeks after your last dose of disulfiram, you may experience blurred vision, chest pain, confusion, dizziness, fainting, flushing, headache, nausea, pounding heartbeat, sweating, vomiting, and weakness. The reaction usually occurs within five to ten minutes of drinking alcohol and can last from half an hour to two hours, depending on the dose of disulfiram and the quantity of alcohol ingested.

• If this drug makes you drowsy, do not take part in any activities that require alertness, such as driving a car or operating potentially dangerous equipment.

• Be sure to tell your doctor if you are pregnant. Birth defects have been reported in both animals and humans whose mothers received disulfiram during pregnancy. It must also be kept in mind that alcohol, even in small amounts, can cause a variety of birth defects when ingested during pregnancy. The risks should be discussed with your doctor. Also, tell your doctor if you are breast-feeding an infant. It is not known whether or not disulfiram passes into breast milk.

Ditan—see phenytoin

Ditropan—see oxybutynin

Diucardin—see hydroflumethiazide

Diulo—see metolazone

Diurese—see trichlormethiazide

Diuril—see chlorothiazide

Diu-Scrip—see hydrochlorothiazide

Dolacet—see acetaminophen and propoxyphene combination

Dolene—see propoxyphene

Dolene AP-65—see acetaminophen and propoxyphene combination

Dolene Compound-65—see aspirin, caffeine, and propoxyphene combination

Dolobid—see diflunisal

Dolo-Pap—see acetaminophen and hydrocodone combination

Dolophine—see methadone

Domeform-HC—see hydrocortisone and iodochlorhydroxyquin combination (topical)

Donnamor—see atropine, scopolamine, hyoscyamine, and phenobarbital combination

Donna-Sed—see atropine, scopolamine, hyoscyamine, and phenobarbital combination

Donnatal—see atropine, scopolamine, hyoscyamine, and phenobarbital combination

Dopar—see levodopa

Doriden—see glutethimide

Doxaphene—see propoxyphene

Doxaphene Compound—see aspirin, caffeine, and propoxyphene combination

---

doxepin

BRAND NAMES (Manufacturers)
Adapin (Pennwalt)
Sinequan (Roerig)

TYPE OF DRUG
Tricyclic anti-depressant (mood elevator)
INGREDIENT
doxepin as the hydrochloride salt
DOSAGE FORMS
Capsules (10 mg, 25 mg, 50 mg, 75 mg, 100 mg, and 150 mg)
Oral concentrate (10 mg per ml)
STORAGE
Doxepin should be stored at room temperature in tightly closed containers. This medication should never be frozen.

USES

Doxepin is used to relieve the symptoms of mental depression. This medication belongs to a group of drugs referred to as the tricyclic anti-depressants. These medicines are thought to relieve depression by increasing the concentration of certain chemicals necessary for nerve transmission in the brain.

TREATMENT

This medication should be taken exactly as your doctor prescribes. You can take it with water or with food to lessen the chance of stomach irritation (unless your doctor tells you to do otherwise).

Each dose of the oral concentrate should be diluted in at least 4 ounces (half a glass) of water, milk, or fruit juice just prior to administration. Measure the correct amount carefully with the dropper provided. DO NOT mix the medication with grape juice or with carbonated beverages, since they may decrease the medicine's effectiveness.

If you miss a dose of this medication, take the missed dose as soon as possible, then return to your regular dosing schedule. If, however, the dose you missed was a once-a-day bedtime dose, do not take that dose in the morning; check with your doctor instead. If the dose is taken in the morning, it may cause some unwanted side effects. Never double the dose.

The effects of therapy with this medication may not become apparent for two or three weeks.

SIDE EFFECTS

Minor. Agitation; anxiety; blurred vision; confusion; constipation; cramps; diarrhea; dizziness; drowsiness; dry mouth; fatigue; indigestion; insomnia; loss of appetite; nausea; peculiar tastes in the mouth; restlessness; sweating; vomiting; weakness; or weight gain or loss. As your body adjusts to the medication, these side effects should disappear.

Dry mouth can be relieved by chewing sugarless gum or by sucking on ice chips or a piece of hard candy.

To relieve constipation, increase the amount of fiber (bran, salads, whole-grain breads, fresh fruits and vegetables) in your diet, and drink more water (unless your doctor directs you to do otherwise).

To avoid dizziness or light-headedness when you stand, contract and relax the muscles of your legs for a few moments before rising. Do this by pushing one foot against the floor while raising the other foot slightly, alternating feet so that you are "pumping" your legs in a pedaling motion.

This medication may cause increased sensitivity to sunlight. You should therefore avoid prolonged exposure to sunlight and sunlamps. Wear protective clothing, and use an effective sunscreen.

Major. Tell your doctor about any side effects that are persistent or particularly bothersome. IT IS ESPECIALLY IMPORTANT TO TELL YOUR DOCTOR about a tendency to bleed or bruise; chest pain; convulsions; difficulty urinating; enlarged or painful breasts (in both sexes); fainting; fever; fluid retention; hair loss; hallucinations; headaches; impotence; mood changes; mouth sores; nervousness; nightmares; numbness in the fingers or toes; palpitations; ringing in the ears; seizures; skin rash; sleep disorders; sore throat; tremors; uncoordinated movements or balance problems; or yellowing of the eyes or skin.

INTERACTIONS

Doxepin interacts with a number of other medications.

1. Extreme drowsiness can occur when this medicine is taken with central nervous system depressants (medicines that slow the activity of the nervous system), such as alco-

hol, antihistamines, barbiturates, benzodiazepine tranquilizers, muscle relaxants, narcotics, pain medications, phenothiazine tranquilizers, and sleeping medications.
2. Doxepin may decrease the effectiveness of antiseizure medications and may block the blood-pressure-lowering effects of clonidine and guanethidine.
3. Oral contraceptives (estrogens) can increase the side effects and reduce the effectiveness of the tricyclic antidepressants (including doxepin).
4. Tricyclic anti-depressants may increase the side effects of thyroid medications and over-the-counter (nonprescription) cough, cold, allergy, asthma, sinus, and diet medications.
5. The concurrent use of tricyclic anti-depressants and monoamine oxidase (MAO) inhibitors should be undertaken very carefully, because the combination may result in fever, convulsions, or high blood pressure.
Before starting to take doxepin, BE SURE TO TELL YOUR DOCTOR if you are already taking any of the medications listed above.

WARNINGS

• Tell your doctor if you have had unusual or allergic reactions to medications, especially to doxepin or any of the other tricyclic anti-depressants (amitriptyline, imipramine, trimipramine, amoxapine, protriptyline, desipramine, maprotiline, or nortriptyline).
• Tell your doctor if you now have, or if you have ever had, asthma, high blood pressure, liver or kidney disease, heart disease, a recent heart attack, circulatory disease, stomach problems, intestinal problems, alcoholism, difficulty urinating, enlarged prostate gland, epilepsy, glaucoma, thyroid disease, mental illness, or electroshock therapy.
• If this drug makes you dizzy or drowsy, do not take part in any activity that requires alertness, such as driving a car or operating potentially dangerous equipment.
• Before having any surgery or other medical or dental treatment, be sure to tell your doctor or dentist that you are taking this medication.
• Do not stop taking this drug suddenly. Abruptly stopping it can cause nausea, headache, stomach upset,

fatigue, or a worsening of your condition. Your doctor may want to reduce the dosage gradually.

• The effects of this medication may last as long as seven days after you have stopped taking it, so continue to observe all precautions during that period.

• Be sure to tell your doctor if you are pregnant. Problems in humans have not been reported; however, studies in animals have shown that this medication can cause side effects to the fetus if given to the mother in large doses during pregnancy. Also, tell your doctor if you are breastfeeding an infant. Small amounts of this drug can pass into breast milk and may cause unwanted effects, such as irritability or sleeping problems, in the nursing infant.

Doxy-Caps—see doxycycline

Doxychel Hyclate—see doxycycline

---

doxycycline

BRAND NAMES (Manufacturers)
Doxy-Caps (Barr and Edwards)
Doxychel Hyclate (Rachelle)
doxycycline (various manufacturers)
Doxy-Lemmon (Lemmon)
Doxy-Tabs (Rachelle)
Vibramycin (Pfizer)
Vibra Tabs (Pfizer)
TYPE OF DRUG
Antibiotic (infection fighter)
INGREDIENT
doxycycline as the hyclate or calcium salt
DOSAGE FORMS
Tablets (100 mg)
Capsules (50 mg and 100 mg)
Oral suspension (25 mg per 5 ml teaspoonful)
Oral syrup (50 mg per 5 ml teaspoonful)
STORAGE
Doxycycline tablets, capsules, oral suspension, and oral syrup should be stored at room temperature in tightly

closed, light-resistant containers. Any unused portion of the suspension should be discarded after 14 days, because the drug loses its potency after that period. This medication should never be frozen.

USES

Doxycycline is used to treat a wide variety of bacterial infections, and to prevent or treat traveler's diarrhea. It acts by inhibiting the growth of bacteria.

Doxycycline kills susceptible bacteria, but it is not effective against viruses or fungi.

TREATMENT

To avoid stomach upset, you can take this medication with food (unless your doctor directs you to do otherwise).

The suspension form of this medication should be shaken well just before measuring each dose. The contents tend to settle on the bottom of the bottle, so it is necessary to shake the container to evenly distribute the ingredients and equalize the doses. Each dose of the oral suspension or oral syrup should be measured carefully with a specially designed, 5 ml measuring spoon. An ordinary kitchen teaspoon is not accurate enough.

The oral syrup form of this medication should not be mixed with any other substance, unless your doctor directs you to do so.

Doxycycline works best when the level of medicine in your bloodstream is kept constant. It is therefore best to take the doses at evenly spaced intervals, day and night. For example, if you are to take four doses a day, the doses should be spaced six hours apart.

If you miss a dose of this medication, take the missed dose immediately. However, if you do not remember to take the missed dose until it is almost time for your next dose, take it; then space the next dose about halfway through the regular interval between doses. Then return to your regular dosing schedule. Try not to skip any doses.

It is important to continue to take this medication for the entire time prescribed by your doctor—even if the symptoms disappear before the end of that period. If you stop taking the drug too soon, resistant bacteria are given a chance to continue growing, and the infection could recur.

SIDE EFFECTS

Minor. Diarrhea; discoloration of the nails; dizziness; loss of appetite; nausea; stomach cramps and upset; and vomiting. These side effects should disappear in several days, as your body adjusts to the medication.

Doxycycline can increase your sensitivity to sunlight. In order to avoid this side effect, limit your exposure to sunlight and sunlamps. Wear protective clothing and sunglasses, and use an effective sunscreen.

Major. Tell your doctor about any side effects that are persistent or particularly bothersome. IT IS ESPECIALLY IMPORTANT TO TELL YOUR DOCTOR about darkened tongue; difficulty breathing; joint pain; mouth irritation· rash; rectal or vaginal itching; sore throat and fever; unusual bleeding or bruising; or yellowing of the eyes or skin. Also, if your symptoms of infection seem to be getting worse rather than improving, you should contact your doctor.

INTERACTIONS

Doxycycline interacts with several other types of medication.

1. It can increase the absorption of digoxin, which may lead to digoxin toxicity.

2. The gastrointestinal side effects (nausea, vomiting, stomach upset) of theophylline may be increased by doxycycline.

3. The dosage of oral anti-coagulants (blood thinners, such as warfarin) may need to be adjusted when this medication is started.

4. Doxycycline may decrease the effectiveness of oral contraceptives (birth control pills), and pregnancy could result. You should therefore use another form of birth control while taking doxycycline. Discuss this with your doctor.

5. Barbiturates, carbamazepine, and phenytoin can lower the blood levels of doxycycline, decreasing its effectiveness.

TELL YOUR DOCTOR if you are currently taking any of the medications listed above.

WARNINGS

- Tell your doctor about unusual or allergic reactions you have had to any medications, especially to doxycycline, oxytetracycline, tetracycline, or minocycline.
- Tell your doctor if you now have, or if you have ever had, kidney or liver disease.
- Doxycycline can affect tests for syphilis; tell your doctor you are taking this medication if you are also being treated for this disease.
- Make sure that your prescription for this medication is marked with the drug's expiration date. The drug should be discarded after the expiration date. If doxycycline is used after it has expired, serious side effects (especially to the kidneys) could result.
- This medication has been prescribed for your current infection only. Another infection later on, or one that someone else has, may require a different medicine. You should not give your medicine to other people, or use it for other infections, unless your doctor specifically directs you to do so.
- Be sure to tell your doctor if you are pregnant or if you are breastfeeding an infant. Doxycycline crosses the placenta and passes into breast milk. If used during their development, this drug can cause permanent discoloration of the teeth and can inhibit tooth and bone growth. In addition, this drug should not be used for infants or for children less than eight years of age.

Doxy-Lemmon—see doxycycline

Doxy-Tabs—see doxycycline

Dralzine—see hydralazine

Dri-Phed with Codeine—see pseudoephedrine, tripolidine, guaifenesin, and codeine combination

Drisdol—see ergocalciferol (vitamin D)

Drize—see phenylpropanolamine and chlorpheniramine combination

Duo-Hist—see pseudoephedrine and dexbrompheniramine combination

Duotrate Plateau Caps—see pentaerythritol tetranitrate

Duradyne DHC—see acetaminophen and hydrocodone combination

Duralex—see pseudoephedrine and chlorpheniramine combination

Duraphyl—see theophylline

Duraquin—see quinidine

Duricef—see cefadroxil

Durrax—see hydroxyzine

Duvoid—see bethanechol

Dyazide—see triamterene and hydrochlorothiazide combination

Dycill—see dicloxacillin

Dymelor—see acetohexamide

Dynapen—see dicloxacillin

Dyrenium—see triamterene

Dyrexan-OD—see phendimetrazine

Easprin—see aspirin

Edecrin—see ethacrynic acid

E.E.S. — see erythromycin

E.E.S. 400 — see erythromycin

Efedra P.A. — see pseudoephedrine and dexbrompheniramine combination

Elavil — see amitriptyline

Eldecort — see hydrocortisone (topical)

Elixicon — see theophylline

Elixomin — see theophylline

Elixophylline — see theophylline

Elmotil — see diphenoxylate and atropine

Emcodeine — see aspirin and codeine combination

Emitrip — see amitriptyline

Empirin with Codeine — see aspirin and codeine combination

Empracet with Codeine — see acetaminophen and codeine combination

E-Mycin — see erythromycin

Endep — see amitriptyline

Enduron — see methyclothiazide

Enovid-E — see oral contraceptives

Enoxa — see diphenoxylate and atropine

Entex L.A. — see phenylpropanolamine and guaifenesin combination

Epifoam—see hydrocortisone (topical)

Epiform-HC—see hydrocortisone and
    iodochlorhydroxyquin combination (topical)

Epifrin—see epinephrine (ophthalmic)

Epinal—see epinephrine (ophthalmic)

---

epinephrine (ophthalmic)

BRAND NAMES (Manufacturers)
Epifrin (Allergan)
Epinal (Alcon)
Epitrate (Ayerst)
Eppy/N (Barnes-Hind/Hydrocurve)
Glaucon (Alcon)
TYPE OF DRUG
Anti-glaucoma ophthalmic solution
INGREDIENT
epinephrine (adrenalin) as the hydrochloride, bitartrate,
    or borate salt
DOSAGE FORM
Ophthalmic solution (0.25%, 0.5%, 1%, and 2%)
STORAGE
Epinephrine solution should be stored at room tempera-
ture in a tightly closed, light-resistant container. This
medication should never be frozen. The solution should
be discarded if it turns brown or cloudy, because this
indicates deterioration and loss of potency.

USES
Epinephrine (ophthalmic) is used to treat glaucoma. It
lowers the pressure in the eye by decreasing the production of aqueous humor (a particular fluid in the eye) and
increasing its removal.

TREATMENT
Wash your hands with soap and water before applying
this medication. In order to avoid contamination of the
eye drops, be careful not to touch the dropper or let it

touch your eye; and DO NOT wipe off or rinse the dropper after use.

To apply the eye drops, tilt your head back and pull down your lower eyelid with one hand to make a pouch below the eye. Drop the prescribed amount of medicine into this pouch and slowly close your eyes. Try not to blink. Keep your eyes closed for a minute or two, and place one finger at the corner of the eye, next to your nose, applying a slight pressure (this is done to prevent loss of the medication into the nose and throat canal). Then wipe away any excess with a clean tissue. Since the drops are somewhat difficult to apply, you may want to have someone else apply them for you.

If you have been prescribed more than one type of eye drop, after applying epinephrine, wait at least five minutes before using any other eye medication (to give the epinephrine time to work). However, if you are also using an eye drop that constricts your pupils, check with your doctor to see which drug should be applied first.

If you miss a dose of epinephrine, apply the missed dose as soon as possible, unless it is almost time for the next dose. In that case, do not apply the missed dose at all; just return to your regular dosing schedule. Do not double the next dose.

SIDE EFFECTS

Minor. Brow ache; headache; or transitory stinging on initial application. These side effects should disappear in several days, as your body adjusts to the medication.

Major. Tell your doctor about any side effects that are persistent or particularly bothersome. IT IS ESPECIALLY IMPORTANT TO TELL YOUR DOCTOR about blurred vision; eye pain; fainting; palpitations; sweating; or trembling.

INTERACTIONS

Epinephrine interacts with other types of medication.

1. Concurrent use of epinephrine and monoamine oxidase (MAO) inhibitors or tricyclic anti-depressants can lead to serious side effects. At least 21 days should therefore separate doses of epinephrine and either of these types of medication.

2. Digoxin can increase the side effects of epinephrine. BE SURE TO TELL YOUR DOCTOR if you are already taking any of the medications listed above

WARNINGS

• Tell your doctor about unusual or allergic reactions you have had to any medications, especially to epinephrine.
• Before starting to take this medication, be sure to tell your doctor if you now have, or if you have ever had, diabetes mellitus (sugar diabetes), heart or blood vessel disease, high blood pressure, stroke, or thyroid disease.
• If this medication blurs your vision, try to avoid activities that require alertness, such as driving a car or operating potentially dangerous equipment.
• Epinephrine can cause discoloration of soft contact lenses. If you currently wear soft contact lenses, you should discuss with your doctor whether your medication or your contact lenses should be changed.
• Be sure to tell your doctor if you are pregnant. Although epinephrine (ophthalmic) appears to be safe during pregnancy, studies in humans have not yet been completed. Also, tell your doctor if you are breastfeeding an infant. It is not known whether or not epinephrine passes into breast milk.

Epitrate—see epinephrine (ophthalmic)

E.P. Mycin—see oxytetracycline

Eppy/N—see epinephrine (ophthalmic)

Equagesic—see meprobamate and aspirin combination

Equanil—see meprobamate

Eramycin—see erythromycin

Ercaf—see ergotamine and caffeine combination

Ercatab—see ergotamine and caffeine combination

Ergo-Caff—see ergotamine and caffeine combination

ergocalciferol (vitamin D)

BRAND NAMES (Manufacturers)
Calciferol (Kremers-Urban)
Deltalin Gelseals (Lilly)
Drisdol (Winthrop)
vitamin D (various manufacturers)
TYPE OF DRUG
Vitamin D
INGREDIENT
ergocalciferol
DOSAGE FORMS
Tablets (50,000 units)
Capsules (25,000 units and 50,000 units)
Oral liquid (8,000 units per ml)
STORAGE
Ergocalciferol tablets, capsules, and liquid should be stored at room temperature in tightly closed, light-resistant containers. This medication should never be frozen.

USES

Ergocalciferol is used to treat rickets, hypophosphatemia (low blood levels of phosphate), and hypoparathyroidism (underactive parathyroid gland). This medication is converted by the liver and kidney to the active form of vitamin D—a vitamin essential to many body systems (including bone and tooth structure, regulation of blood calcium levels, and heart and muscle contraction).

TREATMENT

Ergocalciferol can be taken either on an empty stomach or with food or milk (as directed by your doctor).

Each dose of the oral liquid form of this medication should be measured carefully, with the dropper provided. The liquid can then be taken directly or mixed with fruit juice, cereal, or other foods.

If you miss a dose of this medication, take the missed dose as soon as possible, unless it is almost time for the next dose. In that case, do not take the missed dose at all; just return to your regular dosing schedule. Do not double the next dose.

SIDE EFFECTS
Minor. None, at the dosages normally prescribed.
Major. The side effects associated with ergocalciferol therapy are usually the result of too much medication (vitamin D intoxication). Tell your doctor about any side effects that are persistent or particularly bothersome. IT IS ESPECIALLY IMPORTANT TO TELL YOUR DOCTOR about blurred vision; bone pain; constipation; dry mouth; headache; increased thirst; increased urination; irritability; loss of appetite; metallic taste in the mouth; mental disorders; muscle pain; nausea; palpitations; runny nose; vomiting; weakness; or weight loss.

INTERACTIONS
Cholestyramine, colestipol, and mineral oil can decrease the absorption of ergocalciferol from the gastrointestinal tract, decreasing its effectiveness. BE SURE TO TELL YOUR DOCTOR if you are already taking any of these medications.

WARNINGS
• Tell your doctor about unusual or allergic reactions you have had to any medications, especially to ergocalciferol (vitamin D), calcitriol, calcifediol, or dihydrotachysterol.
• Before starting to take this medication, be sure to tell your doctor if you now have, or if you have ever had, heart or blood vessel disease, hypercalcemia (high blood levels of calcium), hyperphosphatemia (high blood levels of phosphate), vitamin D intoxication, or sarcoidosis.
• Before taking any over-the-counter (non-prescription) products that contain calcium, phosphates, magnesium, or vitamin D, check with your doctor. These ingredients can increase the side effects of ergocalciferol.
• Be sure to tell your doctor if you are pregnant. Although ergocalciferol appears to be safe during pregnancy, extensive studies in humans have not yet been completed. Also, tell your doctor if you are breastfeeding an infant. Small amounts of ergocalciferol may pass into breast milk.

ergoloid mesylates

BRAND NAMES (Manufacturers)
Circanol (Riker)
Deapril-ST (Mead Johnson)
ergoloid mesylates (various manufacturers)
Gerimal (Rugby)
H.E.A. (Vangard)
Hydergine (Sandoz)
Trigot (Squibb)
TYPE OF DRUG
Vasodilator
INGREDIENTS
ergoloid mesylates
DOSAGE FORMS
Oral tablets (1 mg)
Sublingual tablets (0.5 mg and 1 mg)
Oral liquid (1 mg per ml with 30% alcohol)
STORAGE
Ergoloid mesylates tablets and oral liquid should be stored at room temperature in tightly closed, light-resistant containers. This medication should never be frozen.

USES

This medication is used to reduce the symptoms associated with senility. It is not clear how ergoloid mesylates work, but It Is thought that they act by dilating the blood vessels, increasing blood flow to the brain.

TREATMENT

In order to avoid stomach irritation, you can take the oral tablets or oral liquid with food or milk. Be sure to measure the dose of the liquid form of this medication carefully, with the dropper provided.

The sublingual form of this medication must be placed under the tongue, and allowed to dissolve completely. Try not to swallow for as long as possible, because the drug is more completely absorbed through the lining of the mouth than it is from the stomach. Do not drink any liquid, eat, or smoke for at least ten minutes after placing the tablet under the tongue.

If you miss a dose of this medication, take the missed dose as soon as possible, unless it is almost time for the next dose. In that case, do not take the missed dose at all; just return to your regular dosing schedule. Do not double the next dose.

It may take three or four weeks for the effects of this medication to become apparent.

SIDE EFFECTS

Minor. Blurred vision; dizziness; drowsiness; flushing; headache; irritation under the tongue (with the sublingual form only); light-headedness; loss of appetite; nasal congestion; nausea; stomach cramps; and vomiting. These side effects should disappear in several days, as your body adjusts to the medication.

If you feel dizzy or light-headed, sit or lie down awhile; get up slowly, and be careful on stairs.

Major. Tell your doctor about any side effects that are persistent or particularly bothersome. IT IS ESPECIALLY IMPORTANT TO TELL YOUR DOCTOR about a slowed heart rate.

INTERACTIONS

Ergoloid mesylates do not interact with other medications, if they are used according to directions.

WARNINGS

• Tell your doctor about unusual or allergic reactions you have had to any medications, especially to ergoloid mesylates or ergot alkaloids (such as ergonovine, ergotamine, or bromocriptine).

• Before starting to take this medication, be sure to tell your doctor if you now have, or if you have ever had, liver disease, low blood pressure, porphyria, severe mental illness, or a slowed heart rate.

• Ergoloid mesylates may lessen your ability to adjust to the cold. Therefore, do not expose your body to very cold temperatures for prolonged periods.

• Your doctor may want you to take your pulse daily while you are using this medication. Contact your doctor if your pulse becomes slower than normal, or if it drops below 50 beats per minute.

• If this drug makes you dizzy or drowsy, or blurs your vision, do not take part in any activities that require alertness, such as driving a car or operating potentially dangerous machinery.
• Some of these products contain F.D. & C. Yellow Dye No. 5 (tartrazine), which can cause allergic-type symptoms (rash, shortness of breath, or fainting) in certain susceptible individuals.

Ergomar — see ergotamine

---

ergonovine

BRAND NAMES (Manufacturers)
ergonovine maleate (various manufacturers)
Ergotrate Maleate (Lilly)
TYPE OF DRUG
Uterine stimulant
INGREDIENT
ergonovine as the maleate salt
DOSAGE FORM
Tablets (0.2 mg)
STORAGE
Ergonovine should be stored at room temperature, in a tightly closed container.

USES

Ergonovine is used to prevent or treat post-partum (immediately after delivery) or post-abortion uterine bleeding. This medication is usually administered for only a short period of time (usually 48 hours). It acts directly on the uterus to cause contractions and to constrict blood vessels.

TREATMENT

Ergonovine tablets can be taken either on an empty stomach or with food or milk (as directed by your doctor). For more rapid effect, the tablet can also be placed under the tongue to dissolve.

If you miss a dose of this medication, do not take the

missed dose at all; just return to to your regular dosing schedule. Do not double the next dose.

SIDE EFFECTS

Minor. Diarrhea; headache; nausea; and vomiting. These side effects should disappear as your body adjusts to the medication.

Major. Tell your doctor about any side effects that are persistent or particularly bothersome. IT IS ESPECIALLY IMPORTANT TO TELL YOUR DOCTOR about chest pain; confusion; convulsions; excitement; hallucinations; hives; itching; numbness or coldness of the fingers or toes; ringing in the ears; shortness of breath; skin rash; or tingling sensations—even if these side effects appear or continue after you stop taking ergonovine.

INTERACTIONS

Ergonovine does not interact with other medications, if it is used according to directions.

WARNINGS

• Tell your doctor about unusual or allergic reactions you have had to medications, especially to ergonovine, or to any other ergot alkaloid (bromocriptine, ergotamine, or ergoloid mesylates).

• Before starting to take this medication, tell your doctor if you now have, or if you have ever had, hypocalcemia (low blood calcium levels); heart disease; high blood pressure; kidney disease; liver disease; or peripheral vascular disease (poor circulation).

• Be sure to tell your doctor if you are breastfeeding an infant. Ergonovine can pass into breast milk and may cause side effects in the nursing infant. It can also decrease milk production.

ergonovine maleate—see ergonovine

Ergostat—see ergotamine

ergotamine

BRAND NAMES (Manufacturers)
Ergomar (Fisons)
Ergostat (Parke-Davis)
Gynergen (Sandoz)
Medihaler Ergotamine (Riker)
Wigrettes (Organon)
TYPE OF DRUG
Anti migraine (vasoconstrictor)
INGREDIENT
ergotamine as the tartrate salt
DOSAGE FORMS
Oral tablets (1 mg)
Sublingual tablets (2 mg)
Aerosol (0.36 mg per spray)
STORAGE
This medication should be stored at room temperature, in tightly closed, light-resistant containers.

The container of the aerosol form of this medication is pressurized; it should therefore never be punctured or broken. It should also be stored away from heat and direct sunlight.

USES

This medication is used to treat migraine and cluster headaches. These headaches are thought to be caused by an increase in the diameter of the blood vessels in the head, which results in increased blood flow, increased pressure, and pain. Ergotamine acts by constricting the blood vessels, thereby counteracting these effects.

TREATMENT

It is best to take this medication as soon as you notice your migraine headache symptoms. If you wait until the headache becomes severe, the drug takes longer to work and may not be as effective.

After you take any of these forms of ergotamine, you should try to lie down in a quiet, dark room for at least two hours (in order to help the medication work). The drug usually takes effect in 30 to 60 minutes.

It is very important that you understand how often you

can repeat a dose of this medication during an attack (usually every 30 to 60 minutes) and the maximum number of tablets you can take per day (usually six oral tablets or three sublingual tablets). Ten is generally the maximum number of oral tablets (or five sublingual tablets) that can be taken in any one-week period. CHECK WITH YOUR DOCTOR if you have any questions.

The oral tablet form of this medication should be swallowed with liquid. Take one tablet when you first notice your migraine headache symptoms. If necessary, take a second dose 30 to 60 minutes later to relieve your headache.

The sublingual tablets should be placed under your tongue. DO NOT swallow these tablets—they are more efficiently absorbed through the lining of the mouth than from the gastrointestinal tract. Try not to eat, drink, or chew while the tablet is dissolving.

The aerosol form of this medication comes packaged with instructions for use. Read the directions carefully; if you have any questions, check with your doctor or pharmacist. The aerosol can should be shaken well just before each dose is sprayed. The contents tend to settle on the bottom of the container, so it should be shaken to disperse the medication and equalize the doses.

If you are on prolonged treatment with this drug and you miss a dose, take it as soon as you remember. Wait four hours to take the next dose. It is very important that you consult your doctor before you discontinue using this drug. Your doctor may want to reduce your dosage gradually.

SIDE EFFECTS

Minor. Diarrhea; dizziness; headache; nausea; vomiting; sensation of cold hands and feet with MILD numbness or tingling. These side effects should disappear as your body adjusts to the medication.

The aerosol form of ergotamine can cause hoarseness or throat irritation. Gargling or rinsing your mouth out with water after taking the dose may help prevent this side effect.

Major. Tell your doctor about any side effects that are persistent or particularly bothersome. IT IS ESPECIALLY

IMPORTANT TO TELL YOUR DOCTOR about chest pain; confusion; fluid retention; itching; localized swelling; muscle pain; coldness, numbness, pain, tingling, or dark discoloration of fingers or toes; severe abdominal pain and swelling; or unusual weakness.

INTERACTIONS

Ergotamine interacts with several kinds of drugs, including amphetamines, ephedrine, epinephrine (adrenalin), pseudoephedrine, and troleandomycin. Such combinations can lead to increases in blood pressure or increased risk of adverse reaction to ergotamine.

BE SURE TO TELL YOUR DOCTOR if you are already taking any of the medications listed above.

Do not drink alcoholic beverages while you are taking this medication. Since alcohol dilates the blood vessels (makes them larger), drinking will only make your headache worse.

Ergotamine interacts with marijuana to produce cold sensations in the arms and legs, or even persistent chill.

Tobacco (nicotine) and cocaine decrease the effectiveness of ergotamine, and therefore make the headache worse.

The caffeine in tea, coffee, and cola drinks also interacts with this medication. It may actually help to relieve your headache.

WARNINGS

• Tell your doctor about unusual or allergic reactions you have had to any medications, especially to ergotamine, bromocriptine, or any other ergot alkaloid.

• Before starting to take this medication, be sure to tell your doctor if you now have, or if you have ever had, heart or blood vessel disease, high blood pressure, infections, kidney disease, liver disease, or thyroid disease.

• Avoid any foods to which you are allergic—they may make your headache worse.

• If this drug makes you dizzy or drowsy, do not take part in any activity that requires alertness, such as driving a car or operating potentially dangerous equipment.

• Try to avoid exposure to cold. Since this drug acts by constricting blood vessels throughout the body (not just in the head), your hands and feet, especially, may become very sensitive to the cold.

• This medication should not be taken for longer periods or in higher doses than recommended by your doctor. Extended use of this drug can lead to serious side effects. In addition, tolerance can develop—higher doses would be required to obtain the same beneficial effects (at the same time increasing the risk of side effects).

• Be sure to tell your doctor if you are pregnant. Ergotamine can cause contractions of the uterus, which can harm the developing fetus. Also, tell your doctor if you are breastfeeding an infant. Ergotamine passes into breast milk and may cause vomiting, diarrhea, or convulsions in the nursing infant.

MONEY-SAVING TIP

Save the inhaler piece from the aerosol container. Refill units, which are less expensive, are available.

---

ergotamine and caffeine combination

BRAND NAMES (Manufacturers)
Cafergot (Sandoz)
Cafertabs (Three P Products)
Cafertrate (Henry Schein)
Ercaf (Geneva Generics)
Ercatab (Cord)
Ergo-Caff (Rugby)
TYPE OF DRUG
Anti-migraine (vasoconstrictor)
INGREDIENTS
ergotamine as the tartrate salt; caffeine
DOSAGE FORMS
Tablets (1 mg ergotamine, 100 mg caffeine)
Capsules (1 mg ergotamine, 100 mg caffeine)
Suppositories (2 mg ergotamine, 100 mg caffeine)
STORAGE
The tablet and capsule forms of this medication should be stored at room temperature in tightly closed, light-

resistant containers. They should also be stored away from heat and direct sunlight.

The suppository form of this medication should be stored in the refrigerator in a tightly closed container.

USES

This medication is used to treat migraine and cluster headaches. These headaches are thought to be caused by an increase in the diameter of the blood vessels in the head, which results in increased blood flow, increased pressure, and pain. Ergotamine acts by constricting the blood vessels, thereby counteracting these effects. Caffeine helps in both the absorption of the drug from the gastrointestinal tract and in constricting blood vessels.

TREATMENT

It is best to take this medication as soon as you notice your migraine headache symptoms. If you wait until the headache becomes severe, the drug takes longer to work and may not be as effective.

After you take any of these forms of ergotamine and caffeine combination, you should try to lie down in a quiet, dark room for at least two hours (in order to help the medication work). The drug usually takes effect in 30 to 60 minutes.

It is very important that you understand how often you can repeat a dose of this medication during an attack (usually every 30 to 60 minutes) and the maximum number of tablets you can take per day (usually six tablets or capsules). Ten is generally the maximum number of tablets or capsules that can be taken in any one-week period. CHECK WITH YOUR DOCTOR if you have any questions.

The tablet or capsule forms of this medication should be swallowed with liquid. Take one tablet or capsule when you first notice your migraine headache symptoms. If necessary, take a second dose 30 to 60 minutes later to relieve your headache.

To use the suppository form of this medication, first unwrap it and moisten it slightly with water (if the suppository is too soft, run cold water over it or refrigerate it for 30 minutes before you unwrap it). Lie down on your left side, with your right knee bent. Push the suppository well into the rectum with your finger. Try to avoid having a bowel movement for at least an hour, to give the medication time to be absorbed. Insert one suppository when you first notice your migraine symptoms. If necessary, insert a second suppository one hour later for full relief of your migraine headache.

If you are on prolonged treatment with this drug and you miss a dose, take it as soon as you remember. Wait four hours to take the next dose. It is very important that you consult your doctor before you discontinue using this drug. Your doctor may want to reduce your dosage gradually.

SIDE EFFECTS

Minor. Diarrhea; dizziness; headache; nausea; vomiting; sensation of cold hands and feet with MILD numbness or tingling. These side effects should disappear as your body adjusts to the medication.

Major. Tell your doctor about any side effects that are persistent or particularly bothersome. IT IS ESPECIALLY IMPORTANT TO TELL YOUR DOCTOR about chest pain; confusion; fluid retention; itching; localized swelling; muscle pain; coldness, numbness, pain, tingling, or dark discoloration of fingers or toes; severe abdominal pain and swelling; or unusual weakness.

INTERACTIONS

Ergotamine interacts with several kinds of drugs, including amphetamines, ephedrine, epinephrine (adrenalin), pseudoephedrine, and troleandomycin. Such combinations can lead to increases in blood pressure or increased risk of adverse reaction to ergotamine.

BE SURE TO TELL YOUR DOCTOR if you are already taking any of the medications listed above.

Do not drink alcoholic beverages while you are taking this medication. Since alcohol dilates the blood vessels (makes them larger), drinking will only make your headache worse.

Ergotamine interacts with marijuana to produce cold sensations in the arms and legs, or even persistent chill.

Tobacco (nicotine) and cocaine decrease the effectiveness of the ergotamine, and therefore make the headache worse.

The caffeine in tea, coffee, and cola drinks also interacts with this medication. It may actually help to relieve your headache.

WARNINGS

- Tell your doctor about unusual or allergic reactions you have had to medications, especially to ergotamine, caffeine, or to any ergot alkaloid (ergonovine, ergoloid mesylates, or bromocriptine).
- Before starting to take this medication, be sure to tell your doctor if you now have, or if you have ever had, heart or blood vessel disease, high blood pressure, infections, kidney disease, liver disease, or thyroid disease.
- Avoid any foods to which you are allergic—they may make your headache worse.
- If this drug makes you dizzy or drowsy, do not take part in any activity that requires alertness, such as driving a car or operating potentially dangerous equipment.
- Try to avoid exposure to cold. Since this drug acts by constricting blood vessels throughout the body (not just in the head), your hands and feet, especially, may become very sensitive to the cold.
- This medication should not be taken for longer periods or in higher doses than recommended by your doctor. Extended use of this drug can lead to serious side effects. In addition, tolerance can develop—higher doses would be required to obtain the same beneficial effects (at the same time increasing the risk of side effects).
- Be sure to tell your doctor if you are pregnant. This medication can cause contractions of the uterus, which can harm the developing fetus. Also, tell your doctor if you are breastfeeding an infant. This drug combination passes into breast milk and may cause vomiting, diarrhea, irritability, or convulsions in nursing infants.

Ergotrate Maleate—see ergonovine

Eryc—see erythromycin

Erypar—see erythromycin

Ery-Tab—see erythromycin

Erythrocin—see erythromycin

---

erythromycin

BRAND NAMES (Manufacturers)
Bristamycin (Bristol)
Delta-E (Trimen)
E.E.S. (Abbott)
E.E.S. 400 (Abbott)
E-Mycin (Upjohn)
Eramycin (Wesley)
Eryc (Parke-Davis)
Erypar (Parke-Davis)
Ery-Tab (Abbott)
Erythrocin (Abbott)
Ethril (Squibb)
Ilosone (Dista)
Ilotycin (Dista)
Pediamycin (Ross)
Pfizer-E (Pfipharmecs)
Robimycin (Robins)
RP-Mycin (Reid-Provident)
SK-Erythromycin (Smith Kline & French)
Wyamycin S (Wyeth)

TYPE OF DRUG
Antibiotic (infection fighter)

INGREDIENT
erythromycin as the base or as the estolate, ethylsuccinate, or stearate salt

DOSAGE FORMS
Tablets (250 mg, 333 mg, and 500 mg)
Chewable tablets (125 mg, 200 mg, and 250 mg)
Capsules (125 mg and 250 mg)
Oral drops (100 mg per ml)
Oral suspension (100 mg, 125 mg, 200 mg, 250 mg, and 400 mg per 5 ml teaspoonful)

STORAGE
Erythromycin tablets and capsules should be stored at room temperature in tightly closed, light-resistant con-

tainers. Erythromycin oral drops and oral suspension should be stored in the refrigerator in tightly closed, light-resistant containers. Any unused portion of the liquid forms should be discarded after 14 days, because the drug loses its potency after that time. Erythromycin ethylsuccinate liquid does not need to be refrigerated; however, refrigeration helps to preserve the taste. This medication should never be frozen.

USES

Erythromycin is used to treat a wide variety of bacterial infections, including infections of the middle ear, or of the upper and lower respiratory tract, and infections in people allergic to penicillin. It acts by preventing the bacteria from manufacturing protein, which prevents their growth. Erythromycin kills susceptible bacteria, but it is not effective against viruses, parasites, or fungi.

TREATMENT

In order to prevent stomach upset, erythromycin coated tablets and erythromycin estolate or ethylsuccinate can be taken either on an empty stomach or with food or milk. Other erythromycin products should be taken with a full glass of water, preferably on an empty stomach, one hour before a meal, or two hours after a meal.

Each dose of the oral drops should be measured carefully, with the dropper provided.

The oral suspension form of this medication should be shaken well just before measuring each dose. The contents tend to settle on the bottom of the bottle, so it is necessary to shake the container to evenly distribute the ingredients and equalize the doses. Each dose should then be measured carefully with a specially designed, 5 ml measuring spoon. An ordinary kitchen teaspoon is not accurate enough.

In order to prevent gastrointestinal side effects, the coated tablets and capsules should be swallowed whole; do not break, chew, or crush these products.

Erythromycin works best when the level of medicine in your bloodstream is kept constant. It is therefore best to take the doses at evenly spaced intervals, day and night. For example, if you are to take four doses a day, the doses should be spaced six hours apart.

If you miss a dose of this medication, take the missed dose immediately. However, if you do not remember to take the missed dose until it is almost time for your next dose, take it; then space the following dose halfway through the regular interval between doses. Then return to your regular schedule. Try not to skip any doses.

It is important to continue to take this medication for the entire time prescribed by your doctor (usually seven to 14 days), even if the symptoms disappear before the end of that period. If you stop taking this drug too soon, resistant bacteria are given a chance to continue growing, and the infection could recur.

SIDE EFFECTS

Minor. Abdominal cramps; black tongue; cough; diarrhea; fatigue; irritation of the mouth; loss of appetite; nausea; and vomiting. These side effects should disappear in several days, as your body adjusts to the medication.

Major. Tell your doctor about any side effects that are persistent or particularly bothersome. IT IS ESPECIALLY IMPORTANT TO TELL YOUR DOCTOR about fever; hearing loss; rash; rectal or vaginal itching; or yellowing of the eyes or skin. Also, if your symptoms of infection seem to be getting worse rather than improving, you should contact your doctor.

INTERACTIONS

Erythromycin interacts with several other medications. It can decrease the elimination of aminophylline, oxtriphylline, theophylline, digoxin, oral anti-coagulants (blood thinners, such as warfarin), and carbamazepine from the body, which can lead to serious side effects. TELL YOUR DOCTOR if you are already taking any of the medications listed above.

WARNINGS

• Tell your doctor about unusual or allergic reactions you have had to medications, especially to erythromycin.
• Tell your doctor if you now have, or if you have ever had, liver disease.

- This medication has been prescribed for your current infection only. Another infection later on, or one that someone else has, may require a different medicine. You should not give your medicine to other people, or use it for other infections, unless your doctor specifically directs you to do so.
- Before having any surgery or other medical or dental treatment, be sure to tell your doctor or dentist that you are taking erythromycin.
- Not all erythromycin products are chemically equivalent. However, they all produce the same therapeutic effect. Discuss with your doctor or pharmacist which forms of erythromycin are appropriate for you, then choose the least expensive product among those recommended.
- Some of these products contain F.D. & C. Yellow Dye No. 5 (tartrazine), which can cause allergic-type reactions (difficulty breathing, rash, or fainting) in certain susceptible individuals.
- Be sure to tell your doctor if you are pregnant. Although erythromycin appears to be safe during pregnancy, extensive studies in humans have not yet been completed. Also, tell your doctor if you are breastfeeding an infant. Small amounts of this medication pass into breast milk and may temporarily alter the bacteria in the intestinal tract of the nursing infant, resulting in diarrhea.

---

erythromycin and sulfisoxazole combination

BRAND NAME (Manufacturer)
Pediazole (Ross)
TYPE OF DRUG
Antibiotic (infection fighter)
INGREDIENTS
erythromycin as the ethylsuccinate salt; sulfisoxazole
DOSAGE FORM
Oral suspension (200 mg erythromycin and 600 mg sulfisoxazole per 5 ml teaspoonful)

STORAGE

Erythromycin and sulfisoxazole oral suspension should be stored in the refrigerator, in a tightly closed container. Any unused portion of the suspension should be discarded after the expiration date (usually after 14 days), because the drug loses its potency after that time. This medication should never be frozen.

USES

Erythromycin and sulfisoxazole is used to treat acute otitis media (middle ear infection) in children. Erythromycin acts by preventing the bacteria from manufacturing protein, thereby preventing their growth. Sulfisoxazole also acts by preventing production of nutrients that are required for growth of the infecting bacteria. Erythromycin and sulfisoxazole combination kills a wide range of susceptible bacteria, but it is not effective against viruses, parasites, or fungi.

TREATMENT

In order to avoid stomach upset, you can take this medication either with food, or with a full glass or water or milk. You can also take it on an empty stomach.

The oral suspension should be shaken well, just before measuring each dose. The contents tend to settle on the bottom of the bottle, so it is necessary to shake the container to evenly distribute the ingredients and equalize the doses. Each dose should then be measured carefully, with a specially designed, 5 ml measuring spoon. An ordinary kitchen teaspoon is not accurate enough.

This medication works best when the level of medicine in your bloodstream is kept constant. It is best therefore to take the doses at evenly spaced intervals, day and night. For example, if you are to take four doses a day, the doses should be spaced six hours apart.

If you miss a dose of this medication, take the missed dose immediately. However, if you do not remember to take the missed dose until it is almost time for your next dose, take it; then space the next dose about halfway through the regular interval between doses. Then return to your regular schedule. Try not to skip any doses.

It is important to continue to take this medication for

the entire time prescribed by your doctor (usually seven to 14 days), even if the symptoms disappear before the end of that period. If you stop taking the drug too soon, resistant bacteria are given a chance to continue growing, and the infection could recur.

SIDE EFFECTS

Minor. Diarrhea; dizziness; headache; loss of appetite; nausea; sleep disorders; sore mouth or tongue; and vomiting. These side effects should disappear in several days, as your body adjusts to the medication.

If you feel dizzy, sit or lie down awhile; get up slowly, and be careful on stairs.

This medication can cause increased sensitivity to sunlight. It is therefore important to avoid prolonged exposure to sunlight and sunlamps. Wear protective clothing and sunglasses, and use an effective sunscreen. However, sunscreens containing para-aminobenzoic acid (PABA) interfere with the anti-bacterial activity of sulfisoxazole, and should not be used.

Major. Tell your doctor about any side effects that are persistent or particularly bothersome. IT IS ESPECIALLY IMPORTANT TO TELL YOUR DOCTOR about aching, or joint and muscle pain; convulsions; difficult or painful urination; difficulty swallowing; hallucinations; mental depression; loss of hearing; redness, blistering, or peeling of the skin; itching; rash; sore throat and fever; uncoordinated movements; unusual bleeding or bruising; unusual tiredness; or yellowing of the eyes or skin. Also, if your symptoms of infection seem to be getting worse rather than improving, you should contact your doctor.

INTERACTIONS

This medication interacts with several other types of medication.

1. Erythromycin can decrease the elimination of aminophylline, oxtriphylline, theophylline, digoxin, oral anti-coagulants (blood thinners, such as warfarin), and carbamazepine from the body, which can lead to serious side effects.

2. Sulfisoxazole can increase the blood levels of active oral anti-coagulants (blood thinners, such as warfarin),

oral anti-diabetic agents, methotrexate, oxyphenbutazone, phenylbutazone, and phenytoin, which can lead
to serious side effects.
3. Methenamine can increase the side effects to the kidneys caused by sulfisoxazole.
4. Probenecid and sulfinpyrazone can increase the
blood levels of sulfisoxazole.
Before starting to take this medication, BE SURE TO TELL
YOUR DOCTOR if you are already taking any of the
medications listed above.

WARNINGS

• Tell your doctor about unusual or allergic reactions you
have had to medications, especially to erythromycin, sulfisoxazole, or to any other sulfa medication (sulfonamide
antibiotics, diuretics, dapsone, sulfoxone, oral anti-diabetic medicines, or acetazolamide).
• Tell your doctor if you now have, or if you have ever
had, glucose-6-phosphate dehydrogenase (G6PD) deficiency, kidney disease, liver disease, or porphyria.
• This medication has been prescribed for your current
infection only. Another infection later on, or one that
someone else has, may require a different medicine. You
should not give your medicine to other people, or use
it for other infections, unless your doctor specifically
directs you to do so.
• Be sure to tell your doctor if you are pregnant. Small
amounts of erythromycin and sulfisoxazole cross the
placenta. Although these antibiotics appear to be safe
during pregnancy, extensive studies in humans have not
been completed. Also, tell your doctor if you are
breastfeeding an infant. Small amounts of this medication
pass into breast milk and may temporarily alter the bacteria in the intestinal tract of the nursing infant, resulting in
diarrhea. This medication should not be used in an infant
less than two months of age (in order to avoid side effects
involving the liver.)

Esidrix—see hydrochlorothiazide

Eskalith—see lithium

Eskalith CR—see lithium

Estinyl—see ethinyl estradiol

estrogens, conjugated

BRAND NAMES (Manufacturers)
conjugated estrogens (various manufacturers)
Evestrone (Delta Drug)
Premarin (Ayerst)
TYPE OF DRUG
Estrogen (female hormone)
INGREDIENTS
conjugated estrogens
DOSAGE FORM
Tablets (0.3 mg, 0.625 mg, 0.9 mg, 1.25 mg, and 2.5 mg)
STORAGE
These tablets should be stored at room temperature in a
tightly closed container.

USES

Conjugated estrogens are a group of estrogen-like products obtained from natural sources (the urine of pregnant
mares). They are used to treat menopausal symptoms,
prostatic cancer, uterine bleeding, and some cases of
breast cancer. They can also be used in replacement
therapy for women who do not produce enough estrogen
of their own.

TREATMENT

In order to avoid stomach irritation, you can take conjugated estrogens with food or immediately after a meal.

Follow your doctor's instructions carefully when you
take this medication. Often, conjugated estrogens are
prescribed to be taken for three-week periods, with one
week off (in order to reduce potential side effects).

If you miss a scheduled dose of this medication, take
the missed dose as soon as possible, unless it is almost
time for the next dose. In that case, do not take the missed
dose at all; just return to your regular dosing schedule. Do
not double the next dose.

SIDE EFFECTS

Minor. Bloating; change in sexual desire; depression; diarrhea; dizziness; headache; loss of appetite; nausea; and vomiting. These side effects should disappear in several days, as your body adjusts to the medication.

If you feel dizzy or light-headed, sit or lie down awhile; get up slowly, and be careful on stairs.

This medication can increase your sensitivity to sunlight. Avoid prolonged exposure to sunlight and sunlamps. Wear protective clothing and sunglasses, and use an effective sunscreen.

Major. Tell your doctor about side effects that are persistent or particularly bothersome. IT IS ESPECIALLY IMPORTANT TO TELL YOUR DOCTOR about changes in menstrual patterns; chest pain; difficulty breathing; eye pain; loss of coordination; lumps in the breast; painful urination; pain in the calves; skin color changes; slurred speech; sudden, severe headache; swelling of the feet or ankles; vision changes; weight gain or loss; or yellowing of the eyes or skin.

INTERACTIONS

Conjugated estrogens interact with several other types of medication.

1. Estrogens can decrease the effectiveness of oral anticoagulants (blood thinners, such as warfarin).

2. Carbamazepine, ampicillin, phenobarbital, phenytoin, primidone, and rifampin can increase the elimination of estrogen from the body, decreasing its effectiveness.

3. Estrogens can increase the side effects, and decrease the effectiveness, of the tricyclic anti-depressants.

Before starting to take conjugated estrogens, BE SURE TO TELL YOUR DOCTOR if you are already taking any of the medications listed above.

WARNINGS

• Tell your doctor about unusual or allergic reactions you have had to medications, especially to conjugated estrogens or to any other estrogen product.

• Before starting to take this medication, tell your doctor if you now have, or if you have ever had, asthma, blood clot disorders, breast cancer, diabetes mellitus (sugar diabetes), endometriosis, epilepsy, gallbladder disease, heart disease, high blood pressure, hypercalcemia (high blood levels of calcium), kidney disease, liver disease, migraine headaches, porphyria, uterine fibroid tumors, vaginal bleeding, or depression.

• Studies have shown that estrogens increase the risk of certain types of cancer. Ask your pharmacist for the brochure that describes the benefits and risks of estrogen therapy.

• Cigarette smoking increases the risk of serious side effects from estrogens. The risk increases with both age and the amount of smoking.

• If this medication makes you dizzy or light-headed, do not take part in any activity that requires alertness, such as driving a car or operating potentially dangerous equipment.

• Estrogens can change your blood's clotting ability, so be especially careful to avoid injuries.

• Before having any surgery or other medical or dental treatment, be sure to tell your doctor or dentist that you are taking this medication.

• Be sure to tell your doctor if you are pregnant. Several studies have shown that estrogens, taken during pregnancy, can cause birth defects. Also, tell your doctor if you are breastfeeding an infant. Estrogens pass into breast milk.

---

ethacrynic acid

BRAND NAME (Manufacturer)
Edecrin (Merck Sharp & Dohme)
TYPE OF DRUG
Diuretic (water pill) and anti-hypertensive
INGREDIENT
ethacrynic acid
DOSAGE FORM
Tablets (25 mg and 50 mg)
STORAGE
Ethacrynic acid should be stored at room temperature in a tightly closed, light-resistant container.

USES

Ethacrynic acid is prescribed to treat high blood pressure. It is also used to reduce fluid accumulation in the body caused by conditions such as heart failure, cirrhosis of the liver, kidney disease, and the long-term use of some medications. This medication reduces fluid accumulation by increasing the elimination of sodium and water through the kidneys.

TREATMENT

To decrease stomach irritation, you can take ethacrynic acid with a glass of milk or with a meal (unless your doctor directs you to do otherwise). Try to take it at the same time every day. Avoid taking a dose after 6:00 P.M.—this will prevent you from having to get up during the night to urinate.

If you miss a dose of this medication, take the missed dose as soon as possible, unless it is almost time for the next dose. In that case, do not take the missed dose at all; just wait until the next scheduled dose. Do not double the dose.

This medication does not cure high blood pressure, but it will help to control the condition, as long as you continue to take it.

SIDE EFFECTS

Minor. Blurred vision; constipation; cramping; diarrhea; dizziness; headache; itching; loss of appetite; muscle spasm; nausea; sore mouth; stomach upset; vomiting; and weakness. As your body adjusts to the medication, these side effects should disappear.

This medication will cause an increase in the amount of urine or in the frequency of urination when you first begin to take it. It may also cause you to have an unusual feeling of tiredness. These effects should lessen after several days.

This medication can cause increased sensitivity to sunlight. It is therefore important to avoid prolonged exposure to sunlight and sunlamps. Wear protective clothing, and use an effective sunscreen.

To avoid dizziness or light-headedness when you stand, contract and relax the muscles of your legs for a few moments before rising. Do this by pushing one foot against the floor while raising the other foot slightly, alternating feet so that you are "pumping" your legs in a pedaling motion.

Major. Tell your doctor about any side effects that are persistent or particularly bothersome. IT IS ESPECIALLY IMPORTANT TO TELL YOUR DOCTOR about black, tarry stools; confusion; difficulty breathing; dry mouth; fainting; increased thirst; joint pains; loss of appetite; mood changes; muscle cramps; palpitations; rash; ringing in the ears; sore throat; severe abdominal pain; tingling in the fingers and toes; unusual bleeding or bruising; watery diarrhea; or yellowing of the eyes or skin.

INTERACTIONS

Ethacrynic acid interacts with several other types of drugs.

1. It can increase the side effects of alcohol, barbiturates, narcotics, cephalosporin antibiotics, chloral hydrate, cortisone-like steroids (such as cortisone, dexamethasone, hydrocortisone, prednisone, prednisolone), digoxin, digitalis, lithium, amphotericin B, heparin, and warfarin.

2. Probenecid may decrease the effectiveness of this medicine.

3. The effectiveness of anti-gout medications, insulin, and oral anti-diabetic medications may be decreased when combined with ethacrynic acid.

Before taking ethacrynic acid, BE SURE TO TELL YOUR DOCTOR if you are taking any of the medicines listed above.

WARNINGS

• Tell your doctor about unusual or allergic reactions you have had to any medications, especially to diuretics (water pills).

• Before you start taking this medication, tell your doctor if you now have, or if you have ever had, kidney disease or problems with urination, or liver disease.

• This drug can cause potassium loss. Signs of potassium loss include dry mouth; thirst; weakness; muscle pain or cramps; nausea; and vomiting. If you experience any of these symptoms, call your doctor. Your doctor may have blood tests performed periodically in order to monitor your potassium levels. To help avoid potassium loss, take this medication with a glass of fresh or frozen orange or cranberry juice, or eat a banana every day. The use of a salt substitute also helps prevent potassium loss. Do not change your diet, however, before discussing it with your doctor. Too much potassium can also be dangerous.

• To prevent severe water loss (dehydration) while taking this medication, check with your doctor if you have any illness that causes severe or continuous nausea, vomiting, or diarrhea.

• Before having any kind of surgery or other medical or dental treatment, be sure to tell your doctor or dentist that you are taking ethacrynic acid.

• To avoid dizziness, light-headedness, and fainting, get up from a sitting or lying position slowly; and avoid standing for long periods of time, strenuous exercise, and prolonged exposure to hot weather.

• While taking this medication, limit your intake of alcoholic beverages in order to prevent dizziness or light-headedness.

• If you have high blood pressure, do not take any over-the-counter (non-prescription) medication for weight control, or for allergy, asthma, cough, cold, or sinus problems, unless you first check with your doctor.

• Be sure to tell your doctor if you are pregnant. This drug crosses the placenta. Although studies in humans have not yet been completed, adverse effects have been observed on the fetuses of animals who received large doses of this drug during pregnancy. Also, tell your doctor if you are breastfeeding an infant. Small amounts of this drug pass into breast milk.

ethinyl estradiol

BRAND NAMES (Manufacturers)
Estinyl (Schering)
Feminone (Upjohn)
TYPE OF DRUG
Estrogen (female hormone)

INGREDIENT
ethinyl estradiol
DOSAGE FORM
Tablets (0.02 mg, 0.05 mg, and 0.5 mg)
STORAGE
Ethinyl estradiol should be stored at room temperature, in a tightly closed container.

USES

Ethinyl estradiol is a synthetic estrogen that is used to treat menopausal symptoms, certain types of breast cancer, and prostate cancer.

TREATMENT

In order to avoid stomach irritation, you can take ethinyl estradiol with food or with a full glass of milk or water (unless your doctor directs you to do otherwise).

If you miss a dose of this medication, take the missed dose as soon as possible, unless it is almost time for the next dose. In that case, do not take the missed dose at all; just return to your regular dosing schedule. Do not double the next dose.

SIDE EFFECTS

Minor. Abdominal cramping; abnormal vaginal bleeding; bloating; breast tenderness; diarrhea; dizziness; fluid retention; frequent or painful urination; hair loss; headache; itching; nausea; nervousness; skin rash; darkening of the skin; vomiting; and weight gain. These side effects should disappear as your body adjusts to the medication.

If you feel dizzy, sit or lie down awhile; get up slowly, and be careful on stairs.

Eating a full breakfast or having a midmorning snack may help to relieve the nausea and vomiting.

This medication can increase your sensitivity to sunlight. You should therefore try to avoid prolonged exposure to sunlight and sunlamps. Wear protective clothing and sunglasses, and use an effective sunscreen.

Major. Tell your doctor about any side effects that are persistent or particularly bothersome. IT IS ESPECIALLY IMPORTANT TO TELL YOUR DOCTOR about blurred vision; chest pain; convulsions; depression; pain or inflammation of the calves or thighs; shortness of breath; or yellowing of the eyes or skin.

INTERACTIONS

Ethinyl estradiol interacts with other medication.

1. It can decrease the effectiveness of oral anti-coagulants (blood thinners, such as warfarin).

2. Carbamazepine, phenobarbital, phenytoin, primidone, and rifampin can reduce the effectiveness of ethinyl estradiol.

3. Ethinyl estradiol can increase the side effects and decrease the benefits of tricyclic anti-depressants.

BE SURE TO TELL YOUR DOCTOR if you are already taking any of the medications listed above.

WARNINGS

• Tell your doctor about unusual or allergic reactions you have had to medications, especially to ethinyl estradiol, other estrogens, or oral contraceptives.

• Before starting to take this medication, be sure to tell your doctor if you now have, or if you have ever had, asthma, blood clot disorders, breast disease, depression, diabetes mellitus (sugar diabetes), epilepsy, endometriosis, gallstones or gallbladder disease, heart disease, high blood pressure, kidney disease, liver disease, migraine headaches, porphyria, or uterine tumors.

• Some of these products contain F.D. & C. Yellow Dye No. 5 (tartrazine), which can cause allergic-type symptoms (shortness of breath, fainting, rash) in certain susceptible individuals.

• Estrogens can change your blood's clotting ability, so be especially careful to avoid injuries.

• Before having any surgery or other medical or dental treatment, be sure to tell your doctor or dentist that you are taking this medication.

• A package insert entitled "Information for the Patient" should be dispensed with your prescription. It is important that you understand the possible risks and benefits of this medication. If you have any questions, check with your doctor or pharmacist.

• Cigarette smoking can greatly increase the risk of developing heart or blood vessel disorders while taking this medication. The risks increase with the amount of smoking and the age of the smoker.

• Be sure to tell your doctor if you are pregnant. Estrogens have been shown to cause birth defects in the offspring of women who received these medications during pregnancy. Also, tell your doctor if you are breastfeeding an infant. Small amounts of estrogen pass into breast milk. Ethinyl estradiol can also decrease milk production.

Ethon—see methyclothiazide

---

ethosuximide

BRAND NAME (Manufacturer)
Zarontin (Parke-Davis)
TYPE OF DRUG
Anti-convulsant
INGREDIENT
ethosuximide
DOSAGE FORMS
Capsules (250 mg)
Oral syrup (250 mg per 5 ml teaspoonful)
STORAGE
Ethosuximide capsules and oral syrup should be stored at room temperature in tightly closed, light-resistant containers. This medication should never be frozen.

USES

This medication is used to treat absence (petit mal) seizures. Although it is not exactly clear how it does so, ethosuximide seems to prevent seizure activity by decreasing the activity of certain chemicals (nerve transmitters) in the brain.

TREATMENT

In order to avoid stomach irritation, you can take ethosuximide with food or with a full glass of water or milk (unless your doctor directs you to do otherwise).

Each dose of the oral syrup form of this medication should be measured carefully, with a specially designed,

5 ml measuring spoon. An ordinary kitchen teaspoon is not accurate enough.

Ethosuximide works best when the level of medicine in your bloodstream is kept constant. It is therefore best to take the doses at evenly spaced intervals, day and night. For example, if you are to take three doses a day, the doses should be spaced eight hours apart.

It is important to try not to miss any doses of this medication. If you do miss a dose, and you remember within four hours of the scheduled time, take the missed dose immediately, then return to your normal schedule. If more than four hours have passed, do not take the missed dose at all; just return to your regular dosing schedule. Do not double the next dose.

SIDE EFFECTS

Minor. Constipation; diarrhea; dizziness; drowsiness; headache; hiccups; loss of appetite; nausea; stomach upset; and weight loss. These side effects should disappear in several days, as your body adjusts to the medication.

To relieve constipation, increase the amount of fiber in your diet (bran, salads, fresh fruits and vegetables, and whole-grain breads), exercise, and drink more water (unless your doctor directs you to do otherwise).

If you feel dizzy, sit or lie down awhile; get up slowly, and be careful on stairs.

Major. Tell your doctor about any side effects that are persistent or particularly bothersome. IT IS ESPECIALLY IMPORTANT TO TELL YOUR DOCTOR about blurred vision; confusion; depression; difficult or painful urination; false sense of well-being; fatigue; irritability; joint pains; loss of coordination; mental disorders; nervousness; skin rash; swelling of the eyes or tongue; unusual bleeding or bruising; or vaginal bleeding.

INTERACTIONS

Tricyclic anti-depressants, haloperidol, thiothixene, phenothiazine tranquilizers, and alcohol can increase the risk of seizures. Dosage adjustments of ethosuximide may be necessary when any of these medications are started. BE SURE TO TELL YOUR DOCTOR if you are already taking any of the drugs listed above.

WARNINGS

- Tell your doctor about unusual or allergic reactions you have had to any medications, especially to ethosuximide, methsuximide, or phensuximide.
- Before starting to take this medication, be sure to tell your doctor if you now have, or if you have ever had, blood disorders, kidney disease, or liver disease.
- If this drug makes you dizzy or drowsy, do not take part in any activities that require alertness, such as driving a car or operating potentially dangerous equipment. Children should be careful while playing or climbing trees.
- Before having any surgery or other medical or dental treatment, be sure to tell your doctor or dentist that you are taking ethosuximide.
- Do not stop taking this medication unless you first check with your doctor. Stopping the drug abruptly may lead to a worsening of your condition. Your doctor may want to reduce your dosage gradually or start you on another drug when treatment with ethosuximide is stopped.
- Be sure to tell your doctor if you are pregnant. Birth defects have been reported more often in infants whose mothers have seizure disorders. It is unclear if the increased risk of birth defects is associated with the disorder or with the anti-convulsion medications, such as ethosuximide, that are used to treat the condition. The risks and benefits of treatment should be discussed with your doctor. Also, tell your doctor if you are breastfeeding an infant. Ethosuximide passes into breast milk.

Ethril—see erythromycin

Etrafon—see perphenazine and amitriptyline combination

Eutonyl—see pargyline

Evestrone—see estrogens, conjugated

Exna—see benzthiazide

Fastin—see phentermine

Feco-T — see iron supplements

Feldene — see piroxicam

Feminone — see ethinyl estradiol

---

fenfluramine

BRAND NAME (Manufacturer)
Pondimin (Robins)
TYPE OF DRUG
Anorectic (appetite suppressant)
INGREDIENT
fenfluramine as the hydrochloride salt
DOSAGE FORM
Tablets (20 mg)
STORAGE
Fenfluramine should be stored at room temperature in a tightly closed, light-resistant container.

USES
Fenfluramine is used as an appetite suppressant during the first few weeks of dieting to help establish new eating habits. This medication is thought to relieve hunger by altering nerve impulses to the appetite control center in the brain. Its effectiveness lasts only for short periods (three to 12 weeks), however.

TREATMENT
You can take fenfluramine with a full glass of water, one hour before meals (unless your doctor directs you to do otherwise).

If you miss a dose of this medication, take the missed dose as soon as possible, unless it is almost time for your next dose. In that case, don't take the missed dose at all; just return to your regular dosing schedule. Do not double the next dose.

SIDE EFFECTS
Minor. Blurred vision; constipation; diarrhea; dizziness; dry mouth; euphoria; fatigue; insomnia; irritability;

nausea; nervousness; restlessness; stomach pain; sweating; tremors; unpleasant taste in the mouth; and vomiting. These side effects should disappear in several days, as your body adjusts to the medication.

Dry mouth can be relieved by sucking on ice chips or a piece of hard candy, or by chewing sugarless gum.

In order to prevent constipation, increase the amount of fiber in your diet (raw vegetables, fruits, salads, bran, and whole-grain breads), and drink more water (unless your doctor tells you not to do so).

Major. Tell your doctor about any side effects that are persistent or particularly bothersome. IT IS ESPECIALLY IMPORTANT TO TELL YOUR DOCTOR about changes in sexual desire; chest pain; difficulty urinating; enlarged breasts (in both sexes); fever; hair loss; headaches; impotence; menstrual irregularities; mental depression; mood changes; mouth sores; muscle pains; nosebleeds; palpitations; rash; or sore throat.

INTERACTIONS

Fenfluramine interacts with other medication.
1. Concurrent use of it with central nervous system depressants (drugs that slow the activity of the nervous system), including alcohol, antihistamines, barbiturates, muscle relaxants, narcotics, pain medications, and phenothiazine tranquilizers, or with tricyclic antidepressants can cause extreme drowsiness.
2. Fenfluramine may alter insulin and oral anti-diabetic medication dosage requirements in diabetic patients.
3. The blood-pressure-lowering effects of antihypertensive medications, especially guanethidine, reserpine, methyldopa, and diuretics (water pills), may be increased by this medication.
4. Use of fenfluramine within 14 days of a monoamine oxidase (MAO) inhibitor (isocarboxazid, pargyline, phenelzine, and tranylcypromine) can result in high blood pressure and other side effects.
TELL YOUR DOCTOR if you are already taking any of the medications listed above.

WARNINGS

• Tell your doctor about unusual or allergic reactions you

have had to any medications, especially to fenfluramine or other appetite suppressants (such as benzphetamine, phendimetrazine, diethylpropion, phenmetrazine, mazindol, or phentermine), or to epinephrine, norepinephrine, ephedrine, amphetamines, dextroamphetamine, phenylephrine, phenylpropanolamine, pseudoephedrine, albuterol, metaproterenol, or terbutaline.

• Tell your doctor if you have a history of drug abuse, or if you have ever had angina (chest pain); diabetes mellitus (sugar diabetes); emotional disturbances; glaucoma; heart or cardiovascular disease; high blood pressure; thyroid disease; alcoholism; epilepsy; or mental depression.

• Fenfluramine can mask the symptoms of extreme fatigue, and can cause dizziness or light-headedness. Your ability to perform tasks that require alertness, such as driving a car or operating potentially dangerous machinery, may be decreased. Appropriate caution should therefore be taken.

• Before having any surgery or other medical or dental treatment, be sure to tell your doctor or dentist that you are taking this medication.

• Fenfluramine is related to amphetamine and may be habit-forming when taken for long periods of time (both physical and psychological dependence can occur). You should therefore not increase the dose of this medication or take it for longer than 12 weeks, unless you first consult your doctor. It is also important that you not stop taking this medication abruptly. Fatigue, sleep disorders, mental depression, nausea, vomiting, stomach cramps, or pain could occur. Your doctor may want to decrease your dosage gradually in order to prevent these side effects.

• Fenfluramine can alter blood sugar levels in diabetic patients. Therefore, if you are diabetic and starting to take this medication, you should carefully monitor your blood or urine glucose levels for the first several days.

• Be sure to tell your doctor if you are pregnant. Although side effects in humans have not yet been studied, some of the appetite suppressants cause side effects in the fetuses of animals who receive large doses of these drugs during pregnancy. Also, tell your doctor if you are breastfeeding an infant. It is not known whether or not this medication passes into breast milk.

---

fenoprofen

BRAND NAME (Manufacturer)
Nalfon (Dista)
TYPE OF DRUG
Non-steroidal anti-inflammatory analgesic (pain reliever)
INGREDIENT
fenoprofen as the calcium salt
DOSAGE FORMS
Capsules (200 mg and 300 mg)
Tablets (600 mg)
STORAGE
This medication should be stored in tightly closed containers at room temperature, away from heat and direct sunlight.

USES

Fenoprofen is used to treat the pain, swelling, stiffness, and inflammation of certain types of arthritis, gout, bursitis, and tendinitis.

TREATMENT

You should take this medication on an empty stomach 30 to 60 minutes before meals or two hours after meals, so that it gets into your bloodstream quickly. Since fenoprofen can cause stomach irritation, however, your doctor may want you to take this medicine with food or antacids.

If you are taking fenoprofen to relieve arthritis, you must take it regularly, as directed by your doctor. It may take up to three weeks before you feel its full benefits. This medication does not cure arthritis, but it will help to control the condition, as long as you continue to take it.

It is important to take fenoprofen on schedule and not to miss any doses. If you do miss a dose, take it as soon as possible, unless it is almost time for your next dose. In that case, don't take the missed dose at all; just return to your regular dosing schedule. Do not double the next dose.

SIDE EFFECTS

Minor. Bloating; constipation; diarrhea; difficulty sleeping; dizziness; drowsiness; headache; heartburn; indigestion; light-headedness; loss of appetite; nausea; nervousness; soreness of the mouth; unusual sweating; and vomiting. As your body adjusts to the drug, these side effects should disappear.

If you become dizzy, sit or lie down awhile; get up slowly, and be careful on stairs.

Acetaminophen may be helpful in relieving any headaches.

Major. If any side effects are persistent or particularly bothersome, you should report them to your doctor. IT IS ESPECIALLY IMPORTANT TO TELL YOUR DOCTOR about bloody or black, tarry stools; blurred vision; confusion; depression; difficult or painful urination; difficulty breathing; hearing difficulties; palpitations; ringing or buzzing in the ears; skin rash, hives, or itching; stomach pain; swelling of the feet; tightness in the chest; unexplained sore throat and fever; unusual bleeding or bruising; unusual fatigue or weakness; unusual weight gain; or yellowing of the eyes or skin.

INTERACTIONS

Fenoprofen interacts with several types of medication.
1. Anti-coagulants (blood thinners, such as warfarin) can lead to an increase in bleeding complications.
2. Aspirin, salicylates, and other anti-inflammation medications can lead to an increase in stomach irritation.
BE SURE TO TELL YOUR DOCTOR if you are already taking any of these types of medication.

WARNINGS

• Before you take this medication, it is important to tell your doctor if you have ever had unusual or allergic reactions to fenoprofen or any chemically related drug (aspirin or other salicylates, diflunisal, indomethacin, ibuprofen, meclofenamate, mefenamic acid, naproxen, oxyphenbutazone, phenylbutazone, piroxicam, sulindac, tolmetin, and zomepirac).
• Tell your doctor if you now have, or if you have ever had, bleeding problems; colitis, stomach ulcers, or other

stomach problems; epilepsy; heart disease; high blood pressure; asthma; kidney disease; liver disease; mental illness; or Parkinson's disease.

• If this drug makes you dizzy or drowsy, do not take part in any activity that requires alertness, such as driving a car or operating potentially dangerous equipment.

• Before having any surgery or other medical or dental treatment, be sure to tell your doctor or dentist that you are taking fenoprofen.

• Stomach problems are more likely to occur if you take aspirin regularly or drink alcohol while being treated with this medication. These should therefore be avoided (unless your doctor directs you to do otherwise).

• Be sure to tell your doctor if you are pregnant. Although studies in humans have not yet been completed, unwanted side effects (on the heart) have been reported in the offspring of animals who received fenoprofen during pregnancy. Also, tell your doctor if you are breastfeeding an infant. Small amounts of this medication can pass into breast milk.

Fenylhist—see diphenhydramine

Feosol—see iron supplements

Feostat—see iron supplements

Fergon—see iron supplements

Fer-In-Sol—see iron supplements

Fer-Iron—see iron supplements

Ferndex—see dextroamphetamine

Fernisolone-P—see prednisolone (systemic)

Fernisone—see prednisone (systemic)

Fero-Gradumet—see iron supplements

Ferospace—see iron supplements

Ferralet—see iron supplements

Ferralyn Lanacaps—see iron supplements

ferrous fumarate—see iron supplements

ferrous gluconate—see iron supplements

ferrous sulfate—see iron supplements

Fiorinal—see aspirin, caffeine, and butalbital combination

Fiorinal with Codeine—see aspirin, caffeine, butalbital, and codeine combination

Flagyl—see metronidazole

Flexeril—see cyclobenzaprine

Florvite—see vitamins, multiple, with fluoride

Fluidil—see cyclothiazide

---

fluocinolone (topical)

BRAND NAMES (Manufacturers)
fluocinolone acetonide (various manufacturers)
Flurosyn (Rugby)
Synalar (Syntex)
Synalar-HP (Syntex)
Synemol (Syntex)
TYPE OF DRUG
Adrenocorticosteroid hormone
INGREDIENT
fluocinolone as the acetonide salt
DOSAGE FORMS
Cream (0.01%, 0.025% and 0.2%)
Ointment (0.025%)
Solution (0.01%)

STORAGE

Fluocinolone ointment, cream, and solution should be stored at room temperature, in tightly closed containers. This medication should never be frozen.

USES

Your adrenal glands naturally produce certain cortisone-like chemicals. These chemicals are involved in various regulatory processes in the body (such as fluid balance, temperature, and reactions to inflammation). Fluocinolone belongs to a group of drugs known as adrenocorticosteroids (or cortisone-like medications). It is used to relieve the skin inflammation (redness, swelling, itching, and discomfort) associated with conditions such as dermatitis, eczema, and poison ivy. How this drug acts to relieve these disorders is not completely understood.

TREATMENT

Before applying this medication, wash your hands. Then, unless your doctor gives you different instructions, gently wash the area of the skin where the medication is to be applied. With a clean towel, pat the area almost dry; it should be slightly damp when you put the medicine on.

Apply a small amount of fluocinolone to the affected area in a thin layer. Do not bandage the area unless your doctor tells you to do so. If you are to apply an occlusive dressing (like kitchen plastic wrap), be sure you understand the instructions.

If you miss a dose of this medication, apply the dose as soon as possible, unless it is almost time for the next application. In that case, do not apply the missed dose; just return to your regular schedule. Do not put twice as much of the medication on your skin at the next application.

SIDE EFFECTS

Minor. Acne; burning sensation; irritation of the affected area; itching; rash; or skin dryness.

If the affected area is extremely dry or scaling, the skin may be moistened before applying the medication by soaking in water or by applying water with a clean cloth. The ointment form is probably better for dry skin.

A mild, temporary stinging sensation may occur after this medication is applied. If this persists, contact your doctor.

Major. Tell your doctor about any side effects that are persistent or particularly bothersome. IT IS ESPECIALLY IMPORTANT TO TELL YOUR DOCTOR about blistering; increased hair growth; loss of skin color; secondary infection in the area being treated; or thinning of the skin with easy bruising.

INTERACTIONS

This medication does not interact with any other medications, as long as it is used according to directions.

WARNINGS

• Tell your doctor about unusual or allergic reactions you have had to medications, especially to fluocinolone or any other adrenocorticosteroid (such as amcinonide, betamethasone, clocortolone, cortisone, desonide, desoximetasone, dexamethasone, diflorasone, flumethasone, fluocinonide, fluorometholone, fluprednisolone, flurandrenolide, halcinonide, hydrocortisone, methylprednisolone, paramethasone, prednisolone, prednisone, or triamicinolone).

• Tell your doctor if you now have, or if you have ever had, blood vessel disease, chicken pox, diabetes mellitus (sugar diabetes), fungal infection, peptic ulcers, shingles, tuberculosis, tuberculosis of the skin, vaccinia, or any other type of infection, especially at the site currently being treated.

• If irritation develops while using this drug, immediately discontinue its use and notify your doctor.

• This product is not for use in the eyes or mucous membranes. Exposure of this medication to the eye may result in ocular (to the eye) side effects.

• Do not use this product with an occlusive wrap unless your doctor directs you to do so. Systemic absorption of this drug is increased if extensive areas of the body are treated, particularly if occlusive bandages are used. If it is necessary for you to use this drug under a wrap, follow your doctor's instructions exactly; do not leave the wrap in place longer than specified.

- If you are using fluocinolone on a child's diaper area, do not put tight-fitting diapers or plastic pants on the child. This could lead to increased systemic absorption of the drug and a possible increase in side effects.
- Be sure to tell your doctor if you are pregnant. If large amounts of this drug are applied for prolonged periods, some of it will be absorbed and may cross the placenta. Although studies in humans have not yet been completed, birth defects have been observed in the fetuses of animals who were given large doses of this type of drug during pregnancy. Also, tell your doctor if you are breastfeeding an infant. If absorbed through the skin, small amounts of fluocinolone pass into breast milk and may cause growth suppression or a decrease in natural adrenocorticosteroid production in the nursing infant.

fluocinolone acetonide — see fluocinolone (topical)

---

fluocinonide (topical)

BRAND NAMES (Manufacturers)
Lidex (Syntex)
Lidex-E (Syntex)
Topsyn (Syntex)
TYPE OF DRUG
Adrenocorticosteroid hormone
INGREDIENT
fluocinonide
DOSAGE FORMS
Ointment (0.05%)
Cream (0.05%)
Gel (0.05%)
STORAGE
Fluocinonide ointment, cream, and gel should be stored at room temperature, in tightly closed containers. This medication should never be frozen.

USES
Your adrenal glands naturally produce certain cortisone-like chemicals. These chemicals are involved in various regulatory processes in the body (such as fluid balance,

temperature, and reactions to inflammation). Fluocinonide belongs to a group of drugs known as adrenocorticosteroids (or cortisone-like medications). It is used to relieve the skin inflammation (redness, swelling, itching, and discomfort) associated with conditions such as dermatitis, eczema, and poison ivy. How this drug acts to relieve these disorders is not completely understood.

TREATMENT

Before applying this medication, wash your hands. Then, unless your doctor gives you different instructions, gently wash the area of the skin where the medication is to be applied. With a clean towel, pat the area almost dry; it should be slightly damp when you put the medicine on.

Apply a small amount of fluocinonide to the affected area, in a thin layer. Do not bandage the area unless your doctor tells you to do so. If you are to apply an occlusive dressing (like kitchen plastic wrap), be sure you understand the instructions.

If you miss a dose of this medication, apply the dose as soon as possible, unless it is almost time for the next application. In that case, do not apply the missed dose; just return to your regular schedule. Do not put twice as much of the medication on your skin at the next application.

SIDE EFFECTS

Minor. Acne; burning sensation; irritation of the affected area; itching; rash; or skin dryness.

If the affected area is extremely dry or scaling, the skin may be moistened before applying the medication by soaking in water or by applying water with a clean cloth. The ointment form is probably better for dry skin.

A mild, temporary stinging sensation may occur after this medication is applied. If this persists, contact your doctor.

Major. Tell your doctor about any side effects that are persistent or particularly bothersome. IT IS ESPECIALLY IMPORTANT TO TELL YOUR DOCTOR about blistering; increased hair growth; loss of skin color; secondary infection in the area being treated; or thinning of the skin with easy bruising.

INTERACTIONS

This medication does not interact with any other medications, as long as it is used according to directions.

WARNINGS

• Tell your doctor about unusual or allergic reactions you have had to medications, especially to fluocinonide or any other adrenocorticosteroid (such as amcinonide, betamethasone, clocortolone, cortisone, desonide, desoximetasone, dexamethasone, diflorasone, flumethasone, fluocinolone, fluorometholone, fluprednisolone, flurandrenolide, halcinonide, hydrocortisone, methylprednisolone, paramethasone, prednisolone, prednisone, or triamcinolone).

• Tell your doctor if you now have, or if you have ever had, blood vessel disease, chicken pox, diabetes mellitus (sugar diabetes), fungal infection, peptic ulcers, shingles, tuberculosis, tuberculosis of the skin, vaccinia, or any other type of infection, especially at the site currently being treated.

• If irritation develops while using this drug, immediately discontinue its use and notify your doctor.

• This product is not for use in the eyes or mucous membranes. Exposure of this medication to the eye may result in ocular (to the eye) side effects.

• Do not use this product with an occlusive wrap unless your doctor directs you to do so. Systemic absorption of this drug is increased if extensive areas of the body are treated, particularly if occlusive bandages are used. If it is necessary for you to use this drug under a wrap, follow your doctor's instructions exactly; do not leave the wrap in place longer than specified.

• If you are using fluocinonide on a child's diaper area, do not put tight-fitting diapers or plastic pants on the child. This may lead to increased systemic absorption of the drug and a possible increase in side effects.

• Be sure to tell your doctor if you are pregnant. If large amounts of this drug are applied for prolonged periods, some of it will be absorbed and may cross the placenta. Although studies in humans have not yet been completed, birth defects have been observed in the fetuses of animals who were given large doses of this type of drug during pregnancy. Also, tell your doctor if you are breastfeeding an infant. If absorbed through the skin, small amounts of fluocinonide pass into breast milk and may cause growth suppression or a decrease in natural adrenocorticosteroid production in the nursing infant.

Fluoral — see sodium fluoride

Fluorigard — see sodium fluoride

Fluorineed — see sodium fluoride

Fluorinse — see sodium fluoride

Fluoritab — see sodium fluoride

---

fluphenazine

BRAND NAMES (Manufacturers)
Permitil (Schering)
Permitil Chronotabs (Schering)
Prolixin (Squibb)
TYPE OF DRUG
Phenothiazine tranquilizer
INGREDIENT
fluphenazine as the hydrochloride salt
DOSAGE FORMS
Tablets (0.25 mg, 1 mg, 2.5 mg, 5 mg, and 10 mg)
Sustained-release tablets (1 mg)
Oral concentrate (5 mg per ml)
Oral elixir (2.5 mg per 5 ml teaspoonful)
STORAGE
The tablet forms of this medication should be stored at room temperature in tightly closed, light-resistant containers. The oral concentrate and the elixir forms of fluphenazine should be stored in the refrigerator in tightly closed, light-resistant containers. If the oral concentrate or elixir turns to a slight yellow color, the medicine is still effective and can be used. However, if they change color markedly, or have particles floating in them, they should

not be used, but discarded down the sink. This medication should never be frozen.

USES

Fluphenazine is prescribed to treat the symptoms of certain types of mental illness, such as emotional symptoms of psychosis, the manic phase of manic-depressive illness, and severe behavioral problems in children. This medication is thought to relieve the symptoms of mental illness by blocking certain chemicals involved with nerve transmission in the brain.

TREATMENT

To avoid stomach irritation, you can take the tablet or elixir form of this medication with a meal or with a glass of water or milk (unless your doctor directs you to do otherwise).

The sustained-release tablets should be swallowed whole; do not crush, break, or open them. Breaking them releases the medication all at once—defeating the purpose of the sustained release tablets.

Measure the oral suspension carefully, with a specially designed, 5 ml measuring spoon. An ordinary kitchen teaspoon is not accurate enough.

The oral concentrate form of this medication should be measured carefully with the dropper provided, then added to 4 ounces (½ cup) or more of water, milk, juice, or a carbonated beverage, or to applesauce or pudding, immediately prior to administration. To prevent possible loss of effectiveness, the medication should not be diluted in tea, coffee, or apple juice.

Antacids and diarrhea medicine may decrease the absorption of this medication from the gastrointestinal tract. Therefore, at least one hour should separate doses of one of these medicines and fluphenazine.

The full effects of this medication for the control of emotional or mental symptoms may not become apparent for two weeks after starting it.

If you miss a dose of this medication, take the missed dose as soon as possible and return to your regular dosing schedule. If it is almost time for the next dose, however.

skip the one you missed and return to your regular schedule. Do not double the dose (unless your doctor directs you to do so).

SIDE EFFECTS

Minor. Blurred vision; constipation; decreased sweating; diarrhea; discoloration of the urine to red, pink, or red-brown; dizziness; drooling; drowsiness; dry mouth; fatigue; jitteriness; menstrual irregularities; nasal congestion; restlessness; tremors; vomiting; and weight gain. As your body adjusts to the medication, these side effects should disappear.

If you are constipated, increase the amount of fiber in your diet (raw vegetables, fruits, salads, bran, and whole-grain breads), and drink more water (unless your doctor directs you to do otherwise).

Chew sugarless gum, or suck on ice chips or a piece of hard candy, to reduce mouth dryness.

This medication can cause increased sensitivity to sunlight. It is therefore important to avoid prolonged exposure to sunlight and sunlamps. Wear protective clothing, and use an effective sunscreen.

To avoid dizziness or light-headedness when you stand, contract and relax the muscles of your legs for a few moments before rising. Do this by pushing one foot against the floor while raising the other foot slightly, alternating feet so that you are "pumping" your legs in a pedaling motion.

Major. Tell your doctor about any side effects that are persistent or particularly bothersome. IT IS ESPECIALLY IMPORTANT TO TELL YOUR DOCTOR about breast enlargement (in both sexes); chest pain; convulsions; darkened skin; difficulty swallowing or breathing; fainting; fever; impotence; involuntary movements of the face, mouth, jaw, or tongue; palpitations; rash; sleep disorders; sore throat; uncoordinated movements; unusual bleeding or bruising; visual disturbances; or yellowing of the eyes or skin.

INTERACTIONS

Fluphenazine interacts with several other types of drugs.
1. It can cause extreme drowsiness when combined with

alcohol or other central nervous system depressants (drugs that slow the nervous system), such as barbiturates, benzodiazepine tranquilizers, muscle relaxants, narcotics, and pain medication, or with tricyclic antidepressants.

2. Fluphenazine can decrease the effectiveness of amphetamines, guanethidine, anti-convulsants, and levodopa.

3. The side effects of epinephrine, monoamine oxidase (MAO) inhibitors, propranolol, phenytoin, and tricyclic anti-depressants may be increased when combined with this medication.

4. Lithium may increase the side effects, and decrease the effectiveness, of this medication.

Before starting to take fluphenazine, BE SURE TO TELL YOUR DOCTOR if you are already taking any of the medications listed above.

WARNINGS

• Tell your doctor about unusual or allergic reactions you have had to medications, especially to fluphenazine or any other phenothiazine tranquilizers (such as acetophenazine, carphenazine, chlorpromazine, mesoridazine, perphenazine, piperacetazine, prochlorperazine, promazine, thioridazine, trifluoperazine, triflupromazine), or to loxapine.

• Tell your doctor if you now have, or if you have ever had, any blood disease; bone marrow disease; brain disease; breast cancer; blockage of the urinary or digestive tract; alcoholism; drug-induced depression; epilepsy; high or low blood pressure; diabetes mellitus (sugar diabetes); glaucoma; heart or circulatory disease; liver disease; lung disease; Parkinson's disease; peptic ulcers; or an enlarged prostate gland.

• Tell your doctor about any recent exposure to a pesticide or an insecticide. Fluphenazine may increase the side effects from the exposure.

• To prevent over-sedation, avoid drinking alcoholic beverages while taking this medication.

• If this medication makes you dizzy or drowsy, do not take part in any activity that requires alertness, such as driving a car or operating potentially dangerous equipment. Be careful on stairs; and avoid getting up suddenly from a lying or sitting position.

• Before having any kind of surgery or other medical or dental treatment, be sure to tell your doctor or dentist that you are taking this medication.

• Some of the side effects caused by this drug can be prevented by taking an anti-parkinson drug. Discuss this with your doctor.

• Fluphenazine has been reported to cause certain tumors in rats. This effect has not been shown to occur in humans.

• This medication can decrease sweating and heat release from the body. You should therefore avoid getting overheated by strenuous exercise in hot weather, and should avoid hot baths, showers, and saunas.

• Do not stop taking this medication suddenly. If the drug is stopped abruptly you may experience nausea, vomiting, stomach upset, headache, increased heart rate, insomnia, tremulousness, or a worsening of your condition. Your doctor may want to reduce the dosage gradually.

• If you are planning to have a myelogram, or any procedure in which dye will be injected into your spinal cord, tell your doctor that you are taking this medication.

• Avoid spilling the oral concentrate or elixir forms of this medication on your skin or clothing; they may cause redness and irritation of the skin.

• While taking this medication, do not take any over-the-counter (non-prescription) medication for weight control, or for cough, cold, allergy, asthma, or sinus problems, without first checking with your doctor. The combination of these medications may cause high blood pressure.

• Some of these products contain F.D. & C. Yellow Dye No. 5 (tartrazine), which can cause allergic-type reactions (shortness of breath, rash, or fainting) in certain susceptible individuals.

• Be sure to tell your doctor if you are pregnant. Small amounts of this medication cross the placenta. Although there are reports of safe use of this drug during pregnancy, there are also reports of liver disease and tremors in newborn infants whose mothers received this type of medication close to term. Also, tell your doctor if you are breastfeeding an infant. Small amounts of this medication pass into breast milk and may cause unwanted effects in the nursing infant.

Flura—see sodium fluoride

Flura-Drops—see sodium fluoride

Flura-Loz—see sodium fluoride

---

flurandrenolide (topical)

BRAND NAMES (Manufacturers)
Cordran (Dista)
flurandrenolide (various manufacturers)
TYPE OF DRUG
Adrenocorticosteroid hormone
INGREDIENT
flurandrenolide
DOSAGE FORMS
Ointment (0.025% and 0.05%)
Cream (0.025% and 0.05%)
Lotion (0.05%)
Tape (4 mcg per square centimeter of tape)
STORAGE
Flurandrenolide ointment, cream, lotion, and tape should be stored at room temperature, in tightly closed containers. This medication should never be frozen.

USES

Your adrenal glands naturally produce certain cortisone-like chemicals. These chemicals are involved in various regulatory processes in the body (such as fluid balance, temperature, and reactions to inflammation). Flurandrenolide belongs to a group of drugs known as adrenocorticosteroids (or cortisone-like medications). It is used to relieve the skin inflammation (redness, swelling, itching, and discomfort) associated with conditions such as dermatitis, eczema, and poison ivy. How this drug acts to relieve these disorders is not completely understood.

TREATMENT

Before applying this medication, wash your hands. Then, unless your doctor gives you different instructions, gently wash the area of the skin where the medication is to be applied. With a clean towel, pat the area almost dry; it should be slightly damp when you put the medicine on.

If you are using the lotion form of this medication, shake it well before pouring out the medicine. The contents tend to settle on the bottom of the bottle, so it is necessary to shake the container to evenly distribute the ingredients and equalize the doses.

Apply a small amount of the medication to the affected area in a thin layer. Do not bandage the area unless your doctor tells you to do so. If you are to apply an occlusive dressing (like kitchen plastic wrap), be sure you understand the instructions.

To use the tape form of this medication, prepare the skin as described above. The skin should be dried before the tape is applied. Remove the tape from the package and cut a piece slightly larger than the area to be covered. Round off the corners. Pull the white paper from the transparent tape (be careful that the tape does not stick to itself). Press the tape into place, keeping the skin smooth. If ends of the tape loosen prematurely, they may be trimmed off and replaced with fresh tape. The tape should always be cut, never torn.

If you miss a dose of this medication, apply the dose as soon as possible, unless it is almost time for the next application. In that case, do not apply the missed dose; just return to your regular schedule. Do not put twice as much medication on your skin at the next application.

SIDE EFFECTS

Minor. Acne; burning sensation; irritation of the affected area; itching; rash; or skin dryness.

If the affected area is extremely dry or scaling, the skin may be moistened before applying the medication by soaking in water or by applying water with a clean cloth. The ointment form is probably better for dry skin.

A mild, temporary stinging sensation may occur after this medication is applied. If this persists, contact your doctor.

Major. Tell your doctor about any side effects that are persistent or particularly bothersome. IT IS ESPECIALLY IMPORTANT TO TELL YOUR DOCTOR about blistering; increased hair growth; loss of skin color; secondary infection in the area being treated; or thinning of the skin with easy bruising.

INTERACTIONS
This medication does not interact with any other medications, as long as it is used according to directions.

WARNINGS
• Tell your doctor about unusual or allergic reactions you have had to medications, especially to flurandrenolide or any other adrenocorticosteroid (such as amcinonide, betamethasone, clocortolone, cortisone, desonide, desoximetasone, dexamethasone, diflorasone, flumethasone, fluocinolone, fluocinonide, fluorometholone, fluprednisolone, halcinonide, hydrocortisone, methylprednisolone, paramethasone, prednisolone, prednisone, or triamcinolone).
• Tell your doctor if you now have, or if you have ever had, blood vessel disease, chicken pox, diabetes mellitus (sugar diabetes), fungal infection, peptic ulcers, shingles, tuberculosis, tuberculosis of the skin, vaccinia, or any other type of infection, especially at the site currently being treated.
• If irritation develops while using this drug, immediately discontinue its use and notify your doctor.
• This product is not for use in the eyes or mucous membranes. Exposure of this medication to the eye may result in ocular (to the eye) side effects.
• Do not use this product with an occlusive wrap unless your doctor directs you to do so. Systemic absorption of this drug is increased if extensive areas of the body are treated, particularly if occlusive bandages are used. If it is necessary for you to use this drug under a wrap, follow your doctor's instructions exactly; do not leave the wrap in place longer than specified.
• If you are using this medication on a child's diaper area, do not put tight-fitting diapers or plastic pants on the child. This could lead to increased systemic absorption of

the drug and a possible increase in side effects.

• Be sure to tell your doctor if you are pregnant. If large amounts of this drug are applied for prolonged periods, some of it will be absorbed and may cross the placenta. Although studies in humans have not yet been completed, birth defects have been observed in the fetuses of animals who were given large doses of this type of drug during pregnancy. Also, tell your doctor if you are breastfeeding an infant. If absorbed through the skin, small amounts of flurandrenolide pass into breast milk and may cause growth suppression or a decrease in natural adrenocorticosteroid production in the nursing infant.

---

flurazepam

BRAND NAME (Manufacturer)
Dalmane (Roche)
TYPE OF DRUG
Sedative/hypnotic (sleeping aid)
INGREDIENT
flurazepam as the hydrochloride salt
DOSAGE FORM
Capsules (15 mg and 30 mg)
STORAGE
This medication should be stored at room temperature in a tightly closed, light-resistant container.

USES

Flurazepam is prescribed to treat insomnia (including problems falling asleep, waking during the night, and early morning wakefulness). It is not clear exactly how this medicine works, but it may relieve insomnia by acting as a depressant of the central nervous system.

TREATMENT

Flurazepam should be taken 30 to 60 minutes before bedtime. It can be taken with food or a full glass of water if stomach upset occurs. Do not take this medication with a dose of antacids, since they may retard its absorption from the gastrointestinal tract.

Your sleeping problem may improve the first night you take this medication, but it may take two or three nights before the effectiveness of flurazepam is noticed.

If you are taking this medication regularly and you miss a dose, take the missed dose immediately, if you remember within an hour of the scheduled time. If more than an hour has passed, skip the dose you missed and wait for the next scheduled dose. Do not double the dose.

SIDE EFFECTS

Minor. Bitter taste in the mouth; constipation; depression; diarrhea; dizziness; drowsiness (after a night's sleep); dry mouth; excess saliva; fatigue; flushing; headache; heartburn; loss of appetite; nausea; nervousness; sweating; and vomiting. As your body adjusts to the medicine, these side effects should disappear.

Dry mouth can be relieved by chewing sugarless gum or by sucking on ice chips.

If you feel dizzy, sit or lie down awhile; get up slowly, and be careful on stairs.

Major. Tell your doctor about any side effects that are persistent or particularly bothersome. IT IS ESPECIALLY IMPORTANT TO TELL YOUR DOCTOR about blurred or double vision; chest pain; difficulty urinating; fainting; falling; fever; joint pain; hallucinations; mouth sores; nightmares; palpitations; rash; severe depression; shortness of breath; slurred speech; sore throat; uncoordinated movements; unusual excitement; unusual tiredness; or yellowing of the eyes or skin.

INTERACTIONS

Flurazepam interacts with other medications.

1. To prevent over-sedation, this drug should not be taken with alcohol, other sedative drugs, or central nervous system depressants (such as antihistamines, barbiturates, muscle relaxants, pain medicines, narcotics, medicines for seizures, phenothiazine tranquilizers), or with anti-depressants.

2. This medication may decrease the effectiveness of carbamazepine, levodopa, and oral anti-coagulants (blood thinners); and may increase the effects of phenytoin.

3. Disulfiram, isoniazid, and cimetidine can increase the blood levels of flurazepam, which can lead to toxic effects.

4. Concurrent use of rifampin may decrease the effectiveness of flurazepam.

If you are already taking any of the medications listed above, CONSULT YOUR DOCTOR about their use.

WARNINGS

• Tell your doctor about unusual or allergic reactions you have had to any medications, especially to flurazepam or other benzodiazepine tranquilizers (such as alprazolam, chlordiazepoxide, clorazepate, diazepam, halazepam, lorazepam, oxazepam, prazepam, temazepam, or triazolam).

• Tell your doctor if you now have, or if you have ever had, liver disease, kidney disease, epilepsy, lung disease, myasthenia gravis, porphyria, mental depression, or mental illness.

• Flurazepam can cause drowsiness. Avoid tasks that require alertness, such as driving a car or using potentially dangerous machinery.

• This medication has the potential for abuse and must be used with caution. Tolerance may develop quickly; do not increase the dosage of the drug without first consulting your doctor. It is also important not to stop taking this drug suddenly if you have been taking it in large amounts or if you have used it for several weeks. Your doctor may want to reduce the dosage gradually.

• This is a safe drug when used properly. When it is combined with other sedative drugs or with alcohol, however, serious side effects may develop.

• Be sure to tell your doctor if you are pregnant. This type of medicine may increase the chance of birth defects if it is taken during the first three months of pregnancy. In addition, too much use of this medicine during the last six months of pregnancy may result in addiction of the fetus—leading to withdrawal side effects at birth. Also, use of this medicine during the last weeks of pregnancy may cause drowsiness, slowed heartbeat, and breathing difficulties in the infant. Tell your doctor if you are breastfeeding an infant. This medicine can pass into breast milk and cause drowsiness, slowed heartbeat, and breathing difficulties in nursing infants.

Flurosyn—see fluocinolone (topical)

Flutex—see triamcinolone (topical)

Foypromazine—see chlorpromazine

Fulvicin P/G—see griseofulvin

Fumasorb—see iron supplements

Fumerin—see iron supplements

Furadantin—see nitrofurantoin

Furalan—see nitrofurantoin

Furan—see nitrofurantoin

Furanite—see nitrofurantoin

Furatoin—see nitrofurantoin

---

furosemide

BRAND NAMES (Manufacturers)
furosemide (various manufacturers)
Lasix (Hoechst-Roussel)
SK-Furosemide (Smith Kline & French)
TYPE OF DRUG
Diuretic (water pill) and anti-hypertensive
INGREDIENT
furosemide
DOSAGE FORMS
Tablets (20 mg, 40 mg, and 80 mg)
Oral solution (10 mg per ml)
STORAGE
Furosemide tablets should be stored at room temperature in a tightly closed, light-resistant container. The oral solu-

tion should be stored in the refrigerator in a tightly closed, light-resistant container. This medication should never be frozen.

USES

Furosemide is prescribed to treat high blood pressure. It is also used to reduce fluid accumulation in the body caused by conditions such as heart failure, cirrhosis of the liver, kidney disease, and the long-term use of some medications. Furosemide reduces fluid accumulation by increasing the elimination of sodium and water through the kidneys.

TREATMENT

To decrease stomach irritation, you can take furosemide with a glass of milk or with a meal (unless your doctor directs you to do otherwise). Try to take it at the same time every day. Avoid taking a dose after 6:00 P.M.—this will prevent you from having to get up during the night to urinate.

This medication does not cure high blood pressure, but it will help to control the condition, as long as you continue to take it.

If you miss a dose of this medication, take the missed dose as soon as possible, unless it is almost time for the next dose. In that case, do not take the missed dose at all; just wait until the next scheduled dose. Do not double the dose.

SIDE EFFECTS

Minor. Blurred vision; constipation; cramping; diarrhea; dizziness; headache; itching; loss of appetite; muscle spasms; nausea; sore mouth; stomach upset; vomiting; and weakness. As your body adjusts to the medication, these side effects should disappear.

This medication will cause an increase in the amount of urine or in your frequency of urination when you first begin to take it. It may also cause you to have an unusual feeling of tiredness. These effects should subside after several days.

Furosemide can cause increased sensitivity to sunlight. It is therefore important to avoid prolonged exposure to sunlight and sunlamps. Wear protective clothing, and use an effective sunscreen.

To avoid dizziness and light-headedness when you stand, contract and relax the muscles of your legs for a few moments before rising. Do this by pushing one foot against the floor while raising the other foot slightly, alternating feet so that you are "pumping" your legs in a pedaling motion.

Major. Tell your doctor about any side effects that are persistent or particularly bothersome. IT IS ESPECIALLY IMPORTANT TO TELL YOUR DOCTOR about confusion; difficulty breathing; dry mouth; fainting; increased thirst; joint pains; loss of appetite; mood changes; muscle cramps; palpitations; rash; ringing in the ears; severe abdominal pain; sore throat; tingling in the fingers or toes; unusual bleeding or bruising; or yellowing of the eyes or skin.

INTERACTIONS

Furosemide interacts with several other drugs.

1. It can increase the side effects of alcohol, barbiturates, narcotics, cephalosporin antibiotics, chloral hydrate, cortisone-like steroids (such as cortisone, dexamethasone, hydrocortisone, prednisone, prednisolone), digoxin, digitalis, lithium, amphotericin B, clofibrate, aspirin, and theophylline.

2. The effectiveness of anti-gout medications, insulin, and oral anti-diabetic medications may be decreased when combined with furosemide.

3. Phenytoin can decrease the absorption and effectiveness of furosemide.

4. Indomethacin can decrease the diuretic effects of furosemide.

BE SURE TO TELL YOUR DOCTOR if you are taking any of the medicines listed above.

WARNINGS

• Tell your doctor about unusual or allergic reactions you have had to any medications, especially to diuretics (water pills), oral anti-diabetic medicines, or sulfonamide antibiotics.

• Before you start taking this medication, tell your doctor

if you now have, or if you have ever had, kidney disease or problems with urination; diabetes mellitus (sugar diabetes); gout; liver disease; asthma; pancreas disease; or systemic lupus erythematosus (SLE).

• Furosemide can cause potassium loss. Signs of potassium loss include dry mouth; thirst; weakness; muscle pain or cramps; nausea; and vomiting. If you experience any of these symptoms, call your doctor. Your doctor may want to have blood tests performed periodically in order to monitor your blood potassium levels. To help avoid potassium loss, take this medicine with a glass of fresh or frozen orange juice or cranberry juice, or eat a banana every day. The use of a salt substitute also helps to prevent potassium loss. Do not change your diet, however, before discussing it with your doctor. Too much potassium may also be dangerous.

• Before having any kind of surgery or other medical or dental treatment, be sure to tell your doctor or dentist that you are taking furosemide.

• To avoid dizziness, light-headedness, or fainting, get up from a sitting or lying position slowly; and avoid standing for long periods of time. You should also avoid strenuous exercise and prolonged exposure to hot weather.

• Furosemide oral solution contains F.D. & C. Yellow Dye No. 5 (tartrazine), which may cause allergic symptoms (shortness of breath, rash, or fainting) in certain susceptible individuals.

• While taking this medication, limit your intake of alcoholic beverages, in order to prevent dizziness and light-headedness.

• If you have high blood pressure, do not take any over-the-counter (non-prescription) medication for weight control, or for cough, cold, asthma, allergy, or sinus problems, unless you first check with your doctor.

• To prevent severe water loss (dehydration) while taking this medication, check with your doctor if you have any illness that causes severe or continuous nausea, vomiting, or diarrhea.

• This medication can raise blood sugar levels in diabetic patients. Therefore, blood sugar should be monitored carefully with blood or urine tests when this medication is started.

- Be sure to tell your doctor if you are pregnant. This drug crosses the placenta. Although studies in humans have not been completed, adverse effects have been observed on the fetuses of animals who received large doses of this drug during pregnancy. Also, tell your doctor if you are breastfeeding an infant. Small amounts of furosemide pass into breast milk.

Fynex—see diphenhydramine

Gantanol—see sulfonamides

Gantanol DS—see sulfonamides

Gantrisin—see sulfonamides

gemfibrozil

BRAND NAME (Manufacturer)
Lopid (Parke-Davis)
TYPE OF DRUG
Anti-hyperlipidemic (lipid-lowering drug)
INGREDIENT
gemfibrozil
DOSAGE FORM
Capsules (300 mg)
STORAGE
Gemfibrozil capsules should be stored at room temperature in a tightly closed container.

USES
Gemfibrozil is used to treat hyperlipidemia (high blood fat levels) in patients who have not responded to diet, weight reduction, exercise, and control of blood sugar. It is not clear how gemfibrozil lowers blood lipid levels, but it is thought to decrease the body's production of certain fats.

TREATMENT
In order to maximize its effectiveness, gemfibrozil should be taken 30 minutes before meals.

If you miss a dose of this medication, take the missed dose as soon as possible, unless it is almost time for the next dose. In that case, do not take the missed dose at all; just return to your regular dosing schedule. Do not double the next dose.

SIDE EFFECTS

Minor. Constipation; diarrhea; dizziness; dry mouth; gas; headache; insomnia; loss of appetite; nausea; and stomach upset. These side effects should disappear in several days, as your body adjusts to the medication.

To relieve constipation, increase the amount of fiber in your diet (bran, salads, fresh fruits and vegetables, and whole-grain breads), exercise, and drink more water (unless your doctor directs you to do otherwise).

If you feel dizzy, sit or lie down awhile; get up slowly, and be careful on stairs.

To help relieve mouth dryness, chew sugarless gum or suck on ice chips.

Major. Tell your doctor about any side effects that are persistent or particularly bothersome. IT IS ESPECIALLY IMPORTANT TO TELL YOUR DOCTOR about back pain; blurred vision; fatigue; muscle cramps; rash; ringing in the ears; swollen or painful joints; tingling sensations; or yellowing of the eyes or skin.

INTERACTIONS

Gemfibrozil can increase the effects of oral anti-coagulants (blood thinners, such as warfarin), which can lead to bleeding complications. BE SURE TO TELL YOUR DOCTOR if you are already taking a medication of this type.

WARNINGS

• Tell your doctor about unusual or allergic reactions you have had to any medications, especially to gemfibrozil.
• Before starting to take this medication, be sure to tell your doctor if you now have, or if you have ever had, biliary disorders; gallstones or gallbladder disease; kidney disease; or liver disease.
• If this drug makes you dizzy or blurs your vision, do not take part in activities that require alertness, such as driving a car or operating potentially dangerous equipment.

• Do not stop taking this medication unless you first check with your doctor. Stopping the drug abruptly may lead to a rapid increase in blood lipid (fats) and cholesterol levels. Your doctor may therefore want to start you on a special diet or another medication when gemfibrozil is discontinued.

• Large doses of gemfibrozil administered to animals for prolonged periods of time have been associated with benign and malignant cancers. This association has not been observed in humans.

• Be sure to tell your doctor if you are pregnant. Although gemfibrozil appears to be safe during pregnancy, extensive studies in humans have not yet been completed. Also, tell your doctor if you are breastfeeding an infant. It is not known if gemfibrozil passes into breast milk.

Geocillin—see carbenicillin

Gerimal—see ergoloid mesylates

Glaucon—see epinephrine (ophthalmic)

---

glipizide

BRAND NAME (Manufacturer)
Glucotrol (Roerig)
TYPE OF DRUG
Oral anti-diabetic
INGREDIENT
glipizide
DOSAGE FORM
Tablets (5 mg and 10 mg)
STORAGE
This medication should be stored at room temperature in a tightly closed container.

USES

Glipizide is used for the treatment of diabetes mellitus (sugar diabetes), which appears in adulthood and cannot be managed by control of diet alone. This type of diabetes is known as noninsulin-dependent diabetes (sometimes called maturity-onset or Type II diabetes). Glipizide lowers blood sugar levels by increasing the release of insulin from the pancreas.

TREATMENT

This medication should be taken on an empty stomach 30 minutes before a meal (unless your doctor directs you to do otherwise).

It is important to try not to miss any doses of this medication. If you do miss a dose, take it as soon as possible, unless it is almost time for the next dose. In that case, do not take the missed dose at all; just return to your regular dosing schedule. Do not double the next dose. Tell your doctor if you feel any side effects from missing a dose of this drug.

Diabetics who are taking oral anti-diabetic medication may need to be switched to insulin if they develop diabetic coma, have a severe infection, are scheduled for major surgery, or become pregnant.

SIDE EFFECTS

Minor. Diarrhea; headache; heartburn; loss of appetite; nausea; stomach pain; stomach discomfort; or vomiting. These side effects usually go away during treatment, as your body adjusts to the medicine.

Glipizide may increase your sensitivity to sunlight. It is therefore important to use caution during exposure to the sun. Use an effective sunscreen and avoid exposure to sunlamps.

Major. If any side effects are persistent or particularly bothersome, it is important to notify your doctor. IT IS ESPECIALLY IMPORTANT TO TELL YOUR DOCTOR about dark urine; fatigue; itching of the skin; light-colored stools; rash; sore throat and fever; unusual bleeding or bruising; or yellowing of the eyes or skin.

INTERACTIONS

Glipizide interacts with a number of other medications.
1. Chloramphenicol, guanethidine, insulin, monoamine oxidase (MAO) inhibitors, oxyphenbutazone, oxytetracycline, phenylbutazone, probenecid, aspirin or other salicylates, and sulfonamide antibiotics, when combined

with glipizide, can lower blood sugar levels — sometimes to dangerously low levels.

2. Thyroid hormones; dextrothyroxine; epinephrine; phenytoin; thiazide diuretics (water pills); and cortisone-like medications (such as dexamethasone, hydrocortisone, prednisone), combined with glipizide, can actually increase blood sugar levels—just what you are trying to avoid.

3. Anti-diabetic medications can increase the effects of warfarin, which can lead to bleeding complications.

4. Beta-blocking medications (such as atenolol, metoprolol, nadolol, pindolol, propranolol, and timolol), combined with glipizide, can result in either high or low blood sugar levels. Beta-blockers can also mask the symptoms of low blood sugar, which can be dangerous.

BE SURE TO TELL YOUR DOCTOR if you are already taking any of the medications listed above.

WARNINGS

• It is important to tell your doctor if you have ever had any unusual or allergic reaction to this medicine or to any sulfa medication [sulfonamide antibiotics, diuretics (water pills), or other oral anti-diabetics].

• It is also important to tell your doctor if you now have, or if you have ever had, kidney disease, liver disease, severe infection, or thyroid disease.

• Avoid drinking alcoholic beverages while taking this medication (unless otherwise directed by your doctor). Some patients who take this medicine suffer nausea; vomiting; dizziness; stomach pain; pounding headache; sweating; and redness of the face and skin when they drink alcohol. Also, large amounts of alcohol can lower blood sugar to dangerously low levels.

• It is important to follow the special diet that your doctor gave you. This is an important part of controlling your blood sugar and is necessary in order for this medicine to work properly.

• Be sure to tell your doctor or dentist that you are taking this medicine, before having any kind of surgery or other medical or dental treatment.

• Test for sugar in your urine as directed by your doctor. It is a convenient way to determine whether or not your

diabetes is being controlled by this medicine.
• Eat or drink something containing sugar right away if you experience any symptoms of low blood sugar (such as anxiety; chills; cold sweats; cool or pale skin; drowsiness; excessive hunger; headache; nausea; nervousness; rapid heartbeat; shakiness; or unusual tiredness or weakness). It is also important that your family and friends know the symptoms of low blood sugar and what to do if they observe any of these symptoms in you.

Check with your doctor as soon as possible—even if these symptoms are corrected by the sugar. The blood-sugar-lowering effects of this medicine can last for hours, and the symptoms may return during this period. Good sources of sugar are orange juice, corn syrup, honey, sugar cubes, and table sugar. You are at greatest risk of developing low blood sugar if you skip or delay meals, exercise more than usual, cannot eat because of nausea or vomiting, or drink large amounts of alcohol.
• Be sure to tell your doctor if you are pregnant. Studies have not yet been completed in humans, but studies in animals have shown that this medicine can cause birth defects. Also, tell your doctor if you are breastfeeding an infant. Small amounts of glipizide pass into breast milk.

Glucotrol—see glipizide

---

glutethimide

BRAND NAMES (Manufacturers)
Doriden (USV)
glutethimide (various manufacturers)
TYPE OF DRUG
Sedative/hypnotic (sleeping aid)
INGREDIENT
glutethimide
DOSAGE FORMS
Tablets (250 mg and 500 mg)
Capsules (500 mg)
STORAGE
Glutethimide tablets and capsules should be stored at room temperature, in tightly closed containers.

USES
This medication is used for short-term treatment of insomnia. It is not clearly understood how glutethimide works to produce sleep, but it is a central nervous system depressant (a drug that slows the activity of the brain and spinal cord). This drug loses its effectiveness in producing and maintaining sleep after three to seven days of continuous treatment.

TREATMENT
To avoid stomach irritation, you can take glutethimide tablets or capsules either on an empty stomach or with food or milk (unless your doctor directs you to do otherwise). The dose should be taken 15 to 30 minutes before bedtime.

SIDE EFFECTS
Minor. Drowsiness during the daytime; dizziness; a "hangover" feeling; headache; nausea; and vomiting. These side effects should disappear as your body adjusts to the medication.

If you feel dizzy, sit or lie down awhile; change position slowly, and be careful on stairs.

Major. Tell your doctor about any side effects that are persistent or particularly bothersome. IT IS ESPECIALLY IMPORTANT TO TELL YOUR DOCTOR about blurred vision; clumsiness; confusion; convulsions; difficulty breathing; fever; hallucinations; muscle cramps; nightmares; skin rash; slurred speech; sore throat; trembling; unusual bleeding or bruising; or unusual weakness.

INTERACTIONS
Glutethimide interacts with a number of other medications.

1. Concurrent use of it with other central nervous system depressants (such as alcohol, antihistamines, barbiturates, benzodiazepine tranquilizers, muscle relaxants, narcotics, pain medications, phenothiazine tranquilizers, and other sleeping medications) or with tricyclic anti-depressants can lead to extreme drowsiness and can be dangerous.

2. Glutethimide can decrease the blood levels and effec-

tiveness of oral anti-coagulants (blood thinners, such as warfarin).
BE SURE TO TELL YOUR DOCTOR if you are already taking any of the medications listed above.

WARNINGS

• Tell your doctor about unusual or allergic reactions you have had to any medications, especially to glutethimide.

• Before starting to take this medication, be sure to tell your doctor if you now have, or if you have ever had, glaucoma; heart arrhythmias; kidney disease; severe pain; peptic ulcers; enlarged prostate gland; porphyria; or blockage of the intestines or urinary tract.

• If this medication makes you drowsy or dizzy, or blurs your vision, do not take part in any activity that requires alertness, such as driving a car or operating potentially dangerous equipment.

• This medication has the potential for abuse. Therefore, it should not be used in higher doses or for longer periods than recommended by your doctor. If you have been taking glutethimide for longer than several weeks, check with your doctor before discontinuing it. Stopping abruptly can lead to a withdrawal reaction. Your doctor may want to reduce the dosage gradually to prevent this reaction.

• Be sure to tell your doctor if you are pregnant. Extensive studies in pregnant women using glutethimide have not yet been completed. However, it is known that large amounts of the drug taken during the last three months of pregnancy can cause the baby to become dependent on the medication, leading to withdrawal side effects after birth. Also tell your doctor if you are breastfeeding an infant. Small amounts of glutethimide pass into breast milk and can cause extreme drowsiness in the nursing infant.

glyburide

BRAND NAMES (Manufacturers)
Diabeta (Hoechst-Roussel)
Micronase (Upjohn)

TYPE OF DRUG
Oral anti-diabetic
INGREDIENT
glyburide
DOSAGE FORM
Tablets (1.25 mg, 2.5 mg, and 5 mg)
STORAGE
This medication should be stored at room temperature in a tightly closed container.

USES

Glyburide is used for the treatment of diabetes mellitus (sugar diabetes) that appears in adulthood and cannot be managed by control of diet alone. This type of diabetes is known as noninsulin-dependent diabetes (sometimes called maturity-onset or Type II diabetes). Glyburide lowers blood sugar levels by increasing the release of insulin from the pancreas.

TREATMENT

In order for glyburide to work correctly, it must be taken as directed by your doctor. To maintain a constant blood sugar level, it is best to take this medication at the same time(s) each day.

It is therefore important to try not to miss any doses of this medication. If you do miss a dose, take it as soon as possible, unless it is almost time for the next dose. In that case, do not take the missed dose at all; just return to your regular dosing schedule. Do not double the next dose. Tell your doctor if you feel any side effects from missing a dose of this drug.

Diabetics who are taking oral anti-diabetic medication may need to be switched to insulin if they develop diabetic coma, have a severe infection, are scheduled for major surgery, or become pregnant.

SIDE EFFECTS

Minor. Diarrhea; headache; heartburn; loss of appetite; nausea; vomiting; stomach pain; or stomach discomfort. These side effects usually disappear during treatment, as your body adjusts to the medicine.

Glyburide may increase your sensitivity to sunlight. It is

therefore important to use caution during exposure to the sun. You may want to wear protective clothing and sunglasses. Use an effective sunscreen, and avoid exposure to sunlamps.

Major. If any side effects are persistent or particularly bothersome, it is important to notify your doctor. IT IS ESPECIALLY IMPORTANT TO TELL YOUR DOCTOR about dark urine; fatigue; itching of the skin; light-colored stools; rash; sore throat and fever; unusual bleeding or bruising; or yellowing of the eyes or skin.

INTERACTIONS

Glyburide interacts with a number of other medications.

1. Chloramphenicol, guanethidine, insulin, monoamine oxidase (MAO) inhibitors, oxyphenbutazone, oxytetracycline, phenylbutazone, probenecid, aspirin or other salicylates, and sulfonamide antibiotics, when combined with glyburide, can lower blood sugar levels—sometimes to dangerously low levels.

2. Thyroid hormones, dextrothyroxine, epinephrine, phenytoin, thiazide diuretics (water pills), and cortisone-like medications (such as dexamethasone, hydrocortisone, prednisone), combined with glyburide, can actually increase blood sugar levels—just what you are trying to avoid.

3. Anti-diabetic medications can increase the effects of warfarin, which can lead to bleeding complications.

4. Beta-blocking medications (such as atenolol, metoprolol, nadolol, pindolol, propranolol, and timolol) combined with glyburide can result in either high or low blood sugar levels. Beta-blockers can also mask the symptoms of low blood sugar, which can be dangerous.

BE SURE TO TELL YOUR DOCTOR if you are already taking any of the medications listed above.

WARNINGS

• It is important to tell your doctor if you have ever had unusual or allergic reactions to medications, especially to glyburide or to any sulfa medication [sulfonamide antibiotics, diuretics (water pills), or other oral anti-diabetics].

• It is also important to tell your doctor if you now have, or if you have ever had, kidney disease, liver disease, severe infection, or thyroid disease.

- It is important to follow the special diet that your doctor gave you. This is an important part of controlling your blood sugar and is necessary in order for this medicine to work properly.

- Avoid drinking alcoholic beverages while taking this medication (unless otherwise directed by your doctor). Some patients who take this medicine suffer nausea; vomiting; dizziness; stomach pain; pounding headache; sweating; and redness of the face and skin when they drink alcohol. Also, large amounts of alcohol can lower blood sugar to dangerously low levels.

- Be sure to tell your doctor or dentist that you are taking this medication, before having any kind of surgery or other medical or dental treatment.

- Test for sugar in your urine as directed by your doctor. It is a convenient way to determine whether or not your diabetes is being controlled by this medicine.

- Eat or drink something containing sugar right away if you experience any symptoms of low blood sugar (such as anxiety; chills; cold sweats; cool or pale skin; drowsiness; excessive hunger; headache; nausea; nervousness; rapid heartbeat; shakiness; or unusual tiredness or weakness). It is also important that your family and friends know the symptoms of low blood sugar and what to do if they observe any of these symptoms in you.

Check with your doctor as soon as possible—even if these symptoms are corrected by the sugar. The blood-sugar-lowering effects of this medicine can last for hours, and the symptoms may return during this period. Good sources of sugar are orange juice, corn syrup, honey, sugar cubes, and table sugar. You are at greatest risk of developing low blood sugar if you skip or delay meals, exercise more than usual, cannot eat because of nausea or vomiting, or drink large amounts of alcohol.

- Diabeta brand glyburide contains F.D. & C. Yellow Dye No. 5 (tartrazine), which may cause allergic-type reactions (shortness of breath, rash, or fainting) in certain susceptible individuals.

- Be sure to tell your doctor if you are pregnant. Studies have not yet been completed in humans, but studies in animals have shown that this medication can cause birth defects. It is also important to tell your doctor if you are breastfeeding an infant. Small amounts of glyburide may pass into breast milk.

Glyceryl-T—see theophylline and guaifenesin combination

Grifulvin V—see griseofulvin

Grisactin—see griseofulvin

---

griseofulvin

BRAND NAMES (Manufacturers)
Fulvicin P/G (Schering)
Grifulvin V (Ortho)
Grisactin (Ayerst)
griseofulvin (various manufacturers)
Gris-PEG (Sandoz)
TYPE OF DRUG
Anti-fungal
INGREDIENT
griseofulvin
DOSAGE FORMS
Tablets (125 mg, 165 mg, 250 mg, 330 mg, and 500 mg)
Capsules (125 mg and 250 mg)
Oral suspension (125 mg per 5 ml teaspoonful)
STORAGE
Griseofulvin tablets, capsules, and oral suspension should be stored at room temperature in tightly closed containers. This medication should never be frozen.

USES
This medication is used to treat certain fungal infections of the skin and nails. Griseofulvin prevents the multiplication of susceptible fungi. It also enters the cells of skin, hair, and nails, and protects them from fungal invasion.

TREATMENT
In order to avoid stomach irritation, you can take griseofulvin with food or milk.

The oral suspension form of this medication should be shaken well, just before measuring each dose. The contents tend to settle on the bottom of the bottle, so it is necessary to shake the container to evenly distribute the ingredients and equalize the doses. Each dose should then be measured carefully with a specially designed, 5 ml measuring spoon. An ordinary kitchen teaspoon is not accurate enough.

If you miss a dose of this medication, take the missed dose as soon as possible, unless it is almost time for the next dose. In that case, do not take the missed dose at all; just return to your regular dosing schedule. Do not double the next dose.

It is important to continue to take this medication for the entire time prescribed by your doctor (perhaps six months or more), even if the symptoms disappear before the end of that period. If you stop taking this drug too soon, resistant fungi are given a chance to continue growing, and your infection could recur.

SIDE EFFECTS

Minor. Diarrhea; dizziness; fatigue; headache; insomnia; nausea; stomach upset; and vomiting. These side effects should disappear in several days, as your body adjusts to the medication.

If you feel dizzy, sit or lie down awhile; get up slowly, and be careful on stairs.

This medication can increase your sensitivity to sunlight. You should therefore avoid prolonged exposure to sunlight and sunlamps. Wear protective clothing and sunglasses, and use an effective sunscreen.

Major. Tell your doctor about any side effects that are persistent or particularly bothersome. IT IS ESPECIALLY IMPORTANT TO TELL YOUR DOCTOR about confusion; impairment in performance of routine activities; itching; skin rash; sore throat; or a tingling of the hands or feet.

INTERACTIONS

Griseofulvin interacts with several other types of medication.

1. It can increase the effects of alcohol, resulting in flushing and an increased heart rate.

2. Barbiturates can decrease the effectiveness of griseo-fulvin.

3. Griseofulvin can decrease the effectiveness of oral anti-coagulants (blood thinners, such as warfarin).

Before starting to take griseofulvin, TELL YOUR DOCTOR if you are already taking any of these other drugs.

WARNINGS

- Tell your doctor about unusual or allergic reactions you have had to any medications, especially griseofulvin, pencillins, cephalosporin antibiotics, or penicillamine.
- Before starting to take griseofulvin, be sure to tell your doctor if you now have, or if you have ever had, liver disease, porphyria, or systemic lupus erythematosus (SLE).
- If this drug makes you dizzy, do not take part in any activity that requires alertness, such as driving a car or operating potentially dangerous equipment.
- Observe good hygiene to control the source of infection and to prevent reinfection.
- Concurrent use of an appropriate topical anti-fungal medication may be necessary to help clear the infection.
- Be sure to tell your doctor if you are pregnant. Extensive studies in pregnant women have not yet been completed, but birth defects have been reported in animals whose mothers received large doses of griseofulvin during pregnancy. Also, tell your doctor if you are breastfeeding an infant. It is not known whether or not griseofulvin passes into breast milk.

Gris-PEG—see griseofulvin

---

guanabenz

BRAND NAME (Manufacturer)
Wytensin (Wyeth)
TYPE OF DRUG
Anti-hypertensive
INGREDIENT
guanabenz as the acetate salt

DOSAGE FORM
Tablets (4 mg and 8 mg)
STORAGE
Guanabenz should be stored at room temperature in a tightly closed, light-resistant container.

USES
This medication is used to control high blood pressure. It works by decreasing the release of chemicals in the brain that are responsible for increasing blood pressure.

TREATMENT
Guanabenz can be taken either on an empty stomach or, to avoid stomach irritation, with food or milk (as directed by your doctor).

Try to take the doses at the same times each day, so that you become accustomed to taking this medication. Your doctor may want you to take the last dose of the day at bedtime, in order to control blood pressure at night and to reduce daytime drowsiness.

Guanabenz does not cure high blood pressure, but it will help to control the condition, as long as you continue to take it.

If you miss a dose of this medication, take the missed dose as soon as possible, unless it is almost time for your next dose. In that case, do not take the missed dose at all; just return to your regular dosing schedule. Do not double the next dose. If you miss more than two consecutive doses, contact your doctor as soon as possible.

SIDE EFFECTS
Minor Constipation; diarrhea; dizziness; drowsiness; dry mouth; headache; nasal congestion; nausea; sleep disturbances; stomach upset; taste disorders; vomiting; and weakness. These side effects should disappear in several weeks, as your body adjusts to the medication.

To relieve constipation, increase the amount of fiber in your diet (bran, salads, fresh fruits and vegetables, and whole-grain breads), and drink more water (unless your doctor directs you to do otherwise).

If you feel dizzy, sit or lie down awhile; change positions slowly, and be careful on stairs.

To help relieve mouth dryness, chew sugarless gum, or suck on ice chips or a piece of hard candy.

Major. Tell your doctor about any side effects that are persistent or particularly bothersome. IT IS ESPECIALLY IMPORTANT TO TELL YOUR DOCTOR about anxiety; blurred vision; chest pain; depression; disturbances in sexual function; enlarged or painful breasts (in both sexes); increased urination; itching; loss of coordination; muscle aches; palpitations; rapid weight gain (three to five pounds within a week); shortness of breath; or skin rash.

INTERACTIONS

Concurrent use of guanabenz with central nervous system depressants (drugs that slow the activity of the brain and spinal cord), such as alcohol, antihistamines, barbiturates, benzodiazepine tranquilizers, muscle relaxants, narcotics, pain medications, phenothiazine tranquilizers, and sleeping medication, or with tricyclic antidepressants can lead to extreme drowsiness. BE SURE TO TELL YOUR DOCTOR if you are already taking any of these types of medication.

WARNINGS

• Tell your doctor about unusual or allergic reactions you have had to any medications, especially to guanabenz.

• Before starting to take this medication, be sure to tell your doctor if you now have, or if you have ever had, heart or blood vessel disease; or kidney or liver disease.

• If this medication makes you dizzy or drowsy, or blurs your vision, avoid taking part in activities that require alertness, such as driving a car or operating potentially dangerous equipment.

• Before having any surgery or other medical or dental treatment, be sure your doctor or dentist knows that you are taking this medication.

• Do not stop taking guanabenz unless you first check with your doctor. If this drug is stopped abruptly, you may experience nervousness, agitation, headache, and a *rise in blood pressure*. Your doctor may therefore want to decrease your dosage gradually or start you on another drug when this medication is stopped.

• Check with your doctor or pharmacist before taking any over-the-counter (non-prescription) asthma, allergy, cough, cold, diet, or sinus preparations. Some of these products can reduce the effectiveness of guanabenz.

• Be sure to tell your doctor if you are pregnant. Although guanabenz appears to be safe during pregnancy, extensive studies in humans have not yet been completed. Studies on birth defects in animals have produced conflicting results. Also, tell your doctor if you are breastfeeding an infant. It is not known whether or not guanabenz passes into breast milk.

---

guanadrel

BRAND NAME (Manufacturer)
Hylorel (Pennwalt)
TYPE OF DRUG
Anti-hypertensive
INGREDIENT
guanadrel as the sulfate salt
DOSAGE FORM
Tablets (10 mg and 25 mg)
STORAGE
Guanadrel tablets should be stored at room temperature, in a tightly closed container.

USES

Guanadrel is used to control high blood pressure. It works by blocking the action of the body chemicals responsible for increasing blood pressure.

TREATMENT

Guanadrel can be taken either on an empty stomach or, to avoid stomach irritation, with food or milk (as directed by your doctor). Try to take your doses at the same times each day, in order to become accustomed to taking this medication.

This medication does not cure high blood pressure, but it will help to control the condition, as long as you continue to take it.

If you miss a dose of this medication, take the missed

dose as soon as possible, unless it is almost time for your next dose. In that case, do not take the missed dose at all; just return to your regular dosing schedule. Do not double the next dose.

SIDE EFFECTS

Minor. Constipation; diarrhea; dizziness; drowsiness; dry throat or mouth; fatigue; gas pains; headache; loss of appetite; nausea; sleep disorders; stomach upset; and weight gain or loss. These side effects should disappear in several weeks, as your body adjusts to the medication.

To relieve constipation, increase the amount of fiber in your diet (bran, salads, fresh fruits and vegetables, and whole-grain breads), and drink more water (unless your doctor directs you to do otherwise).

If you feel dizzy, sit or lie down awhile; change positions slowly, and be careful on stairs.

To help relieve mouth dryness, chew sugarless gum, or suck on ice chips or a piece of hard candy.

Major. Tell your doctor about any side effects that are persistent or particularly bothersome. IT IS ESPECIALLY IMPORTANT TO TELL YOUR DOCTOR about backache; blurred vision; chest pain; confusion; coughing; depression; fainting; impotence; increased urination; joint pain; leg cramps; mental disorders; mouth sores; palpitations; rapid weight gain (three to five pounds within a week); shortness of breath; or tingling sensations.

INTERACTIONS

Guanadrel interacts with several other types of drugs.
1. Concurrent use of guanadrel and alcohol can lead to fainting and extreme drowsiness.
2. Amphetamines, diet preparations, ephedrine, methylphenidate, phenothiazine tranquilizers, phenylpropanolamine, and tricyclic anti-depressants can decrease the beneficial effects of guanadrel.
3. Use of guanadrel with monoamine oxidase (MAO) inhibitors can lead to serious side effects. At least one week should separate doses of these two types of drugs.
TELL YOUR DOCTOR if you are already taking any of the medications listed above.

WARNINGS

- Tell your doctor about unusual or allergic reactions you have had to any medications, especially to guanadrel.
- Before starting to take this medication, be sure to tell your doctor if you now have, or if you have ever had, asthma, fevers, heart or blood vessel disease, peptic ulcers, pheochromocytoma, or a slowed heartbeat.
- If this drug makes you dizzy or drowsy, or blurs your vision, avoid taking part in activities that require alertness, such as driving a car or operating potentially dangerous equipment.
- Before having any surgery or other medical or dental treatment, be sure your doctor or dentist knows that you are taking this medication.
- Check with your doctor or pharmacist before taking any over-the-counter (non-prescription) asthma, allergy, cough, cold, diet, or sinus preparation. Some of these products can decrease the effectiveness of guanadrel.
- To prevent feeling faint while you are taking guanadrel, you should avoid drinking alcoholic beverages. You should also avoid standing for prolonged periods, excessive exercising, and exposure to hot showers and saunas.
- Be sure to tell your doctor if you are pregnant. Although guanadrel appears to be safe during pregnancy, extensive studies in humans have not yet been completed. Also, tell your doctor if you are breastfeeding an infant. It is not known whether or not guanadrel passes into breast milk.

---

guanethidine

BRAND NAME (Manufacturer)
Ismelin (Ciba)
TYPE OF DRUG
Anti-hypertensive
INGREDIENT
guanethidine as the sulfate salt
DOSAGE FORM
Tablets (10 mg and 25 mg)
STORAGE
Guanethidine should be stored at room temperature, in a tightly closed container.

USES

Guanethidine is used to control high blood pressure. It works by blocking the action of the chemicals responsible for increasing blood pressure.

TREATMENT

Guanethidine can be taken either on an empty stomach or, to avoid stomach irritation, with food or milk (as directed by your doctor). Try to take your doses at the same times each day, to become accustomed to taking it.

This medication does not cure high blood pressure, but it will help to control the condition, as long as you continue to take it.

If you miss a dose of this medication, take the missed dose as soon as possible, unless it is almost time for the next dose. In that case, do not take the missed dose at all; just return to to your regular dosing schedule. Do not double the next dose.

SIDE EFFECTS

Minor. Diarrhea; dizziness; dry mouth; fatigue; nasal congestion; nausea; vomiting; weakness; and weight gain. These side effects should disappear in several weeks, as your body adjusts to the medication.

If you feel dizzy, sit or lie down awhile; change positions slowly, and be careful on stairs.

To help relieve mouth dryness, chew sugarless gum, or suck on ice chips or a piece of hard candy.

Major. Tell your doctor about any side effects that are persistent or particularly bothersome. IT IS ESPECIALLY IMPORTANT TO TELL YOUR DOCTOR about blurred vision; chest pain; decreased sexual ability; depression; drooping eyelids; hair loss; increased urination; itching; muscle pain or tremors; rapid weight gain (three to five pounds within a week); skin rash; shortness of breath; or swollen or tender glands.

INTERACTIONS

Guanethidine interacts with several other types of drugs.
1. Concurrent use of guanethidine and alcohol can lead to fainting or extreme drowsiness.
2. Amphetamines, appetite suppressants, ephedrine,

methylphenidate, phenothiazine tranquilizers, phenyl-propanolamine, and tricyclic anti-depressants can decrease the beneficial effects of guanethidine.

3. Barbiturates, methotrimeprazine, narcotics, fenfluramine, and reserpine can increase the blood-pressure-lowering effects of guanethidine, which can be dangerous.

4. The dosage of oral anti-diabetic medications may need to be adjusted when guanethidine is started.

5. Concurrent use of guanethidine with monoamine oxidase (MAO) inhibitors can lead to serious side effects. At least one week should separate doses of these two types of medication.

BE SURE TO TELL YOUR DOCTOR if you are already taking any of the medications listed above.

WARNINGS

- Tell your doctor about unusual or allergic reactions you have had to any medications, especially to guanethidine.
- Before starting to take this medication, be sure to tell your doctor if you now have, or if you have ever had, asthma, diabetes mellitus (sugar diabetes), fever, heart or blood vessel disease, kidney disease, liver disease, peptic ulcers, pheochromocytoma, or a slowed heart rate.
- If this medication makes you dizzy or drowsy, avoid activities that require alertness, such as driving a car or operating potentially dangerous equipment.
- To prevent fainting while you are taking guanethidine, you should avoid drinking alcoholic beverages. You should also avoid standing for prolonged periods, excessive exercise, and exposure to hot showers and saunas.
- Before having any surgery or other medical or dental treatment, be sure to tell your doctor or dentist that you are taking this medication.
- Check with your doctor or pharmacist before taking any over-the-counter (non-prescription) asthma, allergy, cough, cold, diet, or sinus preparation. Some of these products can reduce the effectiveness of guanethidine.
- Guanethidine 10 mg tablets contain F.D. & C. Yellow Dye No. 5 (tartrazine), which can cause allergic-type symptoms (fainting, shortness of breath, or rash) in certain susceptible individuals.

• Be sure to tell your doctor if you are pregnant. Although guanethidine appears to be safe during pregnancy, extensive studies in humans have not yet been completed. Also, tell your doctor if you are breastfeeding an infant. It is not known whether or not guanethidine passes into breast milk.

Gyne-Lotrimin — see clotrimazole (vaginal)

Gynergen — see ergotamine

---

halazepam

BRAND NAME (Manufacturer)
Paxipam (Schering)
TYPE OF DRUG
Sedative/hypnotic (anti-anxiety medication)
INGREDIENT
halazepam
DOSAGE FORM
Tablets (20 mg and 40 mg)
STORAGE
This medication should be stored at room temperature in a tightly closed, light-resistant container.

USES

Halazepam is prescribed to treat symptoms of anxiety. It is not clear exactly how this medicine works, but it may relieve anxiety by acting as a depressant of the central nervous system. Halazepam is currently used by many people to relieve nervousness. It is effective for this purpose for short periods, but it is important to try to remove the cause of the anxiety as well.

TREATMENT

This medication should be taken exactly as directed by your doctor. It can be taken with food or a full glass of water if stomach upset occurs. Do not take this medication with a dose of antacids, since they may retard its absorption from the gastrointestinal tract.

If you are taking this medication regularly and you miss

a dose, take the missed dose immediately, if you remember within an hour of the scheduled dose. If more than an hour has passed, skip the dose you missed and wait for the next scheduled dose. Do not double the dose.

SIDE EFFECTS

Minor. Bitter taste in mouth; constipation; depression; diarrhea; dizziness; drowsiness (after a night's sleep); dry mouth; excess saliva; fatigue; flushing; headache; heartburn; loss of appetite; nausea; nervousness; sweating; and vomiting. As your body adjusts to the medicine, these effects should disappear.

Dry mouth can be relieved by chewing sugarless gum or by sucking on ice chips.

If you feel dizzy, sit or lie down awhile; get up slowly, and be careful on stairs.

Major. Tell your doctor about any side effects that are persistent or particularly bothersome. IT IS ESPECIALLY IMPORTANT TO TELL YOUR DOCTOR about blurred or double vision; chest pain; severe depression; difficulty urinating; fainting; falling; fever; joint pain; hallucinations; mouth sores; nightmares; palpitations; rash; shortness of breath; slurred speech; sore throat; uncoordinated movements; unusual excitement; unusual tiredness; or yellowing of the eyes or skin.

INTERACTIONS

Halazepam interacts with several other medications.

1. To prevent over-sedation, it should not be taken with alcohol, other sedative drugs, central nervous system depressants (such as antihistamines, barbiturates, muscle relaxants, pain medicines, narcotics, medicines for seizures, phenothiazine tranquilizers), or with anti-depressants.

2. This medication may decrease the effectiveness of carbamazepine, levodopa, and oral anti-coagulants, and may increase the effects of phenytoin.

3. Disulfiram, isoniazid, and cimetidine can increase the blood levels of halazepam, which can lead to toxic effects.

4. Concurrent use of rifampin may decrease the effectiveness of halazepam.

If you are already taking any of the medications listed above, CONSULT YOUR DOCTOR about their use.

WARNINGS

• Tell your doctor about unusual or allergic reactions you have had to medications, especially to halazepam or any other benzodiazepine tranquilizers (such as alprazolam, chlordiazepoxide, clorazepate, diazepam, flurazepam, lorazepam, oxazepam, or triazolam).

• Tell your doctor if you now have, or if you have ever had, liver or kidney disease, epilepsy, lung disease, myasthenia gravis, porphyria, mental depression, or mental illness.

• This medicine can cause drowsiness. You should therefore avoid tasks that require alertness, such as driving a car or using potentially dangerous machinery.

• This medication has the potential for abuse and must be used with caution. Tolerance may develop quickly; do not increase the dose of the drug without first consulting your doctor. It is also important not to stop taking this drug suddenly if you have been taking it in large amounts, or if you have used it for several weeks. Your doctor may want to reduce the dosage gradually.

• This is a safe drug when used properly. When it is combined with other sedative drugs or alcohol, however, serious side effects can develop.

• Be sure to tell your doctor if you are pregnant. This type of medicine may increase the chance of birth defects if it is taken during the first three months of pregnancy. In addition, too much use of this medicine during the last six months of pregnancy may result in addiction of the fetus, leading to withdrawal side effects in the newborn. Also, use of this medicine during the last weeks of pregnancy may cause drowsiness, slowed heartbeat, and breathing difficulties in the infant. Tell your doctor if you are breastfeeding an infant. This medicine can pass into breast milk and cause drowsiness, slowed heartbeat, and breathing difficulties in nursing infants.

Hal-Chlor —see chlorpheniramine

Halciderm —see halcinonide (topical)

halcinonide (topical)

BRAND NAMES (Manufacturers)
Halciderm (Squibb)
Halog (Squibb)
TYPE OF DRUG
Adrenocorticosteroid hormone
INGREDIENT
halcinonide
DOSAGE FORMS
Ointment (0.025%, 0.1%)
Cream (0.025%, 0.1%)
Solution (0.1%)
STORAGE
Halcinonide ointment, cream, and solution should be stored at room temperature, in tightly closed containers. This medication should never be frozen.

USES

Your adrenal glands naturally produce certain cortisone-like chemicals. These chemicals are involved in various regulatory processes in the body (such as fluid balance, temperature, and reactions to inflammation). Halcinonide belongs to a group of drugs known as adrenocorticosteroids (or cortisone-like medications). It is used to relieve the skin inflammation (redness, swelling, itching, and discomfort) associated with conditions such as dermatitis, eczema, and poison ivy. How this drug acts to relieve these disorders is not completely understood.

TREATMENT

Before applying this medication, wash your hands. Then, unless your doctor gives you different instructions, gently wash the area of the skin where the medication is to be applied. With a clean towel, pat the area almost dry; it should be slightly damp when you put the medicine on.

Apply a small amount of the medication to the affected area in a thin layer. Do not bandage the area unless your doctor tells you to do so. If you are to apply an occlusive dressing (like kitchen plastic wrap), be sure you understand the instructions.

If you miss a dose of this medication, apply the dose as

soon as possible, unless it is almost time for the next application. In that case, do not apply the missed dose, just return to your regular schedule. Do not put twice as much of the medication on your skin at the next application.

SIDE EFFECTS

Minor. Acne; burning sensation; irritation of the affected area; itching; rash; and skin dryness.

If the affected area is extremely dry or scaling, the skin may be moistened before applying the medication by soaking in water or by applying water with a clean cloth. The ointment form is probably better for dry skin.

A mild, temporary stinging sensation may occur after this medication is applied. If this persists, contact your doctor.

Major. Tell your doctor about any side effects that are persistent or particularly bothersome. IT IS ESPECIALLY IMPORTANT TO TELL YOUR DOCTOR about blistering; increased hair growth; loss of skin color; secondary infection in the area being treated; or thinning of the skin with easy bruising.

INTERACTIONS

This medication does not interact with any other medications, as long as it is used according to directions.

WARNINGS

• Tell your doctor about unusual or allergic reactions you have had to medications, especially to halcinonide or any other adrenocorticosteroids (such as amcinonide, betamethasone, cortisone, desonide, desoximetasone, dexamethasone, flumethasone, fluocinolone, fluocinonide, fluorometholone, fluprednisolone, flurandrenolide, hydrocortisone, methylprednisolone, paramethasone, prednisolone, prednisone, or triamcinolone).

• Tell your doctor if you now have, or if you have ever had, blood vessel disease, chicken pox, diabetes mellitus (sugar diabetes), fungal infection, peptic ulcers, shingles, tuberculosis, tuberculosis of the skin, vaccinia, or any other type of infection, especially at the site currently being treated.

- If irritation develops while using this drug, immediately discontinue its use, and notify your doctor.
- This product is not for use in the eyes or mucous membranes. Exposure of this medication to the eye may result in ocular (to the eye) side effects.
- Do not use this product with an occlusive wrap unless your doctor directs you to do so. Systemic absorption of this drug is increased if extensive areas of the body are treated, particularly if occlusive bandages are used. If it is necessary for you to use this drug under a wrap, follow your doctor's instructions exactly; do not leave the wrap in place longer than specified.
- If you are using this medication on a child's diaper area, do not put tight-fitting diapers or plastic pants on the child. This may lead to increased systemic absorption of the drug and a possible increase in side effects.
- Be sure to tell your doctor if you are pregnant. If large amounts of this drug are applied for prolonged periods, some of it will be absorbed and may cross the placenta. Although studies in humans have not yet been completed, birth defects have been observed in the fetuses of animals who were given large oral doses of this type of drug during pregnancy. Also, tell your doctor if you are breastfeeding an infant. If absorbed through the skin, small amounts of halcinonide pass into breast milk and may cause growth suppression or a decrease in natural adrenocorticosteroid production in the nursing infant.

Halcion—see triazolam

Haldol—see haloperidol

Halog—see halcinonide (topical)

---

haloperidol

BRAND NAME (Manufacturer)
Haldol (McNeil)
TYPE OF DRUG
Anti-psychotic

INGREDIENT
haloperidol
DOSAGE FORMS
Tablets (0.5 mg, 1 mg, 2 mg, 5 mg, 10 mg, and 20 mg)
Oral concentrate (2 mg per ml)
STORAGE
Haloperidol tablets should be stored at room temperature in a tightly closed, light-resistant container. The oral concentrate should be stored in the refrigerator in a tightly closed, light-resistant container. This medication should never be frozen.

USES

Haloperidol is prescribed to treat the symptoms of certain types of mental illness, such as emotional symptoms of psychosis, the manic phase of manic-depressive illness, Gilles de la Tourette's syndrome, and severe behavioral problems in children. This medication is thought to relieve symptoms of mental illness by blocking certain chemicals involved with nerve transmission in the brain.

TREATMENT

To avoid stomach irritation, you can take haloperidol tablets with a meal or with a glass of water or milk (unless your doctor directs you to do otherwise).

The oral concentrate form of this medication should be measured carefully with the dropper provided, then added to 4 ounces (½ cup) or more of water, milk, juice, or a carbonated beverage, or to applesauce or pudding, immediately prior to administration. To prevent possible loss of effectiveness, haloperidol should not be diluted with tea, coffee, caffeine-containing beverages, or apple juice.

If you miss a dose of this medication and remember within six hours, take the missed dose as soon as possible; then return to your regular schedule. If more than six hours have passed, however, skip the missed dose and return to your regular dosing schedule. Do not double the dose unless your doctor directs you to do so.

The full effects of haloperidol may not become apparent for two weeks after you start to take it.

SIDE EFFECTS

Minor. Blurred vision; confusion; constipation; diarrhea; dizziness; drooling; drowsiness; dry mouth; fatigue; headache; heartburn; impotence; jitteriness; loss of appetite; menstrual irregularities; nausea; restlessness; sleep disorders; sweating; vomiting; and weakness. As your body adjusts to the medication, these side effects should disappear.

If you are constipated, increase the amount of fiber in your diet (raw vegetables, fruits, salads, bran, and whole-grain breads), and drink more water (unless your doctor directs you to do otherwise).

To reduce mouth dryness, chew sugarless gum, or suck on ice chips or a piece of hard candy.

This medication can cause increased sensitivity to sunlight. It is therefore important to avoid prolonged exposure to sunlight and sunlamps. Wear protective clothing, and use an effective sunscreen.

To avoid dizziness or light-headedness when you stand, contract and relax the muscles of your legs for a few moments before rising. Do this by pushing one foot against the floor while raising the other foot slightly, alternating feet so that you are "pumping" your legs in a pedaling motion.

Major. Tell your doctor about any side effects that are persistent or particularly bothersome. IT IS ESPECIALLY IMPORTANT TO TELL YOUR DOCTOR about aching joints and muscles; unusual bleeding or bruising; breast enlargement (in both sexes); chest pain; convulsions; difficulty breathing or swallowing; difficulty urinating; fainting; fever; fluid retention; hair loss; hallucinations; involuntary movements of the mouth, face, neck, or tongue; mouth sores; palpitations; skin darkening; skin rash; sore throat; tremors; or yellowing of the eyes or skin.

INTERACTIONS

Haloperidol interacts with several other types of medication.

1. It can cause extreme drowsiness when combined with alcohol or other central nervous system depressants (drugs that slow the activity of the nervous system), such as antihistamines, barbiturates, benzodiazepine tranquilizers, muscle relaxants, narcotics, and pain medications, or with tricyclic anti-depressants.

2. This medication can decrease the effectiveness of guanethidine and anti-convulsant (anti-seizure) medications.

3. The blood-pressure-lowering effects of anti-hypertensive medications may be dangerously increased when combined with haloperidol.

4. Haloperidol may increase the side effects of epinephrine, lithium, and methyldopa.

5. It is important to note that tea or coffee can reduce the gastrointestinal absorption of haloperidol, decreasing its effectiveness. Therefore, haloperidol should not be taken at the same time as tea or coffee.

Before starting to take haloperidol, BE SURE TO TELL YOUR DOCTOR if you are already taking any of the medicines listed above.

WARNINGS

- Tell your doctor about unusual or allergic reactions you have had to medications, especially to any medicines used to treat mental illness.
- Tell your doctor if you now have, or if you have ever had, any blood disorders, blockage of the urinary tract, drug-induced depression, enlarged prostate gland, epilepsy, glaucoma, heart or circulatory disease, kidney disease, liver disease, lung disease, mental depression, Parkinson's disease, peptic ulcers, or thyroid disease.
- Avoid drinking alcoholic beverages while taking this medication, in order to prevent over-sedation.
- If this medication makes you dizzy or drowsy, do not take part in any activity that requires alertness, such as driving a car or operating potentially dangerous equipment. Be careful on stairs, and avoid getting up suddenly from a lying or sitting position.
- Prior to having surgery or any other medical or dental treatment, be sure your doctor or dentist knows that you are taking this medication.
- Some of the side effects caused by this drug can be prevented by taking an anti-parkinson drug. Discuss this with your doctor.
- Haloperidol has been reported to cause certain tumors

in rats. This effect has not been shown to occur in humans.

• This medication can decrease sweating and heat release from the body. You should therefore avoid getting overheated by strenuous exercise in hot weather, and should avoid taking hot baths, showers, and saunas.

• Do not stop taking this medication suddenly. If the drug is stopped abruptly, you may experience nausea; vomiting; stomach upset; headache; increased heart rate; insomnia; tremulousness, or worsening of your condition. Your doctor may want to reduce the dosage gradually.

• If you are planning to have a myelogram, or any procedure in which dye is injected into the spinal cord, tell your doctor that you are taking this medication.

• Avoid spilling the oral concentrate form of this medication on your skin or clothing; it can cause redness and irritation of the skin.

• While taking haloperidol, do not take any over-the-counter (non-prescription) medication for weight control, or for cough, cold, allergy, asthma, or sinus problems, unless you first check with your doctor. The combination of these medications may cause high blood pressure.

• Be sure to tell your doctor if you are pregnant. Studies in humans evaluating the effects of this medication on offspring have not yet been completed. However, side effects have appeared in newborn animals whose mothers received large doses of this type of medication during pregnancy. Also, tell your doctor if you are breastfeeding an infant. Small amounts of haloperidol pass into breast milk.

HC-Form—see hydrocortisone and iodochlorhydroxyquin combination (topical)

H-Cort—see hydrocortisone (topical)

H.E.A.—see ergoloid mesylates

Hematinic—see iron supplements

Hemocyte—see iron supplements

Hemorrhoidal HC—see hydrocortisone, benzyl benzoate, bismuth resorcin compound, bismuth subgallate, and Peruvian balsam combination (topical)

Hemusol HC—see hydrocortisone, benzyl benzoate, bismuth resorcin compound, bismuth subgallate, and Peruvian balsam combination (topical)

---

heparin

BRAND NAMES (Manufacturers)
Calciparine (American Critical Care)
heparin sodium (various manufacturers)
Lipo-Hepin (Riker)
Liquaemin (Organon)
Panheprin (Abbott)
TYPE OF DRUG
Anti-coagulant (prevents blood from clotting)
INGREDIENT
heparin as the sodium or calcium salt
DOSAGE FORM
Injection solution obtained from beef lung or pig intestine (various concentrations)
STORAGE
Heparin should be stored at room temperature. DO NOT FREEZE. The solution should not be used if it is discolored or if it has particles floating in it.

USES

Heparin decreases the clotting ability of the blood. It does not dissolve blood clots, but prevents clots that are already formed from becoming larger and causing more serious problems. It also prevents the formation of new clots.

This medication is used for the treatment of clotting disorders in the leg, lung, or brain. It is also used to prevent blood clotting during surgery or dialysis. In low doses, heparin has also been used to prevent clots from forming in patients who must remain in bed for prolonged periods of time.

TREATMENT

Heparin is given by injection either directly into a vein or under the layers of the skin. If you are using these injections at home, it is important that you use the correct amount of heparin, on a regular schedule (to obtain the best results without causing serious bleeding).

If you miss a dose, inject it as soon as possible; then return to your regular dosing schedule. However, if it is almost time for your next dose, skip the missed dose and return to your regular dosing schedule. Do not double the next dose. Doubling the dose may cause bleeding.

SIDE EFFECTS

Minor. None.

Major. Abdominal pain; back or rib pain, or unusual hair loss (can occur after six months of therapy); backaches; black, tarry stools; bleeding from the gums; blood in the urine or stools; bruising; chest pains; chills; collection of blood under the skin; coughing up blood or coffee-ground-like material; difficulty breathing; dizziness; fever; frequent or persistent erection; heavy bleeding or oozing from cuts or wounds; heavy or unexpected menstrual bleeding; joint pains; pain at the injection site; pain or blue discoloration of the skin of hands or feet; rash; severe headache; sloughing of the skin; or tingling in the hands or feet. If you notice any of these effects, CONTACT YOUR DOCTOR IMMEDIATELY.

INTERACTIONS

Heparin interacts with several types of drugs, including warfarin; aspirin; anti-inflammatory medications (such as fenoprofen, ibuprofen, indomethacin, naproxen, piroxicam, sulindac, tolmetin); sulfinpyrazone; adrenocorticosteroids (such as cortisone); ethacrynic acid; dipyridamole; hydroxychloroquine; methimazole; and propyl thiouracil. These medications may cause bleeding problems when taken with heparin, SO BE SURE TO TELL YOUR DOCTOR if you are already taking any of them.

WARNINGS

- It is important to tell your doctor if you have had any recent falls or blows to the body, medical or dental surgery, or spinal anesthesia. It is also important to tell your doctor if you have any allergies (especially to heparin or to beef or pork products), blood disease or bleeding problems, colitis, stomach ulcers, diabetes, high blood pressure, kidney disease, or liver disease, or if you have had an intrauterine device (IUD) inserted.

• Before having any surgery or other medical or dental treatment, BE SURE YOUR DOCTOR OR DENTIST KNOWS that you are taking this medication.

• In order to prevent bleeding problems while taking this medication, it is important that you avoid sports and other activities that may cause you to become injured.

• To avoid gum bleeding, use a soft toothbrush. Take special care while shaving. An electric shaver may be safer than a razor blade.

• Avoid taking any product that contains aspirin while using this medication, because aspirin also decreases your clotting ability. Taking the two drugs together can lead to bleeding problems. Check the labels of all the medications you take to see if they contain aspirin.

• Be sure to tell your doctor if you are pregnant. Heparin does not cross the placenta, but it may cause bleeding problems in the mother, especially in the later months of pregnancy. Heparin does not pass into breast milk, but it can cause severe bone problems in a nursing mother.

heparin sodium—see heparin

hetacillin

BRAND NAMES (Manufacturers)
Versapen (Bristol)
Versapen-K (Bristol)
TYPE OF DRUG
Antibiotic (infection fighter)
INGREDIENT
hetacillin
DOSAGE FORMS
Capsules (225 mg)
Oral suspension (112.5 mg and 225 mg per
    5 ml teaspoonful)

STORAGE

Hetacillin capsules should be stored at room temperature in a tightly closed container. The oral suspension should be stored in the refrigerator in a tightly closed container. Any unused portion of the suspension should be discarded after 14 days, because the drug loses its potency after that time. This medication should never be frozen.

USES

Hetacillin is used to treat a wide variety of bacterial infections, including infections in the middle ear, upper and lower respiratory tracts, and the urinary tract. It acts by severely injuring the cell walls of the infecting bacteria, thereby preventing them from growing and multiplying. Hetacillin kills susceptible bacteria, but is not effective against viruses, parasites, or fungi.

TREATMENT

Hetacillin should be taken on an empty stomach or with a glass of water, one hour before or two hours after a meal. This medication should never be taken with fruit juices or carbonated beverages, because the acidity of these drinks destroys the drug in the stomach.

The suspension form of this medication should be shaken well, just before measuring each dose. The contents tend to settle on the bottom of the bottle, so it is necessary to shake the container to evenly distribute the ingredients and equalize the doses. Each dose should then be measured carefully, with a specially designed, 5 ml measuring spoon. An ordinary kitchen teaspoon is not accurate enough.

Hetacillin works best when the level of the medicine in your bloodstream is kept constant. It is best, therefore, to take the doses at evenly spaced intervals, day and night. For example, if you are taking four doses a day, the doses should be spaced six hours apart.

If you miss a dose of this medication, take the missed dose immediately. However, if you do not remember to take the missed dose until it is almost time for your next dose, take it; then space the following dose about halfway through the regular interval between doses. Then return to your regular schedule. Try not to skip any doses.

It is important to continue to take this medication for the entire time prescribed by your doctor (usually seven to 14 days), even if the symptoms of the infection disappear before the end of that period. If you stop taking the drug too soon, resistant bacteria are given a chance to continue growing, and the infection could recur.

SIDE EFFECTS

Minor. Diarrhea; heartburn; nausea; and vomiting. These side effects should disappear in several days, as your body adjusts to the medication.

Major. Tell your doctor about any side effects that are persistent or particularly bothersome. IT IS ESPECIALLY IMPORTANT TO TELL YOUR DOCTOR about bloating; chills; cough; difficulty breathing; fever; irritation of the mouth; muscle aches; rash; rectal or vaginal itching; severe diarrhea; sore throat; or darkened tongue. Also, if your symptoms of infection seem to be getting worse rather than improving, you should contact your doctor.

INTERACTIONS

Hetacillin interacts with other types of medication.

1. Probenecid can increase the blood concentrations of this medication.

2. Hetacillin may decrease the effectiveness of oral contraceptives (birth control pills), and pregnancy could result. You should therefore use another form of birth control while taking this medication. Discuss this with your doctor.

TELL YOUR DOCTOR if you are currently taking either of the medications listed above.

WARNINGS

• Tell your doctor about unusual or allergic reactions you have had to any medications, especially to hetacillin, amoxicillin, ampicillin, or penicillins, or to cephalosporin antibiotics, penicillamine, or griseofulvin.

• Tell your doctor if you now have, or if you have ever had, kidney disease, asthma, or allergies.

• This medication has been prescribed for your current infection only. Another infection later on, or one that someone else has, may require a different medicine. You should not give your medicine to other people or use it for other infections, unless your doctor specifically directs you to do so.

• Diabetics taking hetacillin should know that this drug can cause a false-positive sugar reaction with a Clinitest urine glucose test. To avoid this problem, while taking hetacillin you should switch to Clinistix or Tes-Tape to test your urine sugar.

• Be sure to tell your doctor if you are pregnant. Although hetacillin appears to be safe during pregnancy, extensive studies in humans have not yet been completed. Also, tell your doctor if you are breastfeeding an infant. Small amounts of this medication pass into breast milk, and may temporarily alter the bacteria in the intestinal tract of the nursing infant, resulting in diarrhea.

Hexadrol—see dexamethasone (systemic)

Hi-Cor—see hydrocortisone (topical)

Hiprex—see methenamine

Histarall—see pseudoephedrine and dexbrompheniramine combination

Histatapp TD—see phenylpropanolamine, phenylephrine, and brompheniramine combination

Hournaze—see pseudoephedrine and chlorpheniramine combination

Humulin N—see insulin

Humulin R—see insulin

Hycodaphen—see acetaminophen and hydrocodone combination

Hydergine—see ergoloid mesylates

hydralazine

BRAND NAMES (Manufacturers)
Apresoline (Ciba)
Dralzine (Lemmon)
hydralazine hydrochloride (various manufacturers)
TYPE OF DRUG
Anti-hypertensive
INGREDIENT
hydralazine as the hydrochloride salt
DOSAGE FORM
Tablets (10 mg, 25 mg, 50 mg, and 100 mg)
STORAGE
Hydralazine tablets should be stored at room temperature in a tightly closed, light-resistant container.

USES
This medication is used to treat high blood pressure or heart failure. Hydralazine is a vasodilator that directly relaxes the muscles of the blood vessels, which causes a lowering of the blood pressure.

TREATMENT
In order to avoid stomach irritation, you can take hydralazine with food, or with a glass of water or milk. To become accustomed to taking this medication, try to take it at the same time(s) each day.

Hydralazine does not cure high blood pressure, but it will help to control the condition, as long as you continue to take it.

It may take up to two weeks before the full effects of this medication are observed.

Try not to miss any doses of this medication. If you do miss a dose, take the missed dose as soon as possible, unless it is almost time for the next dose. In that case, do not take the missed dose at all; just return to your regular dosing schedule. Do not double the next dose.

SIDE EFFECTS
Minor. Constipation; diarrhea; dizziness; drowsiness; flushing; headache; light-headedness; loss of appetite; muscle cramps; nasal congestion; nausea; and vomiting.

These side effects should disappear in several weeks, as your body adjusts to the medication.

If you feel dizzy or light-headed, sit or lie down awhile; get up slowly, and be careful on stairs. To avoid dizziness or light-headedness when you stand, contract and relax the muscles of your legs for a few moments before rising. Do this by pushing one foot against the floor while raising the other foot slightly, alternating feet so that you are "pumping" your legs in a pedaling motion.

Major. Tell your doctor about any side effects that are persistent or particularly bothersome. IT IS ESPECIALLY IMPORTANT TO TELL YOUR DOCTOR about anxiety; chest pain; confusion; cramping; depression; difficulty urinating; fever; itching; numbness or tingling in the fingers or toes; palpitations; rapid weight gain (three to five pounds within a week); rash; shortness of breath; sore throat; tenderness in the joints; unusual bleeding or bruising; or yellowing of the eyes or skin. If you do notice a numbness or tingling, your doctor may want you to take vitamin B_6 (pyridoxine).

INTERACTIONS

The combination of alcohol and hydralazine can lead to dizziness and fainting. You should therefore avoid drinking alcoholic beverages while taking this medication.

Hydralazine, used within 14 days of a monoamine oxidase (MAO) inhibitor, can cause severe reactions. Before you start to take hydralazine, BE SURE TO TELL YOUR DOCTOR if you are already taking any medications of this type.

WARNINGS

• Tell your doctor about any unusual or allergic reactions you have had to medications, especially to hydralazine.

• Tell your doctor if you now have, or if you have ever had, angina (chest pain), heart disease, stroke, a heart attack, or kidney disease.

• To avoid dizziness or fainting, try not to stand for long periods of time, and avoid drinking excessive amounts of alcohol. You should also avoid getting overheated by strenuous exercise in hot weather; and should avoid hot baths, showers, and saunas.

- If this drug makes you dizzy or drowsy, avoid taking part in any activities that require alertness, such as driving a car or operating potentially dangerous equipment.
- Before having any surgery or other medical or dental treatment, be sure to tell your doctor or dentist that you are taking this medication.
- Do not take any over-the-counter (non-prescription) allergy, asthma, sinus, cough, cold, or diet products unless you first consult your doctor or pharmacist. Some of these products increase the workload of the heart.
- Some of these products contain F.D. & C. Yellow Dye No. 5 (tartrazine), which can cause allergic-type symptoms (rash, shortness of breath, or fainting) in certain susceptible individuals.
- Do not stop taking this medication until you check with your doctor. If this drug is stopped abruptly, you could experience a sudden rise in blood pressure and other complications. Your doctor may therefore want to decrease your dosage gradually.
- Be sure to tell your doctor if you are pregnant. Hydralazine crosses the placenta, and studies have shown that it causes birth defects in the offspring of animals who received large doses of it during pregnancy. Also, tell your doctor if you are breastfeeding an infant. It is not known whether or not hydralazine passes into breast milk.

hydralazine hydrochloride—see hydralazine

---

hydralazine, hydrochlorothiazide, and reserpine combination

BRAND NAMES (Manufacturers)
Cam-ap-es (Camall)
Hydrap-Es (Lemmon)
Hyserp (Reid-Provident)
R-HCTZ-H (Lederle)
Ser-A-Gen (Generix)

Seralazide (Lannett)
Ser-Ap-Es (Ciba)
Ser Hydra Zine (Three P Products)
Tri-Hydroserpine (Rugby)
Unipres (Reid-Provident)
TYPE OF DRUG
Anti-hypertensive
INGREDIENTS
hydralazine as the hydrochloride salt, hydrochlorothia-
   zide, and reserpine
DOSAGE FORM
Tablets (25 mg hydralazine, 15 mg hydrochlorothiazide,
   and 0.1 mg reserpine)
STORAGE
These tablets should be stored at room temperature, in a
tightly closed, light-resistant container.

USES
This medication is used to treat high blood pressure. Hydralazine is a vasodilator; it relaxes the muscles of the
blood vessels, resulting in a lowering of the blood pressure. Hydrochlorothiazide is a diuretic (water pill), which
reduces body fluid accumulation by increasing the elimination of sodium and water through the kidneys. Reserpine acts by depleting the body of certain chemicals that
are responsible for maintaining high blood pressure.

TREATMENT
In order to avoid stomach irritation, you can take hydralazine, hydrochlorothiazide, and reserpine combination
with food, or with a full glass of water or milk. To become
accustomed to taking this medication, try to take it at the
same time(s) each day. Avoid taking a dose after 6:00 P.M.;
this will prevent you from having to get up during the
night to urinate.
   If you miss a dose of this medication, take the missed
dose as soon as possible, unless it is almost time for your
next dose. In that case, do not take the missed dose; just
return to your regular dosing schedule. Do not double the
next dose.
   This medication does not cure high blood pressure, but

it will help to control the condition, as long as you continue to take it.

The effects of this medication may not become apparent for up to two weeks after you start to take it.

SIDE EFFECTS

Minor. Abdominal pain; constipation; decrease in sexual desire; diarrhea; dizziness; dry mouth; flushing; impotence; itching; loss of appetite; nasal congestion; nausea; tremors; vomiting; and weight gain. These side effects should disappear in several weeks, as your body adjusts to the medication.

To relieve mouth dryness, chew sugarless gum, or suck on ice chips or a piece of hard candy.

If you feel dizzy or light-headed, sit or lie down awhile; get up slowly, and be careful on stairs. To avoid dizziness or light-headedness when you stand, contract and relax the muscles of your legs for a few moments before rising. Do this by pushing one foot against the floor while raising the other foot slightly, alternating feet so that you are "pumping" your legs in a pedaling motion.

This medication can cause an increase in sensitivity to sunlight. You should therefore avoid prolonged exposure to sunlight and sunlamps. Wear protective clothing and sunglasses, and use an effective sunscreen.

Major. Tell your doctor about any side effects that are persistent or particularly bothersome. IT IS ESPECIALLY IMPORTANT TO TELL YOUR DOCTOR about anxiety; blurred vision; breast enlargment (in both sexes); chest pain; depression; difficulty urinating; drowsiness; fainting; fatigue; fever; headaches; hearing loss; joint pain; mood changes; muscle spasms; nervousness; nightmares; palpitations; rapid weight gain (three to five pounds within a week); rash; shortness of breath; sore throat; swelling of the feet, ankles, or lower legs; tingling in the fingers or toes; unusual bleeding or bruising; weakness; or yellowing of the eyes or skin.

INTERACTIONS

This combination medication interacts with several other types of drugs.

1. Concurrent use of it with central nervous system depressants (drugs that slow the activity of the nervous system), such as alcohol, antihistamines, barbiturates, benzodiazapine tranquilizers, muscle relaxants, narcotics, pain medications, phenothiazine tranquilizers, and sleeping medications, or with tricyclic anti-depressants can cause extreme drowsiness.

2. The use of a monoamine oxidase (MAO) inhibitor within 14 days of this medication can lead to a severe reaction.

3. Reserpine combined with methotrimeprazine or tricyclic anti-depressants can lead to a severe drop in blood pressure (which can be dangerous). Reserpine can also decrease the effectiveness of levodopa and can increase the side effects (to the heart) of digoxin and quinidine.

4. Hydrochlorothiazide can decrease the effectiveness of warfarin, anti-gout medications, insulin, oral anti-diabetic medicines, and methenamine.

5. Fenfluramine may increase the blood-pressure-lowering effects of hydrochlorothiazide (which can be dangerous).

6. Indomethacin may decrease the blood-pressure-lowering effects (thereby counteracting the desired effects) of hydrochlorothiazide.

7. This medication should be taken one hour before, or four hours after, a dose of cholestyramine or colestipol (if you have also been prescribed one of these medications), because they can decrease the absorption of hydrochlorothiazide from the gastrointestinal tract.

8. Hydrochlorothiazide may increase the side effects of amphotericin B, calcium, adrenocorticosteroids (cortisone-like drugs), digoxin, lithium, quinidine, sulfonamide antibiotics, and vitamin D.

BE SURE TO TELL YOUR DOCTOR if you are already taking any of the medications listed above.

WARNINGS

• Tell your doctor about unusual or allergic reactions you have had to medications, especially to hydralazine, reserpine, or hydrochlorothiazide, or to any other sulfa drugs (other diuretics, oral anti-diabetic medicines, dapsone, or sulfone).

• Before starting to take this medication, be sure to tell your doctor if you now have, or if you have ever had, anuria; angina (chest pain); a blood disorder; diabetes mellitus (sugar diabetes); epilepsy; electroshock therapy; kidney disease; heart disease; liver disease; depression; gallstones or gallbladder disease; Parkinson's disease; peptic ulcers; stroke; systemic lupus erythematosus (SLE), or ulcerative colitis.

• One of the components of this product, reserpine, causes cancer in rats. It has not been shown to cause cancer in humans.

• If you experience numbness or tingling in your fingers or toes while using this drug, your doctor may recommend that you take vitamin B_6 (pyridoxine) to relieve the symptoms.

• Some of these products contain F.D. & C. Yellow Dye No. 5 (tartrazine), which can cause allergic-type symptoms (rash, shortness of breath, or fainting) in certain susceptible individuals.

• A doctor does not usually prescribe this drug or other "fixed dose" products as the first choice in the treatment of high blood pressure. Generally, the patient first receives each ingredient singly. If the response is adequate to the fixed dose contained in this product, it can then be substituted. The advantage of a combination product is increased convenience.

• This drug can cause potassium loss. Signs of potassium loss include dry mouth, thirst, weakness, muscle pain or cramps, nausea, and vomiting. If you experience any of these symptoms, CONTACT YOUR DOCTOR. To help prevent this problem, your doctor may want to have blood tests performed periodically. To help avoid potassium loss, take this product with a glass of fresh or frozen orange or cranberry juice, or eat a banana every day. The use of a salt substitute also helps prevent potassium loss. Do not change your diet, however, until you discuss it with your doctor. Too much potassium can also be dangerous.

• To prevent severe water loss (dehydration) while taking this medication, check with your doctor if you have any illness that causes severe or continuous nausea, vomiting, or diarrhea.

• Hydrochlorothiazide can raise blood sugar levels in diabetic patients. Blood sugar should therefore be monitored carefully (using blood or urine tests) when this medication is started.

• In order to prevent dizziness or fainting while taking this medication, try not to stand for long periods of time, avoid drinking excessive amounts of alcohol, and avoid getting overheated (strenuous exercise in hot weather; hot baths, showers, and saunas).

• If this drug makes you dizzy or drowsy, avoid taking part in any activities that require alertness, such as driving a car or operating potentially dangerous equipment.

• Before having any surgery or other medical or dental treatment, be sure your doctor or dentist knows that you are taking this medication.

• Before taking any over-the-counter (non-prescription) allergy, asthma, sinus, cough, cold, or diet product, check with your doctor or pharmacist. Some of these products can cause an increase in blood pressure.

• Do not stop taking this medication until you first check with your doctor. If this drug is stopped abruptly, you may experience a sudden rise in blood pressure. Your doctor may therefore want to decrease your dosage gradually.

• Be sure to tell your doctor if you are pregnant. This medication has been associated with birth defects when used during pregnancy. Also, tell your doctor if you are breastfeeding an infant. Small amounts of this drug pass into breast milk and can cause side effects in nursing infants.

Hydrap-Es—see hydralazine, hydrochlorothiazide, and reserpine combination

Hydrex—see benzthiazide

Hydril—see diphenhydramine

hydrochlorothiazide

BRAND NAMES (Manufacturers)
Aquazide H (Western Research)
Chlorzide (Foy)
Diaqua (W.E. Hauck)
Diu-Scrip (Scrip)
Esidrix (Ciba)
hydrochlorothiazide (various manufacturers)
Hydro-Clor (Vortech)
HydroDiuril (Merck Sharp & Dohme)
Hydromal (Mallard)
Hydro-Z (Maynard)
Hyperetic (Elder)
Mictrin (EconoMed)
Oretic (Abbott)
SK-Hydrochlorothiazide (Smith Kline & French)
Thianal (Vangard)
Thiuretic (Parke-Davis)
Zide (Tutag)

TYPE OF DRUG
Diuretic (water pill) and anti-hypertensive

INGREDIENT
hydrochlorothiazide

DOSAGE FORM
Tablets (25 mg, 50 mg, and 100 mg)

STORAGE
This medication should be stored at room temperature in a tightly closed container.

USES
Hydrochlorothiazide is prescribed to treat high blood pressure. It is also used to reduce fluid accumulation in the body caused by conditions such as heart failure, cirrhosis of the liver, kidney disease, and the long-term use of some medications. This medication reduces body fluid accumulation by increasing the elimination of sodium and water through the kidneys.

TREATMENT
To decrease stomach irritation, you can take this medication with a glass of milk or with a meal (unless your doctor

directs you to do otherwise). Try to take it at the same time every day. Avoid taking a dose after 6:00 P.M.—this will prevent you from having to get up during the night to urinate.

If you miss a dose of this medication, take the missed dose as soon as possible, unless it is almost time for the next dose. In that case, do not take the missed dose at all; just wait until the next scheduled dose. Do not double the dose.

This medication does not cure high blood pressure, but it will help to control the condition, as long as you continue to take it.

SIDE EFFECTS

Minor. Constipation; cramps; diarrhea; dizziness; drowsiness; headache; heartburn; itching; loss of appetite; nausea; restlessness; upset stomach; vomiting. As your body adjusts to the medication, these side effects should disappear.

This medication can cause increased sensitivity to sunlight. It is therefore important to avoid prolonged exposure to sunlight and sunlamps. Wear protective clothing, and use an effective sunscreen.

To avoid dizziness or light-headedness when you stand, contract and relax the muscles of your legs for a few moments before rising. Do this by pushing one foot against the floor while raising the other foot slightly, alternating feet so that you are "pumping" your legs in a ped aling motion.

Major. Tell your doctor about any side effects that are persistent or particularly bothersome. IT IS ESPECIALLY IMPORTANT TO TELL YOUR DOCTOR about any unusual bleeding or bruising; blurred vision; confusion; difficulty breathing; dry mouth; excessive thirst; fever; joint pain; mood changes; muscle spasms; palpitations; skin rash; sore throat; tingling in the fingers or toes; excessive weakness; or yellowing of the eyes or skin.

INTERACTIONS

Hydrochlorothiazide interacts with other medication.

1. It can decrease the effectiveness of oral anti-coagulants, anti-gout medications, insulin, oral anti-diabetic medicines, and methenamine.

2. Fenfluramine can increase the blood-pressure-lowering effects of hydrochlorothiazide (which can be dangerous).

3. Indomethacin can decrease the blood-pressure-lowering effects (thereby counteracting the desired effects) of hydrochlorothiazide.

4. Cholestyramine and colestipol decrease the absorption of this medication from the gastrointestinal tract. Hydrochlorothiazide should therefore be taken one hour before, or four hours after, a dose of cholestyramine or colestipol.

5. Hydrochlorothiazide may increase the side effects of amphotericin B, calcium, cortisone-like steroids (such as cortisone, dexamethasone, hydrocortisone, prednisone, prednisolone), digoxin, digitalis, lithium, quinidine, sulfonamide antibiotics, and vitamin D.

BE SURE TO TELL YOUR DOCTOR if you are already taking any of the medicines listed above.

WARNINGS

• Tell your doctor about unusual or allergic reactions you have had to medications, especially to diuretics (water pills), oral anti-diabetic medications, or sulfonamide antibiotics.

• Before you start taking hydrochlorothiazide, tell your doctor if you now have, or if you have ever had, kidney disease or problems with urination, diabetes mellitus (sugar diabetes), gout, liver disease, asthma, pancreas disease, or systemic lupus erythematosus (SLE).

• Hydrochlorothiazide can cause potassium loss. Signs of potassium loss include dry mouth, thirst, weakness, muscle pain or cramps, nausea, and vomiting. If you experience any of these symptoms, call your doctor. To help avoid potassium loss, take this drug with a glass of fresh or frozen orange or cranberry juice, or eat a banana every day. The use of a salt substitute also helps to prevent potassium loss. Do not change your diet, however, before discussing it with your doctor. Too much potassium can also be dangerous. Your doctor may want you to have blood tests performed periodically, in order to monitor your potassium levels.

- Limit your intake of alcoholic beverages while taking this medication, in order to prevent dizziness and light-headedness.
- If you have high blood pressure, do not take any over-the-counter (non-prescription) medications for weight control or for allergy, asthma, cough, cold, or sinus problems, unless your doctor directs you to do so.
- To prevent dehydration (severe water loss) while taking this medication, check with your doctor if you have any illness that causes severe or continuous nausea, vomiting, or diarrhea.
- This medication can raise blood sugar levels in diabetic patients. Therefore, blood sugar should be carefully monitored by blood or urine tests when this medication is started.
- Be sure to tell your doctor if you are pregnant. This drug crosses the placenta. Studies in humans have not yet been completed, but adverse effects have been observed on the fetuses of animals who received large doses of this drug during pregnancy. Also, tell your doctor if you are breastfeeding an infant. Although problems in humans have not been reported, small amounts of this drug can pass into breast milk, so caution is warranted.

Hydro-Clor—see hydrochlorothiazide

---

hydrocortisone (systemic)

BRAND NAMES (Manufacturers)
Cortef (Upjohn)
Cortef Fluid (Upjohn)
hydrocortisone (various manufacturers)
Hydrocortone (Merck Sharp & Dohme)
TYPE OF DRUG
Adrenocorticosteroid hormone
INGREDIENT
hydrocortisone
DOSAGE FORMS
Tablets (5 mg, 10 mg, and 20 mg)
Oral suspension (10 mg per 5 ml teaspoonful, as the cypionate salt)

STORAGE
Hydrocortisone tablets and oral suspension should be stored at room temperature in tightly closed containers.

USES
Your adrenal glands naturally produce certain cortisone-like chemicals. These chemicals are involved in various regulatory processes in the body (such as maintenance of fluid balance, temperature, and reactions to inflammation). Hydrocortisone belongs to a group of drugs known as adrenocorticosteroids (or cortisone-like medications). It is used to treat a variety of disorders, including endocrine and rheumatic disorders; asthma; blood diseases; certain cancers; eye disorders; gastrointestinal disturbances, such as ulcerative colitis; respiratory diseases; and inflammations, such as arthritis, dermatitis, and poison ivy. How this drug acts to relieve these disorders is not completely understood.

TREATMENT
In order to prevent stomach irritation, you can take hydrocortisone with food or milk.

If you are taking only one dose of this medication each day, try to take it before 9:00 A.M. This will mimic the body's normal production of this type of chemical.

The oral suspension form of this medication should be shaken well just before measuring out each dose. The contents tend to settle on the bottom of the bottle, so it is necessary to shake the container to evenly distribute the ingredients and equalize the doses. Each dose should then be measured carefully with a specially designed, 5 ml measuring spoon. An ordinary kitchen teaspoon is not accurate enough.

It is important to try not to miss any doses of hydrocortisone. However, if you do miss a dose of this medication:

1. If you are taking it more than once a day, take the missed dose as soon as possible, then return to your regular schedule. If it is already time for the next dose, double the dose.

2. If you are taking this medication once a day, take the dose you missed as soon as possible, unless you don't remember until the next day. In that case do not take the missed dose at all; just follow your regular schedule. Do not double the next dose.

3. If you are taking this drug every other day, take the missed dose as soon as you remember. If you missed the scheduled time by a whole day, take it when you remember, then skip a day before you take the next dose. Do not double the dose.

If you miss more than one dose, CONTACT YOUR DOCTOR.

SIDE EFFECTS

Minor. Dizziness; false sense of well-being; increased appetite; increased sweating; indigestion; menstrual irregularities; muscle weakness; nausea; reddening of the skin on the face; restlessness; sleep disorders; thinning of the skin; and weight gain. These side effects should disappear in several days, as your body adjusts to the medication.

To help avoid potassium loss while using this drug, take your dose with a glass of fresh or frozen orange juice, or eat a banana each day. The use of a salt substitute also helps prevent potassium loss. Check with your doctor.

Major. Tell your doctor about any side effects that are persistent or particularly bothersome. IT IS ESPECIALLY IMPORTANT TO TELL YOUR DOCTOR about abdominal enlargement; acne or other skin problems; back or rib pain; bloody or black, tarry stools; blurred vision; unusual bruising or bleeding; convulsions; eye pain; fever and sore throat; growth impairment (in children); headaches; impaired healing of wounds; increased thirst and urination; mental depression; mood changes; muscle wasting; nightmares; rapid weight gain (three to five pounds within a week); rash; severe abdominal pain; shortness of breath; or unusual weakness.

INTERACTIONS

Hydrocortisone interacts with other medication.

1. Alcohol, aspirin, and anti-inflammation medications (such as diflunisal, ibuprofen, indomethacin, mefenamic acid, meclofenamate, naproxen, piroxicam, sulindac, tolmetin) aggravate the stomach problems that are common with use of this medication.

2. A change in the dosage requirements of oral anti-coagulants (blood thinners, such as warfarin), oral anti-diabetic drugs, or insulin may be necessary when this medication is started or stopped.

3. The loss of potassium caused by hydrocortisone can lead to serious side effects in individuals taking digoxin. Also, thiazide diuretics (water pills) can increase the potassium loss caused by hydrocortisone.

4. Phenobarbital, phenytoin, rifampin, and ephedrine can increase the elimination of hydrocortisone from the body, thereby decreasing its effectiveness.

5. Oral contraceptives and estrogen-containing drugs may decrease the elimination of this drug from the body, which can lead to an increase in side effects.

6. Hydrocortisone can increase the elimination from the body of aspirin and isoniazid, thereby decreasing the effectiveness of these two medications.

7. Cholestyramine and colestipol can chemically bind this medication in the stomach and gastrointestinal tract and prevent its absorption.

TELL YOUR DOCTOR if you are currently taking any of the medications listed above.

WARNINGS

● Tell your doctor about unusual or allergic reactions you have had to any medications, especially to hydrocortisone or other adrenocorticosteroids (such as betamethasone, cortisone, dexamethasone, fluocinolone, fluprednisolone, methylprednisolone, prednisolone, prednisone, or triamcinolone).

● Tell your doctor if you now have, or if you have ever had, bone disease; diabetes mellitus (sugar diabetes); emotional instability; glaucoma; fungal infections; heart disease; high blood pressure; high cholesterol levels; myasthenia gravis; peptic ulcers; osteoporosis; thyroid disease; tuberculosis; severe ulcerative colitis; kidney disease; or liver disease.

● If you are using this medication for longer than a week, you may need to receive higher dosages if you are subjected to stress, such as serious infections, injury, or surgery. Discuss this with your doctor.

● If you have been taking this drug for more than a week,

do not stop taking it suddenly. If it is stopped suddenly, you may experience abdominal or back pain, dizziness, fainting, fever, muscle or joint pain, nausea, vomiting, shortness of breath, or extreme weakness. Your doctor may therefore want to reduce the dosage gradually. Never increase the dose or take the drug for longer than the prescribed time, unless you first consult your doctor.

• While you are taking this drug, you should not be vaccinated or immunized. This medication decreases the effectiveness of vaccines and can lead to overwhelming infection if a live virus is administered.

• Before having any surgery or other medical or dental treatment, be sure your doctor or dentist knows that you are taking this medication.

• Because this drug can cause glaucoma and cataracts with long-term use, your doctor may want you to have your eyes examined by an ophthalmologist periodically during treatment.

• If you are taking this medication for prolonged periods, you should wear or carry an identification card or notice stating that you are taking an adrenocorticosteroid.

• This medication can raise blood sugar levels in diabetic patients. Blood sugar should therefore be monitored carefully with blood or urine tests when this medication is started.

• Be sure to tell your doctor if you are pregnant. This drug crosses the placenta. Although studies in humans have not yet been completed, birth defects have been observed in the fetuses of animals who were given large doses of this drug during pregnancy. Also, tell your doctor if you are breastfeeding an infant. Small amounts of this drug pass into breast milk and may cause growth suppression or a decrease in natural adrenocorticosteroid production in the nursing infant.

hydrocortisone (topical)

BRAND NAMES (Manufacturers)
Acticort 100 (Baker/Cummins)
Aeroseb-HC (Herbert)
Bactine Hydrocortisone* (Miles)

Caladryl Hydrocortisone* (Parke-Davis)
Cetacort (Owen)
Clinicort* (Johnson & Johnson)
Cortaid* (Upjohn)
Cort-Dome (Miles)
Cortef Acetate (Upjohn)
Cortizone-5* (Thompson)
Cortril (Pfipharmecs)
Cortril* (Pfipharmecs)
Dermacort (Rowell)
DermiCort* (Republic Drug)
Dermolate* (Schering)
Dermtex HC* (Pfeiffer)
Eldecort (Elder)
Epifoam (Reed & Carnrick)
H-Cort (Pharmaceutical Assoc.)
Hi-Cor (C & M Pharmaceuticals)
HyCort* (Elder)
Hydrocortisone Acetate (various manufacturers)
Hydrocortone Acetate (Merck Sharp & Dohme)
Hydro-tex (Syosset)
Hydro-tex* (Syosset)
Hytone (Dermik)
Hytone* (Dermik)
Lanacort* (Combe)
Locoid (Owen)
My Cort (Scrip)
Nutracort (Owen)
Pharma-Cort* (Purepac)
Racet SE (Lemmon)
Racet SE* (Lemmon)
Rhulicort* (Lederle)
Sensacort* (Plough)
Synacort (Syntex)
Texacort (CooperCare)
Ulcort (Ulmer)
Ulcort* (Ulmer)
Westcort (Westwood)
*Hydrocortisone cream, ointment, lotion, and aerosol
 pump spray are also available over-the-counter (non-
 prescription) under a variety of brand names, in con-
 centrations of 0.5% or less.

TYPE OF DRUG
Adrenocorticosteroid hormone
INGREDIENT
hydrocortisone
DOSAGE FORMS
Cream (0.1%, 0.125%, 0.2%, 0.25%, 0.5%, 1%, and 2.5%)
Ointment (1%, 2.5%)
Lotion (0.125%, 0.25%, 0.5%, 1%, and 2.5%)
Gel (1%)
Aerosol pump spray (0.5%)
Aerosol foam (1%)
STORAGE
Hydrocortisone cream, ointment, lotion, gel, and pump spray aerosol should be stored at room temperature, in tightly closed containers. This medication should never be frozen.

The aerosol foam form of this medication is packaged under pressure. It should not be stored near heat or an open flame, or in direct sunlight; and the container should never be punctured.

USES

Your adrenal glands naturally produce certain cortisone-like chemicals. These chemicals are involved in various regulatory processes in the body (such as fluid balance, temperature, and reactions to inflammation). Hydrocortisone belongs to a group of drugs known as adrenocorticosteroids (or cortisone-like medications). It is used to relieve the skin inflammation (redness, swelling, itching, and discomfort) associated with conditions such as dermatitis, eczema, and poison ivy. How this drug acts to relieve these disorders is not completely understood.

TREATMENT

Before applying this medication, wash your hands. Then, unless your doctor gives you different instructions, gently wash the area of the skin where the medication is to be applied. With a clean towel, pat the area almost dry; it should be slightly damp when you put the medicine on.

Apply a small amount of the medication to the affected area in a thin layer. Do not bandage the area unless your doctor tells you to do so. If you are to apply an occlusive dressing (like kitchen plastic wrap), be sure you understand the instructions.

If you are using the aerosol foam form of this medication, shake the can in order to disperse the medication evenly. Hold the can upright six to eight inches from the area to be sprayed, and spray the area for one to three seconds. DO NOT SMOKE while you are using the aerosol foam; the contents are under pressure and may explode when exposed to heat or flames.

If you miss a dose of this medication, apply the dose as soon as possible, unless it is almost time for the next application. In that case, do not apply the missed dose; just return to your regular dosing schedule. Do not put twice as much of the medication on your skin at the next application.

SIDE EFFECTS

Minor. Acne; burning sensation; skin dryness; irritation of the affected area; itching; and rash.

If the affected area is extremely dry or scaling, the skin may be moistened before applying the medication by soaking in water or by applying water with a clean cloth. The ointment form is probably better for dry skin.

A mild, temporary stinging sensation may occur after this medication is applied. If this persists, contact your doctor.

Major. Tell your doctor about any side effects that are persistent or particularly bothersome. IT IS ESPECIALLY IMPORTANT TO TELL YOUR DOCTOR about blistering; increased hair growth; loss of skin color; secondary infection in the area being treated; or thinning of the skin with easy bruising.

INTERACTIONS

This medication does not interact with any other medications, as long as it is used according to directions.

WARNINGS

• Tell your doctor about unusual or allergic reactions you have had to any medications, especially to hydrocortisone or other adrenocorticosteroids (such as amcinonide, betamethasone, clocortolone, cortisone, desonide, desoximetasone, dexamethasone, diflorasone, flumethasone, fluocinolone, fluocinonide, fluprednisolone, flurandrenolide, halcinonide, methylprednisolone, paramethasone, prednisolone, prednisone, or triamcinolone).

• Tell your doctor if you now have, or if you have ever had, blood vessel disease, chicken pox, diabetes mellitus (sugar diabetes), fungal infections, peptic ulcers, shingles, tuberculosis, tuberculosis of the skin, vaccinia, or any other type of infection, especially at the site currently being treated.

• If irritation develops while using this drug, immediately discontinue its use and notify your doctor.

• This product is not for use in the eyes or mucous membranes. Exposure of this medication to the eye may result in ocular (to the eye) side effects.

• Do not use this product with an occlusive wrap unless your doctor directs you to do so. Systemic absorption of hydrocortisone is increased if extensive areas of the body are treated, particularly if occlusive bandages are used. If it is necessary for you to use this drug under a wrap, follow your doctor's instructions exactly; do not leave the wrap in place longer than specified.

• If you are using this medication on a child's diaper area, do not put tight-fitting diapers or plastic pants on the child. This may lead to increased systemic absorption of the drug and a possible increase in side effects.

• In order to avoid freezing skin tissue when using the aerosol form of hydrocortisone, make sure that you do not spray for more than three seconds; and hold the container at least six inches away.

• When using the aerosol form of this medication on the face, cover your eyes, and do not inhale the spray (in order to avoid side effects).

• Be sure to tell your doctor if you are pregnant. If large amounts of this drug are applied for prolonged periods, some of it will be absorbed and may cross the placenta. Although studies in humans have not yet been completed, birth defects have been observed in the fetuses of animals who were given large oral doses of this drug during pregnancy. Also, tell your doctor if you are breastfeeding an infant. If absorbed through the skin, small amounts of hydrocortisone pass into breast milk and may cause growth suppression or a decrease in natural adrenocorticosteroid production in the nursing infant.

Hydrocortisone Acetate—see hydrocortisone (topical)

---

hydrocortisone and iodochlorhydroxyquin combination (topical)

BRAND NAMES (Manufacturers)
Caquin (O'Neal)
Corque (Geneva Generics)
Cortin (C & M)
Domeform-HC (Miles)
Epiform-HC (Delta Drug)
HC-Form (Recsei)
hydrocortisone with iodochlorhydroxyquin (various manufacturers)
Hysone (Mallard)
Iodocort (Ulmer)
Iodosone (Century)
Lanvisone (Lannett)
Mity-Quin (Reid-Provident)
Pedi-Cort V (Pedinol)
Racet-1% (Lemmon)
Vioform-Hydrocortisone (Ciba)
Vytone (Dermik)

TYPE OF DRUG
Adrenocorticosteroid hormone and anti-infective

INGREDIENTS
hydrocortisone and iodochlorhydroxyquin

DOSAGE FORMS
Cream (0.5% hydrocortisone with 1% or 3% iodochlorhydroxyquin; 1% hydrocortisone with 1% or 3% iodochlorhydroxyquin)
Ointment (0.5% or 1% hydrocortisone with 3% iodochlorhydroxyquin)

Lotion (1% hydrocortisone with 3% iodochlorhydroxy-quin)

Jelly (1% hydrocortisone with 3% iodoclorhydroxyquin)

STORAGE

Hydrocortisone and iodochlorhydroxyquin cream, ointment, lotion, and jelly should be stored at room temperature in tightly closed, light-resistant containers. This medication should never be frozen.

USES

Your adrenal glands naturally produce certain cortisone-like chemicals. These chemicals are involved in various regulatory processes in the body (such as fluid balance, temperature, and reactions to inflammation). Hydrocortisone belongs to a group of drugs known as adrenocorticosteroids (or cortisone-like medications). It is used to relieve the skin inflammation (redness, swelling, itching, and discomfort) associated with conditions such as dermatitis and eczema. How this drug acts to relieve these disorders is not completely understood. Iodochlorhydroxyquin is an antibiotic that acts to prevent the growth and multiplication of infecting bacteria.

TREATMENT

Before applying this medication, wash your hands. Then, unless your doctor gives you different instructions, gently wash the area of the skin where the medication is to be applied. With a clean towel, pat the area almost dry; it should be slightly damp when you put the medication on.

If you are using the lotion form of this medication, shake it well before pouring out the medicine. The contents tend to settle on the bottom of the bottle, so it is necessary to shake the container to evenly distribute the ingredients and equalize the doses.

Apply a small amount of the cream, ointment, lotion, or jelly to the affected area in a thin layer. Do not bandage the area unless your doctor tells you to do so. If you are to apply an occlusive dressing (like kitchen plastic wrap), be sure you understand the instructions.

If you miss a dose of this medication, apply the dose as soon as possible, unless it is almost time for the next application. In that case, do not apply the missed dose at all; just return to your regular schedule. Do not put twice as much of the medication on your skin at the next application.

SIDE EFFECTS

Minor. Acne; burning sensation; skin dryness; irritation of the affected area; itching; and rash. These side effects should disappear in several days, as your body adjusts to the medication.

If the affected area is extremely dry or scaling, the skin may be moistened before applying the medication by soaking in water or by applying water with a clean cloth. The ointment form is probably better for dry skin.

A mild, temporary stinging sensation may occur after this medication is applied. If this persists, contact your doctor.

Major. Tell your doctor about any side effects that are persistent or particularly bothersome. IT IS ESPECIALLY IMPORTANT TO TELL YOUR DOCTOR about blistering; increased hair growth; loss of skin color; secondary infection at the affected site; or thinning of the skin with easy bruising.

INTERACTIONS

This medication does not interact with other medications, as long as it is used according to directions.

WARNINGS

• Tell your doctor about unusual or allergic reactions you have had to medications, especially to hydrocortisone or any other adrenocorticosteroid (such as amcinonide, betamethasone, clocortolone, cortisone, desonide, desoximetasone, dexamethasone, diflorasone, flumethasone, fluocinolone, fluocinonide, fluorometholone, flurandrenolide, halcinonide, methylprednisolone, prednisolone, prednisone, or triamcinolone); to iodochlorhydroxyquin; or to iodine.

• Tell your doctor if you now have, or if you have ever had, tuberculosis, or viral or fungal infections of the skin.

• This product may affect the results of thyroid function

tests. If you are scheduled to have such a test, be sure your doctor knows that you are using this medication.

• If additional irritation develops while using this drug, immediately discontinue its use and notify your doctor.

• This product is not for use in the eyes or mucous membranes. Exposure of this medication to the eye may result in ocular (to the eye) side effects.

• Do not use this product with an occlusive wrap unless you doctor directs you to do so. Systemic absorption of this drug is increased if extensive areas of the body are treated, particularly if occlusive bandages are used. If it is necessary for you to use this drug under a wrap, follow your doctor's instructions exactly—do not leave the wrap in place longer than specified.

• If you are using this medication on a child's diaper area, do not put tight-fitting diapers or plastic pants on the child. This may lead to increased systemic absorption of the drug and a possible increase in side effects.

• It is important to continue to take the medication for the entire time prescribed by your doctor, even if the symptoms disappear before the end of that period. If you stop applying the drug too soon, resistant bacteria are given a chance to continue growing, and the infection could recur.

• This medication has been prescribed for your current infection only. Another infection later on, or one that someone else has, may require a different medicine. You should not give your medicine to other people or use it for other infections, unless your doctor specifically directs you to do so.

• Be sure to tell your doctor if you are pregnant. If large amounts of this drug are applied for prolonged periods, some of it will be absorbed and may cross the placenta. Studies in humans have not yet been completed, but birth defects have been observed in the fetuses of animals who were given large oral doses of this drug during pregnancy. Also, tell your doctor if you are breastfeeding an infant. If absorbed through the skin, small amounts of hydrocortisone pass into breast milk and may cause growth suppression or a decrease in natural adrenocorticosteroid production in the nursing infant.

hydrocortisone, benzyl benzoate, bismuth resorcin compound, bismuth subgallate, and Peruvian balsam combination (topical)

BRAND NAMES (Manufacturers)
Anugard-HC (Vangard)
Anusol HC (Parke-Davis)
Hemorrhoidal HC (Rugby)
Hemusol HC (Three P Products)
Rectacort (Century)

TYPE OF DRUG
Adrenocorticosteroid-containing anorectal product

INGREDIENTS
hydrocortisone as the acetate salt; benzyl benzoate; bismuth resorcin compound; bismuth subgallate; and Peruvian balsam

DOSAGE FORMS
Rectal cream (0.5% hydrocortisone, 1.2% benzyl benzoate, 1.75% bismuth resorcin compound, 2.25% bismuth subgallate, and 1.8% Peruvian balsam per gram of cream)

Rectal suppositories (10 mg hydrocortisone, 1.2% benzyl benzoate, 1.75% bismuth resorcin compound, 2.25% bismuth subgallate, and 1.8% Peruvian balsam per suppository)

STORAGE
The rectal cream should be stored at room temperature in a tightly closed container. The rectal suppositories should be stored in a cool, dry place or in the refrigerator. This medication should never be frozen.

USES

This combination medication is used to relieve the pain, itching, and discomfort arising from hemorrhoids and irritated anorectal tissues.

hydrocortisone, benzyl benzoate, bismuth   **537**
resorcin compound, bismuth subgallate, and
Peruvian balsam combination (topical)

Your adrenal glands naturally produce certain cortisone-like chemicals. These chemicals are involved in various regulatory processes in the body (such as fluid balance, temperature, and reactions to inflammation). Hydrocortisone belongs to a group of drugs known as adrenocorticosteroids (or cortisone-like medications). It is used here to relieve inflammation (redness, swelling, itching, and discomfort). How it does so is not completely understood. The other ingredients in the cream and suppository provide a drying and softening effect.

TREATMENT

To apply the rectal cream, first wash and dry the rectal area, then gently rub in a small amount of the cream. If you must insert the cream inside the rectum, attach the applicator tip to the opened tube. Insert the applicator tip into the rectum and squeeze the tube. Remove the applicator from the tube and wash it with hot water and soap, then thoroughly dry it before storing. Be sure to put the top back on the tube.

To insert the suppository, unwrap the suppository and moisten it slightly with water (if the suppository is too soft, run cold water over it or refrigerate it for up to 30 minutes before you unwrap it). Lie down on your left side with your right knee bent. Push the suppository well into the rectum with your finger. Try not to have a bowel movement for at least an hour.

If you miss a dose of this medication, apply the cream or insert the suppository as soon as possible, unless it is almost time for the next application. In that case, do not use the missed dose at all; just return to your regular dosing schedule.

SIDE EFFECTS

Minor. Burning sensation upon application. The burning should disappear in several days, as your body adjusts to the medication.

Major. Tell your doctor about any side effects that are persistent or particularly bothersome. IT IS ESPECIALLY IMPORTANT TO TELL YOUR DOCTOR about any additional inflammation or infection at the site of application; or rectal pain, bleeding, itching, or blistering.

INTERACTIONS

This medication does not interact with any other medications, as long as it is used according to directions.

WARNINGS

• Tell your doctor about unusual or allergic reactions you have had to medications, especially to benzyl benzoate, bismuth resorcin compound, bismuth subgallate, Peruvian balsam, or to hydrocortisone or any other adrenocorticosteroid (such as amcinonide, betamethasone, clocortolone, cortisone, desonide, desoximetasone, dexamethasone, diflorasone, flumethasone, fluocinolone, fluocinonide, fluorometholone, flurandrenolide, halcinonide, methylprednisolone, paramethasone, prednisolone, prednisone, or triamcinolone).

• If additional irritation develops while using this drug, immediately discontinue its use and notify your doctor.

• You should not use this medication for more than seven consecutive days, unless your doctor specifically directs you to do so.

• If this drug stains your clothing, the stain may be removed by washing with laundry detergent.

• Be sure to tell your doctor if you are pregnant. If large amounts of hydrocortisone are applied for prolonged periods, some of it will be absorbed and may cross the placenta. Studies in humans have not yet been completed, but birth defects have been observed in the fetuses of animals who were given large oral doses of this drug during pregnancy. Also, tell your doctor if you are breastfeeding an infant. If absorbed through the skin, small amounts of hydrocortisone pass into breast milk and may cause growth suppression or a decrease in natural adrenocorticosteroid production in the nursing infant.

hydrocortisone, polymyxin B, and neomycin combination (otic)

BRAND NAMES (Manufacturers)
AK-Sporin H.C. Otic (Akorn)
Cortisporin Otic (Burroughs Wellcome)
Ortega-Otic M (Ortega)
Otobione Otic (Schering)
Otocort (Lemmon)
Otoreid-HC (Reid-Provident)

TYPE OF DRUG
Otic adrenocorticosteroid and antibiotic

INGREDIENTS
hydrocortisone, neomycin as the sulfate salt, and polymyxin B as the sulfate salt

DOSAGE FORMS
Otic solution (1% hydrocortisone, 10,000 units polymyxin B, and 5 mg neomycin per ml)
Otic suspension (1% hydrocortisone, 10,000 units
polymyxin B, and 5 mg neomycin per ml)

STORAGE
The otic solution and suspension should be stored at
room temperature in tightly closed, light-resistant containers. This medication should never be frozen.

USES
This medication is used to treat superficial bacterial infections of the outer ear.

Your adrenal glands naturally produce certain cortisone-like chemicals. These chemicals are involved in various regulatory processes in the body (such as reaction to
inflammation). Hydrocortisone belongs to a group of
drugs known as adrenocorticosteroids (or cortisone-like
medications). It is used here to relieve inflammation (redness, swelling, itching, pain). Polymyxin B and neomycin
are antibiotics, which act to prevent the growth and multiplication of the infecting bacteria.

TREATMENT

For accuracy, and to avoid contamination, another person should insert the ear drops whenever possible.

If you wish to warm the drops before administration, roll the bottle back and forth between your hands. DO NOT place the bottle in boiling water; high temperatures destroy the medication.

The suspension form of this medication should be shaken well before inserting into the ear. The contents tend to settle on the bottom of the bottle, so it is necessary to shake the container to evenly distribute the ingredients and equalize the doses.

To administer the ear drops, tilt the head to one side, with the affected ear turned upward. Grasp the earlobe and GENTLY pull it upward and back, to straighten the ear canal. (If administering ear drops to a child, GENTLY pull the earlobe downward and back.) Fill the dropper and place the prescribed number of drops into the ear. Be careful not to touch the dropper to the ear canal, as the dropper can easily become contaminated. Keep the ear tilted upward for about five minutes. Your doctor may want you to put a piece of cotton soaked with the medication into your ear to keep the medicine from leaking out. To avoid contamination, DO NOT wash or wipe the dropper after use.

If you miss a dose of this medication, insert the drops as soon as possible, unless it is almost time for the next dose. In that case, do not use the missed dose at all; just return to your regular schedule.

SIDE EFFECTS

Minor. Burning sensation upon application. The burning should disappear in several days, as your body adjusts to the medication.

Major. Tell your doctor about any side effects that are persistent or particularly bothersome. IT IS ESPECIALLY IMPORTANT TO TELL YOUR DOCTOR about itching, redness, rash, or swelling at the site of application.

INTERACTIONS

This medication does not interact with any other medications, as long as it is used according to directions.

WARNINGS

• Tell your doctor about unusual or allergic reactions you have had to medications, especially to hydrocortisone or any other adrenocorticosteroid (such as amcinonide, betamethasone, clocortolone, cortisone, desonide, desoximetasone, dexamethasone, diflorasone, flumethasone, fluocinolone, fluocinonide, fluorometholone, fluprednisolone, flurandrenolide, halcinonide, methylprednisolone, prednisolone, prednisone, or triamcinolone); to polymyxin B; or to neomycin or any related antibiotic (such as amikacin, colistimethate, colistin, gentamicin, kanamycin, netilmicin, paromycin, streptomycin, tobramycin or viomycin).

• Tell your doctor if you now have, or if you have ever had, viral or fungal infections of the ear, a punctured eardrum, myasthenia gravis, or kidney disease.

• Do not use this medication for longer than ten consecutive days, unless your doctor directs you to do so. If there is no change in your condition within two or three days after starting to take this medication, contact your doctor. The medication may not be effective for the type of infection you have.

• It is important to continue to take this medication for the entire time prescribed by your doctor—even if the symptoms disappear before the end of that period. If you stop using the drug too soon, resistant bacteria are given a chance to continue growing, and the infection could recur.

• This medication has been prescribed for your current infection only. Another infection later on, or one that someone else has, may require a different medicine. You should not give your medicine to other people or use it for other infections, unless your doctor specifically directs you to do so.

• Be sure to tell your doctor if you are pregnant. If large amounts of hydrocortisone are applied for prolonged periods, some of it will be absorbed and may cross the placenta. Studies in humans have not yet been completed, but birth defects have been observed in the fetuses of animals who were given large oral doses of this drug during pregnancy. Also, tell your doctor if you are breastfeeding an infant. If absorbed through the skin, small amounts of the drug pass into breast milk and may cause growth suppression or a decrease in natural adrenocorticosteroid production in the nursing infant.

---

hydrocortisone, polymyxin B, neomycin, and bacitracin combination (ophthalmic)

BRAND NAME (Manufacturer)
Cortisporin Ophthalmic (Burroughs Wellcome)
TYPE OF DRUG
Ophthalmic adrenocorticosteroid and antibiotic
INGREDIENTS
hydrocortisone, polymyxin B as the sulfate salt, neomycin as the sulfate salt, and bacitracin (ointment only)
DOSAGE FORMS
Ophthalmic drops (1% hydrocortisone, 10,000 units polymyxin B, 0.05% neomycin, and 0.001% thimerosal per ml)
Ophthalmic ointment (1% hydrocortisone, 5,000 units polymyxin B, 0.5% neomycin, 400 units bacitracin, and 0.001% thimerosal per gram of ointment)
STORAGE
The ophthalmic drops and ointment should be stored at room temperature in tightly closed containers. This medication should never be frozen. If the drops or ointment change color, do not use the medication. A change in color demonstrates a loss of effectiveness.

USES

This medication is used for the short-term treatment of bacterial infections of the eyes.

Your adrenal glands naturally produce certain cortisone-like chemicals. These chemicals are involved in various regulatory processes in the body (such as fluid balance, temperature, and reactions to inflammation). Hydrocortisone belongs to a group of drugs known as adrenocorticosteroids (or cortisone-like medications). It is used here to relieve inflammation (redness, swelling, itching, and discomfort). How it does so is not completely understood.

Polymyxin B, neomycin, and bacitracin are antibiotics, which act to prevent the growth and multiplication of infecting bacteria. Thimerosal is a preservative.

TREATMENT

Wash your hands with soap and water before using this medication. If you are using the drops, shake the bottle well before measuring out the drops. The contents tend to settle on the bottom of the bottle, so it is necessary to shake the container to evenly distribute the ingredients and equalize the doses.

In order to prevent contamination of the medicine, be careful not to touch the dropper or the end of the tube; and do not let the dropper or tube touch the eye.

Note that the bottle of the eyedrops is not completely full—this is to allow control of the number of drops used.

To apply the drops, tilt your head back and pull down the lower eyelid with one hand, to make a pouch below the eye. Drop the medicine into the pouch and slowly close your eyes. Do not blink. Keep your eyes closed for a minute or two. Place one finger at the corner of the eye, next to your nose, applying a slight pressure (this is done to prevent loss of medication into the nose and throat canal). If you don't think the medicine got into your eye, repeat the process once.

If you are using more than one type of eye drop, wait at least five minutes between doses of the two types of medication.

Follow the same general procedure for applying the ointment. Tilt your head back, pull down the lower eyelid, and squeeze the ointment in a line along the pouch below the eye. Close your eyes, and place your finger at the corner of the eye, near the nose, for a minute or two. Do not rub your eyes. Wipe off excess ointment and the tip of the tube with clean tissues.

Since applying the medication is somewhat difficult to do, you may want someone else to apply the drops or ointment for you.

If you miss a dose of this medication, insert the drops or apply the ointment as soon as possible, unless it is almost time for the next application. In that case, do not use the missed dose at all; just return to your regular dosing schedule.

SIDE EFFECTS

Minor. Blurred vision; burning; and stinging. These side effects should disappear, as your body adjusts to the medication.

Major. Tell your doctor about any side effects that are persistent or particularly bothersome. IT IS ESPECIALLY IMPORTANT TO TELL YOUR DOCTOR about disturbed or reduced vision; eye pain, itching, or swelling; headache; severe irritation; or rash.

INTERACTIONS

This medication does not interact with any other medication, as long as it is used according to directions.

WARNINGS

• Tell your doctor about unusual or allergic reactions you have had to medications, especially to hydrocortisone or other adrenocorticosteroids (such as amcinonide, betamethasone, clocortolone, cortisone, desonide, desoximetasone, dexamethasone, diflorasone, flumethasone, fluocinolone, fluorometholone, fluprednisolone, flurandrenolide, halcinonide, methylprednisolone, prednisolone, prednisone, or triamcinolone); to polymyxin B; neomycin; or to bacitracin or any related antibiotic (amikacin, colistimethate, colistin, gentamicin, kanamycin, neomycin, netilmicin, paromycin, streptomycin, tobramycin, or viomycin).

• Tell your doctor if you now have, or if you have ever had, fungal or viral infections of the eye, inner ear disease, kidney disease, or myasthenia gravis.

• If there is no change in your condition two or three days after starting to take this medication, contact your doctor.

The medication may not be effective for your particular infection.

● It is important to continue to take this medication for the entire time prescribed by your doctor, even if the symptoms disappear before the end of that period. If you stop applying the drug too soon, resistant bacteria are given a chance to continue growing, and the infection could recur.

● Do not use this medication for longer than ten consecutive days, unless your doctor directs you to do so. Prolonged use of this drug may result in glaucoma, secondary infection, cataracts, or eye damage. If you need to take this medication for as long as six weeks, your doctor may want you to have an eye examination by an ophthalmologist.

● This medication has been prescribed for your current infection only. Another infection later on, or one that someone else has, may require a different medicine. You should not give your medicine to other people or use it for other infections, unless your doctor specifically directs you to do so.

● In order to allow your eye infection to clear, do not apply makeup to the affected eye.

● Be sure to tell your doctor if you are pregnant. When large amounts of hydrocortisone are applied for prolonged periods, some of it is absorbed into the bloodstream. It may cross the placenta. Studies in humans have not yet been completed, but birth defects have been observed in the fetuses of animals who were given large oral doses of this drug during pregnancy. Also, tell your doctor if you are breastfeeding an infant. If absorbed through the skin, small amounts of hydrocortisone pass into breast milk and may cause growth suppression or a decrease in natural adrenocorticosteroid production in the nursing infant.

Hydrocortone—see hydrocortisone (systemic)

Hydrocortone Acetate—see hydrocortisone (topical)

HydroDiuril—see hydrochlorothiazide

hydroflumethiazide

BRAND NAMES (Manufacturers)
Diucardin (Ayerst)
hydroflumethiazide (various manufacturers)
Saluron (Bristol)
TYPE OF DRUG
Diuretic (water pill) and anti-hypertensive
INGREDIENT
hydroflumethiazide
DOSAGE FORM
Tablets (50 mg)
STORAGE
This medication should be stored at room temperature in a tightly closed container.

USES
Hydroflumethiazide is prescribed to treat high blood pressure. It is also used to reduce fluid accumulation in the body caused by conditions such as heart failure, cirrhosis of the liver, kidney disease, and the long-term use of some medications. This medication reduces fluid accumulation by increasing the elimination of sodium and water through the kidneys.

TREATMENT
To decrease stomach irritation, you can take this medication with a glass of milk or with a meal (unless your doctor directs you to do otherwise). Try to take it at the same time every day. Avoid taking a dose after 6:00 P.M.—this will prevent you from having to get up during the night to urinate.

If you miss a dose of this medication, take the missed dose as soon as possible, unless it is almost time for the next dose. In that case, do not take the missed dose at all; just wait until the next scheduled dose. Do not double the next dose.

This medication does not cure high blood pressure, but it will help to control the condition, as long as you continue to take it.

SIDE EFFECTS

Minor. Constipation; cramps; diarrhea; dizziness; drowsiness; headache; heartburn; itching; loss of appetite; nausea; restlessness; upset stomach; and vomiting. As your body adjusts to the medication, these side effects should disappear.

This medication can cause increased sensitivity to sunlight. It is therefore important to avoid prolonged exposure to sunlight and sunlamps. Wear protective clothing, and use an effective sunscreen.

To avoid dizziness and light-headedness when you stand, contract and relax the muscles of your legs for a few moments before rising. Do this by pushing one foot against the floor while raising the other foot slightly, alternating feet so that you are "pumping" your legs in a pedaling motion.

Major. Tell your doctor about any side effects that are persistent or particularly bothersome. IT IS ESPECIALLY IMPORTANT TO TELL YOUR DOCTOR about any unusual bleeding or bruising; blurred vision; confusion; difficulty breathing; dry mouth; excessive thirst; fever; joint pain; mood changes; muscle spasms; palpitations; skin rash; sore throat; tingling in the fingers or toes; excessive weakness; or yellowing of the eyes or skin.

INTERACTIONS

Hydroflumethiazide interacts with other medications.

1. It may decrease the effectiveness of oral anti-coagulants, anti-gout medications, insulin, oral anti-diabetic medicines, and methenamine.

2. Fenfluramine can increase the blood-pressure-lowering effects of hydroflumethiazide (which can be dangerous).

3. Indomethacin can decrease the blood-pressure-lowering effects (thereby counteracting the desired effects) of hydroflumethiazide.

4. Cholestyramine and colestipol decrease the absorption of this medication from the gastrointestinal tract. Hydroflumethiazide should be taken one hour before, or four hours after, a dose of cholestyramine or colestipol (if you have also been prescribed one of these medications).

5. The side effects of amphotericin B, calcium, cortisone-like steroids (such as cortisone, dexamethasone, hydrocortisone, prednisone, prednisolone), digoxin, digitalis, lithium, quinidine, sulfonamide antibiotics, and vitamin D may be increased when taken concurrently with hydroflumethiazide.

BE SURE TO TELL YOUR DOCTOR if you are taking any of the medicines listed above.

WARNINGS

• Tell your doctor about unusual or allergic reactions you have had to any medications, especially to diuretics (water pills), oral anti-diabetic medications, or sulfonamide antibiotics.

• Before you start taking hydroflumethiazide, tell your doctor if you now have, or if you have ever had, kidney disease or problems with urination, diabetes mellitus (sugar diabetes), gout, liver disease, asthma, pancreas disease, or systemic lupus erythematosus (SLE).

• Hydroflumethiazide can cause potassium loss. Signs of potassium loss include dry mouth, thirst, weakness, muscle pain or cramps, nausea, and vomiting. If you experience any of these symptoms, call your doctor. To help avoid potassium loss, take this drug with a glass of fresh or frozen orange or cranberry juice, or eat a banana every day. The use of a salt substitute also helps to prevent potassium loss. Do not change your diet, however, before discussing it with your doctor. Too much potassium can also be dangerous. Your doctor may want you to have blood tests performed periodically, in order to monitor your potassium levels.

• Limit your intake of alcoholic beverages while taking this medication, in order to prevent dizziness and light-headedness.

• If you have high blood pressure, do not take any over-the-counter (non-prescription) medications for weight control, or for allergy, asthma, cough, cold, or sinus problems, unless your doctor directs you to do so.

• To prevent dehydration (severe water loss) while taking this medication, check with your doctor if you have any illness that causes severe nausea, vomiting, or diarrhea.

• This medication can raise blood sugar levels in diabetic patients. Therefore, blood sugar should be carefully monitored by blood or urine tests when this medication is started.

• Be sure to tell your doctor if you are pregnant. This drug is able to cross the placenta. Studies in humans have not yet been completed, but adverse effects have been observed on the fetuses of animals who were given large doses of this drug during pregnancy. Also, tell your doctor if you are breastfeeding an infant. Although problems in humans have not been reported, small amounts of this drug can pass into breast milk, so caution is warranted.

Hydrogesic—see acetaminophen and hydrocodone combination

Hydromal—see hydrochlorothiazide

---

hydromorphone

BRAND NAMES (Manufacturers)
Dilaudid (Knoll)
Hydromorphone Hydrochloride (Wyeth)
TYPE OF DRUG
Analgesic (pain reliever)
INGREDIENT
hydromorphone as the hydrochloride salt
DOSAGE FORMS
Tablets (1 mg, 2 mg, 3 mg, and 4 mg)
Suppositories (3 mg)
STORAGE
Hydromorphone tablets should be stored at room temperature in a tightly closed, light-resistant container. The suppositories should be stored in the refrigerator.

USES

Hydromorphone is a narcotic analgesic that acts directly on the central nervous system (brain and spinal cord). It is used to relieve moderate to severe pain.

TREATMENT

In order to avoid stomach upset, you can take hydromorphone tablets with food or milk.

To use the suppository form of this medication, remove the foil wrapper and moisten the suppository with water (if the suppository is too soft to insert, refrigerate it for half an hour or run cold water over it before removing the wrapper). Lie on your left side with your right knee bent. Push the suppository into the rectum, pointed end first. Lie still for a few minutes. Try to avoid having a bowel movement for at least an hour.

Hydromorphone works most effectively if you take it at the onset of pain, rather than waiting until the pain becomes intense.

If you are taking this medication on a regular schedule and you miss a dose, take the missed dose as soon as possible, unless it is almost time for your next dose. In that case, don't take the missed dose at all; just return to your regular dosing schedule. Do not double the next dose.

SIDE EFFECTS

Minor. Constipation; dizziness; drowsiness; dry mouth; false sense of well-being; flushing; light-headedness; loss of appetite; nausea; rash; sweating; and painful or difficult urination. These side effects should disappear in several days, as your body adjusts to the medication.

If you are constipated, increase the amount of fiber in your diet (raw vegetables, fruits, salads, bran, and whole-grain breads), and drink more water (unless your doctor directs you to do otherwise).

Chew sugarless gum, or suck on ice chips or a piece of hard candy, to reduce mouth dryness.

If you feel dizzy, light-headed, or nauseated, sit or lie down awhile; get up from a sitting or lying position slowly, and be careful on stairs.

Major. Tell your doctor about any side effects that are persistent or particularly bothersome. IT IS ESPECIALLY IMPORTANT TO TELL YOUR DOCTOR about anxiety; difficulty breathing; excitation; fatigue; restlessness; sore throat and fever; tremors; or weakness.

INTERACTIONS

Hydromorphone interacts with several other types of medication.

1. Concurrent use of it with other central nervous system depressants (drugs that slow the activity of the nervous system), such as alcohol, antihistamines, barbiturates, benzodiazepine tranquilizers, muscle relaxants, and phenothiazine tranquilizers, or with tricyclic anti-depressants can cause extreme drowsiness.

2. A monoamine oxidase (MAO) inhibitor taken within 14 days of this medication can lead to unpredictable and severe side effects.

3. Cimetidine, combined with this medication, can cause confusion, disorientation, seizures, and shortness of breath.

Before starting to take hydromorphone, TELL YOUR DOCTOR if you are already taking any of the medications listed above.

WARNINGS

• Tell your doctor about unusual or allergic reactions you have had to medications, especially to hydromorphone or to any other narcotic analgesics (such as codeine, hydrocodone, meperidine, methadone, morphine, oxycodone, or propoxyphene).

• Tell your doctor if you now have, or if you have ever had, acute abdominal conditions, asthma, brain disease, colitis, epilepsy, gallstones or gallbladder disease, head injuries, heart disease, kidney disease, liver disease, lung disease, mental illness, emotional disorders, prostate disease, thyroid disease, or urethral stricture.

• If this drug makes you dizzy or drowsy, do not take part in any activity that requires alertness, such as driving a car or operating potentially dangerous equipment.

• Before having any surgery or other medical or dental treatment, be sure to tell your doctor or dentist that you are taking this medication.

• Hydromorphone has the potential for abuse, and must be used with caution. Usually, you should not take it on a regular schedule for longer than ten days (unless your doctor directs you to do so). Tolerance develops quickly; do not increase the dosage or stop taking the drug abruptly, unless you first consult your doctor. If you have been taking large amounts of this medication for long periods, you may experience a withdrawal reaction (muscle aches, diarrhea, gooseflesh, runny nose, nausea,

vomiting, shivering, trembling, stomach cramps, sleep disorders, irritability, weakness, yawning, and sweating). Your doctor may therefore want to reduce the dosage gradually.
● Some of these products contain F.D. & C. Yellow Dye No. 5 (tartrazine), which can cause allergic-type reactions (difficulty breathing; rash; or fainting) in certain susceptible individuals.
● Be sure to tell your doctor if you are pregnant. The effects of this medication during the early stages of pregnancy have not yet been thoroughly studied in humans. However, hydromorphone, used regularly in large doses during pregnancy, can result in addiction of the fetus, leading to withdrawal symptoms (irritability, excessive crying, tremors, fever, vomiting, diarrhea, sneezing, and yawning) at birth. Also, tell your doctor if you are breast-feeding an infant. Small amounts of this medication may pass into breast milk and cause excessive drowsiness in the nursing infant.

Hydromorphone Hydrochloride—see
  hydromorphone

Hydromox—see quinethazone

Hydro-tex—see hydrocortisone (topical)

---

hydroxyzine

BRAND NAMES (Manufacturers)
Anxanil (EconoMed)
Atarax (Roerig)
Atozine (Major)
Durrax (Dermik)
hydroxyzine hydrochloride (various manufacturers)
hydroxyzine pamoate (various manufacturers)
Hy-Pam (Lemmon)
Vamate (Major)
Vistaril (Pfizer)
TYPE OF DRUG
Antihistamine and sedative/hypnotic (sleeping aid)

INGREDIENT

hydroxyzine as the hydrochloride or pamoate salt

DOSAGE FORMS

Tablets (20 mg, 25 mg, 50 mg, and 100 mg)
Capsules (25 mg, 50 mg, and 100 mg)
Oral syrup (10 mg per 5 ml teaspoonful)
Oral suspension (25 mg per 5 ml teaspoonful)

STORAGE

Hydroxyzine tablets, capsules, oral syrup, and oral suspension should be stored at room temperature, in tightly closed, light-resistant containers. This medication should never be frozen.

USES

Hydroxyzine belongs to a group of drugs known as antihistamines (antihistamines block the action of histamine, a chemical that is released by the body during an allergic reaction). It is therefore used to treat or prevent symptoms of allergy. Hydroxyzine is also used as a sleeping aid and can be used to relieve the symptoms of anxiety and tension.

TREATMENT

To avoid stomach upset, you can take hydroxyzine with food or with a full glass of milk or water (unless your doctor directs you to do otherwise).

The oral syrup and suspension forms of this medication should be shaken well just before measuring each dose. The contents tend to settle on the bottom of the bottle, so it is necessary to shake the container to evenly distribute the ingredients and equalize the doses. Each dose should then be measured carefully, with a specially designed, 5 ml measuring spoon. An ordinary kitchen teaspoon is not accurate enough.

If you miss a dose of this medication, take the missed dose as soon as possible, unless it is close to the time for your next dose. In that case, don't take the missed dose at all; just return to your regular dosing schedule. Do not double the next dose.

SIDE EFFECTS

Minor. Drowsiness and dry mouth. These side effects

should disappear in several days, as your body adjusts to the medication.

Dry mouth can be relieved by chewing sugarless gum, or by sucking on ice chips or a piece of hard candy.

Major. Tell your doctor about any side effects that are persistent or particularly bothersome. IT IS ESPECIALLY IMPORTANT TO TELL YOUR DOCTOR about convulsions; feeling faint; rash; or trembling or shakiness.

INTERACTIONS

Hydroxyzine can interact with several other types of drugs. Concurrent use of it with other central nervous system depressants (drugs that slow the activity of the nervous system), such as alcohol, barbiturates, benzodiazepine tranquilizers, muscle relaxants, narcotics, pain medications, and phenothiazine tranquilizers, or with tricyclic anti-depressants can cause extreme drowsiness. TELL YOUR DOCTOR if you are currently taking any of the medications listed above.

WARNINGS

• Tell your doctor about allergic or unusual reactions you have had to medications, especially to hydroxyzine or to any other antihistamine (such as azatadine, bromodiphenhydramine, brompheniramine, carbinoxamine, chlorpheniramine, clemastine, cyproheptadine, dexchlorpheniramine, dimenhydrinate, dimethindene, diphenhydramine, diphenylpyraline, doxylamine, promethazine, pyrilamine, trimeprazine, tripelennamine, or tripolidine).

• Hydroxyzine can cause drowsiness or dizziness. Your ability to perform tasks that require alertness, such as driving a car or operating potentially dangerous machinery, may be decreased. Appropriate caution should therefore be taken.

• Be sure to tell your doctor if you are pregnant. The effects of this medication during pregnancy have not yet been thoroughly studied in humans. Also, tell your doctor if you are breastfeeding an infant. Small amounts of hydroxyzine pass into breast milk and may cause unusual excitement or irritability in nursing infants.

hydroxyzine hydrochloride—see hydroxyzine

hydroxyzine pamoate—see hydroxyzine

Hydro-Z—see hydrochlorothiazide

Hygroton—see chlorthalidone

Hylidone—see chlorthalidone

Hylorel—see guanadrel

Hyosophen—see atropine, scopolamine, hyoscyamine, and phenobarbital combination

Hy-Pam—see hydroxyzine

Hyperetic—see hydrochlorothiazide

Hyrex 105—see phendimetrazine

Hyserp—see hydralazine, hydrochlorothiazide, and reserpine combination

Hysone—see hydrocortisone and iodochlorhydroxyquin combination (topical)

Hytakerol—see dihydrotachysterol

Hytone—see hydrocortisone (topical)

---

ibuprofen

BRAND NAMES (Manufacturers)
Advil* (Whitehall)
Motrin (Upjohn)
Nuprin* (Bristol-Myers)
Rufen (Boots)
*Ibuprofen is also available over-the-counter (non-prescription), as 200 mg tablets.

TYPE OF DRUG
Non-steroidal anti-inflammatory analgesic (pain reliever)
INGREDIENT
ibuprofen
DOSAGE FORM
Tablets (300 mg, 400 mg, and 600 mg)
STORAGE
This medication should be stored in a tightly closed container at room temperature, away from heat and direct sunlight.

USES
Ibuprofen is used to treat the pain, swelling, stiffness, and inflammation of certain types of arthritis, gout, bursitis, and tendinitis. Ibuprofen is also used to treat painful menstruation.

TREATMENT
You should take this medication on an empty stomach 30 to 60 minutes before meals or two hours after meals, so that it gets into your bloodstream quickly. However, to decrease stomach irritation, your doctor may want you to take the medicine with food or antacids.

This medication does not cure arthritis, but it will help to control the condition, as long as you continue to take it.

If you are taking ibuprofen to relieve arthritis, you must take it regularly, as directed by your doctor. It may take up to two weeks before you feel the full effects of this medication.

It is important to take ibuprofen on schedule and not to miss any doses. If you do miss a dose, take it as soon as possible, unless it is almost time for your next dose. In that case, don't take the missed dose at all; just return to your regular dosing schedule. Do not double the next dose.

SIDE EFFECTS
Minor. Bloating; constipation; diarrhea; difficulty sleeping; dizziness; drowsiness; headache; heartburn; indigestion; light-headedness; loss of appetite; nausea; nervousness; soreness of the mouth; unusual sweating; and vomiting. As your body adjusts to the drug, these side

effects should disappear.

If you become dizzy, sit or lie down awhile; get up slowly, and be careful on stairs.

Acetaminophen may be helpful in relieving any headaches.

Major. If any side effects are persistent or particularly bothersome, you should report them to your doctor. IT IS ESPECIALLY IMPORTANT TO TELL YOUR DOCTOR about bloody or black, tarry stools; blurred vision; confusion; depression; difficulty breathing, or wheezing; difficult or painful urination; palpitations; a problem with hearing; ringing or buzzing in your ears; skin rash, hives, or itching; stomach pain; swelling of the feet; tightness in the chest; unexplained sore throat and fever; unusual bleeding or bruising; unusual fatigue or weakness; unusual weight gain; or yellowing of the eyes or skin.

INTERACTIONS

Ibuprofen interacts with other types of medication.

1. Anti-coagulants (blood thinners, such as warfarin) can lead to an increase in bleeding complications.

2. Aspirin, other salicylates, and other anti-inflammation medications can increase stomach irritation.

3. Ibuprofen can interfere with the diuretic effects of furosemide and thiazide-type diuretics (water pills).

BE SURE TO TELL YOUR DOCTOR if you are already taking any of the medications listed above.

WARNINGS

● Before you start to take this medication, it is important to tell your doctor if you have ever had unusual or allergic reactions to ibuprofen, or to any of the other chemically related drugs (aspirin, other salicylates, diflunisal, fenoprofen, indomethacin, meclofenamate, mefenamic acid, naproxen, oxyphenbutazone, phenylbutazone, piroxicam, sulindac, tolmetin, and zomepirac).

● Tell your doctor if you now have, or if you have ever had, bleeding problems; colitis, stomach ulcers, or other stomach problems; epilepsy; heart disease; high blood pressure; asthma; kidney disease; liver disease; mental illness; or Parkinson's disease.

- If ibuprofen makes you dizzy or drowsy, do not take part in any activity that requires alertness, such as driving a car or operating potentially dangerous equipment.
- Because this drug can prolong your bleeding time, it is important to tell your doctor or dentist that you are taking this drug, before having any surgery or other medical or dental treatment.
- Stomach problems are more likely to occur if you take aspirin regularly or drink alcohol while being treated with this medication. These should therefore be avoided (unless your doctor directs you to do otherwise).
- Be sure to tell your doctor if you are pregnant. This type of medication can cause unwanted effects to the heart or blood flow of the fetus. Studies in animals have also shown that this type of medicine, if taken late in pregnancy, may increase the length of pregnancy, prolong labor, or cause other problems during delivery. Also, tell your doctor if you are breastfeeding an infant. Small amounts of ibuprofen can pass into breast milk.

Iletin I—see insulin

Iletin II—see insulin

Ilosone—see erythromycin

Ilotycin—see erythromycin

Ilozyme—see pancrelipase

---

imipramine

BRAND NAMES (Manufacturers)
imipramine hydrochloride (various manufacturers)
Janimine (Abbott)
SK-Pramine (Smith Kline & French)
Tipramine (Major)
Tofranil (Geigy)
Tofranil-PM (Geigy)
TYPE OF DRUG
Tricyclic anti-depressant (mood elevator)

INGREDIENT
imipramine as the hydrochloride or pamoate salt
DOSAGE FORMS
Tablets (10 mg, 25 mg, and 50 mg)
Capsules (75 mg, 100 mg, 125 mg, and 150 mg)
STORAGE
This medication should be stored at room temperature in tightly closed containers.

USES
Imipramine is used to relieve the symptoms of mental depression. This medication belongs to a group of drugs referred to as the tricyclic anti-depressants. These medicines are thought to relieve depression by increasing the concentration of certain chemicals necessary for nerve transmission in the brain. This medication is also used to treat enuresis (bed-wetting) in children 6 to 12 years of age.

TREATMENT
Imipramine should be taken exactly as your doctor prescribes. It can be taken with water or with food to lessen the chance of stomach irritation, unless your doctor tells you to do otherwise.

If you miss a dose of this medication, take the missed dose as soon as possible, then return to your regular dosing schedule. If, however, the dose you missed was a once a day bedtime dose, do not take that dose in the morning; check with your doctor instead. If the dose is taken in the morning, it may cause some unwanted side effects. Never double the dose.

The effects of therapy with this medication may not become apparent for two or three weeks.

SIDE EFFECTS
Minor. Agitation; anxiety; blurred vision; confusion; constipation; cramps; diarrhea; dizziness; drowsiness; dry mouth; fatigue; heartburn; insomnia; loss of appetite; nausea; peculiar tastes in the mouth; restlessness; sweating; vomiting; weakness; or weight gain or loss. As your body adjusts to the medication, these side effects should disappear.

Dry mouth can be relieved by chewing sugarless gum or by sucking on ice chips or a piece of hard candy.

To relieve constipation, increase the amount of fiber (bran, fresh fruits and vegetables, salads, and whole-grain breads) in your diet, exercise, and drink more water (unless your doctor directs you to do otherwise).

To avoid dizziness or light-headedness when you stand, contract and relax the muscles of your legs for a few moments before rising. Do this by pushing one foot against the floor while raising the other foot slightly, alternating feet so that you are "pumping" your legs in a pedaling motion.

This medication may cause increased sensitivity to sunlight. You should therefore avoid prolonged exposure to sunlight and sunlamps. Wear protective clothing, and use an effective sunscreen.

Major. Tell your doctor about any side effects that are persistent or particularly bothersome. IT IS ESPECIALLY IMPORTANT TO TELL YOUR DOCTOR about chest pains; convulsions; difficulty urinating; enlarged or painful breasts (in both sexes); fainting; fever; fluid retention; hair loss; hallucinations; headaches; impotence; mood changes; mouth sores; nervousness; nightmares; numbness in the fingers or toes; palpitations; ringing in the ears; seizures; skin rash; sleep disorders; sore throat; tremors; uncoordinated movements or balance problems; unusual bleeding or bruising; or yellowing of the eyes or skin.

INTERACTIONS

Imipramine interacts with a number of other types of drugs.

1. Extreme drowsiness can occur when this medicine is taken with central nervous system depressants (medicines that slow the activity of the nervous system), including alcohol, antihistamines, barbiturates, benzodiazepine tranquilizers, muscle relaxants, narcotics, pain medications, phenothiazine tranquilizers, and sleeping medications.

2. Imipramine may decrease the effectiveness of anti-seizure medications and may block the blood-pressure-lowering effects of clonidine and guanethidine.

3. Oral contraceptives (estrogens) can increase the side effects, and reduce the effectiveness, of the tricyclic anti-depressants (including imipramine).
4. Tricyclic anti-depressants may increase the side effects of thyroid medication and of over-the-counter (non-prescription) cough, cold, allergy, asthma, sinus, and diet medications.
5. The concurrent use of tricyclic anti-depressants and monoamine oxidase (MAO) inhibitors should be undertaken very carefully, because the combination may result in fever, convulsions, or high blood pressure.
Before starting to take imipramine, BE SURE TO TELL YOUR DOCTOR if you are already taking any of the medications listed above.

WARNINGS

• Tell your doctor if you have had unusual or allergic reactions to medications, especially to imipramine or any of the other tricyclic anti-depressants (such as amitriptyline, doxepin, trimipramine, amoxapine, protriptyline, desipramine, maprotiline, or nortriptyline).
• Tell your doctor if you now have, or if you have ever had, asthma, high blood pressure, liver or kidney disease, heart disease, a recent heart attack, circulatory disease, stomach problems, intestinal problems, alcoholism, difficulty urinating, enlarged prostate gland, epilepsy, glaucoma, thyroid disease, mental illness, or electroshock therapy.
• If this drug makes you dizzy or drowsy, do not take part in any activity that requires alertness, such as driving a car or operating potentially dangerous equipment.
• Before having any surgery or other medical or dental treatment, be sure to tell your doctor or dentist that you are taking this medication.
• Do not stop taking this drug suddenly. Stopping it abruptly can cause nausea, headache, stomach upset, fatigue, or a worsening of your condition. Your doctor may want to reduce the dosage gradually.
• The effects of this medication may last as long as seven days after you stop taking it, so continue to observe all precautions during that period.
• Some of these products contain F.D. & C. Yellow Dye

No. 5 (tartrazine), which can cause allergic-type reactions (difficulty breathing, rash, or fainting) in certain susceptible individuals.

• Be sure to tell your doctor if you are pregnant. Studies in humans have not yet been completed, but adverse effects have been observed on the fetuses of animals who were given large doses of this drug during pregnancy. Also, tell your doctor if you are breastfeeding an infant. Small amounts of this drug can pass into breast milk and may cause unwanted effects, such as irritability or sleeping problems, in nursing infants.

imipramine hydrochloride—see imipramine

Imodium—see loperamide

Imuran—see azathioprine

indapamide

BRAND NAME (Manufacturer)
Lozol (USV)
TYPE OF DRUG
Diuretic (water pill) and anti-hypertensive
INGREDIENT
indapamide
DOSAGE FORM
Tablets (2.5 mg)
STORAGE
This medication should be stored at room temperature in a tightly closed container.

USES
Indapamide is prescribed to treat high blood pressure. It is also used to reduce fluid accumulation in the body caused by conditions such as heart failure, cirrhosis of the liver, kidney disease, and the long-term use of some medications. This medication reduces fluid accumulation by increasing the elimination of sodium and water through the kidneys.

TREATMENT

To decrease stomach irritation, you can take indapamide with a glass of milk or with a meal (unless your doctor directs you to do otherwise). Try to take it at the same time every day. Avoid taking a dose after 6:00 P.M.   this will prevent you from having to get up during the night to urinate.

If you miss a dose of this medication, take the missed dose as soon as possible, unless it is almost time for the next dose. In that case, do not take the missed dose at all; just wait until the next dose. Do not double the dose.

This medication does not cure high blood pressure, but it will help to control the condition, as long as you continue to take it.

SIDE EFFECTS

Minor. Constipation; cramps; diarrhea; dizziness; drowsiness; headache; heartburn; itching; loss of appetite; nausea; restlessness; upset stomach; and vomiting. As your body adjusts to the medication, these side effects should disappear.

This medication can cause increased sensitivity to sunlight. It is therefore important to avoid prolonged exposure to sunlight and sunlamps. Wear protective clothing, and use an effective sunscreen.

To avoid dizziness or light-headedness when you stand, contract and relax the muscles of your legs for a few moments before rising. Do this by pushing one foot against the floor while raising the other foot slightly, alternating feet so that you are "pumping" your legs in a pedaling motion.

Major. Tell your doctor about any side effects that are persistent or particularly bothersome. IT IS ESPECIALLY IMPORTANT TO TELL YOUR DOCTOR about any unusual bleeding or bruising; blurred vision; confusion; difficulty breathing; dry mouth; excessive thirst; fever; joint pain; mood changes; muscle spasms; palpitations; skin rash; sore throat; tingling in the fingers or toes; excessive weakness; or yellowing of the eyes or skin.

INTERACTIONS

Indapamide interacts with other types of medication.

1. It may decrease the effectiveness of oral anti-coagulants, anti-gout medications, insulin, oral anti-diabetic medicines, and methenamine.

2. Fenfluramine can increase the blood-pressure-lowering effects of indapamide (which can be dangerous).

3. Indomethacin can decrease the blood-pressure-lowering effects (thereby counteracting the desired effects) of indapamide.

4. Cholestyramine and colestipol can decrease the absorption of this medication from the gastrointestinal tract. Indapamide should therefore be taken one hour before, or four hours after, a dose of cholestyramine or colestipol (if you have also been prescribed one of these medications).

5. Indapamide may increase the side effects of amphotericin B, calcium, adrenocorticosteroids (such as hydrocortisone or prednisone), digoxin, digitalis, lithium, quinidine, sulfonamide antibiotics, and vitamin D.

BE SURE TO TELL YOUR DOCTOR if you are already taking any of the medicines listed above.

WARNINGS

• Tell your doctor about unusual or allergic reactions you have had to any medications, especially to diuretics (water pills), oral anti-diabetic medications, or sulfonamide antibiotics.

• Before you start taking indapamide, tell your doctor if you now have, or if you have ever had, kidney disease or problems with urination, diabetes mellitus (sugar diabetes), gout, liver disease, asthma, pancreas disease, or systemic lupus erythematosus (SLE).

• Indapamide can cause potassium loss. Signs of potassium loss include dry mouth, thirst, weakness, muscle pain or cramps, nausea, and vomiting. If you experience any of these symptoms, call your doctor. To help avoid potassium loss, take this drug with a glass of fresh or frozen orange juice or cranberry juice, or eat a banana every day. The use of a salt substitute also helps to prevent potassium loss. Do not change your diet, however, before discussing it with your doctor. Too much potassium can also be dangerous. Your doctor may want you to have blood tests performed periodically, in order to monitor your potassium levels.

- In order to avoid dizziness or fainting while taking this medication, try not to stand for long periods of time; avoid drinking excessive amounts of alcohol; and avoid getting overheated (strenuous exercise in hot weather; hot baths, showers, and saunas).
- If you have high blood pressure, do not take any over-the-counter (non-prescription) medications for weight control, or for allergy, asthma, cough, cold, or sinus problems, unless your doctor directs you to do so.
- To prevent dehydration (severe water loss) while taking this medication, check with your doctor if you have any illness that causes severe or continuous nausea, vomiting, or diarrhea.
- This medication can raise blood sugar levels in diabetic patients. Therefore, blood sugar levels should be carefully monitored by blood or urine tests when this medication is started.
- Be sure to tell your doctor if you are pregnant. Studies in humans have not yet been completed, but adverse effects have been observed on the fetuses of animals who received large doses of this drug during pregnancy. Also, tell your doctor if you are breastfeeding an infant. Although problems in humans have not been reported, small amounts of this drug can pass into breast milk, so caution is warranted.

Inderal—see propranolol

Inderal LA—see propranolol

Inderide—see propranolol and hydrochlorothiazide combination

Indocin—see indomethacin

Indocin SR—see indomethacin

indomethacin

BRAND NAMES (Manufacturers)
Indocin (Merck Sharp & Dohme)

Indocin SR (Merck Sharp & Dohme)
indomethacin (Lederle)
TYPE OF DRUG
Non-steroidal anti-inflammatory analgesic (pain reliever)
INGREDIENT
indomethacin
DOSAGE FORMS
Capsules (25 mg and 50 mg)
Extended-release capsules (75 mg)
STORAGE
This medication should be stored in closed containers at
room temperature, away from heat and direct sunlight.

USES
Indomethacin is used to treat the pain, swelling, stiffness,
and inflammation of certain types of arthritis, gout, bursitis, and tendinitis.

TREATMENT
You should take this drug immediately after meals or with
food, in order to reduce stomach irritation. Ask your doctor if you can take indomethacin with an antacid.

Do not chew or crush the extended-release capsules;
they should be swallowed whole. Breaking the capsule
would release the medication all at once—defeating the
purpose of the extended-release capsules.

It is important to take indomethacin on schedule and
not to miss any doses. If you do miss a dose, take the
missed dose as soon as possible, unless more than one
hour has passed. In that case, don't take the missed dose
at all; just return to your regular dosing schedule. Do not
double the next dose.

This medication does not cure arthritis, but it will help
to control the condition, as long as you continue to take it.
It may take up to four weeks before you feel the full benefits of this medication.

SIDE EFFECTS
Minor. Bloating; constipation; diarrhea; difficulty sleeping; dizziness; drowsiness; headache; heartburn; indigestion; light-headedness; loss of appetite; nausea; nervousness; soreness of the mouth; unusual sweating; and

vomiting. As your body adjusts to the drug, these side effects should disappear.

If you become dizzy, sit or lie down awhile; get up slowly, and be careful on stairs.

Acetaminophen may be helpful in relieving any headaches.

Major. If any side effects are persistent or particularly bothersome, you should report them to your doctor. IT IS ESPECIALLY IMPORTANT TO TELL YOUR DOCTOR about bloody or black, tarry stools; blurred vision; confusion; depression; difficult or painful urination; difficulty breathing, or wheezing; palpitations; a problem with hearing; ringing or buzzing in the ears; skin rash, hives, or itching; stomach pain; swelling of the feet; tightness in the chest; unexplained sore throat and fever; unusual bleeding or bruising; unusual fatigue or weakness; unusual weight gain; or yellowing of the eyes or skin.

INTERACTIONS

Indomethacin interacts with several types of medication.
1. Anti-coagulants (blood thinners, such as warfarin) can lead to an increase in bleeding complications.
2. Aspirin, salicylates, and other anti-inflammation medications can cause increased stomach irritation.
3. Indomethacin can decrease the elimination of lithium from the body, resulting in possible lithium toxicity.
4. Indomethacin may interfere with the blood-pressure-lowering effects of beta-blocking medications, such as atenolol, metoprolol, pindolol, and propranolol.
5. Indomethacin can interfere with the diuretic effect of furosemide and thiazide-type diuretics (water pills).
6. Indomethacin can increase the amount of probenecid in the bloodstream when both drugs are being taken.
TELL YOUR DOCTOR if you are already taking any of the medications listed above.

WARNINGS

• Before you take this medication, it is important to tell your doctor if you have ever had any unusual or allergic reactions to indomethacin or any of the other chemically related drugs (including aspirin, other salicylates, diflunisal, fenoprofen, ibuprofen, meclofenamate, mefenamic acid, naproxen, oxyphenbutazone, phenylbutazone, piroxicam, sulindac, tolmetin, and zomepirac).

• Before taking indomethacin, it is important to tell your doctor if you now have, or if you have ever had, bleeding problems; colitis, stomach ulcers, or other stomach problems; epilepsy; heart disease; high blood pressure; asthma; kidney disease; liver disease; mental illness; or Parkinson's disease.

• If indomethacin makes you dizzy or drowsy, do not take part in any activity that requires alertness, such as driving a car or operating potentially dangerous equipment.

• If you will be taking this medication for a long period of time, your doctor may want to have your eyes examined periodically by an ophthalmologist. Some visual problems have been known to occur with long-term indomethacin use. Your doctor might want to keep a careful watch for these.

• Stomach problems are more likely to occur if you take aspirin regularly or drink alcohol while being treated with this medication. These should therefore be avoided (unless your doctor directs you to do otherwise).

• Be sure to tell your doctor if you are pregnant. Studies in animals have shown that indomethacin can cause unwanted effects in offspring, including lower birth weights, slower development of bones, nerve damage, and heart damage. If taken late in pregnancy, the drug can also prolong labor. Studies in humans have not yet been completed. Also, tell your doctor if you are breastfeeding an infant. Small amounts of indomethacin can pass into breast milk.

Insulatard NPH—see insulin

---

insulin

BRAND NAMES (Manufacturers)
Actrapid (Squibb-Novo)
Humulin N (Lilly)
Humulin R (Lilly)
Iletin I (Lilly)

Iletin II (Lilly)
Insulatard NPH (Nordick)
Lentard (Squibb-Novo)
Mixtard (Nordisk)
Monotard (Squibb-Novo)
Semitard (Squibb-Novo)
Ultratard (Squibb-Novo)
Velosulin (Nordisk)

TYPE OF DRUG

Anti-diabetic

INGREDIENTS

insulin (from beef, pork, or recombinant DNA sources)

DOSAGE FORM

Injectable (all types) (40 U [units]/ml and 100 U/ml)
Injectable (regular) (40 U/ml; 100 U/ml; and 500 U/ml)

This drug is available only as an injectable (if insulin is taken orally, it is destroyed by stomach acid). Various types of insulin provide different times of onset and different durations of action. The various types of insulin are listed below:

Insulin Type	Onset (in hours)	Duration (in hours)
Regular insulin	½	6
Insulin zinc suspension, prompt (Semilente)	½	14
Isophane insulin (NPH)	1	24
Insulin zinc suspension (Lente)	1	24
Globin zinc insulin	2	24
Protamine zinc insulin (PZI)	6	36
Insulin zinc suspension, extended (Ultralente)	6	36

STORAGE

This drug is stored in the refrigerator in the pharmacy, but once the bottle has been opened, most forms (except U-500 strength) may be kept at room temperature if the contents are used within six months. Unopened vials should be kept refrigerated. This medication should never be frozen.

USES

Insulin is a hormone that is normally produced by the pancreas; it functions in the regulation of blood sugar levels. This medication is used to treat diabetes mellitus (sugar diabetes)—a disorder that results from an inability of the pancreas to produce enough insulin. Injectable insulin is only used to treat those patients whose blood sugar levels cannot be controlled by diet or by oral anti-diabetic medications.

TREATMENT

Your doctor, nurse, dietician, or pharmacist will show you how to inject yourself with insulin, using a specially marked hypodermic syringe. This medication is packaged with printed instructions that should be carefully followed.

You may prefer to use pre-sterilized disposable needles and syringes, which are used once, then discarded. If you use a glass syringe and metal needle, you must sterilize them before re-use.

Make sure that the insulin you are using is exactly the kind your doctor ordered, and that its expiration date has not passed.

Do not shake the bottle; tip it gently, end to end, to mix.

ALWAYS CHECK THE DOSE in the syringe at least twice before injecting it.

Clean the site of the injection thoroughly with an antiseptic, such as rubbing alcohol.

Change the site of the injection daily, and avoid injecting cold insulin.

NEVER use a vial of insulin if there are solid lumps in it.

Make your insulin injection a regular part of your schedule, so that you do not miss any doses. Ask your doctor what to do if you have to take a dose later than the scheduled time.

SIDE EFFECTS

Minor. Insulin can cause redness and rash at the site of injection. Try to rotate injection sites in order to avoid this reaction.

Major. Tell your doctor about any side effects that are persistent or particularly bothersome. IT IS ESPECIALLY IMPORTANT TO TELL YOUR DOCTOR about skin rash; shortness of breath; sweating; palpitations; and fainting.

Too much insulin can cause hypoglycemia (low blood sugar), which can lead to anxiety; chills; cold sweats; drowsiness; fast heart rate; headache; loss of consciousness; nausea; nervousness; tremors; unusual hunger; or unusual weakness. If you experience these symptoms, eat a quick source of sugar (such as table sugar, orange juice, honey, or a non-diet cola). You should also tell your doctor that you have had this reaction.

Too little insulin can cause symptoms of high blood sugar (hyperglycemia), such as confusion; drowsiness; dry skin; fatigue; flushing; frequent urination; fruit-like breath odor; loss of appetite; or rapid breathing. If you experience any of these symptoms, contact your doctor —he or she may want to modify your dosing schedule or change your insulin dosage.

INTERACTIONS

Insulin interacts with several other types of medication.

1. Insulin can increase the side effects to the heart of digoxin.

2. Oral contraceptives, adrenocorticosteroids (cortisone-like medicines), danazol, dextrothyroxine, furosemide, ethacrynic acid, thyroid hormone, thiazide diuretics (water pills), phenytoin, or nicotine (from smoking) can increase insulin dosing requirements.

3. Monoamine oxidase (MAO) inhibitors, phenylbutazone, large doses of aspirin, guanethidine, disopyramide, sulfinpyrazone, tetracycline, alcohol, or anabolic steroids can increase the effects of insulin, leading to hypoglycemia.

4. Beta-blockers (atenolol, metoprolol, nadolol, pindolol, propranolol, timolol) may prolong the effects of insulin and mask the signs of hypoglycemia.

BE SURE TO TELL YOUR DOCTOR if you are already taking any of the medications listed above.

WARNINGS

• Tell your doctor about unusual or allergic reactions you have had to any medications, especially to insulin.

• Before starting to take this medication, be sure to tell your doctor if you now have, or if you have ever had, high fevers, infections, kidney disease, liver disease, thyroid disease, or nausea and vomiting.

• Make sure that your friends and family are aware of the symptoms of an insulin reaction, and know what to do should they observe any of the symptoms in you.

• Carry a card or wear a bracelet that identifies you as a diabetic.

• Always have insulin and syringes available.

• To avoid the possibility of hypoglycemia (low blood sugar levels), you should eat on a regular schedule, and should avoid skipping meals.

• Before having any surgery or other medical or dental treatment, be sure to tell your doctor or dentist that you are taking insulin.

• Check with your doctor or pharmacist before taking any over-the-counter (non-prescription) cough, cold, diet, allergy, asthma, or sinus medications. Some of these products affect blood sugar levels.

• If you become ill—if you catch a cold or the flu, or become nauseated—your insulin requirements may change. Consult your doctor.

• Be sure to tell your doctor if you are pregnant. Insulin dosing requirements often change during pregnancy.

Intal—see cromolyn sodium (inhalation)

Iodocort—see hydrocortisone and
    iodochlorhydroxyquin combination (topical)

Iodosone—see hydrocortisone and
    iodochlorhydroxyquin combination (topical)

Ionamin—see phentermine

ipecac

BRAND NAME (Manufacturer)
ipecac (various manufacturers)
TYPE OF DRUG
Emetic (vomiting-producer)
INGREDIENT
ipecac
DOSAGE FORM
Oral syrup
STORAGE
Ipecac syrup should be stored at room temperature in a tightly closed container.

USES

Ipecac is for emergency use to treat drug overdose or poisoning. Ipecac works on the stomach and on the vomiting center in the brain to produce vomiting.

TREATMENT

Before administering ipecac, call a physician, poison control center, or emergency room for advice.

It is important to administer ipecac with adequate amounts of water (½ glass for infants less than 1 year old; 1 to 2 glasses for children and adults) to assure that there is adequate fluid in the stomach. If vomiting does not occur within 20 minutes after a second dose has been given, call again IMMEDIATELY for further instructions.

SIDE EFFECTS

Minor. Ipecac can cause diarrhea; drowsiness; or nausea or vomiting that continues for more than 30 minutes. These side effects should disappear within several hours.
Major. Tell your doctor about any side effects that are persistent or particularly bothersome. IT IS ESPECIALLY IMPORTANT TO TELL YOUR DOCTOR about aching or stiffness of the muscles; stomach cramps or pain; difficulty breathing; palpitations; or weakness.

INTERACTIONS

Ipecac should not be administered with milk or carbonated beverages; these fluids may affect how quickly ipecac works. Activated charcoal absorbs ipecac. If both activated charcoal and ipecac are to be used, give the activated charcoal only after successful vomiting has been produced by the ipecac.

WARNINGS

• Vomiting is not the proper treatment in all cases of possible poisoning; ipecac should NOT be used if gasoline, oils, kerosene, acids, alkalies (lye), or strychnine has been swallowed, since vomiting may cause seizures, additional burns to the throat, or pneumonia.

• Ipecac should be used cautiously if the poisoned patient is losing consciousness, has no gag reflex, is in shock, is having seizures, or has heart disease.

• Muscle and heart disorders, and at least one death, have been reported as a result of the chronic use of ipecac by young women who were using it to induce vomiting in order to lose weight.

• Ipecac is available over-the-counter (non-prescription), and can be purchased from most pharmacies. Mothers should have a one-ounce bottle of ipecac for each child under five years of age in the house. Always call a physician, emergency room, or poison control center for instructions BEFORE administering ipecac.

• Be sure to tell your doctor if the overdose or poisoning victim is pregnant. Although ipecac appears to be safe, extensive studies in pregnant women have not yet been completed.

Ircon—see iron supplements

Iromal—see iron supplements

iron supplements

BRAND NAMES (Manufacturers)
Feco-T* (Blaine)
Feosol* (Menley & James)
Feostat* (O'Neal)
Fergon* (Winthrop-Breon)
Fer-In-Sol* (Mead Johnson)

Fer-Iron* (Bay)
Fero-Gradumet* (Abbott)
Ferospace* (Hudson)
Ferralet* (Mission)
Ferralyn Lanacaps* (Lannett)
ferrous fumarate* (various manufacturers)
ferrous gluconate* (various manufacturers)
ferrous sulfate* (various manufacturers)
Fumasorb* (Milhance)
Fumerin⁺ (Laser)
Hematinic* (Mallard)
Hemocyte* (U.S. Chemical)
Ircon* (Key)
Iromal* (Mallard)
Mol-Iron* (Schering)
Palmiron* (Hauck)
Simron* (Merrell Dow)
Slow Fe* (Ciba)
*Note that the products listed above are available over-the-counter (non-prescription).

TYPE OF DRUG
Iron supplement

INGREDIENTS
iron as the fumarate, gluconate, or sulfate salt

DOSAGE FORMS
Tablets; sustained-release tablets; chewable tablets; capsules; sustained-release capsules; liquid; syrup; elixir; and suspension (in various strengths)

STORAGE
Iron supplements should be stored at room temperature in a tightly closed container. This medication should never be frozen.

USES

Iron is an essential mineral. Iron supplements are used to prevent iron deficiency due to such causes as blood loss, pregnancy, or malnutrition.

TREATMENT

In order to increase the absorption of the iron, these supplements should be taken on an empty stomach with a full glass of water or juice, one hour before or two hours after a meal. If iron upsets your stomach, however, check with your doctor to see if you can take it with food.

In order to prevent iron stains on your teeth, dilute the liquid forms in water or juice, use a straw, or place the dose on the back of your tongue.

The sustained-release tablets and capsules should be swallowed whole. Breaking, chewing, or crushing these tablets or capsules destroys their sustained-release activity, and possibly increases the side effects.

Shake the bottle of the suspension form of this medication thoroughly, just before measuring each dose. The contents tend to settle on the bottom of the bottle, so it must be shaken to disperse the iron and equalize the doses. Each dose of the liquid and suspension forms of iron should be measured carefully, with a specially designed, 5 ml measuring spoon or the dropper provided. An ordinary kitchen teaspoon is not accurate enough.

If you miss a dose of this medication, take the missed dose as soon as possible, unless it is almost time for the next dose. In that case, do not take the missed dose at all; just return to your regular dosing schedule. Do not double the next dose.

SIDE EFFECTS

Minor. Abdominal cramps; constipation; diarrhea; heartburn; nausea; and vomiting. These side effects should disappear in several days, as your body adjusts to the medication.

Iron can turn your stools black; this is the result of unabsorbed iron and is a harmless effect.

In order to relieve constipation, increase the amount of fiber in your diet (bran, salads, fresh fruits and vegetables), exercise, and drink more water (unless your doctor directs you to do otherwise).

Major. Tell your doctor about any side effects that are persistent or particularly bothersome. IT IS ESPECIALLY IMPORTANT TO TELL YOUR DOCTOR about bloody or tarry stools; bluish-colored lips, fingernails, or palms of hands; chest pain; clammy skin; drowsiness; palpitations; severe abdominal pain; or unusual weakness.

INTERACTIONS

1. Alcohol can increase the body's storage of iron, leading to serious side effects.

2. Antacids, eggs, milk products, tea, and whole-grain breads and cereals decrease the absorption of iron from the gastrointestinal tract. The dose of iron should therefore be taken one hour before, or two hours after, these foods.

3. Iron can decrease the absorption of tetracycline, leading to decreased effectiveness. Your doctor should be aware of it if you are taking both of these medications.

WARNINGS

- Tell your doctor about unusual or allergic reactions you have had to any medications, especially to iron products.
- Before starting to take this medication, be sure to tell your doctor if you now have, or if you have ever had, infections, inflammation of the gastrointestinal tract, iron overload, liver disease, pancreatitis, or peptic ulcers.

MONEY-SAVING TIP

If you are given a prescription for an iron supplement, ask your doctor if you could use one of the many available over-the-counter brands instead.

Ismelin—see guanethidine

Iso-Bid—see isosorbide dinitrate

Isoclor—see pseudoephedrine and chlorpheniramine combination

Isoclor Timesules—see pseudoephedrine and chlorpheniramine combination

---

isoetharine

BRAND NAMES (Manufacturers)
Arm-A-Med (Armour)

Beta-2 (Nephron)
Bronkometer (Winthrop-Breon)
Bronkosol (Winthrop-Breon)
Dey-Dose Isoetharine (Dey)
Dey-Lute Isoetharine (Dey)
Dispos-a-Med (Parke-Davis)
isoetharine hydrochloride (various manufacturers)

TYPE OF DRUG

Bronchodilator

INGREDIENT

isoetharine as the hydrochloride salt

DOSAGE FORMS

Solutions for nebulization (0.06%, 0.08%, 0.1%,
0.125%, 0.17%, 0.2%, 0.25%, 0.5%, and 1%)
Aerosol (0.61%)

STORAGE

Isoetharine solution should be stored at room temperature in tightly closed, light-resistant containers. The solution should not be used if it turns brown or contains particles; this indicates that the medication is no longer potent. The inhalation aerosol form of this medication should be stored at room temperature, away from direct sunlight and excessive heat—the contents are pressurized and can explode if heated. The container should NEVER be punctured or broken.

USES

Isoetharine is used to relieve wheezing and shortness of breath caused by lung diseases such as asthma, bronchitis, and emphysema. This drug acts directly on the muscles of the bronchi (breathing tubes) to relieve bronchospasm (muscle contractions of the bronchi), which in turn reduces airway resistance, and allows air to move more freely to and from the lungs.

TREATMENT

The aerosol form of isoetharine comes packaged with instructions. Before using this medication, be sure you understand all the directions. If you have any questions, check with your doctor. To obtain the maximum effect, wait at least one minute after inhaling the first dose before inhaling a second dose (if a second dose is needed). Do not take more than two inhalations at any one time (unless your doctor directs you to do so).

If your breathing difficulties do not improve after using this medication, or if your condition worsens, contact your doctor or go to an emergency room immediately.

If you are using the solution form of this medication in a nebulizer, make sure you completely understand how to use it. Check with your doctor if you have any questions.

SIDE EFFECTS

Minor. Difficulty sleeping; dizziness; headache; irritability; nausea; nervousness; or weakness. These side effects should disappear in several days, as your body adjusts to the medication.

If you feel dizzy or light-headed, sit or lie down awhile; change positions slowly, and be careful on stairs.

Major. Tell your doctor about any side effects that are persistent or particularly bothersome. IT IS ESPECIALLY IMPORTANT TO TELL YOUR DOCTOR about chest pains or palpitations.

INTERACTIONS

Beta-adrenergic blockers (atenolol, metoprolol, nadolol, pindolol, propranolol, and timolol) can decrease the effectiveness of isoetharine. TELL YOUR DOCTOR if you are already taking a medication of this type.

WARNINGS

• Tell your doctor about unusual or allergic reactions you have had to medications, especially to isoetharine or to any related drug (such as albuterol, amphetamine, ephedrine, epinephrine, isoproterenol, metaproterenol, norepinephrine, phenylephrine, phenylpropanolamine, pseudoephedrine, or terbutaline).

• Before starting to take this medication, be sure to tell your doctor if you now have, or if you have ever had, heart disease, high blood pressure, or thyroid disease.

• Try to avoid contact of this medication with your eyes. Exposure to the eyes can cause irritation and redness.

• Be sure to tell your doctor if you are pregnant. Although isoetharine appears to be safe during pregnancy, extensive studies in humans have not yet been completed.

Also, tell your doctor if you are breastfeeding an infant. It is not known whether or not isoetharine passes into breast milk.

MONEY-SAVING TIP

Save the inhaler piece from the aerosol container. Refill units, which are less expensive, are available.

isoetharine hydrochloride—see isoetharine

Isogard—see isosorbide dinitrate

Isollyl—see aspirin, caffeine, and butalbital combination

Isollyl with Codeine—see aspirin, caffeine, butalbital, and codeine combination

Isonate—see isosorbide dinitrate

---

isoniazid

BRAND NAMES (Manufacturers)
isoniazid (various manufacturers)
Laniazid (Lannett)
Nydrazid (Squibb)
Teebaconin (CMC)
TYPE OF DRUG
Anti-tubercular
INGREDIENT
isoniazid
DOSAGE FORMS
Tablets (50 mg, 100 mg, and 300 mg)
Oral syrup (50 mg per 5 ml teaspoonful)
STORAGE
Isoniazid tablets and oral syrup should be stored at room temperature in tightly closed, light-resistant containers. This medication should never be frozen.

USES

Isoniazid is used to prevent and treat tuberculosis. It acts by severely injuring the cell walls of tuberculosis bacteria, thereby preventing them from growing and multiplying.

TREATMENT

In order to avoid stomach irritation, you can take isoniazid with food or a full glass of water or milk (unless your doctor directs you to do otherwise).

Antacids prevent the absorption of isoniazid from the gastrointestinal tract, so they should not be taken within an hour of a dose of isoniazid.

Each dose of the oral syrup form of this medication should be measured carefully, with a specially designed, 5 ml measuring spoon. An ordinary kitchen teaspoon is not accurate enough.

It is important to continue to take this medication for the entire time prescribed by your doctor, even if your symptoms disappear before the end of that period. If you stop taking the drug too soon, resistant bacteria are given a chance to continue growing, and your infection could recur.

Try not to miss any doses of this medication. If you do miss a dose, take the missed dose as soon as possible, unless it is almost time for the next dose. In that case, don't take the missed dose at all; just return to your regular dosing schedule. Do not double the next dose.

SIDE EFFECTS

Minor. Abdominal pain; dizziness; heartburn; nausea; and vomiting. These side effects should disappear in several days, as your body adjusts to the medication.

If you feel dizzy, sit or lie down awhile; get up slowly, and be careful on stairs.

Major. Tell your doctor about any side effects that are persistent or particularly bothersome. IT IS ESPECIALLY IMPORTANT TO TELL YOUR DOCTOR about blurred vision; unusual bleeding or bruising; breast enlargement (in both sexes); chills; darkening of the urine; eye pain; fever; malaise; memory impairment; numbness or tingling in the fingers or toes; rash; vision changes; weakness; or yellowing of the eyes or skin.

Your doctor may want to prescribe vitamin B_6 (pyridoxine) to prevent the numbness and tingling.

INTERACTIONS

Isoniazid interacts with several other types of drugs.

1. Concurrent use of isoniazid and alcohol can lead to decreased effectiveness of isoniazid, and increased side effects on the liver.

2. The combination of isoniazid and cycloserine can result in dizziness or drowsiness.

3. The combination of isoniazid and disulfiram can lead to dizziness, loss of coordination, irritability, and insomnia.

4. Isoniazid can increase the blood levels of phenytoin and carbamazepine, which can lead to an increase in side effects.

5. In combination, rifampin and isoniazid can increase the risk of liver damage.

6. The effectiveness of isoniazid may be decreased when administered with adrenocorticosteroids (cortisone-like medicines).

7. The side effects of benzodiazepine tranquilizers may be increased by isoniazid.

Before starting to take isoniazid, BE SURE TO TELL YOUR DOCTOR if you are already taking any of the medications listed above.

WARNINGS

• Tell your doctor about unusual or allergic reactions you have had to any medications, especially to isoniazid, ethionamide, pyrazinamide, or niacin (vitamin B_3).

• Before starting to take this medication, be sure to tell your doctor if you now have, or if you have ever had, alcoholism, kidney disease, liver disease, or seizures.

• If this drug makes you dizzy, avoid tasks that require alertness, such as driving a car or operating potentially dangerous equipment.

• Your doctor may want you to have periodic eye examinations while taking this medication, especially if you begin to have visual symptoms.

• Isoniazid can interact with several foods (fish-skipjack, tuna, yeast extracts, sauerkraut juice, sausages, and cheese), leading to severe reactions. You should therefore avoid eating these foods while being treated with isoniazid.

• Diabetics using Clinitest urine glucose tests may get erroneously high sugar readings while they are taking isoniazid. Temporarily changing to Clinistix or Tes-Tape urine tests avoids this problem.

• Be sure to tell your doctor if you are pregnant. Although isoniazid appears to be safe during pregnancy, it does cross the placenta. Extensive studies in pregnant women have not yet been completed. Also, tell your doctor if you are breastfeeding an infant. Small amounts of isoniazid pass into breast milk.

Isopro T.D. — see prochlorperazine and isopropamide combination

Isoptin — see verapamil

Isopto Carpine — see pilocarpine (ophthalmic)

Isopto Cetamide — see sodium sulfacetamide (ophthalmic)

Isordil Tembids — see isosorbide dinitrate

Isordil Titradose — see isosorbide dinitrate

---

isosorbide dinitrate

BRAND NAMES (Manufacturers)
Dilatrate-SR (Reed & Carnrick)
Iso-Bid (Geriatric)
Isogard (Vangard)
Isonate (Major)
Isordil Tembids (Ives)
Isordil Titradose (Ives)
isosorbide dinitrate (various manufacturers)
Isotrate Timecelles (Hauck)
Onset (Bock)
Sorate (Trimen)
Sorbide T.D. (Mayrand)
Sorbitrate (Stuart)
Sorbitrate SA (Stuart)

TYPE OF DRUG
Anti-anginal
INGREDIENT
isosorbide dinitrate
DOSAGE FORMS
Tablets (5 mg, 10 mg, 20 mg, 30 mg, and 40 mg)
Chewable tablets (5 mg and 10 mg)
Sublingual tablets (2.5 mg, 5 mg, and 10 mg)
Sustained-release tablets (40 mg)
Capsules (40 mg)
Sustained-release capsules (40 mg)
STORAGE
Isosorbide dinitrate tablets and capsules should be stored in a cool, dry place. This medication loses potency when exposed to heat or moisture.

USES
Isosorbide dinitrate is a vasodilator that relaxes the muscles of the blood vessels, leading to an increase in the oxygen supply to the heart. It is used (chewable and sublingual tablets) to relieve or (oral tablets and capsules) to prevent chest pain (angina). The chewable and sublingual tablets act quickly—they can be used to relieve chest pain after it has begun. The oral tablets and capsules do not act quickly—they are used only to prevent angina attacks.

TREATMENT
Take the chewable or sublingual forms of this medication at the first sign of an angina attack. DO NOT WAIT for the attack to become severe. Then sit down. These tablets are absorbed more completely through the lining of the mouth than from the stomach. Your mouth should be empty when you take these tablets. Do not eat, drink, or smoke with a tablet in your mouth. If the pain of an attack continues, you can take another tablet after ten minutes, and a third tablet after another ten minutes. If three tablets provide no relief within 30 minutes, CONTACT YOUR DOCTOR IMMEDIATELY or go to the nearest hospital.

The chewable tablet should be chewed for at least two minutes before swallowing.

Place the sublingual tablet under the tongue or against the cheek and allow it to dissolve—DO NOT CHEW OR

SWALLOW IT. Do not swallow until the drug is dissolved, and do not rinse your mouth for several minutes (this gives a greater opportunity for the drug to be absorbed through the lining of the mouth).

The regular tablets and capsules and the sustained-release forms of this medication should be taken with a full glass of water on an empty stomach. The sustained-release forms should be swallowed whole. Breaking, crushing, or chewing these tablets or capsules destroys their sustained-release activity and possibly increases the side effects.

If you are taking this medication on a regular schedule, try not to miss any doses. If you do miss a dose, however, take the missed dose as soon as possible, unless it is within two hours of the next dose (or six hours for the sustained-release forms). In that case, don't take the missed dose at all; just return to your regular dosage schedule. Do not double the next dose.

SIDE EFFECTS

Minor. Dizziness; flushing; headache; light-headedness; nausea; and vomiting. These side effects should disappear in several days, as your body adjusts to the medication.

If you feel dizzy or light-headed, sit or lie down awhile; get up slowly, and be careful on stairs. To avoid dizziness or light-headedness when you stand, contract and relax the muscles of your legs for a few moments before rising. Do this by pushing one foot against the floor while raising the other foot slightly, alternating feet so that you are "pumping" your legs in a pedaling motion.

Acetaminophen may help relieve headaches caused by this medication.

Major. Tell your doctor about any side effects that are persistent or particularly bothersome. IT IS ESPECIALLY IMPORTANT TO TELL YOUR DOCTOR about fainting spells; palpitations; rash; restlessness; sweating; or unusual weakness.

INTERACTIONS

Isosorbide dinitrate, in combination with alcohol, can lead to dizziness and fainting. Over-the-counter (non-prescription) sinus, allergy, cough, cold, asthma, and diet products can block the anti-angina effects of isosorbide dinitrate. CHECK WITH YOUR DOCTOR OR PHARMACIST before taking any of these medications.

WARNINGS

• Tell your doctor about unusual or allergic reactions you have had to medications, especially to isosorbide dinitrate or to any other nitrate drugs (such as nitroglycerin).

• Before starting to take this medication, tell your doctor if you now have, or if you have ever had, severe anemia, glaucoma, a recent heart attack, or thyroid disease.

• Before using this medication to relieve chest pain, be certain that the pain arises from the heart and is not due to a muscle spasm or to indigestion. If your chest pain is not relieved by use of this drug, or if pain arises from a different location or differs in severity, CONSULT YOUR DOCTOR IMMEDIATELY.

• If this drug makes you dizzy or light-headed, do not take part in any activity that requires alertness, such as driving a car or operating potentially dangerous equipment.

• Before having any surgery or other medical or dental treament, be sure your doctor or dentist knows that you are taking this medication.

• Tolerance may develop to this medication. If the drug begins to lose its effectiveness, contact your doctor.

• Isosorbide dinitrate should not be discontinued unless you first consult your doctor. Stopping the drug abruptly may lead to further chest pain. Your doctor may therefore want to decrease your dosage gradually.

• If you have frequent diarrhea, you may not be absorbing the sustained-release form of this medication. Discuss this with your doctor.

• Be sure to tell your doctor if you are pregnant. Although this drug appears to be safe, extensive studies in pregnant women have not yet been completed. Also, tell your doctor if you are breastfeeding an infant. It is not known whether or not isosorbide dinitrate passes into breast milk.

Isotrate Timecelles—see isosorbide dinitrate

isotretinoin

BRAND NAME (Manufacturer)
Accutane (Roche)
TYPE OF DRUG
Acne preparation
INGREDIENT
isotretinoin
DOSAGE FORM
Capsules (10 mg)
STORAGE
Isotretinoin should be stored at room temperature in a tightly closed, light-resistant container.

USES

This medication is used to treat severe, cystic acne. It is not clearly understood how isotretinoin works, but it decreases the production of sebum (secretions) and dries up the acne lesions.

TREATMENT

An information leaflet is packaged with this product. Be sure to read it carefully.

Isotretinoin should be taken with meals to obtain the maximum benefit.

It may take one to two months before the maximum effects of this medication are observed.

If you miss a dose of this medication, take the missed dose as soon as possible, then return to your regular dosing schedule. However, if you do not remember until it is time for your next dose, double the next dose, then return to your regular dosing schedule.

SIDE EFFECTS

Minor. Changes in skin color; dry lips and mouth; fatigue; fluid retention; headache; indigestion; inflammation of the eyelids; inflammation of the lips; muscle pain; rash; and thinning of the hair. These side effects should disappear in several weeks, as your body adjusts to the medication.

You may notice a worsening of your acne for the first few days of treatment.

To relieve mouth dryness, chew sugarless gum, or suck on ice chips or a piece of hard candy.

This medication can cause an increased sensitivity to sunlight. Avoid prolonged exposure to sunlight and sunlamps. Wear protective clothing and sunglasses, and use an effective sunscreen.

Major. Tell your doctor about any side effects that are persistent or particularly bothersome. IT IS ESPECIALLY IMPORTANT TO TELL YOUR DOCTOR about black, tarry stools; bruising; burning or tingling sensation of the skin; changes in the menstrual cycle; dizziness; hives; peeling of the palms and soles; visual disturbances; or weight loss.

INTERACTIONS

The concurrent use of alcohol and isotretinoin can lead to an increase in blood lipid (fat) levels, which can be dangerous. Vitamin A and isotretinoin can result in additive toxic effects.

WARNINGS

• Tell your doctor about unusual or allergic reactions you have had to any medications, especially to isotretinoin, vitamin A, or the preservative parabens.

• Before starting to take this medication, tell your doctor if you now have, or if you have ever had, diabetes mellitus or hyperlipidemia (high blood lipid levels).

• Be sure to tell your doctor if you are pregnant. Isotretinoin has been shown to cause birth defects in humans. An effective form of birth control should be used by women of child-bearing potential while they are taking this drug, and for at least one month after they stop taking it. Also, tell your doctor if you are breastfeeding an infant. It is not known whether or not this drug passes into breast milk.

---

isoxsuprine

BRAND NAMES (Manufacturers)
isoxsuprine hydrochloride (various manufacturers)
Vasodilan (Mead Johnson)

Voxsuprine (Major)
TYPE OF DRUG
Vasodilator
INGREDIENT
isoxsuprine as the hydrochloride salt
DOSAGE FORM
Tablets (10 mg and 20 mg)
STORAGE
Isoxsuprine should be stored at room temperature, in a tightly closed container.

USES
Isoxsuprine is used to relieve the symptoms of stroke or peripheral vascular disease (poor circulation). It works directly on the muscles of the blood vessels to cause dilation.

TREATMENT
In order to avoid stomach irritation, you can take isoxsuprine with food, milk, or antacids (unless your doctor directs you to do otherwise).

If you miss a dose of this medication, take the missed dose as soon as possible, unless it is almost time for the next dose. In that case, do not take the missed dose at all; just return to your regular dosing schedule. Do not double the next dose.

SIDE EFFECTS
Minor. Dizziness; nausea; nervousness; stomach upset; and vomiting. These side effects should disappear as your body adjusts to the medication.

If you feel dizzy, sit or lie down awhile; get up slowly, and be careful on stairs.

Major. Tell your doctor about any side effects that are persistent or particularly bothersome. IT IS ESPECIALLY IMPORTANT TO TELL YOUR DOCTOR about chest pain; fainting; flushing; palpitations; skin rash; or unusual weakness.

INTERACTIONS
Isoxsuprine does not interact with other medications, if it is used according to directions.

WARNINGS

- Tell your doctor about unusual or allergic reactions you have had to any medications, especially to isoxsuprine.
- Before starting to take this medication, be sure to tell your doctor if you now have, or if you have ever had, bleeding disorders, glaucoma, heart disease, or stroke.
- Before having any surgery or other medical or dental treatment, be sure your doctor or dentist knows that you are taking this medication
- If this medication makes you dizzy, you should avoid activities that require alertness, such as driving a car or operating potentially dangerous equipment.
- Cigarette smoking decreases the effectiveness of this medication (nicotine constricts the blood vessels).
- Be sure to tell your doctor if you are pregnant. Although isoxsuprine appears to be safe during pregnancy, extensive studies in humans have not yet been completed. To avoid bleeding complications, this medication should not be taken by a woman who has just given birth. Also, tell your doctor if you are breastfeeding an infant. It is not known whether or not isoxsuprine passes into breast milk.

isoxsuprine hydrochloride—see isoxsuprine

Janimine—see imipramine

Kaochlor—see potassium chloride

Kaon—see potassium chloride

Karidium—see sodium fluoride

Karigel—see sodium fluoride

Kari-Rinse—see sodium fluoride

Kato—see potassium chloride

Kay Ciel—see potassium chloride

KEFF—see potassium chloride

Keflex—see cephalexin

Kenac—see triamcinolone (topical)

Kenacort—see triamcinolone (systemic)

Kenalog—see triamcinolone (topical)

Kenalog-H—see triamcinolone (topical)

ketoconazole

BRAND NAME (Manufacturer)
Nizoral (Janssen)
TYPE OF DRUG
Anti-fungal
INGREDIENT
ketoconazole
DOSAGE FORM
Tablets (200 mg)
STORAGE
Ketoconazole should be stored at room temperature in a
tightly closed container.

USES

This medication is used to treat fungal infections of the
skin, throat, urinary tract, or lung. Ketoconazole kills the
fungus organisms by interfering with their production of
essential nutrients.

TREATMENT

In order to prevent stomach irritation, you can take ketoconazole with food or milk (unless your doctor directs you
to do otherwise).

Antacids prevent the absorption of ketoconazole from
the gastrointestinal tract. Therefore, at least two hours
should separate doses of these two types of medication.

Try not to miss any doses of this medication. If you do
miss a dose, take the missed dose as soon as possible, un-

less it is almost time for the next dose. In that case, take the missed dose immediately, take the following dose in about 12 hours, then continue with your regular dosing schedule.

It is important to continue taking this medication for the entire time prescribed by your doctor (usually 10 to 14 days, but up to six months for some skin infections), even if your symptoms improve. If you stop taking this medication too soon, your infection could recur.

SIDE EFFECTS

Minor. Diarrhea; dizziness; drowsiness; headache; nausea; sensitivity of the eyes to sunlight; stomach upset; and vomiting. These side effects should disappear in several days, as your body adjusts to the medication.

If you feel dizzy, sit or lie down awhile; get up slowly, and be careful on stairs.

In order to relieve sensitivity of the eyes to light, wear sunglasses and avoid exposure to bright lights.

Major. Tell your doctor about any side effects that are persistent or particularly bothersome. IT IS ESPECIALLY IMPORTANT TO TELL YOUR DOCTOR about breast tenderness (in both sexes); chills; fever; impotence; itching; or yellowing of the eyes or skin.

INTERACTIONS

If you are also taking cimetidine or ranitidine, you should know that they can decrease the absorption of ketoconazole from the gastrointestinal tract. You should therefore take ketoconazole at least two hours before either of these medications. DISCUSS THIS WITH YOUR DOCTOR.

WARNINGS

• Tell your doctor about unusual or allergic reactions you have had to any medications, especially to ketoconazole.
• Before you start to take ketoconazole, be sure to tell your doctor if you now have, or if you have ever had, achlorhydria (reduced stomach acid) or liver disease.
• If this drug makes you dizzy or drowsy, avoid taking part in any activity that requires alertness, such as driving a car or operating potentially dangerous equipment.
• Different types of infections require different durations

of treatment before improvement can be expected. Ask your doctor how long treatment of your infection will take.
● If the symptoms of your infection do not improve within the expected period after starting this medication, or if the condition becomes worse, CHECK WITH YOUR DOCTOR. Ketoconazole may not be effective for your particular infection.
● Ketoconazole has been prescribed for your current infection only. It may not be effective for another infection later on, or one that someone else has. You should not give your medication to other people, or use it for other infections unless your doctor specifically directs you to do so.
● Be sure to tell your doctor if you are pregnant. Birth defects have been reported in animals whose mothers received large doses of ketoconazole during pregnancy. Extensive studies have not yet been completed in humans. Also, tell your doctor if you are breastfeeding an infant. Small amounts of ketoconazole pass into breast milk and can cause liver problems in nursing infants.

Klavikordal—see nitroglycerin (systemic)

K-Lor—see potassium chloride

Klor-Con—see potassium chloride

Klorvess—see potassium chloride

Klotrix—see potassium chloride

K-Lyte-Cl—see potassium chloride

Korostatin—see nystatin

Kronofed-A Kronocaps—see pseudoephedrine and chlorpheniramine combination

Kronofed-A Jr.—see pseudoephedrine and chlorpheniramine combination

K-Tab—see potassium chloride

Ku-Zyme HP—see pancrelipase

Kwell—see lindane

LaBID—see theophylline

Laniazid—see isoniazid

Lanophyllin—see theophylline

Lanophyllin-GG—see theophylline and guaifenesin combination

Lanorinal—see aspirin, caffeine, and butalbital combination

Lanoxicaps—see digoxin

Lanoxin—see digoxin

Lanvisone—see hydrocortisone and iodochlorhydroxyquin combination (topical)

Larodopa—see levodopa

Larotid—see amoxicillin

Lasix—see furosemide

Ledercillin VK—see penicillin VK

Lemiserp—see reserpine

Lentard—see insulin

---

leucovorin

BRAND NAME (Manufacturer)
Wellcovorin (Burroughs Wellcome)
TYPE OF DRUG
Folic acid analog

INGREDIENT
leucovorin as the calcium salt (folinic acid or citrovorum factor)
DOSAGE FORM
Tablets (5 mg and 25 mg)
STORAGE
Leucovorin should be stored at room temperature in a tightly closed, light-resistant container.

USES
Leucovorin is a folic acid derivative that is used to prevent or treat some of the side effects of the folic acid antagonist, methotrexate. It is also used to correct megaloblastic (folic-acid deficiency) anemia.

TREATMENT
Leucovorin tablets can be taken either on an empty stomach or with food or milk (as directed by your doctor).

If you are taking leucovorin to prevent some of the side effects of methotrexate, it is very important that you take this medication EXACTLY as directed.

If you miss a dose of this medication, take the missed dose immediately, then return to your regular dosing schedule.

SIDE EFFECTS
Minor. None, at the dosages normally prescribed.
Major. Tell your doctor about any side effects that are persistent or particularly bothersome. IT IS ESPECIALLY IMPORTANT TO TELL YOUR DOCTOR about hives, itching, rash, or shortness of breath.

INTERACTIONS
Leucovorin interacts with several other medications
1. It can decrease the effectiveness of phenytoin.
2. Phenytoin, primidone, p-aminosalicylic acid, and sulfasalazine can decrease the blood levels and effectiveness of leucovorin.
BE SURE TO TELL YOUR DOCTOR if you are already taking any of these medications.

WARNINGS

● Tell your doctor about unusual or allergic reactions you have had to any medications, especially to leucovorin or folic acid.

● Before starting to take this medication, be sure to tell your doctor if you now have, or if you have ever had, fluid accumulation in the lungs or chest cavity, kidney disease, or vitamin B_{12} deficiency (pernicious anemia).

● Be sure to tell your doctor if you are pregnant. Although leucovorin appears to be safe during pregnancy, extensive studies in humans have not yet been completed. Also, tell your doctor if you are breastfeeding an infant. It is not known whether or not leucovorin passes into breast milk.

Leukeran—see chlorambucil

___

levodopa

BRAND NAMES (Manufacturers)
Dopar (Norwich Eaton)
Larodopa (Roche)
levodopa (various manufacturers)
TYPE OF DRUG
Anti-parkinson
INGREDIENT
levodopa
DOSAGE FORMS
Tablets (100 mg, 250 mg, and 500 mg)
Capsules (100 mg, 250 mg, and 500 mg)
STORAGE
Levodopa tablets and capsules should be stored at room temperature in tightly closed, light-resistant containers.

USES

Levodopa is used to treat the symptoms of Parkinson's disease. It is converted in the body to dopamine, a chemical in the brain that is diminished in patients with Parkinson's disease.

TREATMENT

In order to avoid stomach irritation, you can take levodopa with food or with a full glass of milk or water (unless your doctor directs you to do otherwise). These tablets and capsules should be swallowed whole for maximum effectiveness—do not crush, break, or chew them.

You may not observe significant benefit from this drug for two to three weeks after starting to take it.

If you miss a dose of this medication, take the missed dose as soon as possible, unless it is within two hours of the next scheduled dose. In that case, do not take the missed dose at all; just return to your regular dosing schedule. Do not double the next dose.

SIDE EFFECTS

Minor. Abdominal pain; anxiety; bitter taste in the mouth; burning sensation of the tongue; constipation; diarrhea; dizziness; dry mouth; fatigue; flushing; gas; increased hand tremors; headache; hiccups; hoarseness; increased sexual interest; insomnia; loss of appetite; nausea; offensive body odor; salivation; increased sweating; vision changes; vomiting; weakness; and weight gain. These side effects should disappear in several weeks, as your body adjusts to the medication.

To relieve constipation, increase the amount of fiber in your diet (bran, salads, fresh fruits and vegetables, and whole-grain breads), drink more water, and exercise (unless your doctor directs you to do otherwise).

If you feel dizzy, sit or lie down awhile; get up slowly, and be careful on stairs.

To relieve mouth dryness, chew sugarless gum, or suck on ice chips or a piece of hard candy.

Levodopa can cause a darkening of your urine or sweat. This is a harmless effect.

Major. Tell your doctor about any side effects that are persistent or particularly bothersome. IT IS ESPECIALLY IMPORTANT TO TELL YOUR DOCTOR about confusion; convulsions; bloody or black, tarry stools; depression; fainting; false sense of well-being; loss of hair; loss of coordination; nightmares; painful erection; palpitations; rapid weight gain (3 to 5 pounds within a week); skin rash; visual disturbances; or unusual weakness.

INTERACTIONS

Levodopa interacts with several other types of medication.

1. The dosage of anti-hypertensive drugs and oral anti-diabetic drugs may require adjustment when levodopa is started.

2. The effectiveness of levodopa may be decreased by benzodiazepine tranquilizers, phenothiazine tranquilizers, haloperidol, thiothixene, phenytoin, papaverine, and reserpine.

3. Methyldopa can increase or decrease the side effects of levodopa.

4. Use of levodopa and a monoamine oxidase (MAO) inhibitor within 14 days of each other can lead to severe side effects.

5. Levodopa can increase the side effects of tricyclic antidepressants, ephedrine, and amphetamines.

6. Antacids may alter the absorption of levodopa from the gastrointestinal tract.

7. Pyridoxine (vitamin B_6) can decrease the effectiveness of levodopa.

BE SURE TO TELL YOUR DOCTOR if you are already taking any of the medications listed above.

WARNINGS

● Tell your doctor about unusual or allergic reactions you have had to any medications, especially to levodopa.

● Before starting to take this medication, be sure to tell your doctor if you now have, or if you have ever had, asthma; diabetes mellitus (sugar diabetes); difficulty urinating; epilepsy; glaucoma; heart disease; hormone disorders; kidney disease; liver disease; lung disease; melanoma; mental disorders; or peptic ulcers.

● Some of these products contain F.D. & C. Yellow Dye No. 5 (tartrazine), which can cause allergic-type symptoms (difficulty breathing, faintness, or rash) in certain susceptible individuals.

● If levodopa makes you dizzy or blurs your vision, avoid activities that require alertness, such as driving a car or operating potentially dangerous equipment.

● Before having any surgery or other medical or dental treatment, be sure your doctor or dentist knows that you are taking this medication.

• Levodopa can cause erroneous readings of urine glucose and ketone tests. Diabetic patients should not change their medication dosage, unless they first check with their doctor.

• Pyridoxine (vitamin B$_6$) can decrease the effectiveness of levodopa. Persons taking levodopa should avoid taking this vitamin and should avoid foods rich in pyridoxine (foods that contain it include beans, bacon, avocados, liver, dry skim milk, oatmeal, sweet potatoes, peas, and tuna).

• Be sure to tell your doctor if you are pregnant. Although levodopa appears to be safe in humans, birth defects have been reported in animals whose mothers received large doses during pregnancy. Also, tell your doctor it you are breastfeeding an infant. Levodopa passes into breast milk and can cause side effects in nursing infants.

levodopa and carbidopa combination

BRAND NAME (Manufacturer)
Sinemet (Merck Sharp & Dohme)
TYPE OF DRUG
Anti-parkinson
INGREDIENTS
levodopa and carbidopa
DOSAGE FORM
Tablets (100 mg levodopa and 10 mg or 25 mg carbidopa; 250 mg levodopa and 25 mg carbidopa)
STORAGE
Levodopa and carbidopa combination tablets should be stored at room temperature in a tightly closed, light-resistant container.

USES
This medication is used to treat the symptoms of Parkinson's disease. Levodopa is converted in the body to dopamine, a chemical in the brain that is diminished in patients with Parkinson's disease. Carbidopa increases the amount of dopamine that reaches certain regions of the brain

TREATMENT

In order to prevent stomach irritation, you can take this medication with food or with a full glass of milk or water (unless your doctor directs you to do otherwise).

You may not observe significant benefit from this drug for two to three weeks after starting to take it.

If you miss a dose of this medication, take the missed dose as soon as possible, unless it is within two hours of the next scheduled dose. In that case, do not take the missed dose at all; just return to your regular dosing schedule. Do not double the next dose.

SIDE EFFECTS

Minor. Abdominal pain; agitation; anxiety; bitter taste in the mouth; constipation; diarrhea; dizziness; dry mouth; fatigue; flushing; gas; increased hand tremors; headache; hiccups; hoarseness; increased sexual interest; insomnia; loss of appetite; nausea; offensive body odor; salivation; increased sweating; vision changes; vomiting; and weakness. These side effects should disappear in several weeks, as your body adjusts to the medication.

To relieve constipation, increase the amount of fiber in your diet (bran, salads, fresh fruits and vegetables, and whole-grain breads), drink more water, and exercise (unless your doctor directs you to do otherwise).

If you feel dizzy, sit or lie down awhile; get up slowly, and be careful on stairs.

To relieve mouth dryness, chew sugarless gum, or suck on ice chips or a piece of hard candy.

Levodopa can cause a darkening of your urine or sweat. This is a harmless effect.

Major. Tell your doctor about any side effects that are persistent or particularly bothersome. IT IS ESPECIALLY IMPORTANT TO TELL YOUR DOCTOR about bloody or black, tarry stools; unusual bleeding or bruising; burning sensation of the tongue; confusion; convulsions; difficulty swallowing; difficulty urinating; double vision; fainting; false sense of well-being; grinding of the teeth; hallucinations; involuntary movements; jaw stiffness; loss of hair; loss of balance or coordination; nightmares; numbness; painful erection; palpitations; personality changes; skin rash; tremors; visual disturbances; unusual weakness;

rapid weight gain (three to five pounds within a week); or weight loss.

INTERACTIONS

Levodopa and carbidopa combination interacts with several other types of medication.

1. The dosage of anti-hypertensive drugs and oral anti-diabetic drugs may require adjustment when levodopa is started.

2. The effectiveness of levodopa may be decreased by benzodiazepine tranquilizers, phenothiazine tranquilizers, haloperidol, thiothixene, phenytoin, papaverine, and reserpine.

3. Methyldopa can increase or decrease the side effects of this medication.

4. Use of levodopa and a monoamine oxidase (MAO) inhibitor within 14 days of each other can lead to severe side effects.

5. Levodopa can increase the side effects of tricyclic antidepressants, ephedrine, and amphetamines.

6. Antacids may alter the absorption of levodopa from the gastrointestinal tract.

BE SURE TO TELL YOUR DOCTOR if you are already taking any of the medications listed above.

WARNINGS

• Tell your doctor about unusual or allergic reactions you have had to any medications, especially to levodopa or carbidopa.

• Before starting to take this medication, be sure to tell your doctor if you now have, or if you have ever had, asthma; diabetes mellitus (sugar diabetes); difficulty urinating; epilepsy; glaucoma; heart disease; hormone disorders; kidney disease; liver disease; lung disease; melanoma (a type of skin cancer); mental disorders; or peptic ulcers.

• If levodopa makes you dizzy or blurs your vision, avoid activities that require alertness, such as driving a car or operating potentially dangerous equipment.

• Before having any surgery or other medical or dental treatment, be sure your doctor or dentist knows that you are taking this medication.

• Diabetic patients should know that levodopa and carbidopa combination can cause errors in urine glucose test results. CHECK WITH YOUR DOCTOR before changing your insulin dose.

• Although persons taking levodopa are told to avoid taking vitamin B$_6$ (pyridoxine) and to avoid eating foods rich in this vitamin, it is not necessary for patients taking the levodopa and carbidopa combination to observe this precaution.

• Be sure to tell your doctor if you are pregnant. Although this drug appears to be safe in humans, birth defects have been reported in animals whose mothers received large doses during pregnancy. Also, tell your doctor if you are breastfeeding an infant. Levodopa passes into breast milk and can cause side effects in nursing infants.

Levothroid—see levothyroxine

---

levothyroxine

BRAND NAMES (Manufacturers)
Levothroid (Armour)
Noroxine (Vortech)
Synthroid (Flint)
TYPE OF DRUG
Thyroid hormone
INGREDIENT
levothyroxine as the sodium salt
DOSAGE FORM
Tablets (0.025 mg, 0.05 mg, 0.075 mg, 0.1 mg, 0.125 mg, 0.15 mg, 0.2 mg, and 0.3 mg)
STORAGE
Levothyroxine tablets should be stored at room temperature in a tightly closed, light-resistant container.

USES
Levothyroxine is prescribed to replace natural thyroid hormones that are absent because of a disorder of the thyroid gland. This product is prepared synthetically, but is exactly like the natural hormone produced by the body.

TREATMENT

Levothyroxine tablets should be taken on an empty stomach with a full glass of water. If this medication upsets your stomach, check with your doctor to see if you can take it with food or milk.

In order to get used to taking this medication, try to take it at the same time each day. Try not to miss any doses. If you do miss a dose of this medication, take it as soon as you remember, unless it is almost time for the next dose. In that case, do not take the missed dose at all, just return to your regular dosing schedule. Do not double the next dose. If you miss more than one or two doses of this medication, check with your doctor.

SIDE EFFECTS

Minor. Constipation; dry, puffy skin; fatigue; headache; listlessness; muscle aches; and weight gain. These side effects should disappear in several days, as your body adjusts to the medication.

To relieve constipation, increase the amount of fiber in your diet (bran, fresh fruits and vegetables, salads, and whole-grain breads) and drink more water (unless your doctor directs you to do otherwise).

Major. Tell your doctor about any side effects that are persistent or particularly bothersome. Most of the major side effects associated with this drug are the result of too large a dose. The dosage of this medication may need to be adjusted if you experience any of the following side effects: chest pain; diarrhea; fever; heat intolerance; insomnia; irritability; leg cramps; menstrual irregularities; nervousness; palpitations; shortness of breath; sweating; trembling; or weight loss. CHECK WITH YOUR DOCTOR.

INTERACTIONS

Levothyroxine interacts with several other types of medications.

1. Dosing requirements for insulin or oral anti-diabetic agents may change when levothyroxine is used.

2. The effects of oral anti-coagulants (blood thinners, such as warfarin) may be increased by levothyroxine, which could lead to bleeding complications.

3. Cholestyramine and colestipol chemically bind

levothyroxine in the gastrointestinal tract, preventing its absorption. Therefore, at least four hours should separate doses of levothyroxine and one of these medications.

4. Estrogens (oral contraceptives) may change dosage requirements for levothyroxine.

5. The side effects of digoxin may be increased by levothyroxine.

6. Phenobarbital may decrease the effects of levothyroxine; but phenytoin, tricyclic anti-depressants, and over-the-counter (non-prescription) allergy, asthma, cough, cold, sinus, and diet medications may increase its side effects. BE SURE TO TELL YOUR DOCTOR if you are already taking any of the medications listed above.

WARNINGS

● Tell your doctor about unusual or allergic reactions you have had to any medications, especially to thyroid hormone or levothyroxine.

● Tell your doctor if you now have, or if you have ever had, angina pectoris; diabetes mellitus (sugar diabetes); heart disease; high blood pressure; kidney disease; or an underactive adrenal or pituitary gland.

● If you have an underactive thyroid gland, you may need to take this medication for life. You should not stop taking it unless you first check with your doctor.

● Before having any surgery or other medical or dental treatment, be sure to tell your doctor or dentist that you are taking levothyroxine.

● Over-the-counter (non-prescription) allergy, asthma, cough, cold, sinus, and diet medications can increase the side effects of levothyroxine. Therefore, check with your doctor or pharmacist before taking ANY of these products.

● Although many thyroid products are on the market, they are not all bioequivalent; that is, they may not all be absorbed into the bloodstream at the same rate or have the same overall activity. DON'T CHANGE BRANDS of this drug without first consulting your doctor or pharmacist to make sure you are receiving an equivalent product.

● Some of these products contain F. D. & C. Yellow Dye No. 5 (tartrazine), which can cause allergic-type reactions (difficulty breathing, fainting, and rash) in certain susceptible individuals.

• Be sure to tell your doctor if you are pregnant. Levothyroxine does not readily cross the placenta, and the drug appears to be safe during pregnancy. However, your dosing requirements of levothyroxine may change during pregnancy.

Librax—see chlordiazepoxide and clidinium combination

Libritabs—see chlordiazepoxide

Librium—see chlordiazepoxide

Lidex—see fluocinonide (topical)

Lidex-E—see fluocinonide (topical)

Limbitrol—see chlordiazepoxide and amitriptyline combination

Limit—see phendimetrazine

---

lindane

BRAND NAMES (Manufacturers)
Kwell (Reed & Carnrick)
lindane (various manufacturers)
Scabene (Stiefel)
TYPE OF DRUG
Pediculocide and scabicide
INGREDIENTS
lindane (formerly known as gamma benzene hexachloride)
DOSAGE FORMS
Cream (1%)
Lotion (1%)
Shampoo (1%)
STORAGE
Lindane cream, lotion, and shampoo should be stored at room temperature in tightly closed containers. This medication should never be frozen.

USES

This medication is used to eliminate crab lice, head lice, and scabies. Lindane is a central nervous system (brain and spinal cord) stimulant, which causes convulsions and death of the parasites (at the dosage generally used, it is not harmful to humans).

TREATMENT

Complete directions for the use of these products are supplied by the manufacturers. Ask your pharmacist for these directions, and follow the instructions carefully.

If you are applying this medication to another person, you should wear plastic or rubber gloves on your hands, in order to avoid absorption of this drug through the skin

The lotion form of this medication should be shaken well before each dose is measured. The contents tend to settle on the bottom of the bottle, so it must be shaken to evenly distribute the medication and equalize the doses.

Be sure to rinse off this product according to the directions. If it is not rinsed off COMPLETELY, too much of the medication will be absorbed.

SIDE EFFECTS

Minor. You may experience a rash or skin irritation when this medication is applied.

Major. Tell your doctor about any side effects that are persistent or particularly bothersome. The serious side effects associated with this medication (clumsiness; unsteadiness; unusual nervousness; restlessness; irritability; vomiting; muscle cramps; convulsions; and palpitations) are due to absorption of this drug through the skin. This should not happen if the product is used according to directions. If you experience any of these symptoms, CONTACT YOUR DOCTOR.

INTERACTIONS

Do not use other skin preparations (lotions, ointments, or oils). They increase the absorption of this product through the skin, which can lead to serious side effects.

WARNINGS

• Tell your doctor about unusual or allergic reactions you

have had to any medications, especially to lindane.
- This product should NOT be used on the face. If you do get lindane in your eyes, it should be flushed out immediately. In order to decrease the amount of drug absorbed through the skin, avoid using this product on any open wounds, cuts, or sores.
- Lice are easily transmitted from one person to another. All family members (and sexual partners) should be carefully examined. Personal items (clothing, towels) should be machine washed using the "hot" temperature cycle, then dried. No unusual cleaning measures are required. Combs, brushes, and other washable items may be soaked in boiling water for one hour.
- After each application you must remove the dead nits (eggs). Use a fine-toothed comb to remove them from your hair, or mix a solution of equal parts of water and vinegar and apply it to the affected area. Rub the solution in well. After several minutes, shampoo with your regular shampoo, then brush your hair. This process should remove all nits.
- Be sure to tell your doctor if you are pregnant. Lindane is absorbed through the skin and may cause central nervous system side effects in the mother and in the developing fetus. Also, tell your doctor if you are breastfeeding an infant. Because it probably passes into breast milk, lindane may cause side effects in nursing infants.

Lioresal—see baclofen

Lioresal DS—see baclofen

liothyronine

BRAND NAME (Manufacturer)
Cytomel (Smith Kline & French)
TYPE OF DRUG
Thyroid hormone
INGREDIENT
liothyronine
DOSAGE FORM
Tablets (5 mcg, 25 mcg, and 50 mcg)

STORAGE
Liothyronine should be stored at room temperature in a tightly closed container.

USES
Liothyronine is a synthetic form of natural thyroid hormone. It has all of the pharmacologic activities of the natural substance. This medication is used to replace thyroid hormone in patients who cannot produce enough of their own

TREATMENT
Liothyronine can be taken either on an empty stomach or with food or a full glass of water or milk, as directed by your doctor.

Because liothyronine is replacing natural thyroid hormone, you may need to take this medication for the rest of your life.

In order for you to become accustomed to taking this medication, try to take it at the same time each day.

If you miss a dose of this medication, take the missed dose as soon as possible, unless it is almost time for the next dose. In that case, do not take the missed dose at all; just return to your regular dosing schedule. Do not double the next dose.

SIDE EFFECTS
Minor. Abdominal cramps; diarrhea; headache; insomnia; and nausea. These side effects should disappear in several days, as your body adjusts to the medication.

Major. Tell your doctor about any side effects that are persistent or particularly bothersome. Most of the serious side effects of this medication are the result of too high a dose—these include chest pain; intolerance to heat; fever; menstrual irregularities; nervousness; palpitations; skin rash; sweating; tremors; and weight loss. CONTACT YOUR DOCTOR if you experience any of these symptoms.

INTERACTIONS
Liothyronine interacts with other types of medication.
1. It can increase the effects of oral anti-coagulants (blood

thinners, such as warfarin), which can lead to bleeding complications.

2. The dosage of insulin or oral anti-diabetic medicines may require adjustment when liothyronine is started.

3. Cholestyramine decreases the absorption of liothyronine from the gastrointestinal tract. Therefore, at least 4 to 5 hours should separate doses of these medications.

4. Liothyronine may increase the side effects of digoxin and tricyclic anti-depressants.

Before starting to take this medication, BE SURE TO TELL YOUR DOCTOR if you are already taking any of the medications listed above.

WARNINGS

• Tell your doctor about unusual or allergic reactions you have had to any medications, especially to liothyronine, thyroid hormone, or levothyroxine.

• Before starting to take this medication, be sure to tell your doctor if you now have, or if you have ever had, an underactive adrenal gland, diabetes mellitus (sugar diabetes), heart or blood vessel disease, or an underactive pituitary gland.

• Before having any surgery or other medical or dental treatment, be sure your doctor or dentist knows that you are taking this medication.

• Do not stop taking this medication unless you first check with your doctor. Stopping this medication may result in a worsening of your condition.

• Do not take any over-the-counter (non-prescription) cough, cold, allergy, asthma, sinus, or diet medication without first checking with your doctor or pharmacist. Some of these products can increase the side effects of liothyronine.

• Be sure to tell your doctor if you are pregnant. Your dosage of liothyronine may need to be adjusted during pregnancy. Also, tell your doctor if you are breastfeeding an infant. Small amounts of liothyronine pass into breast milk.

Lipo-Hepin—see heparin

Lipo-Gantrisin—see sulfonamides

Lipoxide—see chlordiazepoxide

Liquaemin—see heparin

Liquaphylline—see theophylline

Liquid Pred—see prednisone (systemic)

Lithane—see lithium

---

lithium

BRAND NAMES (Manufacturers)
Cibalith-S (Ciba)
Eskalith (Smith Kline & French)
Eskalith CR (Smith Kline & French)
Lithane (Miles Pharmaceutical)
lithium carbonate (various manufacturers)
lithium citrate (various manufacturers)
Lithobid (Ciba)
Lithonate (Rowell)
Lithotabs (Rowell)
TYPE OF DRUG
Anti-manic (mood stabilizer)
INGREDIENT
lithium as either the citrate or carbonate salt
DOSAGE FORMS
Capsules (300 mg)
Tablets (300 mg)
Extended-release tablets (300 mg and 450 mg)
Syrup (300 mg per 5 ml teaspoonful)
STORAGE
Lithium tablets, capsules, and syrup should be stored at room temperature, away from heat and direct sunlight. The syrup should not be frozen. Do not store the medication in the bathroom cabinet, because moisture may cause the breakdown of lithium. Do not keep these medications beyond the expiration date.

USES
Lithium is a medication used to control the manic phase

of manic-depressive illness. Manic-depressive patients often experience unstable emotions ranging from excitement to hostility to depression. The mechanism of lithium's mood-stabilizing effect is unknown, but it appears to work on the central nervous system to control emotions.

TREATMENT

Lithium should be taken exactly as directed by your doctor. The effectiveness of this medication depends upon the amount of lithium in your blood. Therefore, the medication should be taken every day in regularly spaced doses, in order to keep a constant amount of lithium in your blood.

If you miss a dose of this medication, take it as soon as possible. However, if it is within two hours (six hours for extended-release tablets) of your next scheduled dose, skip the missed dose and return to your regular schedule. Do not take more than one dose at a time.

An improvement in your condition may not be observed for up to several weeks after starting this medication.

SIDE EFFECTS

Minor. Diarrhea; increased frequency of urination; increased thirst; nausea; trembling of the hands; drowsiness; weight gain; weakness or tiredness; bloating; and acne.

Major. Blurred vision; clumsiness; confusion; convulsions; difficulty breathing; dizziness; fainting; palpitations; slurred speech; and severe trembling are possible effects of too much drug in the bloodstream. Dry, rough skin; hair loss; hoarseness; swelling of the feet or lower legs; swelling of the neck; unusual sensitivity to the cold; unusual tiredness; and unusual weight gain may be the result of low thyroid function caused by the medication. CHECK WITH YOUR DOCTOR IMMEDIATELY if any of these side effects appear.

INTERACTIONS

Lithium interacts with a number of other drugs.

1. Aminophylline, caffeine, dyphylline, oxtriphylline, and theophylline can increase the elimination of lithium from the body.

2. Diuretics (water pills), especially hydrochlorothiazide, chlorothiazide, chlorthalidone, triamterene and hydrochlorothiazide combination, and furosemide, may cause lithium toxicity by delaying lithium elimination from the body.

3. Chlorpromazine, other phenothiazine tranquilizers, and indomethacin can also slow lithium elimination.

4. Lithium can increase the side effects of haloperidol.

5. Drinking large amounts of caffeine-containing coffees, teas, or colas may reduce the effectiveness of lithium by increasing its elimination from the body through the urine.

BE SURE TO TELL YOUR DOCTOR if you are already taking any of these drugs.

WARNINGS

● Tell your doctor about unusual or allergic reactions you have had to any medications, especially to lithium.

● Tell your doctor if you now have, or if you have ever had, diabetes mellitus, epilepsy, heart disease, kidney disease, Parkinson's disease, or thyroid disease.

● Elderly patients may be more sensitive to lithium's side effects.

● In order to maintain a constant level of lithium in your blood, it is important to drink 2 or 3 quarts of water or other fluid each day, and to not change the amount of salt in your diet, unless your doctor directs you to do so.

● The loss of large amounts of body fluid (from prolonged vomiting or diarrhea, or from heavy sweating due to hot weather, fever, exercise, saunas, or hot baths) can result in increased lithium levels in the blood, which can lead to an increase in side effects.

● The toxic dose of lithium is very close to the therapeutic dose, so it is very important to follow your correct dosing schedule.

● Lithium is not recommended for use during pregnancy, especially during the first three months, because of possible effects on the thyroid and heart of the developing fetus. Be sure to tell your doctor if you are breastfeeding an infant. Lithium also passes into breast milk and may cause side effects in the nursing infant.

lithium carbonate—see lithium

lithium citrate—see lithium

Lithobid—see lithium

Lithonate—see lithium

Lithotabs—see lithium

Lixaminol—see aminophylline

Lixolin—see theophylline

Locoid—see hydrocortisone (topical)

Lodrane—see theophylline

Loestrin—see oral contraceptives

Lofene—see diphenoxylate and atropine

Lomotil—see diphenoxylate and atropine

lomustine

BRAND NAME (Manufacturer)
CeeNU (Bristol)
TYPE OF DRUG
Anti-neoplastic (anti-cancer drug)
INGREDIENT
lomustine
DOSAGE FORM
Capsules (10 mg, 40 mg, and 100 mg)
STORAGE
Lomustine should be stored at room temperature in a tightly closed container.

USES
This medication belongs to a group of drugs known as nitrosourea alkylating agents. It is used to treat a variety of cancers. Lomustine is thought to work by binding to the

rapidly growing cancer cells, preventing their multiplication and growth.

TREATMENT

To help prevent nausea, you should take lomustine on an empty stomach (unless your doctor directs you to do otherwise).

The patient is usually required to take this medication as a single dose once a week. The total weekly dose consists of a number of capsules of different strengths and colors, which are all taken at the same time. The timing of each weekly dose is very important; be sure you completely understand your doctor's instructions on how and when this medication should be taken.

SIDE EFFECTS

Minor. Nausea and vomiting may occur three to six hours after taking a dose of lomustine—these symptoms usually last less than 24 hours. Lomustine also causes hair loss, which is reversible when the medication is stopped.

Major. Tell your doctor about any side effects that are persistent or particularly bothersome. IT IS ESPECIALLY IMPORTANT TO TELL YOUR DOCTOR about unusual bleeding or bruising; chills; confusion; difficult or painful urination; disorientation; fever; uncoordination; itching; loss of appetite; lethargy; mouth sores; sore throat; weakness; or yellowing of the eyes or skin. These side effects may even appear several weeks after the last dose is taken.

INTERACTIONS

Lomustine does not interact with other medications, if it is used according to directions.

WARNINGS

● Tell your doctor about unusual or allergic reactions you have had to any medications, especially to lomustine, carmustine, or streptozocin.

● Before starting to take this medication, be sure to tell your doctor if you now have, or if you have ever had, blood disorders, chronic or recurrent infections, or kidney disease.

● Before having any surgery or other medical or dental

treatment, be sure your doctor or dentist knows that you are taking this medication.

● You should not receive any immunizations or vaccinations while taking this medication. Lomustine blocks the effectiveness of vaccines, which could result in an overwhelming infection if a live virus is administered.

● Lomustine can lower your platelet count, which can decrease your body's ability to form blood clots. You should therefore be especially careful while brushing your teeth, flossing, or using toothpicks, razors, or fingernail scissors. Try to avoid falls and other injuries.

● Lomustine can decrease fertility in both men and women.

● Be sure to tell your doctor if you are pregnant. Lomustine has been reported to cause birth defects in both humans and animals whose mothers received the drug during pregnancy. The risks should be discussed with your doctor. Also, tell your doctor if you are breastfeeding an infant. Small amounts of lomustine pass into breast milk.

Loniten—see minoxidil

Lonox—see diphenoxylate and atropine

Lo-Ovral—see oral contraceptives

---

loperamide

BRAND NAME (Manufacturer)
Imodium (Janssen)
TYPE OF DRUG
Anti-diarrheal
INGREDIENT
loperamide as the hydrochloride salt
DOSAGE FORMS
Capsules (2 mg)
Oral liquid (2 mg per 5 ml teaspoonful)
STORAGE
Loperamide capsules and liquid should be stored at room temperature in tightly closed containers. This medication should never be frozen.

USES

Loperamide is used to treat acute and chronic diarrhea and to reduce the volume of discharge in patients who have ileostomies. It acts by slowing the movement of the gastrointestinal tract and decreasing water and electrolyte (small molecules) passage into the bowel.

TREATMENT

In order to avoid stomach upset, you can take loperamide with food, or with a full glass of water or milk.

The oral liquid form of this medication should be measured carefully, with a special dropper or with a specially designed, 5 ml measuring spoon. An ordinary kitchen teaspoon is not accurate enough.

If you miss a dose of this medication, do not take the missed dose at all; just return to your regular dosing schedule. Do not double the next dose.

SIDE EFFECTS

Minor. Constipation; dizziness; drowsiness; dry mouth; fatigue; loss of appetite; nausea; and vomiting. These side effects should disappear in several days, as your body adjusts to the medication.

Chew sugarless gum, or suck on ice chips or a piece of hard candy, to reduce mouth dryness.

If you feel dizzy or light-headed, sit or lie down awhile; get up from a sitting or lying position slowly, and be careful on stairs.

Major. Tell your doctor about any side effects that are persistent or particularly bothersome. IT IS ESPECIALLY IMPORTANT TO TELL YOUR DOCTOR about abdominal bloating or pain; fever; rash; or sore throat.

INTERACTIONS

Loperamide is not known to interact with any other medications.

WARNINGS

• Tell your doctor about unusual or allergic reactions you have had to any medications, especially to loperamide.
• Tell your doctor if you now have, or if you have ever

had, colitis, diarrhea caused by infectious organisms, drug-induced diarrhea, liver disease, dehydration, or conditions in which constipation must be avoided (such as hemorrhoids, diverticulitis, heart or blood vessel disorders, or blood clotting disorders).

• If this drug makes you dizzy or drowsy, do not take part in any activity that requires alertness, such as driving a car or operating potentially dangerous equipment.

• Before having any surgery or other medical or dental treatment, be sure to tell your doctor or dentist that you are taking this medication.

• Check with your doctor if your diarrhea does not subside within two to three days. Unless your doctor prescribes otherwise, do not take this drug for more than ten days at a time.

• While taking this medication, drink lots of fluids to replace those lost with the diarrhea.

• Be sure to tell your doctor if you are pregnant. Although loperamide has been shown to be safe in animals, the effects of this medication during pregnancy have not yet been thoroughly studied in humans. Also, tell your doctor if you are breastfeeding an infant. It is not known whether or not loperamide passes into breast milk.

Lopid—see gemfibrozil

Lopressor—see metoprolol

Lopurin—see allopurinol

---

lorazepam

BRAND NAME (Manufacturer)
Ativan (Wyeth)
TYPE OF DRUG
Sedative/hypnotic (anti-anxiety medication)
INGREDIENT
lorazepam
DOSAGE FORM
Tablets (0.5 mg, 1 mg, and 2 mg)

STORAGE
This medication should be stored at room temperature in a tightly-closed, light-resistant container.

USES
Lorazepam is prescribed to treat symptoms of anxiety, and anxiety associated with depression. It is not clear exactly how this medicine works, but it may relieve anxiety by acting as a depressant of the central nervous system. This drug is currently used by many people to relieve nervousness. It is effective for this purpose for short periods, but it is important to try to remove the cause of the anxiety as well.

TREATMENT
Lorazepam should be taken exactly as your doctor directs. It can be taken with food or a full glass of water if stomach upset occurs. Do not take this medication with a dose of antacids, since they may retard its absorption.

If you are taking this medication regularly and you miss a dose, take the missed dose immediately, if you remember within an hour of the scheduled time. If more than an hour has passed, skip the dose you missed and wait for the next scheduled dose. Do not double the dose.

SIDE EFFECTS
Minor. Bitter taste in mouth; constipation; depression; diarrhea; dizziness; drowsiness (after a night's sleep); dry mouth; fatigue; flushing; headache; heartburn; excess saliva; loss of appetite; nausea; nervousness; sweating; and vomiting. As your body adjusts to this medicine, these side effects should disappear.

Dry mouth can be relieved by chewing sugarless gum or by sucking on ice chips.

If you feel dizzy, sit or lie down awhile; get up slowly, and be careful on stairs.

Major. Tell your doctor about any side effects that are persistent or particularly bothersome. IT IS ESPECIALLY IMPORTANT TO TELL YOUR DOCTOR about blurred or double vision; chest pain; severe depression; difficulty urinating; fainting; falling; fever; joint pain; hallucinations; mouth sores; nightmares; palpitations; rash; shortness of breath; slurred speech; sore throat; uncoordinated movements; unusual excitement; unusual tiredness; or yellowing of the eyes or skin

INTERACTIONS

Lorazepam interacts with a number of other medications
1. To prevent over-sedation, this drug should not be taken with alcohol, other sedative drugs, or central nervous system depressants, such as antihistamines, barbiturates, muscle relaxants, pain medicines, narcotics, medicines for seizures, and phenothiazine tranquilizers, or with anti-depressants.
2. This medication may decrease the effectiveness of carbamazepine, levodopa, and oral anti-coagulants (blood thinners), and may increase the effects of phenytoin.
3. Disulfiram and isoniazid can increase the blood levels of lorazepam, which can lead to toxic effects.
4. Concurrent use of rifampin may decrease the effectiveness of lorazepam.
If you are currently taking any of the medications listed above, CONSULT YOUR DOCTOR about their use.

WARNINGS

• Tell your doctor about unusual or allergic reactions you have had to any medications, especially to lorazepam or other benzodiazepine tranquilizers (such as alprazolam, chlordiazepoxide, clorazepate, diazepam, flurazepam, halazepam, oxazepam, prazepam, temazepam, or triazolam).
• Tell your doctor if you now have, or if you have ever had, liver disease, kidney disease, epilepsy, lung disease, myasthenia gravis, porphyria, mental depression, or mental illness.
• This medicine can cause drowsiness. Avoid tasks that require alertness, such as driving a car or using potentially dangerous equipment.
• This medication has the potential for abuse and must be used with caution. Tolerance may develop quickly; do not increase the dose of the drug without first consulting your doctor. It is also important not to stop this drug suddenly if you have been taking it in large amounts or if you have used it for several weeks. Your doctor may want to re-

duce the dosage gradually.
- This is a safe drug when used properly. When it is combined with other sedative drugs or alcohol, however, serious side effects can develop.
- Be sure to tell your doctor if you are pregnant. This medicine may increase the chance of birth defects if it is taken during the first three months of pregnancy. In addition, too much use of this medicine during the last six months of pregnancy may cause the fetus to become dependent on it, resulting in withdrawal side effects in the newborn. Also, use of this medicine during the last weeks of pregnancy may cause drowsiness, slowed heartbeat, and breathing difficulties in the newborn. Tell your doctor if you are breastfeeding an infant. This medicine can pass into the breast milk and cause drowsiness, slowed heartbeat, and breathing difficulties in the nursing infant.

Lorelco—see probucol

Lortab—see acetaminophen and hydrocodone combination

Lotrimin—see clotrimazole (topical)

Lo-Trol—see diphenoxylate and atropine

Low-Quel—see diphenoxylate and atropine

---

loxapine

BRAND NAMES (Manufacturers)
Loxitane (Lederle)
Loxitane C (Lederle)
TYPE OF DRUG
Anti-psychotic
INGREDIENT
loxapine as the hydrochloride or succinate salt
DOSAGE FORMS
Capsules (5 mg, 10 mg, 25 mg, and 50 mg)
Oral concentrate (25 mg per ml)

STORAGE

Loxapine capsules and oral concentrate should be stored at room temperature in tightly closed containers. This medication should never be frozen. If the oral concentrate turns to a slight yellow color, the medicine is still effective and can be used. However, if the oral concentrate changes color markedly, or has particles floating in it, it should not be used, but discarded down the sink.

USES

Loxapine is prescribed to treat the symptoms of mental illness, such as the emotional symptoms of psychosis. This medication is thought to relieve the symptoms of mental illness by blocking certain chemicals involved with nerve transmission in the brain.

TREATMENT

To avoid stomach irritation, you can take the tablet form of loxapine with a meal or with a glass of water or milk (unless your doctor directs you to do otherwise).

The oral concentrate form of this medication should be measured carefully with the dropper provided, and diluted in 8 ounces (a full cup) or more of orange or grapefruit juice immediately prior to administration.

If you miss a dose of this medication, take the missed dose as soon as possible and return to your regular dosing schedule. If it is almost time for the next dose, however, skip the one you missed and return to your regular schedule. Do not double the dose unless your doctor directs you to do so.

Antacids and diarrhea medicine can decrease the absorption of this medication from the gastrointestinal tract. Therefore, at least one hour should separate doses of one of these medicines and loxapine.

The full effects of this medication for the control of emotional or mental symptoms may not become apparent for two weeks after starting to take it.

SIDE EFFECTS

Minor. Blurred vision; constipation; decreased sweating; diarrhea; dizziness; drooling; drowsiness; dry mouth; fatigue; jitteriness; menstrual irregularities; nasal congestion; restlessness; tremors; vomiting; and weight gain. As your body adjusts to the medication, these side effects should disappear.

If you are constipated, increase the amount of fiber in your diet (raw vegetables, fruits, salads, bran, and whole-grain breads), and drink more water (unless your doctor directs you to do otherwise).

To reduce mouth dryness, chew sugarless gum, or suck on ice chips or a piece of hard candy.

This medication can cause increased sensitivity to sunlight. It is therefore important to avoid prolonged exposure to sunlight and sunlamps. Wear protective clothing, and use an effective sunscreen.

To avoid dizziness or light-headedness when you stand, contract and relax the muscles of your legs for a few moments before rising. Do this by pushing one foot against the floor while raising the other foot slightly, alternating feet so that you are "pumping" your legs in a pedaling motion.

Major. Tell your doctor about any side effects that are persistent or particularly bothersome. IT IS ESPECIALLY IMPORTANT TO TELL YOUR DOCTOR about unusual bleeding or bruising; breast enlargement (in both sexes); chest pain; convulsions; darkened skin; difficulty swallowing or breathing; fainting; fever; impotence; involuntary movements of the face, mouth, jaw, or tongue; palpitations; rash; sleep disorders; sore throat; uncoordinated movements; visual disturbances; or yellowing of the eyes or skin.

INTERACTIONS

Loxapine interacts with several other types of medication.
1. It can cause extreme drowsiness when combined with alcohol or other central nervous system depressants (drugs that slow the activity of the nervous system), such as barbiturates, benzodiazepine tranquilizers, muscle relaxants, narcotics, and pain medications, or with tricyclic anti-depressants.
2. This medication can decrease the effectiveness of amphetamines, guanethidine, anti-convulsants, and levodopa.
3. The side effects of epinephrine, monoamine oxidase

(MAO) inhibitors, and tricyclic anti-depressants may be increased when combined with this medication.

Before starting to take loxapine, BE SURE TO TELL YOUR DOCTOR if you are taking any of the medications listed above.

WARNINGS

● Tell your doctor about any unusual or allergic reactions you have had to medications, especially to loxapine.

● TELL YOUR DOCTOR if you now have, or if you have ever had, alcoholism, heart or circulatory disease, epilepsy, glaucoma, liver disease, Parkinson's disease, enlarged prostate gland, or blockage of the urinary tract.

● Avoid drinking alcoholic beverages while taking this medication, in order to prevent over-sedation.

● If this medication makes you dizzy or drowsy, do not take part in any activity that requires alertness, such as driving a car or operating potentially dangerous equipment. Be careful on stairs and avoid getting up suddenly from a lying or sitting position.

● Prior to having surgery or any other medical or dental treatment, be sure to tell your doctor or dentist that you are taking loxapine.

● Some of the side effects caused by this drug can be prevented by taking an anti-parkinson drug. Discuss this with with your doctor.

● This type of medication has been reported to cause certain tumors in rats. This effect has not been shown to occur in humans.

● This medication can decrease sweating and heat release from the body. Therefore, avoid getting overheated by strenuous exercise in hot weather, and avoid taking hot baths, showers, and saunas.

● Do not stop taking this medication suddenly. If the drug is stopped abruptly you may experience nausea; vomiting; stomach upset; headache; increased heart rate; insomnia; tremulousness; or worsening of your condition. Your doctor may want to reduce the dosage gradually.

● If you are planning to have a myelogram, or any procedure in which dye is injected into the spinal cord, tell your doctor that you are taking this medication.

● Avoid spilling the oral concentrate form of this medication on your skin or clothing; it can cause redness and irritation of the skin.

● While taking this medication, do not take any over-the-counter (non-prescription) medication for weight control, or for cough, cold, asthma, allergy, or sinus problems, unless you first check with your doctor. The combination of these two types of medications can cause high blood pressure.

● Be sure to tell your doctor if you are pregnant. Small amounts of this medication will cross the placenta. Although there are reports of safe use of this type of drug during pregnancy, there are also reports of liver disease and tremors in newborn infants whose mothers received this type of medication close to term. Also, tell your doctor if you are breastfeeding an infant. Small amounts of this medication pass into breast milk and may cause unwanted effects in the nursing infant.

Loxitane—see loxapine

Loxitane C—see loxapine

Lozol—see indapamide

Ludiomil—see maprotiline

Luminal Ovoids—see phenobarbital

Luride—see sodium fluoride

Luride Lozi-Tabs—see sodium fluoride

Lysodren—see mitotane

Macrodantin—see nitrofurantoin

Malatal—see atropine, scopolamine, hyoscyamine, and phenobarbital combination

Mallergan-VC Expectorant with Codeine—see phenylephrine, potassium guaiacolsulfonate, promethazine, and codeine combination

Mandelamine—see methenamine

---

maprotiline

BRAND NAME (Manufacturer)
Ludiomil (Ciba)
TYPE OF DRUG
Tetracyclic anti-depressant (mood elevator)
INGREDIENT
maprotiline as the hydrochloride salt
DOSAGE FORM
Tablets (25 mg, 50 mg, and 75 mg)
STORAGE
This medication should be stored at room temperature in a tightly closed container.

USES

Maprotiline is used to relieve the symptoms of mental depression. This medication is a tetracyclic anti-depressant. It is related to a group of drugs referred to as the tricyclic anti-depressants. These medicines are thought to relieve depression by increasing the concentration of certain chemicals necessary for nerve transmission in the brain.

TREATMENT

This medication should be taken exactly as your doctor prescribes. It can be taken with water or food to lessen the chance of stomach irritation, unless your doctor tells you to do otherwise.

If you miss a dose of this medication, take the missed dose as soon as possible, then return to your regular dosing schedule. However, if the dose you missed was a once-a-day bedtime dose, do not take that dose in the morning; check with your doctor instead. If the dose is taken in the morning, it may cause some unwanted side effects. Never double the dose.

The effects of therapy with this medication may not be apparent for two or three weeks.

SIDE EFFECTS

Minor. Agitation; anxiety; blurred vision; confusion; constipation; cramps; diarrhea; dizziness; drowsiness; dry mouth; fatigue; heartburn; insomnia; loss of appetite; nausea; peculiar tastes in the mouth; restlessness; sweating; vomiting; weakness; or weight gain or loss. As your body adjusts to the medication, these side effects should disappear.

Dry mouth can be relieved by chewing sugarless gum or by sucking on ice chips or a piece of hard candy.

To relieve constipation, increase the amount of fiber (bran, salads, whole-grain breads, fresh vegetables and fruits) in your diet, and drink more water (unless your doctor directs you to do otherwise).

To avoid dizziness or light-headedness when you stand, contract and relax the muscles of your legs for a few moments before rising. Do this by pushing one foot against the floor while raising the other foot slightly, alternating feet so that you are "pumping" your legs in a pedaling motion.

This medication may cause increased sensitivity to sunlight. Therefore, avoid prolonged exposure to sunlight and sunlamps. Wear protective clothing, and use an effective sunscreen.

Major. Tell your doctor about any side effects that are persistent or particularly bothersome. IT IS ESPECIALLY IMPORTANT TO TELL YOUR DOCTOR about chest pain; convulsions; difficulty urinating; enlarged or painful breasts (in both sexes); fainting; fever; fluid retention; hair loss; hallucinations; headaches; impotence; mood changes; mouth sores; nervousness; nightmares; numbness in the fingers or toes; palpitations; ringing in the ears; seizures; skin rash; sleep disorders; sore throat; tremors; uncoordinated movements or balance problems; unusual bleeding or bruising; or yellowing of the eyes or skin.

INTERACTIONS

Maprotiline can interact with a number of other types of medicines.

1. Extreme drowsiness can occur when this medicine is taken with central nervous system depressants (medicines that slow the activity of the central nervous system), including alcohol, antihistamines, barbiturates, benzodiazepine tranquilizers, muscle relaxants, narcotics, pain medications, phenothiazine tranquilizers, and sleeping medications, or with other anti-depressants.

2. Maprotiline may decrease the effectiveness of anti-seizure medications and block the blood-pressure-lowering effects of clonidine and guanethidine.

3. Oral contraceptives (estrogens) can increase the side effects and reduce the effectiveness of the tetracyclic anti-depressants (including maprotiline).

4. Tetracyclic anti-depressants may increase the side effects of thyroid medication and over-the-counter (non-prescription) allergy, cough, cold, asthma, sinus, and diet medications.

5. The concurrent use of tetracyclic anti-depressants and monoamine oxidase (MAO) inhibitors should be undertaken very carefully, because the combination may result in fever, convulsions, or high blood pressure.

Before starting to take maprotiline, BE SURE TO TELL YOUR DOCTOR if you are already taking any of the medications listed above.

WARNINGS

● Tell your doctor if you have had unusual or allergic reactions to medications, especially to maprotiline or any of the tricyclic anti-depressants (such as amitriptyline, imipramine, doxepin, trimipramine, amoxapine, protriptyline, desipramine, or nortriptyline).

● Tell your doctor if you now have, or if you have ever had, asthma, high blood pressure, liver or kidney disease, heart disease, a recent heart attack, circulatory disease, stomach problems, intestinal problems, alcoholism, difficulty urinating, enlarged prostate gland, epilepsy, glaucoma, thyroid disease, mental illness, or electroshock therapy.

● If this drug makes you dizzy or drowsy, do not take part in any activity that requires alertness, such as driving a car or operating potentially dangerous equipment.

● Before having any surgery or other medical or dental treatment, be sure to tell your doctor or dentist that you are taking this medication.

● Do not stop taking this drug suddenly. Abruptly stopping it can cause nausea, headache, stomach upset, fatigue, or a worsening of your condition. Your doctor may want to reduce the dosage gradually.

• The effects of this medication may last as long as seven days after you have stopped taking it, so continue to observe all precautions during that period.

• Be sure to tell your doctor if you are pregnant. Problems in humans have not been reported; however, studies in animals have shown that this type of medication can cause side effects to the fetus if given to the mother in large doses during pregnancy. Also, tell your doctor if you are breastfeeding an infant. Small amounts of this drug can pass into breast milk and may cause unwanted effects, such as irritability or sleeping problems, in the nursing infant.

Marazide——see benzthiazide

Marbaxin——see methocarbamol

Marnal——see aspirin, caffeine, and butalbital combination

Matulane——see procarbazine

Mazanor——see mazindol

---

mazindol

BRAND NAMES (Manufacturers)
Mazanor (Wyeth)
Sanorex (Sandoz)
TYPE OF DRUG
Anorectic (appetite suppressant)
INGREDIENT
mazindol
DOSAGE FORM
Tablets (1 mg and 2 mg)
STORAGE
Mazindol should be stored at room temperature in a tightly closed, light-resistant container.

USES

Mazindol is used as an appetite suppressant during the first few weeks of dieting, to help establish new eating habits. This medication is thought to relieve hunger by altering nerve impulses to the appetite control center in the brain. Its effectiveness lasts only for short periods (three to 12 weeks), however.

TREATMENT

Mazindol can be taken with a full glass of water one hour before meals (unless your doctor directs you to do otherwise).

If you miss a dose of this medication, take the missed dose as soon as possible, unless it is almost time for your next dose. In this case, don't take the missed dose at all; just return to your regular dosing schedule. Do not double the next dose.

In order to avoid difficulty falling asleep, the last dose of this medication each day should be taken four to six hours before bedtime (for the 1 mg tablet) or ten to 14 hours before bedtime (for the 2 mg tablet).

SIDE EFFECTS

Minor. Blurred vision; constipation; diarrhea; dizziness; dry mouth; false sense of well-being; fatigue; insomnia; irritability; nausea; nervousness; restlessness; stomach pain; sweating; tremors; unpleasant taste in the mouth; and vomiting. These side effects should disappear in several days, as your body adjusts to the medication.

Dry mouth can be relieved by sucking on ice chips or a piece of hard candy, or by chewing sugarless gum.

In order to prevent constipation, increase the amount of fiber in your diet (raw vegetables, fruits, salads, bran, and whole-grain breads), and drink more water (unless your doctor tells you not to do so).

Major. Tell your doctor about any side effects that are persistent or particularly bothersome. IT IS ESPECIALLY IMPORTANT TO TELL YOUR DOCTOR about changes in sexual desire; chest pain; difficulty urinating; enlarged breasts (in either sex); fever; hair loss; headaches; impotence; menstrual irregularities; mental depression; mood changes; mouth sores; muscle pains; palpitations; rash; sore throat; or unusual bleeding or bruising.

INTERACTIONS

Mazindol interacts with other types of medications.

1. Use of this medication within 14 days of a monoamine oxidase (MAO) inhibitor (such as isocarboxazid, pargyline, phenelzine, tranylcypromine) can result in high blood pressure and other side effects.

2. Barbiturate medications and phenothiazine tranquilizers (especially chlorpromazine) can antagonize (act against) the appetite suppressant activity of this medication.

3. Mazindol can decrease the blood-pressure-lowering effects of anti-hypertensive medications (especially guanethidine); and may alter insulin and oral anti-diabetic medication dosage requirements in diabetic patients.

4. The side effects of other central nervous system stimulants, such as caffeine, over-the-counter (non-prescription) appetite suppressants, or sinus, cough, cold, asthma, and allergy preparations, may be increased by this medication. Before starting to take mazindol, BE SURE TO TELL YOUR DOCTOR if you are already taking any of the medications listed above.

WARNINGS

● Tell your doctor about unusual or allergic reactions you have had to any medications, especially to mazindol or other appetite suppressants (such as benzphetamine, phendimetrazine, diethylpropion, fenfluramine, phenmetrazine, or phentermine), or to epinephrine, norepinephrine, ephedrine, amphetamines, dextroamphetamine, phenylephrine, phenylpropanolamine, pseudoephedrine, albuterol, metaproterenol, or terbutaline.

● Tell your doctor if you now have, or if you have ever had, angina (chest pain); diabetes mellitus (sugar diabetes); emotional disturbances; glaucoma; heart or cardiovascular disease; high blood pressure; a history of drug abuse; or thyroid disease.

● Mazindol can mask the symptoms of extreme fatigue and can cause dizziness or light-headedness. Your ability to perform tasks that require alertness, such as driving a car or operating potentially dangerous machinery, may be decreased. Appropriate caution should therefore be taken.

● Before having any surgery or other medical or dental treatment, be sure to tell your doctor or dentist that you are taking this medication.

● Mazindol is related to amphetamine and may be habit-forming when taken for long periods of time (both physical and psychological dependence can occur). Therefore, you should not increase the dose of this medication or take it for longer than 12 weeks, unless you first consult your doctor. It is also important that you not stop taking this medication abruptly. Fatigue, sleep disorders, mental depression, nausea or vomiting, or stomach cramps or pain can occur while your body adjusts to discontinuing this medication. Your doctor may want to decrease the dosage gradually in order to prevent these side effects.

● Be sure to tell your doctor if you are pregnant. Although side effects in humans have not yet been studied, some of the appetite suppressants cause side effects in the offspring of animals who receive large doses of these drugs during pregnancy. Also, tell your doctor if you are breastfeeding an infant. It is not known whether or not this medication passes into breast milk.

M-Cillin B—see penicillin G

---

meclizine

BRAND NAMES (Manufacturers)
Antivert (Roerig)
Bonine* (Pfipharmecs)
Dizmiss* (Bowman)
meclizine hydrochloride (various manufacturers)
Motion Cure* (Wisconsin)
Wehvert* (Hauck)
*Meclizine is also available over-the-counter (non-prescription), under various brand names.
TYPE OF DRUG
Anti-emetic (anti-nauseant)
INGREDIENT
meclizine as the hydrochloride salt

DOSAGE FORMS
Tablets (12.5 mg and 25 mg)
Chewable tablets (25 mg)
STORAGE
Meclizine should be stored at room temperature in a tightly closed container.

USES
Meclizine is used to provide symptomatic relief of dizziness due to ear infections, or to prevent or relieve dizziness, nausea, and vomiting due to motion sickness. It is thought to relieve dizziness and vomiting by altering nerve transmission in the balance and vomiting centers in the brain.

TREATMENT
To avoid stomach upset, you can take meclizine with food or with a full glass of milk or water (unless your doctor directs you to do otherwise).

The chewable tablets should be chewed for at least two minutes, in order to obtain the full benefit of this medication.

If you are taking meclizine to prevent motion sickness, you should take it one hour before traveling.

If you miss a dose of this medication, take the missed dose as soon as possible, unless it is almost time for your next dose. In that case, don't take the missed dose at all; just return to your regular dosing schedule. Do not double the next dose.

SIDE EFFECTS
Minor. Blurred vision; confusion; constipation; diarrhea; difficult or painful urination; dizziness; dry mouth, throat, or nose; headache; irritability; loss of appetite; nausea; restlessness; ringing or buzzing in the ears; rash; stomach upset; and unusual increase in sweating. These side effects should disappear in several days, as your body adjusts to the medication.

If you are constipated, increase the amount of fiber in your diet (raw vegetables, fruits, salads, bran, and whole-grain breads), and drink more water (unless your doctor tells you not to do so).

Chew sugarless gum, or suck on ice chips or a piece of hard candy, to reduce mouth dryness.

Major. Tell your doctor about any side effects that are persistent or particularly bothersome. IT IS ESPECIALLY IMPORTANT TO TELL YOUR DOCTOR about unusual bleeding or bruising; change in menstruation; clumsiness; feeling faint; flushing of the face; hallucinations; sleeping disorders; seizures; shortness of breath; sore throat or fever; palpitations; tightness in the chest; or unusual tiredness or weakness.

INTERACTIONS

Meclizine interacts with several other types of medication. Concurrent use of it with other central nervous system depressants (drugs that slow the activity of the nervous system), such as barbiturates, benzodiazepine tranquilizers, muscle relaxants, narcotics, pain medications, phenothiazine tranquilizers, and alcohol, or with tricyclic antidepressants can cause extreme drowsiness. TELL YOUR DOCTOR if you are already taking any of the medications listed above.

WARNINGS

• Tell your doctor about allergic or unusual reactions you have had to any medications, especially to meclizine, cyclizine, or buclizine.

• Tell your doctor if you now have, or if you have ever had, asthma, blood vessel disease, glaucoma, high blood pressure, kidney disease, peptic ulcers, enlarged prostate gland, or thyroid disease.

• Meclizine can cause drowsiness or dizziness. Your ability to perform tasks that require alertness, such as driving a car or operating potentially dangerous machinery, may be decreased. Appropriate caution should therefore be taken.

• Be sure to tell your doctor if you are pregnant. The effects of this medication during pregnancy have not yet been thoroughly studied in humans. Also, tell your doctor if you are breastfeeding an infant. Small amounts of meclizine pass into breast milk and may cause unusual excitement or irritability in nursing infants.

meclizine hydrochloride—see meclizine

meclofenamate

BRAND NAME (Manufacturer)
Meclomen (Parke-Davis)
TYPE OF DRUG
Non-steroidal anti-inflammatory analgesic (pain reliever)
INGREDIENT
meclofenamate as the sodium salt
DOSAGE FORM
Capsules (50 mg and 100 mg)
STORAGE
This medication should be stored in a tightly closed container at room temperature, away from heat and direct sunlight.

USES
Meclofenamate is used to treat the inflammation (pain, swelling, stiffness) of certain types of arthritis, gout, bursitis, and tendinitis.

TREATMENT
If this medication upsets your stomach, you can take it with food, milk, or antacids (unless your doctor recommends otherwise). If stomach irritation continues, check with your doctor.

It is important to take meclofenamate on schedule and not to miss any doses. If you do miss a dose, take it as soon as possible, unless it is almost time for your next dose. In that case, don't take the missed dose at all; just return to your regular dosing schedule. Don't double the dose.

If you are taking meclofenamate to relieve arthritis, you must take it regularly, as directed by your doctor. It may take up to three weeks before you feel the full benefits of this medication.

This medication does not cure arthritis, but it will help to control the condition, as long as you keep taking it.

SIDE EFFECTS
Minor. Bloating; constipation; diarrhea; difficulty sleeping; dizziness; drowsiness; headache; heartburn; indigestion; light-headedness; loss of appetite; nausea; nervousness; soreness of the mouth; unusual sweating;

and vomiting. As your body adjusts to the drug, these side effects should disappear.

If you become dizzy, sit or lie down awhile; get up slowly, and be careful on stairs.

Acetaminophen may be helpful in relieving any headaches.

Major. If any side effects are persistent or particularly bothersome, you should report them to your doctor. IT IS ESPECIALLY IMPORTANT TO TELL YOUR DOCTOR about bloody or black, tarry stools; blurred vision; confusion; depression; difficult or painful urination; palpitations; a problem with hearing; ringing or buzzing in the ears; severe diarrhea; skin rash, hives, or itching; stomach pain; swelling of the feet; tightness in the chest, shortness of breath, difficulty breathing, or wheezing; unexplained sore throat and fever; unusual bleeding or bruising; unusual fatigue or weakness; unusual weight gain; or yellowing of the eyes or skin.

INTERACTIONS

Meclofenamate interacts with several other medications.

1. Anti-coagulants (blood thinners, such as warfarin) can lead to an increase in bleeding complications.

2. Aspirin, salicylates, or other anti-inflammation medication can increase stomach irritation.

BE SURE TO TELL YOUR DOCTOR if you are already taking any of the medicines listed above.

WARNINGS

• Tell your doctor if you have ever had unusual or allergic reactions to meclofenamate or any of the other chemically related drugs (aspirin, other salicylates, diflunisal, fenoprofen, ibuprofen, indomethacin, mefenamic acid, naproxen, oxyphenbutazone, phenylbutazone, piroxicam, sulindac, tolmetin, and zomepirac).

• Before taking meclofenamate, it is important to tell your doctor if you now have, or if you have ever had, bleeding problems; colitis, stomach ulcers, or other stomach problems; epilepsy; heart disease; high blood pressure; asthma; kidney disease; liver disease; mental illness; or Parkinson's disease.

• If this drug makes you dizzy or drowsy, do not take part

in any activity that requires alertness, such as driving a car or operating potentially dangerous equipment.

● Because this drug can prolong your bleeding time, it is important to tell your doctor or dentist that you are taking this drug, before having any surgery or other medical or dental treatment.

● Stomach problems are more likely to occur if you take aspirin regularly or drink alcohol while being treated with this medication. These should therefore be avoided (unless your doctor directs you to do otherwise).

● Be sure to tell your doctor if you are pregnant. Studies have shown that meclofenamate can cause unwanted effects (including slower development of bones, and heart damage) in the offspring of animals who received this drug during pregnancy. If taken late in pregnancy, meclofenamate can also prolong labor. Studies in humans have not yet been completed. Also, tell your doctor if you are breastfeeding an infant. Small amounts of meclofenamate pass into breast milk.

Meclomen—see meclofenamate

Medihaler Ergotamine—see ergotamine

Medrol—see methylprednisolone (systemic)

---

medroxyprogesterone

BRAND NAMES (Manufacturers)
Amen (Carnrick)
Curretab (Reid-Provident)
Provera (Upjohn)
TYPE OF DRUG
Progesterone (female hormone)
INGREDIENT
medroxyprogesterone
DOSAGE FORM
Tablets (2.5 mg and 10 mg)
STORAGE
These tablets should be stored at room temperature in a tightly closed container.

USES

Medroxyprogesterone is a synthetic progesterone (progesterone is a female hormone, which is naturally produced by the body) that is used to treat abnormal menstrual bleeding, difficult menstruation, or lack of menstruation.

TREATMENT

In order to avoid stomach irritation, you can take medroxyprogesterone with food or immediately after a meal.

If you miss a dose of this medication, take the missed dose as soon as possible, unless it is almost time for the next dose. In that case, do not take the missed dose at all; just return to your regular dosing schedule. Do not double the next dose.

SIDE EFFECTS

Minor. Acne; dizziness; hair growth; headache; nausea; and vomiting. These side effects should disappear in several weeks, as your body adjusts to the medication.

If you feel dizzy or light-headed, sit or lie down awhile; get up slowly, and be careful on stairs.

This medication can increase your sensitivity to sunlight. Avoid prolonged exposure to sunlight and sunlamps. Wear protective clothing and sunglasses, and use an effective sunscreen.

Major. Tell your doctor about any side effects that are persistent or particularly bothersome. IT IS ESPECIALLY IMPORTANT TO TELL YOUR DOCTOR about breast tenderness; change in menstrual patterns; chest pain; depression; fainting; hair loss; itching; pain in the calves; rash; spotting, breakthrough, or unusual vaginal bleeding; slurred speech; sudden, severe headache; swelling of the feet or ankles; weight gain; or yellowing of the eyes or skin.

INTERACTIONS

Medroxyprogesterone does not interact with other medications, if it is used according to directions.

WARNINGS

• Tell your doctor about unusual or allergic reactions you have had to any medications, especially to medroxypro-

gesterone, progestin, or progesterone.
● Before starting to take this medication, be sure to tell your doctor if you now have, or if you have ever had, cancer of the breast or genitals; clotting disorders; diabetes mellitus (sugar diabetes); depression; epilepsy; gallbladder disease; asthma; heart disease; kidney disease; liver disease; migraine headaches; porphyria; stroke; or vaginal bleeding.
● A package insert should be included with this drug. Read it carefully, and consult your doctor if you have any questions.
● If this drug makes you dizzy or drowsy, do not take part in any activities that require alertness, such as driving a car or operating potentially dangerous equipment.
● Be sure to tell your doctor if you are pregnant. Medroxyprogesterone should not be used during the first four months of pregnancy because it has been shown to cause birth defects. Since hormones have long-term effects on the body, medroxyprogesterone should be stopped at least three months prior to becoming pregnant. Also, tell your doctor if you are breastfeeding an infant. Small amounts of medroxyprogesterone pass into breast milk.

mefenamic acid

BRAND NAME (Manufacturer)
Ponstel (Parke-Davis)
TYPE OF DRUG
Non-steroidal anti-inflammatory analgesic (pain reliever)
INGREDIENT
mefenamic acid
DOSAGE FORM
Capsules (250 mg)
STORAGE
This medication should be stored in a tightly closed container at room temperature, away from heat and direct sunlight.

USES
Mefenamic acid is used to treat painful menstruation.

TREATMENT

Mefenamic acid should be taken with food or antacids to lessen stomach irritation (unless your doctor recommends otherwise). Take this medication only as directed by your doctor. Do not take more of it, or take it more often; and do not take it for longer than seven days at a time, unless your doctor tells you to do so. Taking too much of this medicine, or using it for long periods of time, may increase your chances of experiencing serious side effects.

It is important to take mefenamic acid on schedule and not to miss any doses. If you do miss a dose, take it as soon as possible, unless it is almost time for your next dose. In that case, don't take the missed dose at all; just return to your regular dosing schedule. Do not double the next dose.

SIDE EFFECTS

Minor. Bloating; constipation; diarrhea; difficulty sleeping; dizziness; drowsiness; headache; heartburn; indigestion; light-headedness; loss of appetite; nausea; nervousness; soreness of the mouth; unusual sweating; and vomiting. As your body adjusts to the drug, these side effects should disappear.

If you become dizzy, sit or lie down awhile; get up slowly, and be careful on stairs.

Acetaminophen may be helpful in relieving any headaches.

Major. If any side effects are persistent or particularly bothersome, you should report them to your doctor. IT IS ESPECIALLY IMPORTANT TO TELL YOUR DOCTOR about bloody or black, tarry stools; blurred vision; confusion; depression; difficult or painful urination; palpitations; a problem with hearing; ringing or buzzing in the ears; severe diarrhea; skin rash, hives, or itching; stomach pain; swelling of the feet; tightness in the chest, shortness of breath, or wheezing; unexplained sore throat and fever; unusual bleeding or bruising; unusual fatigue or weakness; unusual weight gain; or yellowing of the eyes or skin.

INTERACTIONS

Mefenamic acid interacts with several types of medication.

1. Anti-coagulants (blood thinners, such as warfarin) can lead to an increase in bleeding complications.

2. Aspirin, salicylates, or other anti-inflammation medication can increase stomach irritation.

BE SURE TO TELL YOUR DOCTOR if you are already taking any of these medications.

WARNINGS

● Tell your doctor if you have ever had unusual or allergic reactions to mefenamic acid or to any of the other chemically related drugs (aspirin, other salicylates, diflunisal, fenoprofen, ibuprofen, meclofenamate, indomethacin, naproxen, oxyphenbutazone, phenylbutazone, piroxicam, sulindac, tolmetin, and zomepirac).

● Before taking mefenamic acid, it is important to tell your doctor if you now have, or if you have ever had, asthma; bleeding problems; colitis, stomach ulcers, or other stomach problems; epilepsy; heart disease; high blood pressure; kidney disease; liver disease; mental illness; or Parkinson's disease.

● If this drug makes you dizzy or drowsy, do not take part in any activity that requires alertness, such as driving a car or operating potentially dangerous equipment.

● Because mefenamic acid can prolong your bleeding time, it is important to tell your doctor or dentist that you are taking this drug, before having any surgery or other medical or dental treatment.

● If you experience severe diarrhea while taking this medication, check with your doctor immediately. Do not take this medication again unless you first check with your doctor, because severe diarrhea can occur each time you take it.

● Stomach problems are more likely to occur if you take aspirin regularly or drink alcohol while being treated with this medication. These should therefore be avoided (unless your doctor directs you to do otherwise).

● Be sure to tell your doctor if you are pregnant. This type of medication may cause unwanted effects on the heart or blood flow in the unborn infant. Also, studies in animals have shown that this type of medicine, if taken late in pregnancy, can increase the length of pregnancy, prolong labor, and cause other problems during delivery. Mefenamic acid has not been shown to cause birth defects in animals; however, studies in humans have not yet been completed. Also, tell your doctor if you are breastfeeding an infant. Small amounts of mefenamic acid pass into breast milk.

Melfiat—see phendimetrazine

Mellaril—see thioridazine

Menadione—see vitamin K

---

meperidine

BRAND NAMES (Manufacturers)
Demerol (Winthrop)
meperidine hydrochloride (various manufacturers)
Pethadol (Halsey)
TYPE OF DRUG
Analgesic (pain reliever)
INGREDIENT
meperidine as the hydrochloride salt
DOSAGE FORMS
Tablets (50 mg and 100 mg)
Syrup (50 mg per 5 ml teaspoonful)
STORAGE
Meperidine tablets and syrup should be stored at room temperature, in tightly closed, light-resistant containers. This medication should never be frozen.

USES
Meperidine is a narcotic analgesic that acts directly on the central nervous system (brain and spinal cord). It is used to relieve moderate to severe pain.

TREATMENT
In order to avoid stomach upset, you can take meperidine with food or milk. It works most effectively if you take it at the onset of pain, rather than waiting until the pain becomes intense.

Measure the syrup form of this medication carefully, with a specially designed, 5 ml measuring spoon. An ordinary kitchen teaspoon is not accurate enough. Each dose of the syrup should be diluted in 4 ounces (half a glass) of water, in order to avoid the numbness to the mouth and throat that this medication can cause.

If you are taking this medication on a regular schedule and you miss a dose, take the missed dose as soon as possible, unless it is almost time for your next dose. In that case, don't take the missed dose at all; just return to your regular dosing schedule. Do not double the next dose.

SIDE EFFECTS

Minor. Constipation; dizziness; drowsiness; dry mouth; false sense of well-being; flushing; light-headedness; loss of appetite; nausea; rash; sweating; and painful or difficult urination. These side effects should disappear in several days, as your body adjusts to the medication.

If you are constipated, increase the amount of fiber in your diet (raw vegetables, fruits, salads, bran, and whole-grain breads), and drink more water (unless your doctor directs you to do otherwise).

If you feel dizzy, light-headed, or nauseated; sit or lie down awhile; get up from a sitting or lying position slowly, and be careful on stairs.

Major. Tell your doctor about any side effects that are persistent or particularly bothersome. IT IS ESPECIALLY IMPORTANT TO TELL YOUR DOCTOR about anxiety; breathing difficulties; excitation; fatigue; restlessness; sore throat and fever; tremors; or weakness.

INTERACTIONS

Meperidine interacts with several other types of drugs.

1. Concurrent use of this medication with other central nervous system depressants (drugs that slow the activity of the nervous system), such as antihistamines, barbiturates, benzodiazepine tranquilizers, muscle relaxants, phenothiazine tranquilizers, and alcohol, or with tricyclic anti-depressants can cause extreme drowsiness.

2. A monoamine oxidase (MAO) inhibitor taken within 14 days of this medication can lead to unpredictable and severe side effects.

3. Cimetidine, combined with meperidine, can cause

confusion, disorientation, seizures, and shortness of breath.

TELL YOUR DOCTOR if you are currently taking any of the medications listed above.

WARNINGS

• Tell your doctor about unusual or allergic reactions you have had to medications, especially to meperidine or to any other narcotic analgesic (such as codeine, hydrocodone, hydromorphone, methadone, morphine, oxycodone, or propoxyphene).

• Tell your doctor if you now have, or if you have ever had, acute abdominal conditions; asthma; brain disease; colitis; epilepsy; gallstones or gallbladder disease; head injuries; heart disease; kidney disease; liver disease; lung disease; mental illness; emotional disorders; enlarged prostate gland; thyroid disease; or urethral stricture.

• If this drug makes you dizzy or drowsy, do not take part in any activity that requires alertness, such as driving a car or operating potentially dangerous equipment.

• Before having any surgery or other medical or dental treatment, be sure to tell your doctor or dentist that you are taking this medication.

• Because this product contains meperidine, it has the potential for abuse, and must be used with caution. Usually, it should not be taken on a regular schedule for longer than ten days (unless your doctor directs you to do so). Tolerance develops quickly; do not increase the dosage or stop taking the drug abruptly, unless you first consult your doctor. If you have been taking large amounts of this medication or have been taking it for a long period of time, you may experience a withdrawal reaction (muscle aches, diarrhea, gooseflesh, runny nose, nausea, vomiting, shivering, trembling, stomach cramps, sleep disorders, irritability, weakness, yawning, and sweating) when you stop taking it. Your doctor may therefore want to reduce your dosage gradually.

• Be sure to tell your doctor if you are pregnant. The effects of this medication during pregnancy have not yet been thoroughly studied in humans. Meperidine, used regularly in large doses during pregnancy, can result in addiction of the fetus, leading to withdrawal symptoms (irritability, excessive crying, tremors, fever, vomiting, diarrhea, sneezing, and yawning) at birth. Also, tell your doctor if you are breastfeeding an infant. Small amounts of this medication may pass into breast milk and cause excessive drowsiness in the nursing infant.

meperidine hydrochloride—see meperidine

Mephyton—see vitamin K

Mepriam—see meprobamate

---

meprobamate

BRAND NAMES (Manufacturers)
Equanil (Wyeth)
Mepriam (Lemmon)
meprobamate (various manufacturers)
Meprospan (Wallace)
Miltown (Wallace)
Neuramate (Halsey)
Neurate-400 (Trimen)
Sedabamate (Mallard)
SK-Bamate (Smith Kline & French)
Tranmep (Reid-Provident)
TYPE OF DRUG
Sedative/hypnotic (anti-anxiety)
INGREDIENT
meprobamate
DOSAGE FORMS
Tablets (200 mg, 400 mg, and 600 mg)
Capsules (400 mg)
Sustained-release capsules (200 mg and 400 mg)
STORAGE
Meprobamate tablets and capsules should be stored at room temperature, in tightly closed containers.

USES
Meprobamate is used to relieve anxiety or tension, and is also prescribed as a sleeping aid. It is not exactly clear how

meprobamate works, but it is thought to act as a central nervous system depressant (a drug that slows the activity of the brain and spinal cord).

TREATMENT

In order to avoid stomach irritation, you can take meprobamate with food, or with a full glass of water or milk.

The sustained-release capsules should be swallowed whole. Breaking, chewing, or crushing these capsules destroys their sustained-release activity.

If you are taking this medication on a regular schedule and you miss a dose, take the missed dose immediately (if you remember within an hour or so), then return to your regular schedule. If more than an hour has passed, do not take the missed dose at all; just continue with your regular dosing schedule. Do not double the next dose.

SIDE EFFECTS

Minor. Blurred vision; diarrhea; dizziness; drowsiness; dry mouth; headache; nausea; vomiting; and weakness. These side effects should disappear in several days, as your body adjusts to the medication.

If you feel dizzy, sit or lie down awhile; get up slowly, and be careful on stairs.

To relieve mouth dryness, chew sugarless gum, or suck on ice chips or a piece of hard candy.

Major. Tell your doctor about any side effects that are persistent or particularly bothersome. IT IS ESPECIALLY IMPORTANT TO TELL YOUR DOCTOR about clumsiness; confusion; convulsions; difficulty breathing; difficult or painful urination; fainting; false sense of well-being; fever; nightmares; numbness or tingling; palpitations; rapid weight gain (3 to 5 pounds within a week); rash; slurred speech; sore throat; unusual bleeding or bruising; or unusual weakness.

INTERACTIONS

Concurrent use of meprobamate with other central nervous system depressants (such as alcohol, antihistamines, barbiturates, benzodiazepine tranquilizers, muscle relaxants, narcotics, pain medications, phenothiazine tranquilizers, and sleeping medications) or with tricyclic

anti-depressants can cause extreme drowsiness.
TELL YOUR DOCTOR if you are already taking one of
these medications.

WARNINGS

● Tell your doctor about any unusual or allergic reactions
you have had to medications, especially to meprobamate,
carbromal, carisoprodol, mebutamate, or tybamate.
● Before starting to take this medication, be sure to tell
your doctor if you now have, or if you have ever had, a history of drug abuse; epilepsy; kidney disease; liver disease,
or porphyria.
● If this drug causes dizziness or drowsiness, avoid tasks
that require alertness, such as driving a car or operating
potentially dangerous equipment.
● This drug has the potential for abuse and must be used
with caution. Tolerance develops quickly; do not increase
the dose unless you first consult your doctor.
● Do not stop taking this drug abruptly if you have been
taking it for two or three months. Stopping abruptly can
lead to a withdrawal reaction. Your doctor may therefore
want to reduce your dosage gradually.
● Some of these products contain F.D. & C. Yellow Dye
No. 5 (tartrazine), which can cause allergic-type symptoms (rash, fainting, shortness of breath) in certain susceptible individuals.
● Be sure to tell your doctor if you are pregnant. Meprobamate has been reported to cause birth defects when
taken during the first three months of pregnancy. Also, tell
your doctor if you are breastfeeding an infant. Meprobamate passes into breast milk and can cause excessive
drowsiness in the nursing infant.

---

meprobamate and aspirin combination

BRAND NAMES (Manufacturers)
Equagesic (Wyeth)
Micrainin (Wallace)

TYPE OF DRUG
Sedative and analgesic (pain reliever)
INGREDIENTS
meprobamate and aspirin
DOSAGE FORM
Tablets (200 mg meprobamate and 325 mg aspirin)
STORAGE
Meprobamate and aspirin tablets should be stored at room temperature in a tightly closed, light-resistant container. Moisture can cause aspirin to decompose.

USES
Meprobamate and aspirin is used to relieve tension headaches, or pain in muscles or joints accompanied by tension and/or anxiety. It is unclear exactly how meprobamate works to relieve anxiety and tension, but it appears to be a central nervous system depressant (a drug that slows the activity of the brain and spinal cord).

TREATMENT
In order to avoid stomach irritation, you can take meprobamate and aspirin with food or with a full glass of water or milk (unless your doctor directs you to do otherwise).

If you are taking this medication on a regular schedule and you miss a dose, take the missed dose as soon as possible, unless it is almost time for the next dose. In that case, do not take the missed dose at all; just return to your regular dosing schedule. Do not double the next dose.

SIDE EFFECTS
Minor. Abdominal pain; blurred vision; dizziness; drowsiness; fatigue; light-headedness; nausea; and vomiting. These side effects should disappear in several days, as your body adjusts to the medication.

If you feel dizzy or light-headed, sit or lie down awhile; get up slowly, and be careful on stairs.

Major. Tell your doctor about any side effects that are persistent or particularly bothersome. IT IS ESPECIALLY IMPORTANT TO TELL YOUR DOCTOR about buzzing in the ears; chest tightness; fainting; fever; headache; loss of coordination; mental depression; palpitations; shortness of breath; skin rash; or sore throat.

INTERACTIONS

Meprobamate and aspirin interacts with several other types of medication.

1. Concurrent use of meprobamate with other central nervous system depressants (such as alcohol, antihistamines, barbiturates, benzodiazepine tranquilizers, muscle relaxants, narcotics, pain medications, phenothiazine tranquilizers, and sleeping medications) or with tricyclic anti-depressants may cause extreme drowsiness.

2. Aspirin can increase the effects of warfarin, thereby leading to an increase in bleeding complications.

3. The anti-gout effects of probenecid and sulfinpyrazone may be blocked by aspirin.

4. Aspirin can increase the gastrointestinal side effects of anti-inflammation medications, alcohol, phenylbutazone, and adrenocorticosteroids (cortisone-like medicines).

5. Ammonium chloride, methionine, and furosemide can increase the side effects of aspirin; and acetazolamide, methazolamide, antacids, and phenobarbital can decrease the effectiveness of aspirin.

6. Aspirin can increase the side effects of methotrexate, penicillin, thyroid hormone, phenytoin, sulfinpyrazone, naproxen, valproic acid, insulin, and oral anti-diabetic medicines; and can decrease the effects of spironolactone. BE SURE TO TELL YOUR DOCTOR if you are already taking any of the medications listed above.

WARNINGS

● Tell your doctor about unusual or allergic reactions you have had to any medications, especially to meprobamate, carbromal, carisoprodol, mebutamate, tybamate, aspirin, methyl salicylate (oil of wintergreen), fenoprofen, ibuprofen, indomethacin, meclofenamate, mefenamic acid, naproxen, piroxicam, sulindac, or tolmetin.

● Before starting to take meprobamate and aspirin combination, be sure to tell your doctor if you now have, or if you have ever had, asthma, bleeding disorders, congestive heart failure, diabetes, epilepsy, glucose-6-phosphate dehydrogenase (G6PD) deficiency, gout, hemophilia, high blood pressure, kidney disease, liver disease, nasal polyps, peptic ulcers, porphyria, or thyroid disease.

● Before having any surgery or other medical or dental

treatment, be sure to tell your doctor or dentist that you are taking aspirin. Treatment with aspirin is usually discontinued five to seven days before surgery, to prevent bleeding complications.

• If this drug makes you dizzy or drowsy, avoid taking part in any activity that requires alertness, such as driving a car or operating potentially dangerous equipment.

• Diabetic patients should know that large doses of aspirin (greater than eight 325 mg tablets per day) can cause false readings on urine glucose tests. Diabetics should therefore check with their doctor before changing their insulin dosage while they are taking this medication.

• Meprobamate is potentially habit-forming. It should therefore be used with caution. If this drug is being used for several months, tolerance may develop. Do not stop taking the drug unless you first consult your doctor. A withdrawal reaction could result from stopping this medication abruptly. Your doctor may therefore want to reduce your dosage gradually.

• Be sure to tell your doctor if you are pregnant. Meprobamate can cause birth defects if taken during the first three months of pregnancy. In addition, large doses of aspirin taken close to term may prolong labor and may cause bleeding complications in the mother and heart problems in the infant. Also, tell your doctor if you are breastfeeding an infant. Both meprobamate and aspirin pass into breast milk.

Meprospan—see meprobamate

---

mesoridazine

BRAND NAME (Manufacturer)
Serentil (Boehringer Ingelheim)
TYPE OF DRUG
Phenothiazine tranquilizer
INGREDIENT
mesoridazine as the besylate salt
DOSAGE FORMS
Tablets (10 mg, 25 mg, 50 mg, and 100 mg)
Oral concentrate (25 mg per ml)

STORAGE

The tablet form of this medicine should be stored at room temperature in a tightly closed, light-resistant container. The oral concentrate form of this medication should be stored in the refrigerator in a tightly closed, light-resistant container. If the oral concentrate or suspension turns to a slight yellow color, the medicine is still effective and can be used. However, if the oral concentrate or suspension changes color markedly, or has particles floating in it, it should not be used, but discarded down the sink. This medication should never be frozen.

USES

Mesoridazine is prescribed to treat the symptoms of certain types of mental illness, such as emotional symptoms of psychosis, the manic phase of manic-depressive illness, and severe behavioral problems in children. This medication is thought to relieve the symptoms of mental illness by blocking certain chemicals involved with nerve transmission in the brain. Mesoridazine may also be used to treat anxiety.

TREATMENT

To avoid stomach irritation, you can take the tablet form of this medication with a meal or with a glass of water or milk (unless your doctor directs you to do otherwise).

The oral concentrate form of this medication should be measured carefully with the dropper provided, then added to 4 ounces (1/2 cup) or more of water, milk, juice, or a carbonated beverage, or to applesauce or pudding, immediately prior to administration. To prevent possible loss of effectiveness, the medication should not be diluted in tea, coffee, or apple juice.

If you miss a dose of this medication, take the missed dose as soon as possible and return to your regular dosing schedule. If it is almost time for the next dose, however, skip the one you missed and return to your regular schedule. Do not double the dose (unless your doctor directs you to do so).

The full effects of this medication for the control of emotional or mental symptoms may not become apparent for two weeks after you start to take it.

SIDE EFFECTS

Minor. Blurred vision; constipation; decreased sweating; diarrhea; discoloration of the urine to red, pink, or red-brown; dizziness; drooling; drowsiness; dry mouth; fatigue; jitteriness; menstrual irregularities; nasal congestion; restlessness; tremors; vomiting; and weight gain. As your body adjusts to the medication, these side effects should disappear.

If you are constipated, increase the amount of fiber in your diet (raw vegetables, fruits, salads, bran, and whole-grain breads), and drink more water (unless your doctor directs you to do otherwise).

Chew sugarless gum, or suck on ice chips or a piece of hard candy, to reduce mouth dryness.

This medication can cause increased sensitivity to sunlight. Therefore, it is important to avoid prolonged exposure to sunlight or sunlamps. Wear protective clothing, and use an effective sunscreen.

To avoid dizziness when you stand, contract and relax the muscles of your legs for a few moments before rising. Do this by pushing one foot against the floor while raising the other foot slightly, alternating feet so that you are "pumping" your legs in a pedaling motion.

Major. Tell your doctor about any side effects that are persistent or particularly bothersome. IT IS ESPECIALLY IMPORTANT TO TELL YOUR DOCTOR about unusual bleeding or bruising; breast enlargement (in both sexes); chest pain; convulsions; darkened skin; difficulty swallowing or breathing; fainting; fever; impotence; involuntary movements of the face, mouth, jaw, or tongue; palpitations; rash; sleep disorders; sore throat; uncoordinated movements; visual disturbances; or yellowing of the eyes or skin.

INTERACTIONS

Mesoridazine interacts with several other types of drugs.
1. It can cause extreme drowsiness when combined with alcohol; other central nervous system depressants (drugs that slow the activity of the nervous system), such as barbiturates, benzodiazepine tranquilizers, muscle relaxants, narcotics, and pain medications; or with tricyclic anti-depressants.

2. Mesoridazine can decrease the effectiveness of amphetamines, guanethidine, anti-convulsants, and levodopa.

3. The side effects of ephinephrine, monoamine oxidase (MAO) inhibitors, propranolol, phenytoin, and tricyclic anti-depressants may be increased when combined with this medication.

4. Lithium may increase the side effects and decrease the effectiveness of this medication.

5. Antacids and anti-diarrhea medicines may decrease the absorption of mesoridazine from the gastrointestinal tract. Therefore, at least one hour should separate doses of one of these medicines and mesoridazine.

Before starting to take mesoridazine, BE SURE TO TELL YOUR DOCTOR if you are already taking any of the medications listed above.

WARNINGS

● Tell your doctor about unusual or allergic reactions you have had to medications, especially to any phenothiazine tranquilizers (such as acetophenazine, carphenazine, chlorpromazine, fluphenazine, mesoridazine, perphenazine, piperacetazine, prochlorperazine, promazine, thioridazine, trifluoperazine, triflupromazine), or to loxapine.

● Tell your doctor if you now have, or if you have ever had, any blood disease, bone marrow disease, brain disease, breast cancer, blockage in the urinary or digestive tracts, alcoholism, drug-induced depression, epilepsy, severe high or low blood pressure, diabetes mellitus (sugar diabetes), glaucoma, heart or circulatory disease, liver disease, lung disease, Parkinson's disease, peptic ulcers, or an enlarged prostate gland.

● Tell your doctor about any recent exposure to a pesticide or an insecticide. Mesoridazine may increase the side effects from the exposure.

● To prevent over-sedation, avoid drinking alcoholic beverages while taking this medication.

● If this medication makes you dizzy or drowsy, do not take part in any activity that requires alertness, such as driving a car or operating potentially dangerous equipment. Be careful on stairs, and avoid getting up suddenly from a lying or sitting position.

• Prior to having surgery or any other medical or dental treatment, be sure your doctor or dentist knows that you are taking this medication.

• Some of the side effects caused by this drug can be prevented by taking an anti-parkinson drug. Discuss this with your doctor.

• This type of drug has been reported to cause certain tumors in rats. This effect has not been shown to occur in humans.

• Mesoridazine can decrease sweating and heat release from the body. You should therefore avoid getting overheated by strenuous exercise in hot weather, and should avoid hot baths, showers, and saunas.

• Do not stop taking this medication suddenly. If the drug is stopped abruptly you may experience nausea, vomiting, stomach upset, headache, increased heart rate, insomnia, tremulousness, or a worsening of your condition. Your doctor may want to reduce the dosage gradually.

• If you are planning to have a myelogram, or any procedure in which dye is injected into your spinal cord, tell your doctor that you are taking this medication.

• Avoid spilling the oral concentrate form of this medication on your skin or clothing; it may cause redness and irritation of the skin.

• While taking this medication, do not take any over-the-counter (non-prescription) medication for weight control, or for cough, cold, allergy, asthma, or sinus problems, without first checking with your doctor. The combination of these medications may cause high blood pressure.

• Be sure to tell your doctor if you are pregnant. Small amounts of this medication cross the placenta. Although there are reports of safe use of this drug during pregnancy, there are also reports of liver disease and tremors in newborn infants whose mothers received this type of medication close to term. Also, tell your doctor if you are breastfeeding an infant. Small amounts of this medication pass into breast milk and may cause unwanted effects in the nursing infant.

Metahydrin—see trichlormethiazide

Metandren—see methyltestosterone

Metaprel—see metaproterenol

---

metaproterenol

BRAND NAMES (Manufacturers)
Alupent (Boehringer Ingelheim)
Metaprel (Dorsey)
TYPE OF DRUG
Bronchodilator
INGREDIENT
metaproterenol as the sulfate salt
DOSAGE FORMS
Tablets (10 mg and 20 mg)
Oral syrup (10 mg per 5 ml teaspoonful)
Inhalation aerosol (each spray delivers 0.65 mg)
Solution for nebulization (0.6% and 5%)
STORAGE
Metaproterenol tablets and oral syrup should be stored at room temperature in tightly closed, light-resistant containers. The solution for nebulization should be stored in the refrigerator. The inhalation aerosol should be stored at room temperature, away from excessive heat—the contents are pressurized and the container can explode if heated. Metaproterenol syrup and solution should not be used if they turn brown or contain particles—such changes indicate that the drug has lost its effectiveness.

USES
Metaproterenol is used to relieve wheezing and shortness of breath caused by lung diseases such as asthma, bronchitis, and emphysema. This drug acts directly on the muscles of the bronchi (breathing tubes) to relieve bronchospasm (muscle contractions of the bronchi), thereby reducing airway resistance, and allowing air to move more freely to and from the lungs—making breathing easier.

TREATMENT
In order to lessen stomach upset, you can take metaproterenol tablets or oral syrup with food (unless your doctor

directs you to do otherwise).

The oral syrup form of this medication should be measured carefully, with a specially designed, 5 ml measuring spoon. An ordinary kitchen teaspoon is not accurate enough.

The inhalation aerosol form of this medication is usually packaged with an instruction sheet. Read the directions carefully before using this medication. The container should be shaken well just before each use. The contents tend to settle on the bottom, so it is necessary to shake the container to evenly distribute the ingredients and equalize the doses. If more than one inhalation is necessary, wait at least one full minute between doses, so that you receive the full benefit of the first dose.

If you miss a dose of this medication and it is within an hour of your regular dosage schedule, take it when you remember, then follow your regular schedule for the next dose. If you miss the dose by more than an hour or so, just wait until the next scheduled dose. Do not double the dose.

SIDE EFFECTS

Minor. Anxiety; dizziness; headache; flushing; irritability; insomnia; loss of appetite; muscle cramps; nausea; nervousness; restlessness; sweating; tremors; vomiting; weakness; and dryness or irritation of the mouth or throat (from the inhalation aerosol). These side effects should disappear in several days, as your body adjusts to the medication.

To help prevent dryness and irritation of the mouth or throat, rinse your mouth with water after each dose of the inhalation aerosol.

In order to avoid difficulty in falling asleep, check with your doctor to see if you can take the last dose of this medication several hours before bedtime each day.

If you feel dizzy, sit or lie down awhile; get up from a sitting or lying position slowly, and be careful on stairs.

Major. Tell your doctor about any side effects that are persistent or particularly bothersome. IT IS ESPECIALLY IMPORTANT TO TELL YOUR DOCTOR about chest pain; difficult or painful urination; palpitations; or pounding heartbeat.

INTERACTIONS

Metaproterenol interacts with other types of medication.

1. Beta-blockers (atenolol, metoprolol, nadolol, pindolol, propranolol, timolol) antagonize (act against) this medication, decreasing its effectiveness.

2. Monoamine oxidase (MAO) inhibitors, tricyclic antidepressants, antihistamines, levothyroxine, and over-the-counter (non-prescription) cough, cold, allergy, asthma, diet, and sinus medications may increase the side effects of metaproterenol.

3. There may be a change in the dosage requirements of insulin or oral anti-diabetic medications when metaprotrenol is started.

4. The blood-pressure-lowering effects of guanethidine may be decreased by this medication.

TELL YOUR DOCTOR if you are already taking any of the medications listed above.

WARNINGS

• Tell your doctor about unusual or allergic reactions you have had, especially to metaprotrenol or any related drug (such as albuterol, amphetamines, ephedrine, epinephrine, isoproterenol, norepinephrine, phenylephrine, phenylpropanolamine, pseudoephedrine, or terbutaline).

• Tell your doctor if you now have, or if you have ever had, diabetes, glaucoma, high blood pressure, epilepsy, heart disease, enlarged prostate gland, or thyroid disease.

• This medication can cause dizziness. Your ability to perform tasks that require alertness, such as driving a car or operating potentially dangerous machinery, may be decreased. Appropriate caution should therefore be taken.

• Before having any surgery or other medical or dental treatment, be sure to tell your doctor or dentist that you are taking this medication.

• Do not exceed the recommended dosage of this medication; excessive use may lead to an increase in side effects or a loss of effectiveness.

• Try to avoid contact of the aerosol inhalation with your eyes.

• Do not puncture, break, or burn the aerosol inhalation container. The contents are under pressure and may explode.

• Contact your doctor if you do not respond to the usual dose of this medication. It may be a sign of worsening asthma, which may require additional therapy.
• Be sure to tell your doctor if you are pregnant. The effects of this medication during pregnancy have not yet been thoroughly studied in humans, but it has caused side effects in offspring of animals who received large doses during pregnancy. Also, tell your doctor if you are breast-feeding an infant. It is not known whether or not this drug passes into breast milk.

methadone

BRAND NAMES (Manufacturers)
Dolophine (Lilly)
methadone hydrochloride (various manufacturers)
TYPE OF DRUG
Analgesic (pain reliever)
INGREDIENT
methadone as the hydrochloride salt
DOSAGE FORMS
Tablets (5 mg and 10 mg)
Oral solution (5 mg and 10 mg per 5 ml teaspoonful with 8% alcohol)
STORAGE
Methadone should be stored at room temperature in tightly closed, light-resistant containers.

USES
Methadone is a narcotic analgesic that acts directly on the central nervous system (brain and spinal cord). It is used to relieve moderate to severe pain. It is also used to detoxify narcotic addicts and to provide temporary maintenance treatment.

TREATMENT
In order to avoid stomach upset, you can take methadone with food or milk. It works most effectively if you take it at the onset of pain, rather than waiting until the pain becomes intense.

Measure the dose of the solution form of this medication carefully, with a specially designed, 5 ml measuring spoon. An ordinary kitchen teaspoon is not accurate enough.

If you are taking this medication on a regular schedule and you miss a dose, take the missed dose as soon as possible, unless it is almost time for your next dose. In that case, don't take the missed dose at all; just return to your regular dosing schedule. Do not double the next dose.

SIDE EFFECTS

Minor. Constipation; dizziness; drowsiness; dry mouth; false sense of well-being; flushing; light-headedness; loss of appetite; nausea; rash; sweating; and painful or difficult urination. These side effects should disappear in several days, as your body adjusts to the medication.

If you are constipated, increase the amount of fiber in your diet (raw vegetables, fruits, salads, bran, and whole-grain breads), and drink more water (unless your doctor directs you to do otherwise).

Chew sugarless gum, or suck on ice chips or a piece of hard candy, to reduce mouth dryness.

If you feel dizzy, light-headed, or nauseated, sit or lie down awhile; get up from a sitting or lying position slowly, and be careful on stairs.

Major. Tell your doctor about any side effects that are persistent or particularly bothersome. IT IS ESPECIALLY IMPORTANT TO TELL YOUR DOCTOR about anxiety; breathing difficulties; excitation; fainting; fatigue; pounding heartbeat; restlessness; sore throat and fever; tremors; or weakness.

INTERACTIONS

Methadone interacts with several other types of drugs.

1. Concurrent use of it with other central nervous system depressants (drugs that slow the activity of the nervous system), such as alcohol, antihistamines, barbiturates, benzodiazepine tranquilizers, muscle relaxants, and phenothiazine tranquilizers, or with tricyclic anti-depressants can cause extreme drowsiness.

2. A monoamine oxidase (MAO) inhibitor taken within 14 days of this medication can lead to unpredictable and severe side effects.

3. Rifampin and phenytoin can decrease the blood levels and effectiveness of methadone.

4. Cimetidine, combined with this medication, can cause confusion, disorientation, seizures, and shortness of breath.

TELL YOUR DOCTOR if you are currently taking any of the medications listed above.

WARNINGS

• Tell your doctor about unusual or allergic reactions you have had to medications, especially to methadone or to any other narcotic analgesic (such as codeine, hydrocodone, hydromorphone, meperidine, morphine, oxycodone, or propoxyphene).

• Tell your doctor if you now have, or if you have ever had, acute abdominal conditions, asthma, brain disease, colitis, epilepsy, gallstones or gallbladder disease, head injuries, heart disease, kidney disease, liver disease, lung disease, mental illness, emotional disorders, enlarged prostate gland, thyroid disease, or urethral stricture.

• If this drug makes you dizzy or drowsy, do not take part in any activity that requires alertness, such as driving a car or operating potentially dangerous equipment.

• Before having any surgery or other medical or dental treatment, be sure to tell your doctor or dentist that you are taking this medication.

• Methadone has the potential for abuse, and must be used with caution. Usually, it should not be taken on a regular schedule for longer than ten days (unless your doctor directs you to do so). Tolerance develops quickly; do not increase the dosage or stop taking the drug abruptly, unless you first consult your doctor. If you have been taking large amounts of this medication or if you have been taking it for long periods of time, you may experience a withdrawal reaction (muscle aches, diarrhea, gooseflesh, runny nose, nausea, vomiting, shivering, trembling, stomach cramps, sleep disorders, irritability, weakness, yawning, and sweating) when you stop taking it. Your doctor may therefore want to reduce the dosage gradually.

• Be sure to tell your doctor if you are pregnant. The effects of this medication during the early stages of pregnancy have not yet been thoroughly studied in humans.

However, methadone, used regularly in large doses during the later stages of pregnancy, can result in addiction of the fetus, leading to withdrawal symptoms (irritability, excessive crying, tremors, fever, vomiting, diarrhea, sneezing, and yawning) at birth. Also, tell your doctor if you are breastfeeding an infant. Small amounts of this medication may pass into breast milk and cause excessive drowsiness in the nursing infant.

methadone hydrochloride—see methadone

Methampex—see methamphetamine

---

methamphetamine

BRAND NAMES (Manufacturers)
Desoxyn (Abbott)
Desoxyn Gradumets (Abbott)
Methampex (Lemmon)
TYPE OF DRUG
Amphetamine (central nervous system stimulant)
INGREDIENT
methamphetamine as the hydrochloride salt
DOSAGE FORMS
Tablets (5 mg and 10 mg)
Sustained-release capsules (5 mg, 10 mg, and 15 mg)
STORAGE
Methamphetamine should be stored at room temperature in tightly closed containers.

USES

This medication is a central nervous system stimulant that increases mental alertness and decreases fatigue. It is used to treat narcolepsy (problems in staying awake) and abnormal behavioral syndrome in children (hyperkinetic syndrome or attention deficit disorder). The way this medication acts to control abnormal behavioral syndrome in children is not clearly understood.

Methamphetamine is also used as an appetite suppressant during the first few weeks of dieting (while you are trying to establish new eating habits). It is thought to relieve hunger by altering nerve impulses to the appetite control center in the brain. Its effectiveness as an appetite suppressant lasts only for short periods (three to 12 weeks), however.

TREATMENT

In order to avoid stomach upset, you can take methamphetamine with food or with a full glass of milk or water (unless your doctor directs you to do otherwise).

If this medication is being used to treat narcolepsy or abnormal behavioral syndrome in children, the first dose each day should be taken soon after awakening. Subsequent doses should be spaced at four- to six-hour intervals.

If this medication has been prescribed as a diet aid, it should be taken one hour before each meal.

The sustained-release form of this medication should be swallowed whole. Breaking, chewing, or crushing these capsules destroys their sustained-release activity, and may increase the side effects.

In order to avoid difficulty in falling asleep, the last dose of this medication each day should be taken four to six hours before bedtime (tablets) or ten to 14 hours before bedtime (sustained-release capsules).

If you miss a dose of this medication, take the missed dose as soon as possible, unless it is almost time for your next dose. In that case, don't take the missed dose at all; just return to your regular dosing schedule. Do not double the next dose.

SIDE EFFECTS

Minor. Abdominal cramps; constipation; diarrhea; dry mouth; false sense of well-being; dizziness; insomnia; loss of appetite; irritability; nausea; overstimulation; restlessness; unpleasant taste; and vomiting. These side effects should disappear in several days, as your body adjusts to the medication.

In order to prevent constipation, increase the amount of fiber in your diet (fresh fruits and vegetables, salads, bran, whole-grain cereals and breads), drink more water, and increase your exercise (unless your doctor directs you to do otherwise).

Dry mouth can be relieved by sucking on ice chips or a piece of hard candy, or by chewing sugarless gum.

If you feel dizzy, sit or lie down awhile; get up from a sitting or lying position slowly, and be careful on stairs.

Major. Tell your doctor about any side effects that are persistent or particularly bothersome. IT IS ESPECIALLY IMPORTANT TO TELL YOUR DOCTOR about blurred vision; confusion; fatigue; headaches; impotence; mental depression; palpitations; rash; sweating; tightness in the chest; tremors; or uncoordinated movements.

INTERACTIONS

Methamphetamine interacts with several other types of medication.

1. Use of it within 14 days of a monoamine oxidase (MAO) inhibitor (isocarboxazid, pargyline, phenelzine, tranylcypromine) can result in high blood pressure and other side effects.

2. Barbiturate medications, phenothiazine tranquilizers (especially chlorpromazine), and tricyclic anti-depressants can antagonize (act against) this medication.

3. Amphetamines (such as methamphetamine) can decrease the blood-pressure-lowering effects of anti-hypertensive medication (especially guanethidine), and may alter insulin and oral anti-diabetic medication dosage requirements in diabetic patients.

4. The side effects of other central nervous system stimulants, such as caffeine, over-the-counter (non-prescription) appetite suppressants, and asthma, allergy, cough, sinus, or cold preparations, may be increased by methamphetamine.

5. Acetazolamide and sodium bicarbonate can decrease the elimination of methamphetamine from the body, thereby prolonging its action, and increasing the risk of side effects.

TELL YOUR DOCTOR if you are currently taking any of the medications listed above.

WARNINGS

● Tell your doctor about unusual or allergic reactions you have had to any medications, especially to methamphetamine or other central nervous system stimulants (such as albuterol, amphetamine, dextroamphetamine, ephedrine, isoproterenol, metaproterenol, norepinephrine, phenylephrine, phenylpropanolamine, pseudoephedrine, or terbutaline).

● Tell your doctor if you have a history of drug abuse, or if you have ever had problems with agitation, diabetes mellitus (sugar diabetes), glaucoma, heart or blood vessel disease, high blood pressure, or thyroid disease.

● Methamphetamine can mask the symptoms of extreme fatigue and can cause dizziness. Your ability to perform tasks that require alertness, such as driving a car or operating potentially dangerous machinery, may be decreased. Appropriate caution should therefore be taken.

● Before having any surgery or other medical or dental treatment, be sure to tell your doctor or dentist that you are taking this medication.

● Methamphetamine is related to amphetamine and may be habit-forming when taken for long periods of time (both physical and psychological dependence can occur). Therefore, you should not increase the dose of this medication or take it for longer than 12 weeks, unless you first consult your doctor. It is also important that you not stop taking this medication abruptly—fatigue; sleep disorders; mental depression; or nausea, vomiting, stomach cramps, or pain could occur. Your doctor may therefore want to reduce your dosage gradually.

● Some of these products contain F.D. & C. Yellow Dye No. 5 (tartrazine), which can cause allergic-type reactions (difficulty breathing, rash, or fainting) in certain susceptible individuals.

● Be sure to tell your doctor if you are pregnant. Although side effects in humans have not yet been studied, some of the amphetamines can cause heart, brain, and biliary tract abnormalities in the fetuses of animals who receive large doses of these drugs during pregnancy. Also, tell your doctor if you are breastfeeding an infant. Small amounts of this type of drug pass into breast milk, and can cause excessive stimulation in nursing infants.

methenamine

BRAND NAMES (Manufacturers)
Hiprex (Merrell Dow)
Mandelamine* (Parke-Davis)
methenamine mandelate (various manufacturers)
Urex (Riker)
*Note that methenamine is also available over-the-counter
(non-prescription).

TYPE OF DRUG
Antibiotic (infection fighter)

INGREDIENT
methenamine as the hippurate or mandelate salt

DOSAGE FORMS
Tablets (500 mg and 1,000 mg)
Enteric-coated tablets (250 mg, 500 mg, and 1,000 mg)
Oral suspension (250 mg and 500 mg per
  5 ml teaspoonful)
Oral granules (500 mg and 1000 mg packets)

STORAGE
Methenamine tablets, oral suspension, and granules
should be stored at room temperature in tightly closed
containers. This medication should never be frozen.

USES
Methenamine is used to prevent and treat bacterial infections of the urinary tract. It is chemically converted in the
bladder to ammonia and formaldehyde, which kills ac-
tively growing bacteria.

TREATMENT
In order to avoid stomach irritation, you should take
methenamine with food or with a full glass of water or
milk (unless your doctor directs you to do otherwise).

The oral suspension form of this medication should be
shaken well, just before measuring each dose. The contents tend to settle on the bottom of the bottle, so it is necessary to shake the container to evenly distribute the
ingredients and equalize the doses. Each dose should then
be measured carefully, with a specially designed, 5 ml
measuring spoon. An ordinary kitchen teaspoon is not accurate enough.

The enteric-coated tablets should be swallowed whole. Breaking, crushing, or chewing these tablets increases their gastrointestinal side effects.

If you are taking the oral granules, the contents of the packet should be dissolved in 2 to 4 ounces of water, just before you take the dose.

Methenamine works best when the level of medicine in your bloodstream and urine is kept constant. It is best, therefore, to take the doses at evenly spaced intervals, day and night. For example, if you are to take four doses a day, the doses should be spaced six hours apart.

Try not to miss any doses of this medication. If you do miss a dose, take it immediately. Even if you do not remember to take the missed dose until it is almost time for your next dose, take the missed dose immediately. Space the following dose about halfway through the regular interval between doses. Then continue with your regular dosing schedule.

It is important to continue to take this medication for the entire time prescribed by your doctor (usually seven to 14 days), even if the symptoms disappear before the end of that period. If you stop taking the drug too soon, resistant bacteria are given a chance to continue growing, and the infection could recur.

SIDE EFFECTS

Minor. Abdominal cramps; diarrhea; headache; loss of appetite; nausea; and vomiting. These side effects should disappear in several days, as your body adjusts to the medication.

Major. Tell your doctor about any side effects that are persistent or particularly bothersome. IT IS ESPECIALLY IMPORTANT TO TELL YOUR DOCTOR about difficulty breathing; difficult or painful urination; itching; mouth sores; rapid weight gain (3 to 5 pounds within a week); shortness of breath; or skin rash.

INTERACTIONS

Methenamine interacts with several other medications.
1. Sodium bicarbonate, antacids, acetazolamide, and diuretics can decrease the effectiveness of methenamine by preventing its conversion to formaldehyde.

2. Methenamine can increase the side effects (to the kidneys) of sulfonamide antibiotics.

Before starting to take methenamine, TELL YOUR DOCTOR if you are already taking any of these other medications.

WARNINGS

• Tell your doctor about unusual or allergic reactions you have had to any medications, especially to methenamine.
• Before starting to take methenamine, be sure to tell your doctor if you now have, or if you have ever had, dehydration, kidney disease, or liver disease.
• Some of these products contain F.D. & C. Yellow Dye No. 5 (tartrazine), which can cause allergic-type symptoms (shortness of breath, fainting, rash) in certain susceptible individuals.
• This medication has been prescribed for your current infection only. Another infection later on, or one that someone else has, may require a different medicine. You should not give your medicine to other people, or use it for other infections, unless your doctor specifically directs you to do so.
• If the symptoms of your infection do not improve in several days, CONTACT YOUR DOCTOR. This medication may not be effective for your infection.
• In order for this medication to work properly it is necessary that your urine remain acidic. You should therefore avoid foods that cause the urine to become alkaline (nonacidic), such as citrus fruits and milk products. Your doctor may also want you to take vitamin C (ascorbic acid) to help keep the urine acidic.
• Be sure to tell your doctor if you are pregnant. Although methenamine appears to be safe during pregnancy, it does cross the placenta, and extensive studies have not yet been completed. Also, tell your doctor if you are breastfeeding an infant. Small amounts of methenamine pass into breast milk.

methenamine mandelate—see methenamine

Metho-500—see methocarbamol

methocarbamol

BRAND NAMES (Manufacturers)
Delaxin (Ferndale)
Marbaxin (Vortech)
Metho-500 (Mallard)
methocarbamol (various manufacturers)
Robaxin (Robins)
SK-Methocarbamol (Smith Kline & French)

TYPE OF DRUG
Muscle relaxant

INGREDIENT
methocarbamol

DOSAGE FORM
Tablets (500 mg and 750 mg)

STORAGE
Methocarbamol should be stored at room temperature in a tightly closed container.

USES
This medication is used to relieve the discomfort of painful muscle aches and spasms. It should be used in conjunction with rest, physical therapy, and other measures that your doctor may prescribe. It is not clear exactly how methocarbamol works, but it is thought to relieve muscle spasms by acting as a central nervous system depressant (a drug that slows the activity of the brain and spinal cord).

TREATMENT
Methocarbamol can be taken either on an empty stomach, or with food or a full glass of water or milk (as directed by your doctor). These tablets can be crushed and mixed with food or liquid if you have trouble swallowing them.

If you miss a dose of this medication and remember within an hour of the scheduled time, take the missed dose immediately. If more than an hour has passed, do not take the missed dose; just return to your regular dosing schedule. Do not double the next dose.

SIDE EFFECTS
Minor. Dizziness; drowsiness; headache; light-headed-

ness; metallic taste in the mouth; nausea; nasal congestion; and stomach upset. These side effects should disappear in several days, as your body adjusts to the medication.

If you feel dizzy or light-headed, sit or lie down awhile; get up slowly, and be careful on stairs.

This medication can cause the urine to darken to brown, black, or green. This is a harmless effect.

Major. Tell your doctor about any side effects that are persistent or particularly bothersome. IT IS ESPECIALLY IMPORTANT TO TELL YOUR DOCTOR about fainting; fatigue; fever; flushing; uncoordinated movements; skin rash; or visual disturbances.

INTERACTIONS

Methocarbamol interacts with several other types of medication.

1. Concurrent use of methocarbamol with other central nervous system depressants (such as alcohol, antihistamines, barbiturates, benzodiazepine tranquilizers, muscle relaxants, narcotics, pain medications, phenothiazine tranquilizers, and sleeping medications) or with tricyclic anti-depressants can cause extreme drowsiness.

2. Methocarbamol can decrease the effectiveness of pyridostigmine.

Before starting to take methocarbamol, BE SURE TO TELL YOUR DOCTOR if you are already taking any of these medications.

WARNINGS

• Tell your doctor about unusual or allergic reactions you have had to any medications, especially to methocarbamol.

• Before starting to take this medication, be sure to tell your doctor if you now have, or if you have ever had, brain disease.

• If this drug makes you dizzy or drowsy, avoid taking part in any activity that requires mental alertness, such as driving a car or operating potentially dangerous equipment.

• Be sure to tell your doctor if you are pregnant. Although methocarbamol appears to be safe, extensive studies in humans have not yet been completed. Also, tell your doctor if you are breastfeeding an infant. Small amounts of methocarbamol pass into breast milk.

---

methotrexate

BRAND NAME (Manufacturer)
Methotrexate (Lederle)
TYPE OF DRUG
Anti-neoplastic (anti-cancer drug)
INGREDIENT
methotrexate
DOSAGE FORM
Tablets (2.5 mg)
STORAGE
Methotrexate should be stored at room temperature, in a tightly closed container.

USES

Methotrexate is used to treat certain types of cancers and severe psoriasis. It works by slowing cell growth (multiplication) in rapidly growing cells.

TREATMENT

In order to avoid stomach irritation, you can take methotrexate with food or with a full glass of water or milk (unless your doctor directs you to do otherwise).

Try not to miss any doses of this medication. If you do miss a dose, take the missed dose as soon as possible, unless it is almost time for the next dose. In that case, do not take the missed dose at all; just return to your regular dosing schedule. Do not double the next dose. If you miss more than two doses in a row, CONTACT YOUR DOCTOR.

SIDE EFFECTS

Minor. Abdominal distress; fatigue; loss of appetite; nasal congestion; nausea; and vomiting. These side effects should disappear in several weeks, as your body adjusts to the medication. Methotrexate also causes hair loss, which is reversible when the medication is stopped.

This medication can increase your sensitivity to sunlight. Avoid prolonged exposure to sunlight and sunlamps. Wear protective clothing and sunglasses, and use an effective sunscreen.

Major. Tell your doctor about any side effects that are persistent or particularly bothersome. IT IS ESPECIALLY IMPORTANT TO TELL YOUR DOCTOR about unusual bleeding or bruising; back pain; blurred vision; convulsions; skin color changes; diarrhea; drowsiness; fever; headache; itching; difficult or painful urination; menstrual changes; mouth sores; rash; severe abdominal pain; or yellowing of the eyes or skin.

INTERACTIONS

Methotrexate interacts with a number of other medications.

1. Concurrent use of alcohol and methotrexate can lead to an increased risk of liver damage.

2. Methotrexate can block the effectiveness of anti-gout medications.

3. Phenylbutazone, probenecid, phenytoin, tetracycline, aspirin, chloramphenicol, and sulfonamide antibiotics can increase the blood levels of methotrexate, which can lead to an increase in side effects.

4. Methotrexate can increase the effects of warfarin, which can lead to bleeding complications.

Before starting to take methotrexate, BE SURE TO TELL YOUR DOCTOR if you are already taking any of the medications listed above.

WARNINGS

• Tell your doctor about unusual or allergic reactions you have had to any medications, especially to methotrexate.

• Before starting to take this medication, be sure to tell your doctor if you now have, or if you have ever had, blood disorders, gout, infection, kidney disease, liver disease, or inflammation of the gastrointestinal tract.

• If this drug makes you dizzy or drowsy, do not take part in any activity that requires alertness, such as driving a car or operating potentially dangerous equipment.

• While you are taking methotrexate, you should drink plenty of fluids, so that you urinate often (unless your doctor directs you to do otherwise). This helps prevent kidney and bladder problems.

● You should not be immunized or vaccinated while taking methotrexate. The vaccine or immunization will not be effective, and may lead to an infection.

● Methotrexate is a potent medication that can cause serious side effects. Your doctor will therefore want to monitor your therapy carefully with blood tests.

● Be sure to tell your doctor if you are pregnant. Methotrexate has been shown to cause birth defects or death of the fetus. Effective contraception should be used during treatment and for at least eight weeks after treatment with the drug is stopped. Also, tell your doctor if you are breast-feeding an infant. Methotrexate passes into breast milk and can cause side effects in nursing infants.

---

methyclothiazide

BRAND NAMES (Manufacturers)
Aquatensen (Wallace)
Enduron (Abbott)
Ethon (Major)
methyclothiazide (various manufacturers)
TYPE OF DRUG
Diuretic (water pill) and anti-hypertensive
INGREDIENT
methyclothiazide
DOSAGE FORM
Tablets (2.5 mg and 5 mg)
STORAGE
This medication should be stored at room temperature in a tightly closed container.

USES

Methyclothiazide is prescribed to treat high blood pressure. It is also used to reduce fluid accumulation in the body caused by conditions such as heart failure, cirrhosis of the liver, kidney disease, and the long-term use of some medications. This medication reduces fluid accumulation by increasing the elimination of sodium and water through the kidneys.

TREATMENT

This medication can be taken with a glass of milk or with a meal to decrease stomach irritation (unless your doctor directs you to do otherwise). Try to take it at the same time every day. Avoid taking a dose after 6:00 P.M.—this will prevent you from having to get up during the night to urinate.

If you miss a dose of this medication, take the missed dose as soon as possible, unless it is almost time for the next dose. In that case, do not take the missed dose at all; just wait until the next scheduled dose. Do not double the dose.

This medication does not cure high blood pressure, but it will help to control the condition, as long as you continue to take it.

SIDE EFFECTS

Minor. Constipation; cramps; diarrhea; dizziness; drowsiness; headache; heartburn; itching; loss of appetite; nausea; restlessness; upset stomach; and vomiting. As your body adjusts to the medication, these side effects should disappear.

This medication can cause increased sensitivity to sunlight. It is therefore important to avoid prolonged exposure to sunlight or sunlamps. Wear protective clothing, and use an effective sunscreen.

To avoid dizziness or light-headedness when you stand, contract and relax the muscles of your legs for a few moments before rising. Do this by pushing one foot against the floor while raising the other foot slightly, alternating the feet so that you are "pumping" your legs in a pedaling motion.

Major. Tell your doctor about any side effects that are persistent or particularly bothersome. IT IS ESPECIALLY IMPORTANT TO TELL YOUR DOCTOR about unusual bleeding or bruising; blurred vision; confusion; difficulty breathing; dry mouth; fainting; fever; mood changes; muscle spasms; palpitations; skin rash; excessive thirst; sore throat; joint pain; tingling in the fingers or toes; excessive weakness; or yellowing of the eyes or skin.

INTERACTIONS

Methyclothiazide can interact with other medications.

1. It may decrease the effectiveness of oral anti-coagulants, anti-gout medications, insulin, oral anti-diabetic medicines, and methenamine.

2. Fenfluramine can increase the blood-pressure-lowering effects of methyclothiazide (which can be dangerous).

3. Indomethacin can decrease the blood-pressure-lowering effects (thereby counteracting the desired effects) of methyclothiazide.

4. Cholestyramine and colestipol decrease the absorption of this medication from the gastrointestinal tract. Methyclothiazide should therefore be taken one hour before, or four hours after, a dose of cholestyramine or colestipol (if you have also been prescribed one of these medications).

5. The side effects of amphotericin B, calcium, cortisone-like steroids (such as cortisone, dexamethasone, hydrocortisone, prednisone, prednisolone), digoxin, digitalis, lithium, quinidine, sulfonamide antibiotics, and vitamin D may be increased when taken concurrently with methyclothiazide.

BE SURE TO TELL YOUR DOCTOR if you are taking any of the medicines listed above.

WARNINGS

● Tell your doctor about unusual or allergic reactions you have had to any medications, especially to diuretics (water pills), oral anti-diabetic medications, or sulfonamide antibiotics.

● Before you start taking methyclothiazide, tell your doctor if you now have, or if you have ever had, kidney disease or problems with urination, diabetes mellitus (sugar diabetes), gout, liver disease, asthma, pancreas disease, or systemic lupus erythematosus (SLE).

● Methyclothiazide can cause potassium loss. Signs of potassium loss include dry mouth, thirst, weakness, muscle pain or cramps, nausea, and vomiting. If you experience any of these symptoms, call your doctor. To help avoid potassium loss, take this drug with a glass of fresh or frozen orange juice or cranberry juice, or eat a banana every day. The use of a salt substitute also helps to prevent potassium loss. Do not change your diet, however, before discussing it with your doctor. Too much potassium can also be dangerous. Your doctor may want you to have blood tests performed periodically, in order to monitor your potassium levels.

• In order to avoid dizziness or fainting while taking this medication, try not to stand for long periods of time; avoid drinking excessive amounts of alcohol; and avoid getting overheated (strenuous exercise in hot weather; hot baths, showers, and saunas).

• Do not take any over-the-counter (non-prescription) medications for weight control or for cough, cold, allergy, asthma, or sinus problems, unless your doctor directs you to do so. Some of these products can cause an increase in blood pressure.

• To prevent dehydration (severe water loss) while taking this medication, check with your doctor if you have any illness that causes severe nausea, vomiting, or diarrhea.

• This medication can raise blood sugar in diabetic patients. Therefore, blood sugar levels should be carefully monitored by blood or urine tests when this medication is started.

• Be sure to tell your doctor if you are pregnant. This drug is able to cross the placenta. Although studies in humans have not been completed, adverse effects have been observed in the fetuses of animals who were given large doses of this drug during pregnancy. Also, tell your doctor if you are breastfeeding an infant. Although problems in humans have not been reported, small amounts of this drug can pass into breast milk, so caution is warranted.

---

methyldopa

BRAND NAME (Manufacturer)
Aldomet (Merck Sharp & Dohme)
TYPE OF DRUG
Anti-hypertensive
INGREDIENT
methyldopa
DOSAGE FORMS
Tablets (125 mg, 250 mg, and 500 mg)
Oral suspension (250 mg per 5 ml teaspoonful, with 1% alcohol)

STORAGE

Methyldopa tablets and oral suspension should be stored at room temperature in tightly closed, light-resistant containers. This medication should never be frozen.

USES

Methyldopa is used to treat high blood pressure. It is not clear exactly how methyldopa works, but it is thought to act on the central nervous system (brain and spinal cord) to prevent the release of chemicals responsible for maintaining high blood pressure.

TREATMENT

In order to prevent stomach irritation, you can take methyldopa with food or with a full glass of water or milk. In order to become accustomed to taking this medication, try to take it at the same time(s) each day (unless your doctor directs you to do otherwise).

The oral suspension should be shaken well before each dose is measured. The contents tend to settle to the bottom of the bottle, so the bottle should be shaken to evenly distribute the medication and equalize the doses. Each dose should then be measured carefully, with a specially designed, 5 ml measuring spoon. An ordinary kitchen teaspoon is not accurate enough.

Methyldopa does not cure high blood pressure, but it will help to control the condition, as long as you continue to take it.

If you miss a dose of this medication, take the missed dose as soon as possible, unless it is almost time for the next dose. In that case, do not take the missed dose at all; just return to your regular dosing schedule. Do not double the next dose.

SIDE EFFECTS

Minor. Bloating; blurred vision; confusion; constipation; decreased sexual ability; diarrhea; dizziness; drowsiness; dry mouth; gas; headache; inflamed salivary glands; lightheadedness; nasal congestion; nausea; sore or "black" tongue; tremors; vomiting; and weakness. These side effects should disappear in several weeks, as your body adjusts to the medication.

To relieve constipation, increase the amount of fiber in your diet (bran, salads, fresh fruits and vegetables, and whole-grain breads), and drink more water (unless your doctor directs you to do otherwise).

If you feel dizzy or light-headed, sit or lie down awhile; get up slowly, and be careful on stairs. To avoid dizziness or light-headedness when you stand, contract and relax the muscles of your legs for a few moments before rising. Do this by pushing one foot against the floor while raising the other foot slightly, alternating feet so that you are "pumping" your legs in a pedaling motion.

Major. Tell your doctor about any side effects that are persistent or particularly bothersome. IT IS ESPECIALLY IMPORTANT TO TELL YOUR DOCTOR about abdominal distention; unusual bleeding or bruising; breast enlargement (in both sexes); difficulty breathing; chest pain; depression; fainting; fatigue; fever; insomnia; loss of appetite; nightmares; numbness or tingling; rapid weight gain (three to five pounds within a week); severe stomach cramps; sore joints; swelling of the feet or ankles; unusual body movements; or yellowing of the eyes or skin.

INTERACTIONS

Methyldopa interacts with several other types of drugs.

1. It can increase or decrease the anti-parkinson effects of levodopa.

2. The use of a monoamine oxidase (MAO) inhibitor within 14 days of methyldopa can cause headaches, severe hypertension, and hallucinations.

3. The combination of methyldopa and methotrimeprazine can cause irritability; methyldopa and phenoxybenzamine can cause urinary retention; and methyldopa and alcohol can cause dizziness and fainting.

4. Methyldopa can also increase the side effects of tolbutamide and lithium.

Before starting to take methyldopa, BE SURE TO TELL YOUR DOCTOR if you are already taking any of the medications listed above.

WARNINGS

• Tell your doctor about any unusual or allergic reactions

you have had to medications, especially to methyldopa.

• Before starting to take this medication, be sure to tell your doctor if you now have, or if you have ever had, anemia, angina (chest pain), kidney disease, liver disease, mental depression, Parkinson's disease, or stroke.

• In order to avoid dizziness or fainting while you are taking this medication, try not to stand for long periods of time; avoid drinking excessive amounts of alcohol; and avoid getting overheated (strenuous exercise in hot weather; hot baths, showers, and saunas).

• If this drug makes you dizzy or drowsy, avoid taking part in any activities that require alertness, such as driving a car or operating potentially dangerous equipment.

• Before having any surgery or other medical or dental treatment, be sure your doctor or dentist knows that you are taking this medication.

• Before taking any over-the-counter (non-prescription) allergy, asthma, sinus, cough, cold, or diet product, check with your doctor or pharmacist. Some of these products can cause an increase in blood pressure.

• Do not stop taking this medication unless you first check with your doctor. If this drug is stopped abruptly, you could experience a sudden rise in blood pressure. Your doctor may therefore want to decrease your dosage gradually.

• If you have an unexplained fever, especially during the first two or three weeks after starting to take this medication, CONTACT YOUR DOCTOR. Fever can be a sign of a serious reaction to methyldopa.

• Occasionally, tolerance to this drug develops, usually during the second or third month of therapy. If you notice a decrease in effectiveness of methyldopa, contact your doctor.

• Before donating any blood or receiving a blood transfusion, be sure that the doctor knows you are taking this medication. It can cause changes in your blood cells.

• Be sure to tell your doctor if you are pregnant. Although this drug appears to be safe, extensive studies in women during pregnancy have not yet been completed. Also, tell your doctor if you are breastfeeding an infant. Small amounts of methyldopa pass into breast milk.

methyldopa and hydrochlorothiazide combination

BRAND NAME (Manufacturer)
Aldoril (Merck Sharp & Dohme)
TYPE OF DRUG
Anti-hypertensive
INGREDIENTS
methyldopa and hydrochlorothiazide
DOSAGE FORM
Tablets
   (250 mg methyldopa and 15 mg hydrochlorothiazide;
   250 mg methyldopa and 25 mg hydrochlorothiazide;
   500 mg methyldopa and 30 mg hydrochlorothiazide;
   500 mg methyldopa and 50 mg hydrochlorothiazide)
STORAGE
These tablets should be stored at room temperature in a tightly closed container.

USES
Methyldopa and hydrochlorothiazide combination is used to treat high blood pressure. It is not exactly clear how methyldopa works, but it is thought to act on the central nervous system (brain and spinal cord) to prevent the release of chemicals responsible for maintaining high blood pressure. Hydrochlorothiazide is a diuretic (water pill), which reduces body fluid accumulation by increasing the elimination of sodium and water through the kidneys.

TREATMENT
To avoid stomach irritation, you can take methyldopa and hydrochlorothiazide with food or with a full glass of water or milk (unless your doctor directs you to do otherwise). In order to become accustomed to taking this medication, try to take it at the same time(s) each day. Avoid taking a dose after 6:00 P.M., to prevent having to get up during the night to urinate.

This medication does not cure high blood pressure, but it will help to control the condition, as long as you continue to take it.

If you miss a dose of this medication, take the missed dose as soon as possible, unless it is almost time for the next dose. In that case, do not take the missed dose at all; just return to your regular dosing schedule. Do not double the next dose.

SIDE EFFECTS

Minor. Bloating; blurred vision; confusion; constipation; decreased sexual ability; diarrhea; dizziness; drowsiness; dry mouth; gas; headache; inflamed salivary glands; light-headedness; nasal congestion; nausea; sore or "black" tongue; tremors; increased urination; vomiting; and weakness. These side effects should disappear in several weeks, as your body adjusts to the medication.

Chew sugarless gum, or suck on ice chips or a piece of hard candy, to relieve mouth dryness.

If you feel dizzy or light-headed, sit or lie down awhile; get up slowly, and be careful on stairs. To avoid dizziness or light-headedness when you stand, contract and relax the muscles of your legs for a few moments before rising. Do this by pushing one foot against the floor while raising the other foot slightly, alternating feet so that you are "pumping" your legs in a pedaling motion.

This medication can cause increased sensitivity to sunlight. You should therefore avoid prolonged exposure to sunlight and sunlamps. Wear protective clothing and sunglasses, and use an effective sunscreen.

Major. Tell your doctor about any side effects that are persistent or particularly bothersome. IT IS ESPECIALLY IMPORTANT TO TELL YOUR DOCTOR about abdominal distention; unusual bleeding or bruising; breast enlargement (in both sexes); chest pain; depression; difficulty breathing; fainting; fatigue; fever; insomnia; loss of appetite; joint pains; nightmares; numbness or tingling; rapid weight gain (three to five pounds within a week); severe stomach cramps; swelling of the feet or ankles; unusual body movements; or yellowing of the eyes or skin.

INTERACTIONS

Methyldopa and hydrochlorothiazide combination interacts with several other types of drugs.

1. Methyldopa can either increase or decrease the antiparkinson effects of levodopa.

2. The use of a monamine oxidase (MAO) inhibitor within 14 days of methyldopa can cause headaches, severe hypertension, and hallucinations.

3. The combination of methyldopa and methotrimeprazine can cause a severe drop in blood pressure; methyldopa and haloperidol can cause irritability; methyldopa and phenoxybenzamine can cause urinary retention; and methyldopa and alcohol can cause dizziness and fainting.

4. Methyldopa can increase the side effects of tolbutamide and lithium.

5. Hydrochlorothiazide can decrease the effectiveness of oral anti-coagulants (blood thinners, such as warfarin), anti-gout medications, insulin, oral anti-diabetic medications, and methenamine.

6. Fenfluramine may increase the blood-pressure-lowering effects of hydrochlorothiazide; and indomethacin may decrease its blood-pressure-lowering effects.

7. Cholestyramine and colestipol can decrease the absorption of hydrochlorothiazide from the gastrointestinal tract. Therefore, this medication should be taken one hour before, or four hours after, a dose of either of these other medications.

8. The side effects of amphotericin B, calcium, adrenocorticosteroids (cortisone-like medicines), digoxin, lithium, quinidine, sulfonamide antibiotics, and vitamin D may be increased when taken concurrently with hydrochlorothiazide.

Before starting to take methyldopa and hydrochlorothiazide combination, BE SURE TO TELL YOUR DOCTOR if you are already taking any of the medications listed above.

WARNINGS

● Tell your doctor about unusual or allergic reactions you have had to medications, especially to methyldopa or hydrochlorothiazide, or to any other sulfa medication (diuretics, oral anti-diabetic medicines, sulfonamide antibiot-

ics, dapsone, or sulfone).
- Before starting to take this medication, be sure to tell your doctor if you now have, or if you have ever had, anemia, diabetes mellitus (sugar diabetes), gout, kidney disease, liver disease, mental depression, Parkinson's disease, pancreatitis, or stroke.
- A doctor generally does not prescribe this drug or other "fixed dose" products as the first choice in the treatment of high blood pressure. The patient should initially receive each ingredient singly. If the response is adequate to the dose contained in this product, it can then be substituted. The advantage of a combination product is its increased convenience.
- This drug can cause potassium loss. Signs of potassium loss include dry mouth, thirst, weakness, muscle pain or cramps, nausea, and vomiting. If you experience any of these symptoms, CONTACT YOUR DOCTOR. To help prevent this problem, your doctor may want you to have blood tests performed periodically to monitor your potassium levels. To help avoid potassium loss, take this medication with a glass of fresh or frozen orange juice or cranberry juice, or eat a banana every day. The use of a salt substitute also helps prevent potassium loss. Do not change your diet, however, until you discuss it with your doctor. Too much potassium can also be dangerous.
- To prevent severe water loss (dehydration) while taking hydrochlorothiazide, check with your doctor if you have any illness that causes severe or continuous nausea, vomiting, or diarrhea.
- Hydrochlorothiazide can raise blood sugar levels in diabetic patients. Blood sugar should therefore be monitored carefully when this medication is started.
- In order to avoid dizziness or fainting while taking this medication, try not to stand for long periods of time; avoid drinking excessive amounts of alcohol; and avoid getting overheated (strenuous exercise in hot weather; hot baths, showers, and saunas).
- If this drug makes you dizzy or drowsy, avoid taking part in any activity that requires alertness, such as driving a car or operating potentially dangerous equipment.

• Before having any surgery or other medical or dental treatment, be sure your doctor or dentist knows you are taking this medication.

• Before taking any over-the-counter (non-prescription) allergy, asthma, sinus, cough, cold, or diet product, check with your doctor or pharmacist. Some of these products can cause an increase in blood pressure.

• Do not stop taking this medication unless you first check with your doctor. If this drug is stopped abruptly, you could experience a sudden rise in blood pressure. Your doctor may therefore want to decrease your dosage gradually.

• If you have an unexplained fever, especially during the first two to three weeks after starting to take this medication, CONTACT YOUR DOCTOR. Fever can be a sign of a serious reaction to methyldopa.

• Occasionally, tolerance to this medication develops, usually during the second or third month of therapy. If you notice a decrease in effectiveness of this medication, contact your doctor.

• Before donating any blood or receiving a blood transfusion, be sure the doctor knows that you are taking this medication. Methyldopa can cause a change in the blood cells.

• Be sure to tell your doctor if you are pregnant. Methyldopa and hydrochlorothiazide cross the placenta. Although studies in pregnant women have not yet been completed, birth defects have been observed in the fetuses of animals who were given large doses of hydrochlorothiazide during pregnancy. Also, tell your doctor if you are breastfeeding an infant. Small amounts of both of these drugs pass into breast milk.

---

methylphenidate

BRAND NAMES (Manufacturers)
methylphenidate hydrochloride (various manufacturers)
Ritalin (Ciba)
Ritalin-SR (Ciba)

TYPE OF DRUG
Adrenergic (central nervous system stimulant)
INGREDIENT
methylphenidate as the hydrochloride salt
DOSAGE FORMS
Tablets (5 mg, 10 mg, and 20 mg)
Sustained-release tablets (20 mg)
STORAGE
Methylphenidate should be stored at room temperature in tightly closed, light-resistant containers.

USES
Methylphenidate is a central nervous system stimulant that increases mental alertness and decreases fatigue. It is used in the treatment of narcolepsy (problems in staying awake), mild depression, and abnormal behavioral syndrome in children (hyperkinetic syndrome or attention deficit disorder). The way this medication works in abnormal behavioral syndrome in children is not clearly understood.

TREATMENT
In order to avoid stomach upset, you can take methylphenidate with food or with a full glass of water or milk (unless your doctor directs you to do otherwise).

If methylphenidate is being used to treat narcolepsy or abnormal behavioral syndrome in children, the first dose should be taken soon after awakening. Subsequent doses of the regular tablets should then be spaced at four- to six-hour intervals (eight-hour intervals for the sustained-release tablets).

In order to avoid difficulty in falling asleep, the last dose of the regular tablets should be taken four to six hours before bedtime each day (the sustained-release tablets should be taken at least eight hours before bedtime).

The sustained-release tablets should be swallowed whole. Chewing, crushing, or breaking these tablets destroys their sustained-release activity, and may increase the side effects.

If you miss a dose of this medication, take the missed dose as soon as possible, unless it is almost time for your next dose. In that case, don't take the missed dose at all; just return to your regular dosing schedule. Do not double the next dose.

SIDE EFFECTS

Minor. Abdominal pain; dizziness; drowsiness; dry mouth; headache; insomnia; loss of appetite; nausea; nervousness; vomiting; and weakness. These side effects should disappear in several days, as your body adjusts to the medication.

Dry mouth can be relieved by sucking on ice chips or a piece of hard candy, or by chewing sugarless gum.

If you feel dizzy, sit or lie down awhile; get up from a sitting or lying position slowly, and be careful on stairs.

Major. Tell your doctor about any side effects that are persistent or particularly bothersome. IT IS ESPECIALLY IMPORTANT TO TELL YOUR DOCTOR about unusual bleeding or bruising; chest pain; fever; hair loss; hallucinations; hives; joint pain; mood changes; palpitations; rash; seizures; sore throat; or uncoordinated movements.

INTERACTIONS

Methylphenidate interacts with several other types of medication.

1. Use of it within 14 days of a monoamine oxidase (MAO) inhibitor (such as isocarboxazid, pargyline, phenelzine, tranylcypromine) can result in severe high blood pressure.

2. Methylphenidate can decrease the blood-pressure-lowering effects of anti-hypertension medications (especially guanethidine).

3. Acetazolamide and sodium bicarbonate can decrease the elimination of methylphenidate from the body, thereby prolonging its action and increasing the risk of side effects.

4. Methylphenidate can decrease the elimination from the body and increase the side effects of oral anti-coagulants (blood thinners, such as warfarin); tricyclic anti-depressants (such as amitriptyline, desipramine, imipramine, or nortriptyline); anti-convulsants (such as phenytoin, phenobarbital, or primidone); and phenylbutazone.

BE SURE TO TELL YOUR DOCTOR if you are already taking any of the medications listed above.

WARNINGS

- Tell your doctor about unusual or allergic reactions you have had to any medications, especially to methylphenidate.
- Tell your doctor if you now have, or if you have ever had, epilepsy; glaucoma; high blood pressure; motor tics; Tourette's syndrome; or anxiety, agitation, depression, or tension.
- Methylphenidate can mask the symptoms of extreme fatigue and can cause dizziness. Your ability to perform tasks that require alertness, such as driving a car or operating potentially dangerous machinery, may be decreased. Appropriate caution should therefore be taken. A child taking methylphenidate should be careful while riding a bicycle or climbing a tree.
- Before having any surgery or other medical or dental treatment, be sure to tell your doctor or dentist that you are taking this medication.
- Methylphenidate is related to amphetamine and may be habit-forming when taken for long periods of time (both physical and psychological dependence can occur). You should not increase the dosage of this medication or take it for longer than the prescribed time unless you first consult your doctor. It is also important that you not stop taking this medication abruptly—fatigue, sleep disorders, mental depression, nausea or vomiting, or stomach cramps or pain could occur. Your doctor may want to decrease the dosage gradually in order to prevent these side effects.
- Methylphenidate can slow growth in children. Therefore, if this medication is being taken by a child, your doctor may recommend drug-free periods during school holidays and summer vacations. Growth spurts often occur during these drug-free periods.
- Be sure to tell your doctor if you are pregnant. Effects of this drug during pregnancy have not yet been thoroughly studied in either humans or animals. Also, tell your doctor if you are breastfeeding an infant. Small amounts of methylphenidate may pass into breast milk.

methylphenidate hydrochloride—see methylphenidate

methylprednisolone (systemic)

BRAND NAMES (Manufacturers)
Medrol (Upjohn)
methylprednisolone (various manufacturers)
TYPE OF DRUG
Adrenocorticosteroid hormone
INGREDIENT
methylprednisolone
DOSAGE FORM
Tablets (2 mg, 4 mg, 8 mg, 16 mg, 24 mg, and 32 mg)
STORAGE
Methylprednisolone tablets should be stored at room temperature, in a tightly closed container.

USES

Your adrenal glands naturally produce certain cortisone-like chemicals. These chemicals are involved in various regulatory processes in the body (such as maintenance of fluid balance, temperature, and reactions to inflammation). Methylprednisolone belongs to a group of drugs known as adrenocorticosteroids (or cortisone-like medications). It is used to treat a variety of disorders, including endocrine and rheumatic disorders; asthma; blood diseases; certain cancers; eye disorders; gastrointestinal disturbances such as ulcerative colitis; respiratory diseases; and inflammations such as arthritis, dermatitis, and poison ivy. How this drug acts to relieve these disorders is not completely understood.

TREATMENT

In order to prevent stomach irritation, you can take methylprednisolone with food or milk.

If you are taking only one dose of this medication each day, try to take it before 9:00 A.M. This will mimic the body's normal production of this type of chemical.

It is important to try not to miss any doses of methylprednisolone. However, if you do miss a dose:
1. If you are taking it more than once a day, take the missed dose as soon as possible and return to your regular schedule. If it is already time for the next dose, double the dose.

2. If you are taking this medication once a day, take the dose you missed as soon as possible, unless you don't remember until the next day. In that case do not take the missed dose at all; just follow your regular schedule. Do not double the next dose.

3. If you are taking this drug every other day, take it as soon as you remember. If you missed the scheduled time by a whole day, take it when you remember, then skip a day before you take the next dose. Do not double the dose.

If you miss more than one dose, CONTACT YOUR DOCTOR.

SIDE EFFECTS

Minor. Dizziness; false sense of well-being; increased appetite; increased susceptibility to infections; increased sweating; indigestion; menstrual irregularities; muscle weakness; nausea; reddening of the skin on the face; restlessness; sleep disorders; thinning of the skin; and weight gain. These side effects should disappear in several days, as your body adjusts to the medication.

Major. Tell your doctor about any side effects that are persistent or particularly bothersome. IT IS ESPECIALLY IMPORTANT TO TELL YOUR DOCTOR about abdominal enlargement; abdominal pain; acne or other skin problems; back or rib pain; blurred vision; unusual bruising or bleeding; convulsions; eye pain; fever and sore throat; growth impairment (in children); headaches; impaired healing of wounds; increased thirst and urination; mental depression; mood changes; muscle wasting; nightmares; rapid weight gain (three to five pounds within a week); rash; shortness of breath; unusual weakness; and bloody or black, tarry stools.

INTERACTIONS

Methylprednisolone interacts with several other types of medication.

1. Alcohol, aspirin, and anti-inflammation medications (diflunisal, ibuprofen, indomethacin, mefenamic acid, meclofenamate, naproxen, piroxicam, sulindac, tolmetin) aggravate the stomach problems that are common with use of this medication.

2. A change in the dosage requirements of oral anti-coagulants (blood thinners, such as warfarin), oral anti-diabetic drugs, or insulin may be necessary when this medication is started or stopped.

3. The loss of potassium caused by methylprednisolone can lead to serious side effects in individuals taking digoxin. Thiazide diuretics (water pills) can increase the potassium loss caused by methylprednisolone.

4. Phenobarbital, phenytoin, rifampin, and ephedrine can increase the elimination of methylprednisolone from the body, thereby decreasing its effectiveness.

5. Oral contraceptives and estrogen-containing drugs may decrease the elimination of this medication from the body, which can lead to an increase in side effects.

6. Methylprednisolone can increase the elimination of aspirin and isoniazid, thereby decreasing the effectiveness of these two medications.

7. Cholestyramine and colestipol can chemically bind this medication in the stomach and gastrointestinal tract, and prevent its absorption.

TELL YOUR DOCTOR if you are currently taking any of the medications listed above.

WARNINGS

• Tell your doctor about unusual or allergic reactions you have had to any medications, especially to methylprednisolone or other adrenocorticosteroids (such as betamethasone, cortisone, dexamethasone, fluprednisolone, hydrocortisone, paramethasone, prednisolone, prednisone, or triamcinolone).

• Tell your doctor if you now have, or if you have ever had, bone disease; diabetes mellitus (sugar diabetes); emotional instability; glaucoma; fungal infections; heart disease; high blood pressure; high cholesterol levels; myasthenia gravis; peptic ulcers; osteoporosis; thyroid disease; tuberculosis; severe ulcerative colitis; kidney disease; or liver disease.

• To help avoid potassium loss while using this drug, take your dose with a glass of fresh or frozen orange juice, or eat a banana each day. The use of a salt substitute also helps prevent potassium loss. Check with your doctor.

• If you are using this medication for longer than a week,

you may need to have your dosage adjusted if you are subjected to stress, such as serious infections, injury, or surgery. Discuss this with your doctor.

● If you have been taking this drug for more than a week, do not stop taking it suddenly. If it is stopped suddenly, you may experience abdominal or back pain; dizziness; fainting; fever; muscle or joint pain; nausea; vomiting; shortness of breath; or extreme weakness. Your doctor may therefore want to reduce the dosage gradually. Never increase the dose or take the drug for longer than the prescribed time, unless you first consult your doctor.

● While you are taking methylprednisolone, you should not be vaccinated or immunized. This medication decreases the effectiveness of vaccines and can lead to overwhelming infection if a live virus is administered.

● Before having any surgery or other medical or dental treatment, be sure your doctor or dentist knows that you are taking this medication.

● Because this drug can cause glaucoma and cataracts with long-term use, your doctor may want you to have your eyes examined by an ophthalmologist periodically during treatment.

● If you are taking this medication for prolonged periods, you should wear or carry a notice or identification card stating that you are taking an adrenocorticosteroid.

● This medication can raise blood sugar levels in diabetic patients. Blood sugar should therefore be monitored carefully with blood or urine tests when this medication is started.

● Some of these products contain F.D. & C. Yellow Dye No. 5 (tartrazine), which can cause allergic-type reactions (shortness of breath, rash, wheezing, or fainting) in certain susceptible individuals.

● Be sure to tell your doctor if you are pregnant. This drug crosses the placenta. Although studies in humans have not yet been completed, birth defects have been observed in the fetuses of animals who were given large doses of this type of drug during pregnancy. Also, tell your doctor if you are breastfeeding an infant. Small amounts of methylprednisolone pass into breast milk and may cause growth suppression or a decrease in natural adrenocorticosteroid production in the nursing infant.

methyltestosterone

BRAND NAMES (Manufacturers)
Android (Brown)
Metandren (Ciba)
methyltestosterone (various manufacturers)
Oreton Methyl (Schering)
Testred (ICN)
Virilon (Star)
TYPE OF DRUG
Androgen (male hormone)
INGREDIENT
methyltestosterone
DOSAGE FORMS
Oral tablets (10 mg and 25 mg)
Buccal tablets (5 mg and 10 mg)
Capsules (10 mg)
STORAGE
Methyltestosterone should be stored at room temperature, in tightly closed containers.

USES

This medication is a synthetic androgen (male hormone) that is used to treat conditions such as delayed puberty, eunuchism, or impotence in males who can not produce enough testosterone on their own.

TREATMENT

In order to avoid stomach irritation, you can take methyltestosterone oral tablets or capsules with food or with a full glass of water or milk (unless your doctor directs you to do otherwise).

The buccal tablet form of methyltestosterone is meant to be absorbed through the lining of the mouth, rather than swallowed. The tablet should be placed between your gum and cheek and allowed to dissolve slowly. Do not eat, drink, chew, or smoke while the tablet is dissolving.

If you miss a dose of this medication, take the missed dose as soon as possible, unless it is almost time for the next dose. In that case, do not take the missed dose at all; just return to your regular dosing schedule. Do not double the next dose.

SIDE EFFECTS

Minor. Diarrhea; headache; loss of appetite; nausea; decrease or increase in sexual desire; stomach irritation; sleeping difficulties; and vomiting. These side effects should disappear as your body adjusts to the medication.
Major. Tell your doctor about any side effects that are persistent or particularly bothersome. IT IS ESPECIALLY IMPORTANT TO TELL YOUR DOCTOR about acne; breast enlargement or tenderness; black, tarry, or bloody stools; unusual bleeding or bruising; flushing; frequent or continuous erection; hair loss or growth; hoarseness or deepening of the voice; increased urination; shortness of breath; skin rash; swelling of the hands or feet; sore throat; tiredness; or yellowing of the eyes or skin.

INTERACTIONS

Methyltestosterone interacts with several other types of medication.
1. It can increase the effects of oral anti-coagulants (blood thinners, such as warfarin), which can lead to bleeding complications.
2. Diabetic patients should know that methyltestosterone can lower blood sugar levels. The dosage of oral anti-diabetic medication or insulin may therefore require adjustment when this medication is started.
3. Concurrent use of methyltestosterone and adrenocorticosteroids (cortisone-like medications) can lead to fluid retention.
Before starting to take methyltestosterone, BE SURE TO TELL YOUR DOCTOR if you are already taking any of the medications listed above.

WARNINGS

• Tell your doctor about unusual or allergic reactions you have had to medications, especially to methyltestosterone or to any other androgen (such as fluoxymesterone or testosterone).
• Before starting to take this medication, be sure to tell your doctor if you now have, or if you have ever had, breast cancer, fluid retention, heart disease, hypercalcemia (high blood calcium levels), kidney disease, liver disease, or prostate disorders.

- Although androgens have been used by athletes to increase muscle strength, there is no conclusive evidence that these drugs increase athletic performance. There is also some question as to their safety.
- Some of these products contain F.D. & C. Yellow Dye No. 5 (tartrazine), which can cause allergic-type symptoms (shortness of breath, fainting, rash) in certain susceptible individuals.
- Be sure to tell your doctor if you are pregnant. If methyltestosterone is taken by a pregnant woman, it can cause masculine characteristics in the developing fetus, such as increased body hair (Note: this does NOT affect the sex of the fetus, which is determined at conception). Also, tell your doctor if you are breastfeeding an infant. Methyltestosterone passes into breast milk and can cause masculinization of the nursing infant.

Meticorten—see prednisone (systemic)

---

metoclopramide

BRAND NAME (Manufacturer)
Reglan (Robins)
TYPE OF DRUG
Dopamine antagonist and anti-emetic
INGREDIENT
metoclopramide as the hydrochloride salt
DOSAGE FORMS
Tablets (100 mg)
Oral syrup (5 mg per 5 ml teaspoonful)
STORAGE
Metoclopramide tablets and syrup should be stored at room temperature in tightly closed containers.

USES

This medication is used to relieve the symptoms associated with diabetic gastric stasis or gastric reflux, and to prevent nausea and vomiting. Metoclopramide acts directly on the vomiting center in the brain to prevent nausea and vomiting. It also increases the movement of the stomach and intestines.

TREATMENT

To obtain the best results, you should take metoclopramide tablets or syrup 30 minutes before a meal.

Each dose of the syrup should be measured carefully, with a specially designed, 5 ml measuring spoon. An ordinary kitchen teaspoon is not accurate enough.

If you miss a dose of this medication, take the missed dose as soon as possible, unless it is almost time for the next dose. In that case, do not take the missed dose at all; just return to your regular dosing schedule. Do not double the next dose.

SIDE EFFECTS

Minor. Diarrhea; dizziness; drowsiness; dry mouth; fatigue; headache; insomnia; nausea; restlessness; and weakness. These side effects should disappear in several days, as your body adjusts to the medication.

If you feel dizzy or light-headed, sit or lie down awhile; get up slowly, and be careful on stairs.

To relieve mouth dryness, chew sugarless gum, or suck on ice chips or a piece of hard candy.

Major. Tell your doctor about any side effects that are persistent or particularly bothersome. IT IS ESPECIALLY IMPORTANT TO TELL YOUR DOCTOR about anxiety; confusion; depression; disorientation; involuntary movements of the eyes, face, or limbs; muscle spasms; rash; or trembling of the hands.

INTERACTIONS

Metoclopramide interacts with several other types of drugs.

1. Concurrent use of metoclopramide with other central nervous system depressants (drugs that slow the activity of the nervous system), such as alcohol, antihistamines, barbiturates, muscle relaxants, narcotics, pain medications, phenothiazine tranquilizers, benzodiazepine tranquilizers, and sleeping medications, or with tricyclic anti-depressants can cause extreme drowsiness.

2. Narcotic analgesics may block the effectiveness of metoclopramide.

3. Metoclopramide can block the effectiveness of bromocriptine. It can also decrease the absorption of cimetidine and digoxin from the gastrointestinal tract, decreasing their effectiveness.

4. Metoclopramide can increase the absorption of acetaminophen, tetracycline, levodopa, and alcohol.

5. Diabetic patients should know that dosage requirements of insulin may change when metoclopramide is started.

Before starting to take metoclopramide, BE SURE TO TELL YOUR DOCTOR if you are already taking any of the medications listed above.

WARNINGS

- Tell your doctor about unusual or allergic reactions you have had to any medications, especially to metoclopramide, procaine, or procainamide.
- Before starting to take metoclopramide, be sure to tell your doctor if you now have, or if you have ever had, epilepsy, kidney disease, liver disease, intestinal bleeding or blockage, Parkinson's disease, or pheochromocytoma.
- If this drug makes you dizzy or drowsy, do not take part in any activities that require alertness, such as driving a car or operating potentially dangerous equipment.
- Be sure to tell your doctor if you are pregnant. Although this drug appears to be safe, extensive studies in women during pregnancy have not yet been completed. Also, tell your doctor if you are breastfeeding an infant. It is not known whether or not metoclopramide passes into breast milk.

---

metolazone

BRAND NAMES (Manufacturers)
Diulo (Searle)
Zaroxolyn (Pennwalt)
TYPE OF DRUG
Diuretic (water pill) and anti-hypertensive
INGREDIENT
metolazone
DOSAGE FORM
Tablets (2.5 mg, 5 mg, and 10 mg)

STORAGE

This medication should be stored at room temperature in a tightly closed container.

USES

Metolazone is prescribed to treat high blood pressure. It is also used to reduce fluid accumulation in the body caused by conditions such as heart failure, cirrhosis of the liver, kidney disease, and the long-term use of some medications. Metolazone reduces fluid accumulation by increasing the elimination of sodium and water through the kidneys.

TREATMENT

To decrease stomach irritation, you can take this medication with a glass of milk or with a meal (unless your doctor directs you to do otherwise). Try to take it at the same time every day. Avoid taking a dose after 6:00 P.M.—this will prevent you from having to get up during the night to urinate.

If you miss a dose of this medication, take the missed dose as soon as possible, unless it is almost time for the next dose. In that case, do not take the missed dose at all, just wait until the next scheduled dose. Do not double the dose.

This medication does not cure high blood pressure, but it will help to control the condition, as long as you continue to take it.

SIDE EFFECTS

Minor. Constipation; cramps; diarrhea; dizziness; drowsiness; headache; heartburn; itching; loss of appetite; nausea; restlessness; upset stomach; and vomiting. As your body adjusts to the medication, these side effects should disappear.

This medication can cause increased sensitivity to sunlight. It is therefore important to avoid prolonged exposure to sunlight or sunlamps. Wear protective clothing and use an effective sunscreen.

To avoid dizziness or light-headedness when you stand, contract and relax the muscles of your legs for a few moments before rising. Do this by pushing one foot against the floor while raising the other foot slightly, alternating feet so that you are "pumping" your legs in a pedaling motion.

Major. Tell your doctor about any side effects that are persistent or particularly bothersome. IT IS ESPECIALLY IMPORTANT TO TELL YOUR DOCTOR about any unusual bleeding or bruising; blurred vision; confusion; difficulty breathing; dry mouth; fever; mood changes; muscle spasms; palpitations; skin rash; excessive thirst; sore throat; joint pain; tingling in the fingers or toes; excessive weakness; or yellowing of the eyes or skin.

INTERACTIONS

Metolazone can interact with several other types of medication.

1. It may decrease the effectiveness of oral anti-coagulants, anti-gout medications, insulin, oral anti-diabetic medicines, and methenamine.

2. Fenfluramine can increase the blood-pressure-lowering effects of metolazone (which can be dangerous).

3. Indomethacin can decrease the blood-pressure-lowering effects (thereby counteracting the desired effects) of metolazone.

4. Cholestyramine and colestipol decrease the absorption of this medication from the gastrointestinal tract. Metolazone should therefore be taken one hour before, or four hours after, a dose of cholestyramine or colestipol (if you have also been prescribed one of these medications).

5. The side effects of amphotericin B, calcium, cortisone-like steroids (such as cortisone, dexamethasone, hydrocortisone, prednisone, prednisolone), digoxin, digitalis, lithium, quinidine, sulfonamide antibiotics, and vitamin D may be increased when taken concurrently with metolazone.

Before taking metolazone, BE SURE TO TELL YOUR DOCTOR if you are taking any of the medicines listed above.

WARNINGS

• Tell your doctor about unusual or allergic reactions you have had to any medications, especially to diuretics (water pills), oral anti-diabetic medications, or sulfonamide antibiotics.

• Before you start taking metolazone, tell your doctor if you now have, or if you have ever had, kidney disease or problems with urination, diabetes mellitus (sugar diabetes), gout, liver disease, asthma, pancreas disease, or systemic lupus erythematosus (SLE).

• Metolazone can cause potassium loss. Signs of potassium loss include dry mouth, thirst, weakness, muscle pain or cramps, nausea, and vomiting. If you experience any of these symptoms, call your doctor. To help avoid potassium loss, take this drug with a glass of fresh or frozen orange juice or cranberry juice, or eat a banana every day. The use of a salt substitute also helps to prevent potassium loss. Do not change your diet, however, before discussing it with your doctor. Too much potassium can also be dangerous. Your doctor may want to have blood tests performed periodically, in order to monitor your potassium levels.

• Limit your intake of alcoholic beverages while taking this medication, in order to prevent dizziness and light-headedness.

• Do not take any over-the-counter (non-prescription) medications for weight control or for cough, cold, allergy, asthma, or sinus problems, unless your doctor directs you to do so. Some of these products can cause an increase in blood pressure.

• To prevent dehydration (severe water loss) while taking this medication, check with your doctor if you have any illness that causes severe or continuous nausea, vomiting, or diarrhea.

• This medication can raise blood sugar levels in diabetic patients. Therefore, blood sugar should be carefully monitored by blood or urine tests when this medication is started.

• Be sure to tell your doctor if you are pregnant. This drug is able to cross the placenta. Studies in humans have not been completed, but adverse effects have been observed on the fetuses of animals who were given large doses of this drug during pregnancy. Also, tell your doctor if you are breastfeeding an infant. Although problems in humans have not been reported, small amounts of this drug can pass into breast milk, so caution is warranted.

metoprolol

BRAND NAME (Manufacturer)
Lopressor (Geigy)
TYPE OF DRUG
Beta-adrenergic blocking agent
INGREDIENT
metoprolol
DOSAGE FORM
Tablets (50 mg and 100 mg)
STORAGE
Metoprolol should be stored at room temperature in a tightly closed, light-resistant container.

USES

Metoprolol is used to treat high blood pressure and to prevent additional heart attacks in heart attack patients. Metoprolol belongs to a group of medicines known as beta-adrenergic blocking agents or, more commonly, beta-blockers. These drugs work by controlling nerve impulses along certain nerve pathways.

TREATMENT

Metoprolol can be taken with a glass of water, with meals, immediately following meals, or on an empty stomach, depending on your doctor's instructions. Try to take the medication at the same time(s) each day.

Try not to miss any doses of this medicine. If you do miss a dose, take the missed dose as soon as possible. However, if the next scheduled dose is within eight hours (if you are taking this medicine only once a day) or within four hours (if you are taking this medicine more than once a day), do not take the missed dose at all; just return to your regular dosing schedule. Do not double the next dose.

It is important to remember that metoprolol does not cure high blood pressure, but it will help to control the condition, as long as you continue to take it.

SIDE EFFECTS

Minor. Diarrhea; drowsiness; dryness of the eyes, mouth and skin; nausea; numbness or tingling of the fingers or toes; cold hands or feet (due to decreased blood circulation to skin, fingers, and toes); tiredness; weakness; anxiety; nervousness; constipation; decreased sexual ability; headache; stomach discomfort; and difficulty sleeping. These side effects should disappear during treatment, as your body adjusts to the medicine.

If you are extra-sensitive to the cold, be sure to dress warmly during cold weather.

Plain, non-medicated eye drops (artificial tears) may help to relieve eye dryness.

Sucking on ice chips or chewing sugarless gum may help to relieve mouth and throat dryness.

Major. Tell your doctor about any side effects that are persistent or particularly bothersome. IT IS ESPECIALLY IMPORTANT TO TELL YOUR DOCTOR about breathing difficulty or wheezing; confusion; dizziness; fever and sore throat; hair loss; hallucinations; light-headedness; mental depression; nightmares; rapid weight gain (three to five pounds within a week); reduced alertness; swelling; skin rash; or unusual bleeding or bruising.

INTERACTIONS

Metoprolol interacts with a number of other medications.
1. Indomethacin, aspirin, or other salicylates may decrease the blood-pressure-lowering effects of beta-blockers.
2. Concurrent use of beta-blockers and calcium channel blockers (diltiazem, nifedipine, and verapamil) can potentially lead to heart failure or very low blood pressure.
3. Cimetidine can increase the blood concentrations of metoprolol, which can result in greater side effects.
4. Side effects may also be increased if beta-blockers are taken with clonidine, digoxin, epinephrine, phenylephrine, phenylpropanolamine, phenothiazine tranquilizers, reserpine, or monoamine oxidase (MAO) inhibitors. At least 14 days should separate the use of a beta-blocker and an MAO inhibitor.
5. Beta-blockers may antagonize (work against) the effects of theophylline, aminophylline, albuterol, metaproterenol, and terbutaline.
6. Beta-blockers can also interact with insulin or oral antidiabetic agents—raising or lowering blood sugar levels and masking the symptoms of low blood sugar.

BE SURE TO TELL YOUR DOCTOR if you are currently taking any of the medicines listed above.

WARNINGS

• Before starting to take this medication, it is important to tell your doctor if you have ever had unusual or allergic reactions to any beta-blocker (atenolol, metoprolol, nadolol, pindolol, propranolol, and timolol).

• Tell your doctor if you now have or have ever had allergies, asthma, hay fever, eczema, slow heartbeat, bronchitis, diabetes mellitus (sugar diabetes), emphysema, heart or blood vessel disease, kidney disease, liver disease, thyroid disease, or poor circulation in the fingers or toes.

• You may want to check your pulse while taking this medication. If your pulse is much slower than your usual rate (or if it is less than 50 beats per minute), check with your doctor. A pulse rate that is too slow may cause circulation problems.

• This medicine may affect your body's response to exercise. Make sure you discuss with your doctor a safe amount of exercise for your medical condition.

• It is important that you do not stop taking this medicine without first checking with your doctor. Some conditions may become worse when the medicine is stopped suddenly, and the danger of a heart attack is increased in some patients. Your doctor may want you to gradually reduce the amount of medicine you take, before stopping completely. Make sure that you have enough medicine on hand to last through vacations, holidays, and weekends.

• Before having any surgery or any other medical or dental treatment, tell your doctor or dentist that you are taking metoprolol. Often, this medication will be discontinued 48 hours prior to any major surgery.

• Metoprolol can cause dizziness, drowsiness, lightheadedness, or decreased alertness. Therefore, exercise caution while driving a car or using any potentially dangerous machinery.

• While taking this medicine, do not use any over-the-counter (non-prescription) allergy, asthma, cough, cold, sinus or diet preparation without first checking with your pharmacist or doctor. Some of these medicines can result in high blood pressure and slow heartbeat when taken at the same time as a beta-blocker.

● Be sure to tell your doctor if you are pregnant. Animal studies have shown that some beta-blockers, when used in very high doses, can cause problems in pregnancy. Adequate studies have not been completed in humans, but there has been some association between beta-blockers used during pregnancy and low birth rate, as well as breathing problems and slow heart rate in the newborn infants. However, other reports have shown no effects on newborn infants. Also, tell your doctor if you are breast-feeding an infant. Although this medicine has not been shown to cause problems in breast-fed infants, some of the medicine may pass into breast milk, so caution is warranted.

Metra—see phendimetrazine

---

metronidazole

BRAND NAMES (Manufacturers)
Flagyl (Searle)
metronidazole (various manufacturers)
Metryl (Lemmon)
Protostat (Ortho)
Satric (Savage)
TYPE OF DRUG
Antibiotic and anti-parasitic (infection fighter)
INGREDIENT
metronidazole
DOSAGE FORM
Tablets (250 mg and 500 mg)
STORAGE
Metronidazole should be stored at room temperature in a tightly closed, light-resistant container.

USES

Metronidazole is used to treat a wide variety of infections, including infections of the vagina, urinary tract, lower respiratory tract, bones, joints, intestinal tract, and skin. It acts by blocking production of essential nutrients, leading to the death of the infecting bacteria or parasites.

TREATMENT

In order to avoid stomach irritation, you should take metronidazole with food or with a full glass of water or milk (unless your doctor directs you to do otherwise).

Metronidazole works best when the level of the medicine in your bloodstream is kept constant. It is best therefore to take the doses at evenly spaced intervals, day and night. For example, if you are to take three doses a day, the doses should be spaced eight hours apart.

Try not to miss any doses of this medication. If you do miss a dose, take the missed dose as soon as possible, unless it is almost time for the next dose. In that case, don't take the missed dose at all; just return to your regular dosing schedule. Do not double the next dose.

It is important to continue to take this medication for the entire time prescribed by your doctor (usually seven to 14 days), even if the symptoms disappear before the end of that period. If you stop taking the drug too soon, resistant bacteria and parasites are given a chance to continue growing, and the infection could recur.

SIDE EFFECTS

Minor. Abdominal cramps; constipation; decreased sexual interest; diarrhea; dizziness; dry mouth; headache; insomnia; irritability; joint pain; loss of appetite; metallic taste in the mouth; nasal congestion; nausea; restlessness; and vomiting. These side effects should disappear in several days, as your body adjusts to the medication.

If you are constipated, increase the amount of fiber in your diet (raw vegetables, fruits, salads, bran, and whole-grain breads), exercise, and drink more water (unless your doctor directs you to do otherwise).

If you feel dizzy, sit or lie down awhile; get up slowly, and be careful on stairs.

To relieve mouth dryness, chew sugarless gum, or suck on ice chips or a piece of hard candy.

Major. Tell your doctor about any side effects that are persistent or particularly bothersome. IT IS ESPECIALLY IMPORTANT TO TELL YOUR DOCTOR about confusion; convulsions; flushing; hives; itching; loss of bladder control; mouth sores; numbness or tingling in the fingers or toes; rash; sense of pressure inside your abdomen; unexplained sore throat and fever; or unusual weakness. Also, if your symptoms of infection seem to be getting worse, rather than improving, you should contact your doctor.

INTERACTIONS

Metronidazole interacts with several other types of drugs.
1. Concurrent use of alcohol and metronidazole can lead to a severe reaction (abdominal cramps, nausea, vomiting, headache, and flushing), the severity of which is dependent upon the amount of alcohol ingested.
2. Concurrent use of disulfiram and metronidazole can lead to confusion.
3. The effects of oral anti-coagulants (blood thinners, such as warfarin) may be increased by metronidazole, which can lead to bleeding complications.
BE SURE TO TELL YOUR DOCTOR if you are already taking any of these medications.

WARNINGS

● Tell your doctor about unusual or allergic reactions you have had to any medications, especially to metronidazole.
● Before starting to take this medication, be sure to tell your doctor if you now have, or if you have ever had, blood disorders, a central nervous system (brain or spinal cord) disease, or liver disease.
● When metronidazole is used to treat a vaginal infection, sexual partners should receive concurrent therapy, in order to prevent reinfection.
● This medication has been prescribed for your current infection only. Another infection later on, or one that someone else has, may require a different medicine. You should not give your medicine to other people, or use it for other infections, unless your doctor specifically directs you to do so.
● If this drug makes you dizzy, avoid tasks that require alertness, such as driving a car or operating potentially dangerous equipment.
● Before having any surgery or other medical or dental treatment, be sure your doctor or dentist knows that you are taking this medication.
● Be sure to tell your doctor if you are pregnant. Although metronidazole appears to be safe, it does cross the

placenta, and extensive studies in pregnant women have not yet been completed. Also, tell your doctor if you are breastfeeding an infant. Metronidazole passes into breast milk.

Metryl—see metronidazole

---

miconazole (vaginal)

BRAND NAME (Manufacturer)
Monistat 7 (Ortho)
TYPE OF DRUG
Vaginal anti-fungal agent
INGREDIENT
miconazole as the nitrate salt
DOSAGE FORMS
Vaginal cream (2%)
Vaginal suppositories (100 mg)
STORAGE
Miconazole (vaginal) should be stored at room temperature in tightly closed containers.

USES

Miconazole is used to treat fungal infections of the vagina. This medication is an anti-fungal agent that prevents the growth and multiplication of the fungus or yeast *Candida*.

TREATMENT

Miconazole vaginal cream and suppositories are packaged with detailed directions for use. Follow these instructions carefully. An applicator will probably be provided for inserting the medication into the vagina.

You should wash the area carefully prior to inserting the cream or suppository into the vagina.

If you begin to menstruate while you are being treated with miconazole, continue with your regular dosing schedule.

If you miss a dose of this medication, insert the missed dose as soon as possible. However, if you do not remember until the following day, do not insert the missed dose at all; just return to your regular dosing schedule. Do

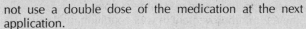

not use a double dose of the medication at the next application.

It is important to continue to insert this medication for the entire time prescribed by your doctor, even if the symptoms disappear before the end of that time. If you stop using the drug too soon, resistant fungus is given a chance to continue growing, and your infection could recur.

Usually, one seven-day course of miconazole is sufficient. However, the treatment may be repeated if your doctor determines that *Candida* is still causing your infection.

SIDE EFFECTS

Minor. You may experience vaginal burning, itching, or irritation when this drug is inserted. This sensation should disappear in several days, as your body adjusts to the medication.

Do not treat any side effects that occur in the area of the infection, unless you first consult your doctor.

Major. Tell your doctor about any side effects that are persistent or particularly bothersome. IT IS ESPECIALLY IMPORTANT TO TELL YOUR DOCTOR about headache, hives, pelvic cramps, or skin rash.

INTERACTIONS

Miconazole (vaginal) does not interact with other medications, if it is used to according to directions.

WARNINGS

• Tell your doctor about unusual or allergic reactions you have had to any medications, especially to miconazole.

• Tell your doctor if you have had other vaginal infections, especially if they have been resistant to treatment.

• In order to prevent reinfection, avoid sexual intercourse, or ask your partner to use a condom, until treatment is complete.

• There may be some vaginal drainage while using this medication; therefore, you may want to use a sanitary napkin or panty liner to prevent the staining of clothing.

• Wear cotton panties rather than those made of nylon or other non-porous materials while being treated for a vaginal fungus infection. Also, in order to prevent reinfection,

always wear freshly laundered underclothes.
- If there is no improvement in your condition, or if irritation in the area continues after several days of treatment, CONTACT YOUR DOCTOR. This medication may be causing an allergic reaction, or it may not be effective against the organism causing your infection.
- This medication has been prescribed for your current infection only. Another infection later on, or one that someone else has, may require a different medication. You should not give your medication to other women, or use it for other infections, unless your doctor specifically directs you to do so.
- Be sure to tell your doctor if you are pregnant. Small amounts of miconazole are absorbed from the vagina, so caution should be used, especially during the first three months of pregnancy. In addition, your doctor may want to change the instructions on how you are to insert this medication if you are pregnant. Also, tell your doctor if you are breastfeeding an infant. It is not known whether or not miconazole passes into breast milk.

Micrainin—see meprobamate and aspirin combination

Micro-K—see potassium chloride

Micronase—see glyburide

Microsul—see sulfonamides

Microsulfon—see sulfonamides

Mictrin—see hydrochlorothiazide

Midamor—see amiloride

Midatane Expectorant—see phenylephrine, phenylpropanolamine, brompheniramine, and guaifenesin combination

Midatap—see phenylpropanolamine, phenylephrine, and brompheniramine combination

Millazine—see thioridazine

Miltown—see meprobamate

Minipress see prazosin

---

minocycline

BRAND NAME (Manufacturer)
Minocin (Lederle)
TYPE OF DRUG
Antibiotic (infection fighter)
INGREDIENT
minocycline
DOSAGE FORM
Capsules (150 mg and 300 mg)
STORAGE
Minocycline capsules should be stored at room temperature in a tightly closed, light-resistant container.

USES
Minocycline is used to treat a wide range of bacterial infections, and to prevent meningococcal meningitis. It acts by preventing the growth of bacteria. This drug kills susceptible bacteria, but is not effective against viruses or fungi.

TREATMENT
To avoid stomach upset, you can take this medication with food (unless your doctor directs you to do otherwise).

Minocycline works best when the level of medicine in your bloodstream is kept constant. It is best therefore to take the doses at evenly spaced intervals, day and night. For example, if you are to take four doses a day, the doses should be spaced six hours apart.

If you miss a dose of this medication, take the missed dose immediately. However, if you do not remember to take the missed dose until it is almost time for your next dose, take it; space the following dose about halfway through the regular interval between doses; then return to your regular dosing schedule. Try not to skip any doses.

It is important to continue to take this medication for the entire time prescribed by your doctor, even if the symptoms disappear before the end of that period. If you stop taking the drug too soon, resistant bacteria are given a chance to continue growing, and the infection could recur.

SIDE EFFECTS

Minor. Diarrhea; dizziness; headache; light-headedness; loss of appetite; nausea; stomach cramps and upset; vomiting; and discoloration of the nails. These side effects should disappear in several days, as your body adjusts to the medication.

Minocycline can increase your sensitivity to sunlight. In order to avoid this side effect, limit your exposure to sunlight and sunlamps. Wear protective clothing and sunglasses, and use an effective sunscreen.

If you feel dizzy or light-headed, sit or lie down awhile; get up from a sitting or lying position slowly, and be careful on stairs.

Major. Tell your doctor about any side effects that are persistent or particularly bothersome. IT IS ESPECIALLY IMPORTANT TO TELL YOUR DOCTOR about unusual bleeding or bruising; darkened tongue; difficulty breathing; joint pain; mouth irritation; rash; rectal or vaginal itching; sore throat and fever; or yellowing of the eyes or skin. Also, if your symptoms of infection seem to be getting worse, rather than improving, you should contact your doctor.

INTERACTIONS

Minocycline interacts with several other types of medication.

1. It can increase the absorption of digoxin, which may lead to digoxin toxicity.

2. The gastrointestinal side effects (nausea, vomiting, stomach upset) of theophylline may be increased by minocycline.

3. The dosage of oral anti-coagulants (blood thinners, such as warfarin) may need to be adjusted when this medication is started.

4. Minocycline may decrease the effectiveness of oral

contraceptives (birth control pills)—pregnancy could result. You should therefore use another form of birth control while taking minocycline. Discuss this with your doctor.

TELL YOUR DOCTOR if you are currently taking any of the medications listed above.

WARNINGS

• Tell your doctor about unusual or allergic reactions you have had to any medications, especially to minocycline or to oxytetracycline, doxycycline, or tetracycline.

• Tell your doctor if you now have, or if you have ever had, kidney or liver disease.

• Minocycline can cause dizziness or light-headedness. Your ability to perform tasks that require alertness, such as driving a car or operating potentially dangerous machinery, may be decreased. Appropriate caution should therefore be taken.

• Minocycline can affect tests for syphilis; tell your doctor you are taking this medication if you are also being treated for this disease.

• Make sure that your prescription for this medication is marked with the drug's expiration date. The drug should be discarded after the expiration date. If the drug is used after it has expired, serious side effects (especially to the kidneys) could result.

• This medication has been prescribed for your current infection only. Another infection later on, or one that someone else has, may require a different medicine. You should not give your medicine to other people, or use it for other infections, unless your doctor specifically directs you to do so.

• Be sure to tell your doctor if you are pregnant or if you are breastfeeding an infant. Minocycline crosses the placenta and passes into breast milk. If used during their development, this drug can cause permanent discoloration of the teeth and can inhibit tooth and bone growth. In addition, it should not be used for infants or for children less than eight years of age.

Minocin—see minocycline

minoxidil

BRAND NAME (Manufacturer)
Loniten (Upjohn)
TYPE OF DRUG
Anti-hypertensive
INGREDIENT
minoxidil
DOSAGE FORM
Tablets (2.5 mg and 10 mg)
STORAGE
Minoxidil should be stored at room temperature, in a tightly closed container.

USES

Minoxidil is used to treat high blood pressure. It lowers blood pressure by dilating (increasing the size of) the blood vessels in the body.

TREATMENT

Minoxidil can be taken either on an empty stomach or with food or a full glass of water or milk (as directed by your doctor).

In order to become accustomed to taking this medication, try to take it at the same time(s) each day.

Minoxidil does not cure high blood pressure, but it will help to control the condition, as long as you continue to take it.

If you miss a dose of this medication, take the missed dose as soon as possible, unless it is almost time for your next dose. In that case, do not take the missed dose at all; just return to your regular dosing schedule. Do not double the next dose.

SIDE EFFECTS

Minor. Fatigue; flushing; headache; nausea; and vomiting. These side effects should disappear in several days, as your body adjusts to the medication.
Major. Tell your doctor about any side effects that are persistent or particularly bothersome. IT IS ESPECIALLY IMPORTANT TO TELL YOUR DOCTOR about abnormal hair

growth; unusual bleeding or bruising; breast tenderness (in both sexes); chest pain; difficult or painful urination; darkening of the skin; palpitations; rapid weight gain (three to five pounds within a week); or skin rash.

INTERACTIONS

Concurrent use of minoxidil and guanethidine can cause a severe drop in blood pressure. BE SURE TO TELL YOUR DOCTOR if you are already taking guanethidine.

WARNINGS

● Tell your doctor about unusual or allergic reactions you have had to any medications, especially to minoxidil.
● Before starting to take this medication, be sure to tell your doctor if you now have, or if you have ever had, angina pectoris (chest pain), heart failure, a heart attack, kidney disease, pericardial effusions, pheochromocytoma, or a stroke.
● Do not take any over-the-counter (non-prescription) cough, cold, allergy, asthma, sinus, or diet medication unless you first check with your doctor or pharmacist. Some of these products can increase your blood pressure.
● Do not stop taking minoxidil unless you first check with your doctor. Stopping the drug abruptly may lead to a worsening of your high blood pressure. Your doctor may therefore want to reduce your dosage gradually or start you on another medication when you stop taking minoxidil.
● Minoxidil is being studied investigationally for the treatment of alopecia (male-pattern baldness). For this purpose, your doctor might prescribe it to be topically applied (as a skin lotion) to the affected areas.
● Be sure to tell your doctor if you are pregnant. Birth defects have been reported in animals whose mothers received large doses of minoxidil during pregnancy. Extensive studies in humans have not yet been completed. Also, tell your doctor if you are breastfeeding an infant. It is not known whether or not minoxidil passes into breast milk, but it is generally recommended that a woman who is taking this medication not nurse.

mitotane

BRAND NAME (Manufacturer)
Lysodren (Bristol)
TYPE OF DRUG
Anti-neoplastic (anti-cancer drug)
INGREDIENT
mitotane
DOSAGE FORM
Tablets (500 mg)
STORAGE
Mitotane should be stored at room temperature in a tightly closed, light-resistant container.

USES

This medication is used to treat adrenal gland cancer and Cushing's syndrome (overactive adrenal gland) in patients on whom surgery cannot be performed. Mitotane directly suppresses the activity of the adrenal gland.

TREATMENT

Initial therapy with mitotane often occurs in the hospital until the dosage is stabilized. Mitotane is potent medication. The dosage is usually adjusted to an individual's needs and tolerance. Be sure you understand your doctor's instructions on how this medication should be taken.

Mitotane tablets can be taken either on an empty stomach or, to reduce stomach irritation, with food or milk (unless your doctor directs you to do otherwise).

Try not to miss any doses of this medication. If you do miss a dose, take the missed dose as soon as possible, unless it is almost time for the next dose. In that case, do not take the missed dose at all; just return to your regular dosing schedule. Do not double the next dose.

SIDE EFFECTS

Minor. Diarrhea; dizziness; drowsiness; loss of appetite; nausea; and vomiting. These side effects should disappear as your body adjusts to the medication. However, it is important to continue taking this medication despite the nausea and vomiting that may occur.

Mitotane can also cause hair loss (which is reversible

when the medication is discontinued).

If you feel dizzy, sit or lie down awhile; get up slowly, and be careful on stairs.

Major. Tell your doctor about any side effects that are persistent or particularly bothersome. IT IS ESPECIALLY IMPORTANT TO TELL YOUR DOCTOR about blurred vision; depression; difficult or painful urination; fainting; flushing; lethargy; muscle aches; or skin rash.

INTERACTIONS

Mitotane interacts with several other types of medication.
1. Concurrent use of it with central nervous system depressants (drugs that slow the activity of the brain and spinal cord), such as alcohol, antihistamines, barbiturates, benzodiazepine tranquilizers, muscle relaxants, narcotics, pain medications, phenothiazine tranquilizers, and sleeping medications, or with tricyclic anti-depressants can cause extreme drowsiness.
2. Mitotane can decrease the effectiveness of adrenocorticosteroids (cortisone-like medications).
BE SURE TO TELL YOUR DOCTOR if you are already taking any of these types of medication.

WARNINGS

• Tell your doctor about unusual or allergic reactions you have had to any medications, especially to mitotane.
• Tell your doctor if you now have, or if you have ever had, chronic infections or liver disease.
• If this drug makes you dizzy or drowsy, do not take part in any activity that requires alertness, such as driving a car or operating potentially dangerous equipment.
• Do not stop taking this medication unless you first check with your doctor. The effects of mitotane on the adrenal gland last several weeks after the drug is stopped. Mitotane can impair your body's response to trauma, stress, and infection. If you experience trauma, stress, or infection while taking this medication, or shortly after you stop taking it (within several weeks), check with your doctor. You may need to take supplemental adrenal hormone during this period.
• Contact your doctor immediately if you get an injury, infection, or any illness. This medication can decrease

your body's ability to respond to stressful situations.

● Before having any surgery or other medical or dental treatment, be sure your doctor or dentist knows that you are taking this medication.

● Be sure to tell your doctor if you are pregnant. Extensive studies of mitotane in pregnant women have not yet been completed. The risks should be discussed with your doctor. Also, tell your doctor if you are breastfeeding an infant. It is not known whether or not mitotane passes into breast milk.

Mity-Quin—see hydrocortisone and iodochlorhydroxyquin combination (topical)

Mixtard—see insulin

Modicon—see oral contraceptives

Moduretic—see amiloride and hydrochlorothiazide combination

Mol-Iron—see iron supplements

Monistat 7—see miconazole (vaginal)

Mono-Press—see trichlormethiazide

Monotard—see insulin

---

morphine

BRAND NAMES (Manufacturers)
morphine sulfate (various manufacturers)
RMS Uniserts (Upsher-Smith)
Roxanol (Roxane)
TYPE OF DRUG
Analgesic (pain reliever)
INGREDIENT
morphine as the sulfate salt
DOSAGE FORMS
Tablets (15 mg and 30 mg)

Oral solution (10 mg and 20 mg per 5 ml teaspoonful with
   10% alcohol; 20 mg per ml)
Rectal suppositories (5 mg, 10 mg, and 20 mg)

STORAGE

Morphine tablets and oral solution should be stored at
room temperature in tightly closed, light-resistant containers. The rectal suppositories should be stored in the
refrigerator.

USES

Morphine is a narcotic analgesic that acts directly on the
central nervous system (brain and spinal cord). It is used to
relieve moderate to severe pain.

TREATMENT

In order to avoid stomach upset, you can take morphine
with food or milk. This medication works most effectively
if you take it at the onset of pain, rather than waiting until
the pain becomes intense.

The solution form of this medication can be mixed with
fruit juices to improve the taste. Measure each dose carefully, with a specially designed, 5 ml measuring spoon or
with the dropper provided. An ordinary kitchen teaspoon
is not accurate enough.

To use the suppository form of this medication, remove
the foil wrapper and moisten the suppository with water (if
the suppository is too soft to insert, refrigerate it for half an
hour or run cold water over it before removing the wrapper). Lie on your left side with your right knee bent. Push
the suppository into the rectum, pointed end first. Lie still
for a few minutes. Try to avoid having a bowel movement
for at least an hour (to give the medication time to be absorbed).

If you are taking this medication on a regular schedule
and you miss a dose, take the missed dose as soon as possible, unless it is almost time for your next dose. In that
case, don't take the missed dose at all; just return to your
regular dosing schedule. Do not double the next dose.

SIDE EFFECTS

Minor. Constipation; dizziness; drowsiness; dry mouth;
false sense of well-being; flushing; light-headedness; loss

of appetite; nausea; rash; sweating; and painful or difficult urination. These side effects should disappear in several days, as your body adjusts to the medication.

If you are constipated, increase the amount of fiber in your diet (raw vegetables, fruits, salads, bran, and whole-grain breads), and drink more water (unless your doctor directs you to do otherwise).

Chew sugarless gum, or suck on ice chips or a piece of hard candy, to reduce mouth dryness.

If you feel dizzy, light-headed, or nauseated, sit or lie down awhile; get up from a sitting or lying position slowly, and be careful on stairs.

Major. Tell your doctor about any side effects that are persistent or particularly bothersome. IT IS ESPECIALLY IMPORTANT TO TELL YOUR DOCTOR about anxiety; difficulty breathing; excitation; fainting; fatigue; palpitations; restlessness; sore throat and fever; tremors; or weakness.

INTERACTIONS

Morphine interacts with several other types of drugs.

1. Concurrent use of it with other central nervous system depressants (drugs that slow the activity of the nervous system), such as alcohol, antihistamines, barbiturates, benzodiazepine tranquilizers, muscle relaxants, and phenothiazine tranquilizers, or with tricyclic anti-depressants can cause extreme drowsiness.

2. A monoamine oxidase (MAO) inhibitor taken within 14 days of this medication can lead to unpredictable and severe side effects.

3. The depressant effects of morphine can be dangerously increased by chloral hydrate, glutethimide, beta-blockers, and furazolidone.

4. Cimetidine, combined with this medication, can cause confusion, disorientation, seizures, and shortness of breath.

TELL YOUR DOCTOR if you are currently taking any of the medications listed above.

WARNINGS

• Tell your doctor about unusual or allergic reactions you have had to any medications, especially to morphine or to other narcotic analgesics (such as codeine, hydrocodone, hydromorphone, meperidine, methadone, oxycodone, or propoxyphene).

● Tell your doctor if you now have, or if you have ever had, acute abdominal conditions; asthma; brain disease; colitis; epilepsy; gallstones or gallbladder disease; head injuries; heart disease; kidney disease; liver disease; lung disease; mental illness; emotional disorders; enlarged prostate gland; thyroid disease; or urethral stricture.

● If this drug makes you dizzy or drowsy, do not take part in any activity that requires alertness, such as driving a car or operating potentially dangerous equipment.

● Before having any surgery or other medical or dental treatment, be sure to tell your doctor or dentist that you are taking this medication.

● Morphine has the potential for abuse, and must be used with caution. Usually, it should not be taken on a regular schedule for longer than ten days (unless your doctor directs you to do so). Tolerance develops quickly; do not increase the dosage or stop taking the drug abruptly, unless you first consult your doctor. If you have been taking large amounts of this medication, or if you have been taking it for long periods of time, you may experience a withdrawal reaction (muscle aches, diarrhea, gooseflesh, runny nose, nausea, vomiting, shivering, trembling, stomach cramps, sleep disorders, irritability, weakness, yawning, and sweating) when you stop taking it. Your doctor may therefore want to reduce the dosage gradually.

● Be sure to tell your doctor if you are pregnant. The effects of this medication during pregnancy have not yet been thoroughly studied in humans. Morphine, used regularly in large doses during pregnancy, can result in addiction of the fetus, leading to withdrawal symptoms (irritability, excessive crying, tremors, fever, vomiting, diarrhea, sneezing, and yawning) at birth. Also, tell your doctor if you are breastfeeding an infant. Small amounts of this medication may pass into breast milk and cause drowsiness in the nursing infant.

morphine sulfate—see morphine

Motrin—see ibuprofen

multiple sulfonamides—see sulfonamides

Murcil—see chlordiazepoxide

Mycelex—see clotrimazole (topical)

Mycelex-G—see clotrimazole (vaginal)

Mychel—see chloramphenicol (systemic)

Mycolog—see triamcinolone, neomycin, nystatin, and gramicidin combination (topical)

My Cort—see hydrocortisone (topical)

Mycostatin—see nystatin

Myco Triacet—see triamcinolone, neomycin, nystatin, and gramicidin combination (topical)

Myidone—see primidone

Myleran—see busulfan

Myobid—see papaverine

Myotonachol—see bethanechol

Mysoline—see primidone

Mytrex—see triamcinolone, neomycin, nystatin, and gramicidin combination (topical)

---

nadolol

BRAND NAME (Manufacturer)
Corgard (Squibb)
TYPE OF DRUG
Beta-adrenergic blocking agent
INGREDIENT
nadolol

DOSAGE FORM
Tablets (40 mg, 80 mg, 120 mg, and 160 mg)

STORAGE
Nadolol should be stored at room temperature in a tightly closed, light-resistant container.

USES
Nadolol is used to treat high blood pressure and angina pectoris (chest pain). It belongs to a group of medicines known as beta-adrenergic blocking agents or, more commonly, beta-blockers. These drugs work by controlling nerve impulses along certain nerve pathways.

TREATMENT
Nadolol can be taken with a glass of water, with meals, immediately following meals, or on an empty stomach, depending on your doctor's instructions. Try to take the medication at the same time(s) each day.

Try not to miss any doses of this medicine. If you do miss a dose, take the missed dose as soon as possible. However, if the next scheduled dose is within eight hours (if you are taking this medicine only once a day) or within four hours (if you are taking this medicine more than once a day), do not take the missed dose at all; just return to your regular dosing schedule. Do not double the next dose.

It is important to remember that nadolol does not cure high blood pressure, but it will help to control the condition, as long as you continue to take it.

SIDE EFFECTS
Minor. Diarrhea; drowsiness; dryness of the eyes, mouth, and skin; nausea; numbness or tingling of the fingers or toes; cold hands or feet (due to decreased blood circulation to skin, fingers, and toes); tiredness; weakness; anxiety; nervousness; constipation; decreased sexual ability; headache; stomach discomfort; and difficulty sleeping. These side effects should disappear during treatment, as your body adjusts to the medication.

If you are extra-sensitive to the cold, be sure to dress warmly during cold weather.

Plain, non-medicated eye drops (artificial tears) may help to relieve eye dryness.

Sucking on ice chips or chewing sugarless gum helps to relieve mouth or throat dryness.

Major. Tell your doctor about any side effects that are persistent or particularly bothersome. IT IS ESPECIALLY IMPORTANT TO TELL YOUR DOCTOR about breathing difficulty or wheezing; confusion; dizziness; fever and sore throat; hair loss; hallucinations; light-headedness; mental depression; nightmares; rapid weight gain (three to five pounds within a week); reduced alertness; swelling; skin rash; or unusual bleeding or bruising.

INTERACTIONS

Nadolol interacts with a number of other medications.

1. Indomethacin, aspirin, or other salicylates may decrease the blood-pressure-lowering effects of beta-blockers.

2. Concurrent use of beta-blockers and calcium channel blockers (diltiazem, nifedipine, and verapamil) can potentially lead to heart failure or very low blood pressure.

3. Side effects may also be increased when beta-blockers are taken with clonidine, digoxin, epinephrine, phenylephrine, phenylpropanolamine, phenothiazine tranquilizers, reserpine, or monoamine oxidase (MAO) inhibitors. At least 14 days should separate the use of a beta-blocker and an MAO inhibitor.

4. Beta-blockers may antagonize (work against) the effects of theophylline, aminophylline, albuterol, metaproterenol, and terbutaline.

5. Beta-blockers can also interact with insulin or oral antidiabetic agents—raising or lowering blood sugar levels or masking the symptoms of low blood sugar.

BE SURE TO TELL YOUR DOCTOR if you are currently taking any of the medicines listed above.

WARNINGS

• Before starting to take this medication, it is important to tell your doctor if you have ever had unusual or allergic reactions to any beta-blocker (atenolol, metoprolol, nadolol, pindolol, propranolol, and timolol).

• Tell your doctor if you now have, or if you have ever had, allergies, asthma, hay fever, eczema, slow heartbeat, bronchitis, diabetes mellitus (sugar diabetes), emphysema, heart or blood vessel disease, kidney disease, liver disease, thyroid disease, or poor circulation in the fingers or toes.

● You may want to check your pulse while taking this medication. If your pulse is much slower than your usual rate (or if it is less than 50 beats per minute), check with your doctor. A pulse rate that is too slow may cause circulation problems.

● This medicine may affect your body's response to exercise. Make sure you discuss with your doctor a safe amount of exercise for your medical condition.

● It is important that you do not stop taking this medicine without first checking with your doctor. Some conditions may become worse when the medicine is stopped suddenly, and the danger of a heart attack is increased in some patients. Your doctor may want you to gradually reduce the amount of medicine you take, before stopping completely. Make sure that you have enough medicine on hand to last through vacations, holidays, and weekends.

● Before having any surgery or other medical or dental treatment, tell the physician or dentist in charge that you are taking this medicine. Often, this medication will be discontinued 48 hours prior to any major surgery.

● Nadolol can cause dizziness, drowsiness, light-headedness, or decreased alertness. You should therefore use caution while driving a car or operating any potentially dangerous machinery.

● While taking this medicine, do not use any over-the-counter (non-prescription) allergy, asthma, cough, cold, sinus, or diet preparation, without first checking with your pharmacist or doctor. Some of these medicines can result in high blood pressure and slow heartbeat when combined with a beta-blocker.

● Be sure to tell your doctor if you are pregnant. Animal studies have shown that some beta-blockers can cause problems in pregnancy when used at very high doses. Adequate studies have not been completed in humans, but there has been some association between beta-blockers used during pregnancy and low birth rate, as well as breathing problems and slow heart rate in the newborn infants. However, other reports have shown no effects on newborn infants. Also, tell your doctor if you are breastfeeding an infant. Although this medicine has not been shown to cause problems in breast-fed infants, some of the medicine may pass into breast milk, so caution is warranted.

nafcillin

BRAND NAME (Manufacturer)
Unipen (Wyeth)
TYPE OF DRUG
Antibiotic (infection fighter)
INGREDIENT
nafcillin as the sodium salt
DOSAGE FORMS
Tablets (500 mg)
Capsules (250 mg)
Oral solution (250 mg per 5 ml teaspoonful)
STORAGE
Nafcillin tablets and capsules should be stored at room temperature in tightly closed containers. The oral solution should be stored in the refrigerator in a tightly closed container. Any unused portion of the solution should be discarded after 14 days, because the drug loses its potency after that time. This medication should never be frozen.

USES
Nafcillin is used to treat a wide variety of bacterial infections, usually involving the *Staphylococcus* bacteria. It acts by severely injuring the cell walls of the infecting bacteria, thereby preventing them from growing and multiplying.

Nafcillin kills susceptible bacteria, but is not effective against viruses, parasites, or fungi.

TREATMENT
Nafcillin should be taken on an empty stomach or with a glass of water, one hour before or two hours after a meal. This medication should never be taken with fruit juices or carbonated beverages, because the acidity of these drinks destroys the drug in the stomach.

The oral solution should be measured carefully, with a

specially designed, 5 ml measuring spoon. An ordinary kitchen teaspoon is not accurate enough.

Nafcillin works best when the level of medicine in your bloodstream is kept constant. It is best therefore to take the doses at evenly spaced intervals, day and night. For example, if you are taking four doses a day, the doses should be spaced six hours apart.

If you miss a dose of this medication, take the missed dose immediately. However, if you do not remember to take the missed dose until it is almost time for your next dose, take it; then space the following dose about halfway through the regular interval between doses. Then return to your regular dosing schedule. Try not to skip any doses.

It is important to continue to take this medication for the entire time prescribed by your doctor (usually seven to 14 days), even if the symptoms of the infection disappear before the end of that period. If you stop taking the drug too soon, resistant bacteria are given a chance to continue growing, and the infection could recur.

SIDE EFFECTS

Minor. Diarrhea; heartburn; nausea; and vomiting. These side effects should disappear in several days, as your body adjusts to the medication.

Major. Tell your doctor about any side effects that are persistent or particularly bothersome. IT IS ESPECIALLY IMPORTANT TO TELL YOUR DOCTOR about bloating; chills; cough; difficulty breathing; fever; irritation of the mouth; muscle aches; rash; rectal or vaginal itching; severe diarrhea; sore throat; or darkened tongue. Also, if your symptoms of infection seem to be getting worse rather than improving, you should contact your doctor.

INTERACTIONS

Nafcillin interacts with several other types of medication.

1. Probenecid can increase the blood concentrations of this medication.

2. Nafcillin may decrease the effectiveness of oral contraceptives (birth control pills), and pregnancy could result. You should therefore use another form of birth control while taking this medication. Discuss this with your doctor.

BE SURE TO TELL YOUR DOCTOR if you are currently taking either of the medications listed above.

WARNINGS

• Tell your doctor about unusual or allergic reactions you have had to any medications, especially to nafcillin, penicillins, cephalosporin antibiotics, penicillamine, or griseofulvin.

• Tell your doctor if you now have, or if you have ever had, kidney disease, asthma, or allergies.

• This medication has been prescribed for your current infection only. Another infection later on, or one that someone else has, may require a different medicine. You should not give your medicine to other people or use it for other infections, unless your doctor specifically directs you to do so.

• Diabetics taking nafcillin should know that this drug can cause a false-positive sugar reaction with a Clinitest urine glucose test. To avoid this problem, while taking nafcillin you should switch to Clinistix or Tes-Tape to test your urine sugar.

• Be sure to tell your doctor if you are pregnant. Although nafcillin appears to be safe during pregnancy, extensive studies in humans have not yet been completed. Also, tell your doctor if you are breastfeeding an infant. Small amounts of this medication pass into breast milk and may temporarily alter the bacteria in the intestinal tract of the nursing infant, resulting in diarrhea.

Naldecon—see phenylpropanolamine, phenylephrine, chlorpheniramine, and phenyltoloxamine combination

Nalfon—see fenoprofen

nalidixic acid

BRAND NAME (Manufacturer)
NegGram (Winthrop)
TYPE OF DRUG
Antibiotic (infection fighter)

INGREDIENT
nalidixic acid
DOSAGE FORMS
Tablets (250 mg, 500 mg, and 1,000 mg)
Suspension (250 mg per 5 ml teaspoonful)
STORAGE
Nalidixic acid tablets and suspension should be stored at room temperature in tightly closed containers. This medication should never be frozen.

USES
Nalidixic acid is an antibiotic that is used to treat bacterial urinary tract infections. It works by preventing the growth and multiplication of susceptible bacteria. This medication is not effective against viruses, parasites, or fungi.

TREATMENT
In order to avoid stomach irritation, you can take nalidixic acid with food or with a full glass of water or milk (unless your doctor directs you to do otherwise).

The suspension form of this medication should be shaken well, just before measuring each dose. The contents tend to settle on the bottom of the bottle, so it is necessary to shake the container to evenly distribute the ingredients and equalize the doses. Each dose should then be measured carefully, with a specially designed, 5 ml measuring spoon. An ordinary kitchen teaspoon is not accurate enough.

Nalidixic acid works best when the level of the medicine in your bloodstream and urine is kept constant. It is best therefore to take the doses at evenly spaced intervals, day and night. For example, if you are to take four doses a day, the doses should be spaced six hours apart.

Try not to miss any doses of this medication. If you do miss a dose, take it as soon as you remember. If it is almost time for your next dose, take the missed dose immediately; space the following dose halfway through the regular dosing interval (in three hours, if you are taking the drug every six hours); then continue with your regular dosing schedule.

It is important to continue to take this medication for the entire time prescribed by your doctor (usually seven to 14

days), even if the symptoms disappear before the end of
that period. If you stop taking the drug too soon, resistant
bacteria are given a chance to continue growing, and your
infection could recur.

SIDE EFFECTS

Minor. Abdominal pain; diarrhea; dizziness; drowsiness;
headache; nausea; vomiting; and weakness. These side effects should disappear in several days, as your body adjusts to the medication.

If you feel dizzy, sit or lie down awhile; get up slowly,
and be careful on stairs.

This medication can increase your sensitivity to sunlight. You should therefore avoid prolonged exposure to
sunlight and sunlamps. Wear protective clothing and sunglasses, and use an effective sunscreen.

Major. Tell your doctor about any side effects that are persistent or particularly bothersome. IT IS ESPECIALLY IM-
PORTANT TO TELL YOUR DOCTOR about any unusual
bleeding or bruising; convulsions; itching; joint pain; skin
rash; tingling sensations; visual disturbances; or yellowing
of the eyes or skin.

INTERACTIONS

Nalidixic acid can increase the effects of oral anti-coagulants (blood thinners, such as warfarin), which can lead to
bleeding complications. Nitrofurantoin can reduce the effectiveness of nalidixic acid.

BE SURE TO TELL YOUR DOCTOR if you are already taking any of these medications.

WARNINGS

- Tell your doctor about unusual or allergic reactions you
have had to any medications, especially to nalidixic acid
or cinoxacin.
- Before starting to take this medication, be sure to tell
your doctor if you now have, or if you have ever had, brain
disorders, epilepsy, kidney disease, or liver disease.
- If this drug makes you dizzy or drowsy, do not take part
in activities that require alertness, such as driving a car or
operating potentially dangerous equipment.
- This medication has been prescribed for your current

infection only. Another infection later on, or one that someone else has, may require a different medicine. You should not give your medication to other people, or use it for other infections, unless your doctor specifically directs you to do so.

• Diabetic patients should know that nalidixic acid can cause false-positive readings of Clinitest urine glucose tests. Temporarily changing to Clinistix or Tes-Tape urine glucose tests avoids this problem. CHECK WITH YOUR DOCTOR before adjusting the dosage of your anti-diabetic medication.

• If the symptoms of your infection do not improve within several days after starting this medication, CHECK WITH YOUR DOCTOR. Nalidixic acid may not be effective against the organism causing your infection.

• Be sure to tell your doctor if you are pregnant. Although nalidixic acid may cross the placenta, it appears to be safe during pregnancy. However, extensive studies in humans have not yet been completed. Also, tell your doctor if you are breastfeeding an infant. Small amounts of nalidixic acid pass into breast milk.

Naprosyn—see naproxen

---

naproxen

BRAND NAMES (Manufacturers)
Anaprox (Syntex)
Naprosyn (Syntex)
TYPE OF DRUG
Non-steroidal anti-inflammatory analgesic (pain reliever)
INGREDIENT
naproxen (Naprosyn)
naproxen as the sodium salt (Anaprox)
DOSAGE FORM
Tablets (250 mg, 375 mg, and 500 mg—Naprosyn);
   (275 mg—Anaprox)
STORAGE
This medication should be stored in a tightly closed container at room temperature, away from heat and direct sunlight.

USES

Naproxen is used to treat the pain, swelling, stiffness, and inflammation of certain types of arthritis, gout, bursitis, and tendinitis. Naproxen is also used to treat painful menstruation.

TREATMENT

You should take this medication on an empty stomach 30 to 60 minutes before meals or two hours after meals, so that it gets into your bloodstream quickly. However, to decrease stomach irritation, your doctor may want you to take the medicine with food or antacids.

It is important to take naproxen on schedule and not to miss any doses. If you do miss a dose, take it as soon as possible, unless it is almost time for your next dose. In that case, don't take the missed dose at all; just return to your regular dosing schedule. Do not double the next dose.

If you are taking naproxen to relieve arthritis, you must take it regularly, as directed by your doctor. It may take up to four weeks before you feel the full benefits of this medication. This medication does not cure arthritis, but it will help to relieve the condition, as long as you continue to take it.

SIDE EFFECTS

Minor. Bloating; constipation; diarrhea; difficulty sleeping; dizziness; drowsiness; headache; heartburn; indigestion; light-headedness; loss of appetite; nausea; nervousness; soreness of the mouth; unusual sweating; and vomiting. As your body adjusts to the drug, these side effects should disappear.

If you become dizzy, sit or lie down awhile; and be careful on stairs.

Acetaminophen may be helpful in relieving any headaches.

Major. If any side effects are persistent or particularly bothersome, you should report them to your doctor. IT IS ESPECIALLY IMPORTANT TO TELL YOUR DOCTOR about ringing or buzzing in the ears or a problem with hearing; bloody or black, tarry stools; stomach pain; skin rash, hives, or itching; tightness in the chest, shortness of breath, or wheezing; pounding heartbeat; swelling of the feet; unexplained sore throat and fever; unusual bleeding or bruising; unusual weight gain; blurred vision; confusion; depression; unusual fatigue or weakness; difficult or painful urination; or yellowing of the eyes or skin.

INTERACTIONS

Naproxen interacts with several types of medication.

1. Anti-coagulants (blood thinners, such as warfarin) can lead to an increase in bleeding complications.

2. Aspirin, salicylates, or other anti-inflammation medication can cause increased stomach irritation.

3. Naproxen can decrease the elimination of lithium from the body, resulting in possible lithium toxicity.

4. Naproxen may interfere with the blood-pressure-lowering effects of beta-blocking medications (such as atenolol, metoprolol, pindolol, and propranolol).

5. This medication can also interfere with the diuretic effects of furosemide and thiazide-type diuretics (water pills).

6. Naproxen can increase the amount of probenecid in the bloodstream when both drugs are being taken.

BE SURE TO TELL YOUR DOCTOR if you are already taking any of the medications listed above.

WARNINGS

• Before you take this medication, it is important to tell your doctor if you have ever had unusual or allergic reactions to medications, especially to naproxen or any of the other chemically related drugs (including aspirin, other salicylates, diflunisal, fenoprofen, meclofenamate, mefenamic acid, indomethacin, oxyphenbutazone, phenylbutazone, piroxicam, sulindac, tolmetin, and zomepirac).

• Before taking this medication, it is important to tell your doctor if you now have, or if you have ever had, bleeding problems; colitis; stomach ulcers or other stomach problems; asthma; epilepsy; heart disease; high blood pressure; kidney disease; liver disease; mental illness; or Parkinson's disease.

• If naproxen makes you dizzy or drowsy, do not take part in any activity that requires alertness, such as driving a car or operating potentially dangerous equipment.

• Because this drug can prolong your bleeding time, it is

important to tell your doctor or dentist that you are taking this drug before having any surgery or other medical or dental treatment.

• Stomach problems are more likely to occur if you take aspirin regularly or drink alcohol while being treated with this medication. These should therefore be avoided (unless your doctor tells you otherwise).

• Be sure to tell your doctor if you are pregnant. Naproxen may cause unwanted effects on the heart or blood flow of the fetus. Studies in animals have shown that naproxen, taken late in pregnancy, may increase the length of pregnancy, prolong labor, or cause other problems during delivery. Also, tell your doctor if you are breastfeeding an infant. Naproxen can pass into breast milk in small amounts.

Naptrate—see pentaerythritol tetranitrate

Naqua—see trichlormethiazide

Nardil—see phenelzine

Nasalcrom—see cromolyn sodium (nasal)

Naturetin—see bendroflumethiazide

Navane—see thiothixene

ND Clear T.D.—see pseudoephedrine and chlorpheniramine combination

NegGram—see nalidixic acid

Nembutal—see pentobarbital

Neomycin, Polymyxin B, and Gramicidin—see neomycin, bacitracin, polymyxin B, and gramicidin combination (ophthalmic)

neomycin, bacitracin, polymyxin B, and gramicidin combination (ophthalmic)

BRAND NAMES (Manufacturers)
AK-Sporin (Akorn)
Neomycin, Polymyxin B, and Gramicidin (Rugby)
Neosporin (Burroughs Wellcome)
Neotal (Mallard)

TYPE OF DRUG
Ophthalmic antibiotic

INGREDIENTS
neomycin as the sulfate salt, polymyxin B as the sulfate salt, bacitracin (ointment only), and gramicidin (solution only)

DOSAGE FORMS
Ophthalmic drops (1.75 mg neomycin, 10,000 units polymyxin B, and 0.025 mg gramicidin per ml)
Ophthalmic ointment (3.5 mg neomycin, 10,000 units polymyxin B, and 400 units bacitracin per gram of ointment)

STORAGE
These ophthalmic drops and ointment should be stored at room temperature in tightly closed containers. This medication should never be frozen.

USES

This medication is used to treat bacterial infections of the eye. It is an antibiotic combination that is effective against a wide range of bacteria. These antibiotics act by preventing the production of nutrients that are required for growth of the infecting bacteria. This medication is not effective against infections caused by viruses or fungi.

TREATMENT

Wash your hands with soap and water before using this medication. In order to prevent contamination of the medication, be careful not to touch the dropper or the end of the tube, and do not let the dropper or tube touch your eye.

Note that the bottle of the eye drops is not completely full. This is to allow control of the number of drops dispensed. To apply the eye drops, tilt your head back and pull down the lower eyelid with one hand to make a pouch below the eye. Drop the medicine into this pouch and slowly close your eyes. Do not blink. Keep your eyes closed, and place one finger at the corner of the eye next to your nose, applying a slight pressure for a minute or two (this is done to prevent loss of medication into the nose and throat canal). If you don't think the medicine got into the eye, repeat the process once. If you are using more than one kind of eye drop, wait at least five minutes before applying the other medication(s).

Follow the same general procedure for the ointment. Tilt your head back, pull down your lower eyelid, and squeeze the ointment in a line along the pouch below the eye. Close the eye and place your finger at the corner of the eye near the nose for a minute or two. Do not rub your eyes. Wipe off excess ointment and the tip of the tube with clean tissues.

Since this medication is somewhat difficult to apply, you may prefer to have someone else apply the drops or ointment for you.

If you miss a dose of this medication, insert the drops or apply the ointment as soon as possible, unless it is almost time for the next application. In that case, do not use the missed dose at all; just return to your regular dosing schedule.

It is important to continue to take this medication for the entire time prescribed by your doctor, even if the symptoms disappear before the end of that period. If you stop applying the drug too soon, resistant bacteria are given a chance to continue growing and the infection could recur.

SIDE EFFECTS

Minor. Blurred vision; burning; and stinging. These side effects should disappear in several days, as your body adjusts to the medication.

Major. Tell your doctor about any side effects that are persistent or particularly bothersome. IT IS ESPECIALLY IMPORTANT TO TELL YOUR DOCTOR about disturbed or reduced vision; or itching, rash, redness, or swelling in or around your eyes (other than the original symptoms of your infection). Also, if your symptoms of infection seem to be getting worse rather than improving, you should contact your doctor.

INTERACTIONS

This medication does not interact with any other medications, as long as it is used according to directions.

WARNINGS

• Tell your doctor about unusual or allergic reactions you have had to medications, especially to neomycin, bacitracin, polymyxin B, gramicidin, or any related antibiotics (such as amikacin, colistimethate, colistin, gentamicin, kanamycin, netilmicin, paromycin, streptomycin, tobramycin, or viomycin).

• Tell your doctor if you now have, or if you have ever had, kidney disease; an injured cornea; inner ear disease; or myasthenia gravis.

• Do not use this medication for longer than ten consecutive days, unless your doctor directs you to do so. Prolonged use of this drug may result in eye damage. If you need to use this medication for six weeks or longer, your doctor may want you to have an eye examination by an ophthalmologist.

• This medication has been prescribed for your current infection only. Another infection later on, or one that someone else has, may require a different medicine. You should not give your medicine to other people or use it for other infections, unless your doctor specifically directs you to do so.

• In order to allow your eye infection to clear, do not apply makeup to the affected eye.

• Be sure to tell your doctor if you are pregnant. The effects of this medication during pregnancy have not yet been thoroughly studied in humans.

Neoquess—see atropine, scopolamine, hyoscyamine, and phenobarbital combination

Neosporin—see neomycin, bacitracin, polymyxin B, and gramicidin combination (ophthalmic)

Neotal—see neomycin, bacitracin, polymyxin B, and gramicidin combination (ophthalmic)

Neotrizine—see sulfonamides

Neuramate—see meprobamate

Neurate-400—see meprobamate

N-G-C—see nitroglycerin (systemic)

NGT—see triamcinolone, neomycin, nystatin, and gramicidin combination (topical)

Niazide—see trichlormethiazide

Nicorette—see nicotine gum

---

nicotine gum

BRAND NAME (Manufacturer)
Nicorette (Merrell Dow)
TYPE OF DRUG
A "stop smoking" aid
INGREDIENT
nicotine
DOSAGE FORM
Chewing gum (2 mg)
STORAGE
This medication should be kept in its original, child-resistant packaging until it is ready to be chewed.

USES
Nicotine gum is used as a temporary aid for smoking cessation programs. It helps control the symptoms of nicotine withdrawal (irritability, headache, fatigue, and insomnia), and thus helps you to concentrate on overcoming the psychological and social aspects of your smoking habit.

TREATMENT

Use nicotine gum when you feel the urge to smoke. Keep the gum with you at all times. Place it where you usually keep your cigarettes. Whenever you feel that you want to smoke, put one piece of gum into your mouth. Chew the gum very slowly, until you taste it or feel a slight tingling in your mouth. As soon as you get the taste of the gum, stop chewing. After the taste or tingling is almost gone (after about one minute), chew slowly again until you taste the gum. Then stop chewing again. The gum should be chewed slowly for 30 minutes to release most of the nicotine. You should not expect the gum to give you the same quick satisfaction that smoking does.

Most people find that ten to 12 pieces of gum per day are enough to control their urge to smoke. Depending on your needs, you can adjust the rate of chewing and the time between pieces. Do not chew more than 30 pieces per day (unless your doctor directs you to do so).

The risk of smoking again is highest in the first months, so it is important that you follow your smoking cessation program, and continue to use nicotine gum as directed during this period. As the urge to smoke decreases, you will find that you use less and less gum.

SIDE EFFECTS

Minor. Because of its nicotine content, the gum does not taste like ordinary chewing gum. It has a peppery taste. During the first several days of chewing the nicotine gum, you may experience mouth sores, jaw muscle aches, headaches, and an increased amount of saliva in the mouth. These side effects should disappear as you continue to use the gum.

If you chew the gum too fast, you may feel effects similar to those people experience when they inhale a cigarette for the first time or when they smoke too fast. These effects include dizziness; light-headedness; nausea; vomiting; constipation; throat and mouth irritation; hoarseness; dry mouth; coughing; sneezing; hiccups; stomach pain; redness of the face; insomnia; gas pains; and stomach upset. Most of these side effects can be controlled by chewing the gum more slowly.

Major. If any of the side effects are persistent or particularly bothersome, report them to your doctor. IT IS ESPE-CIALLY IMPORTANT TO TELL YOUR DOCTOR about signs of too much nicotine (cold sweats; disturbed hearing or vision; confusion; marked weakness; faintness; difficulty breathing; seizures; and palpitations).

If you accidently swallow a piece of gum, you should not experience adverse effects. The nicotine is released by chewing and is absorbed primarily in the mouth.

INTERACTIONS

Smoking cessation, with or without nicotine gum, may affect blood levels of certain medications (including caffeine, glutethimide, imipramine, pentazocine, phenacetin, propoxyphene, and theophylline).

Nicotine can reduce the diuretic effects of furosemide and lessen the blood-pressure-lowering effects of beta-blockers such as propranolol.

BE SURE TO TELL YOUR DOCTOR if you are already taking any of the medications listed above.

WARNINGS

• Tell your doctor if you have recently had a heart attack. It is also important to tell your doctor if you now have, or if you have ever had, heart palpitations or arrhythmias; angina pectoris (chest pain); active temporomandibular joint (jaw) disease; cardiovascular disease; endocrine (hormone) disease; thyroid problems; pheochromocytoma; diabetes mellitus (sugar diabetes); high blood pressure; peptic ulcers; mouth or throat inflammation; or dental problems.

• Be sure to tell your doctor if you are pregnant. Nicotine (from the gum or from cigarette smoke) can cause fetal harm. Also, tell your doctor if you are breastfeeding an infant. Small amounts of nicotine can pass into breast milk.

---

nifedipine

BRAND NAME (Manufacturer)
Procardia (Pfizer)
TYPE OF DRUG
Anti-anginal (calcium channel blocker)

INGREDIENT
nifedipine
DOSAGE FORM
Capsules (10 mg)
STORAGE
Nifedipine capsules should be stored at room temperature in a tightly closed, light-resistant container.

USES

This medication is used to treat various types of angina (chest pain). Nifedipine belongs to a group of drugs known as calcium channel blockers. By blocking calcium, nifedipine relaxes and prevents spasms of the blood vessels of the heart and reduces the oxygen needs of the heart muscle.

TREATMENT

Nifedipine should be taken on an empty stomach with a full glass of water, one hour before or two hours after a meal (unless your doctor directs you to do otherwise). These capsules should be swallowed whole, in order to obtain the maximum benefit.

If you miss a dose of this medication, take the missed dose as soon as possible, unless it is within two hours of your next scheduled dose. In that case, do not take the missed dose at all; just return to your regular dosing schedule. Do not double the next dose.

SIDE EFFECTS

Minor. Bloating; blurred vision; cough; dizziness; flushing; gas; giddiness; headache; heartburn; heat sensation; muscle cramps; nasal congestion; nausea; nervousness; sleep disturbances; sweating; tremors; and weakness. These side effects should disappear in several days, as your body adjusts to the medication.

If you feel dizzy or light-headed, sit or lie down awhile; get up slowly, and be careful on stairs. To avoid dizziness or light-headedness when you stand, contract and relax the muscles of your legs for a few moments before rising. Do this by pushing one foot against the floor while raising the other foot slightly, alternating feet so that you are "pumping" your legs in a pedaling motion.

Major. Tell your doctor about any side effects that are persistent or particularly bothersome. IT IS ESPECIALLY IMPORTANT TO TELL YOUR DOCTOR about chills; confusion; difficulty breathing; fainting; fever; fluid retention; impotence; mood changes; palpitations; or sore throat.

INTERACTIONS

Nifedipine interacts with several other types of drugs.

1. Nifedipine can increase the active blood levels of digoxin, warfarin, phenytoin, and quinine, which can lead to an increase in side effects.

2. The combination of nifedipine and beta-blockers (atenolol, metoprolol, nadolol, pindolol, propranolol, timolol) can lead to a severe drop in blood pressure.

3. Nifedipine can lower quinidine blood levels, which can decrease its effectiveness.

Before starting to take nifedipine, BE SURE TO TELL YOUR DOCTOR if you are already taking any of the medications listed above.

WARNINGS

• Tell your doctor about unusual or allergic reactions you have had to any medications, especially to nifedipine.

• Tell your doctor if you now have, or if you have ever had, heart disease, kidney disease, low blood pressure, or liver disease.

• If this drug makes you dizzy or drowsy, do not take part in any activities that require alertness, such as driving a car or operating potentially dangerous equipment.

• Before having any surgery or other medical or dental treatment, be sure your doctor or dentist knows that you are taking this medication.

• Do not stop taking this medication unless you first consult your doctor. Stopping this medication abruptly may lead to severe chest pain. Your doctor may therefore want to decrease your dosage gradually.

• Be sure to tell your doctor if you are pregnant. Nifedipine has been shown to cause birth defects in the offspring of animals who received large doses of it during pregnancy. This medication has not yet been extensively studied in pregnant women. Also, tell your doctor if you are breastfeeding an infant. It is not known whether or not nifedipine passes into breast milk.

Nilstat—see nystatin

Niong—see nitroglycerin (systemic)

Nitro-Bid—see nitroglycerin (topical)

Nitro-Bid Plateau Caps—see nitroglycerin (systemic)

Nitrocap T.D.—see nitroglycerin (systemic)

Nitrodisc—see nitroglycerin (topical)

Nitro-Dur—see nitroglycerin (topical)

Nitrofan—see nitrofurantoin

---

nitrofurantoin

BRAND NAMES (Manufacturers)
Furadantin (Norwich-Eaton)
Furalan (Lannett)
Furan (American Urologicals)
Furanite (Major)
Furatoin (Vortech)
Macrodantin (Norwich-Eaton)
Nitrofan (Major)
nitrofurantoin (various manufacturers)
TYPE OF DRUG
Antibiotic (infection fighter)
INGREDIENT
nitrofurantoin
DOSAGE FORMS
Tablets (50 mg and 100 mg)
Capsules (25 mg, 50 mg, and 100 mg)
Oral suspension (25 mg per 5 ml teaspoonful)
STORAGE
Nitrofurantoin tablets, capsules, and oral suspension

should be stored at room temperature in tightly closed, light-resistant containers. This medication should never be frozen.

USES

Nitrofurantoin is used to treat bacterial infections of the urinary tract (bladder and kidneys). It kills susceptible bacteria by breaking down their cell walls and interfering with their production of vital nutrients.

TREATMENT

In order to avoid stomach irritation and to increase this drug's effectiveness, you can take it with a meal or with a glass of water or milk.

The tablets and capsules should be swallowed whole to obtain maximum benefit.

The oral suspension form of this medication should be shaken well just before measuring each dose. The contents tend to settle on the bottom of the bottle, so it is necessary to shake the container to evenly distribute the ingredients and equalize the doses. Each dose should then be measured carefully, with a specially designed, 5 ml measuring spoon. An ordinary kitchen teaspoon is not accurate enough. You can then dilute the dose with water, milk, fruit juice, or infant's formula to mask the drug's unpleasant taste.

Nitrofurantoin works best when the level of the medicine in your urine is kept constant. It is best therefore to take the doses at evenly spaced intervals, day and night. For example, if you are to take three doses a day, the doses should be spaced eight hours apart.

If you miss a dose of this medication, take the missed dose immediately. However, if you do not remember to take the missed dose until it is almost time for your next dose, take the missed dose; space the following dose about halfway through the regular interval between doses; then return to your regular dosing schedule. Try not to skip any doses.

It is important to continue to take this medication for the entire time prescribed by your doctor (usually seven to 14 days), even if the symptoms disappear before the end of that period. If you stop taking the drug too soon, resistant bacteria are given a chance to continue growing, and the infection could recur.

SIDE EFFECTS

Minor. Abdominal cramps; diarrhea; dizziness; drowsiness; headache; loss of appetite; nausea; and vomiting. These side effects should disappear in several days, as your body adjusts to the medication.

If this drug makes you dizzy, sit or lie down awhile; get up slowly, and be careful on stairs.

Nitrofurantoin can cause your urine to change color (to rust-yellow or brown). This is a harmless effect, but it may stain your underclothing. The color change will disappear after you stop taking the drug.

The oral suspension can cause a temporary staining of the teeth. Rinsing your mouth out with water immediately after taking each dose will prevent this effect.

Major. Tell your doctor about any side effects that are persistent or particularly bothersome. IT IS ESPECIALLY IMPORTANT TO TELL YOUR DOCTOR about unusual bleeding or bruising; chest pain; chills; cough; difficulty breathing; fainting; fever; hair loss; irritation of the mouth; muscle aches; numbness or tingling; rash; rectal or vaginal itching; weakness; or yellowing of the eyes or skin. Also, if your symptoms of infection seem to be getting worse rather than improving, you should contact your doctor.

INTERACTIONS

Nitrofurantoin interacts with several other types of medication.

1. Nalidixic acid can antagonize (act against) nitrofurantoin, decreasing its effectiveness.

2. Probenecid and sulfinpyrazone can decrease the effectiveness and increase the side effects of nitrofurantoin.

3. Magnesium trisilicate can decrease the absorption of nitrofurantoin from the gastrointestinal tract.

Before starting to take nitrofurantoin, BE SURE TO TELL YOUR DOCTOR if you are already taking any of the medications listed above.

WARNINGS

• Tell your doctor about any unusual or allergic reactions

you have had to medications, especially to nitrofurantoin, nitrofurazone, or furazolidone.

● Before starting to take this medication, be sure to tell your doctor if you now have, or if you have ever had, anemia, diabetes mellitus (sugar diabetes), electrolyte abnormalities, glucose-6-phosphate dehydrogenase (G6PD) deficiency, kidney disease, lung disease, nerve damage, or vitamin B deficiencies.

● If this drug makes you dizzy or drowsy, do not take part in any activities that require alertness, such as driving a car or operating potentially dangerous equipment.

● Before having any surgery or other medical or dental treatment, be sure your doctor or dentist knows that you are taking nitrofurantoin.

● Diabetics should know that nitrofurantoin can cause false-positive results with some urine sugar tests (Clinitest)—Tes-Tape is not affected. Be sure to check with your doctor before adjusting your insulin dose.

● This medication has been prescribed for your current infection only. Another infection later on, or one that someone else has, may require a different medicine. You should not give your medicine to other people, or use it for other infections, unless your doctor specifically directs you to do so.

● Be sure to tell your doctor if you are pregnant. Although nitrofurantoin appears to be safe during the early stages of pregnancy, it should not be used close to term. It may cause anemia in the newborn infant. Nitrofurantoin should not be used in an infant less than one month of age. Also, tell your doctor if you are breastfeeding an infant. Nitrofurantoin passes into breast milk.

---

nitroglycerin (systemic)

BRAND NAMES (Manufacturers)
Ang-O-Span (Scrip)
Klavikordal (U.S. Ethicals)
N-G-C (Kay)
Niong (U.S. Ethicals)
Nitro-Bid Plateau Caps (Marion)
Nitrocap T.D. (Vortech)

Nitroglycerin (Lilly)
Nitroglyn (Key)
Nitrolin (Henry Schein)
Nitro-Long (Major)
Nitronet (U.S. Ethicals)
Nitrong (Wharton)
Nitrospan (USV)
Nitrostat (Parke-Davis)
Trates Granucaps (Reid-Provident)

TYPE OF DRUG
Anti-anginal
INGREDIENT
nitroglycerin
DOSAGE FORMS
Sustained-release tablets (2.6 mg, 6.5 mg, and 9 mg)
Sustained-release capsules (2.5 mg, 6.5 mg, and 9 mg)
Sublingual tablets (0.15 mg, 0.3 mg, 0.4 mg, and 0.6 mg)
STORAGE
Nitroglycerin should be stored in a tightly capped bottle in a cool, dry place.

The sublingual tablets should be kept in their original glass container. NEVER store them in a metal box or plastic vial, or in the refrigerator or the bathroom medicine cabinet, because the drug may lose its potency.

USES

This medication is used to treat angina (chest pain). Nitroglycerin is a vasodilator that relaxes the muscles of the blood vessels, causing an increase in the oxygen supply to the heart.

The oral tablets and capsules do not act quickly; they are used to prevent chest pain. The sublingual tablets act quickly and can be used to relieve chest pain after it has started.

TREATMENT

You should take the sustained-release tablets or capsules with a full glass of water on an empty stomach, one hour before or two hours after a meal. The tablets and capsules should be swallowed whole. Chewing, crushing, or breaking them destroys their sustained-release activity, and possibly increases the side effects.

NEVER chew or swallow the sublingual tablets. In this form, the drug is absorbed directly through the lining of the mouth. It should be allowed to dissolve under the tongue or against the cheek. Take one tablet at the first sign of chest pain. Sit down while you are waiting for the medicine to take effect. Do not eat, drink, or smoke while nitroglycerin is in your mouth. Try not to swallow while nitroglycerin is dissolving, and do not rinse your mouth afterward. Sublingual nitroglycerin should start working in one to three minutes. If there is no relief, take another tablet in five minutes. IF YOU TAKE THREE TABLETS WITHOUT ANY SIGN OF IMPROVEMENT, CALL A DOCTOR IMMEDIATELY OR GO TO A HOSPITAL EMERGENCY ROOM. As a preventive measure, take a nitroglycerin sublingual tablet five or ten minutes before an activity that is likely to trigger an attack, such as heavy exercise, emotional stress, or exposure to high altitudes or extreme cold. Be sure to carry some nitroglycerin sublingual tablets with you at ALL times.

If you miss a dose of the sustained-release tablets or capsules, take the missed dose as soon as possible, unless it is more than halfway through the interval between doses. In that case, do not take the missed dose at all; just return to your regular dosing schedule. Do not double the dose.

SIDE EFFECTS

Minor. Dizziness; flushing of the face; headache; lightheadedness; nausea; vomiting; and weakness. These side effects should disappear in several days, as your body adjusts to the medication.

Acetaminophen may help to relieve headaches.

If you feel dizzy or light-headed, sit or lie down awhile; get up slowly, and be careful on stairs. To avoid dizziness or light-headedness when you stand, contract and relax the muscles of your legs for a few moments before rising. Do this by pushing one foot against the floor while raising the other foot slightly, alternating feet so that you are "pumping" your legs in a pedaling motion.

Major. Tell your doctor about any side effects that are persistent or particularly bothersome. IT IS ESPECIALLY IMPORTANT TO TELL YOUR DOCTOR about fainting; palpitations; rash; or sweating.

INTERACTIONS

The combination of alcohol and nitroglycerin can lead to dizziness and fainting. Nitroglycerin can increase the side effects of the tricyclic anti-depressants.

BE SURE TO TELL YOUR DOCTOR if you are already taking one of these medications.

WARNINGS

● Tell your doctor about unusual or allergic reactions you have had to any medications, especially to nitroglycerin or isosorbide dinitrate.

● Before starting to take this medication, be sure to tell your doctor if you now have, or if you have ever had, anemia, glaucoma, head injury, low blood pressure, a recent heart attack, or thyroid disease.

● If this drug makes you dizzy or light-headed, do not take part in any activity that requires alertness, such as driving a car or operating potentially dangerous equipment.

● Before having any surgery or other medical or dental treatment, be sure your doctor or dentist knows that you are taking this medication.

● Tolerance may develop to this medication within one to three months. If it seems to lose its effectiveness, contact your doctor.

● You should not discontinue use of nitroglycerin (if you have been taking it on a regular basis) unless you first consult your doctor. Stopping the drug abruptly may lead to further chest pain. Your doctor may therefore want to decrease your dosage gradually.

● If you have frequent diarrhea, you may not be absorbing the sustained-release form of this medication. Discuss this with your doctor.

● While taking this medication, do not take any over-the-counter (non-prescription) asthma, allergy, sinus, cough, cold, or diet preparations without first checking with your doctor or pharmacist. Some of these drugs decrease the effectiveness of nitroglycerin.

● The sublingual tablet should cause a slight stinging sensation when it is placed under the tongue. If this does not occur, it indicates a loss of potency—a new bottle of tablets is necessary.

- The cotton plug should be removed when the bottle is first opened; it should NOT be replaced (the cotton absorbs some of the medication, decreasing its potency).
- Nitroglycerin is highly flammable. Do not use it in places where it might be ignited.
- Be sure to tell your doctor if you are pregnant. Although this drug appears to be safe, extensive studies in pregnant women have not yet been completed. Also, tell your doctor if you are breastfeeding an infant. It is not known whether or not nitroglycerin passes into breast milk.

---

nitroglycerin (topical)

BRAND NAMES (Manufacturers)
Nitro-Bid (Marion)
Nitrodisc (Searle)
Nitro-Dur (Key)
nitroglycerin (various manufacturers)
Nitrol (Kremers-Urban)
Nitrong (Wharton)
Nitrostat (Parke-Davis)
Transderm-Nitro (Ciba)

TYPE OF DRUG
Anti-anginal

INGREDIENT
nitroglycerin

DOSAGE FORMS
Ointment (2%)
Transdermal system (the patch delivers 2.5 mg, 5 mg, 7.5 mg, 10 mg, or 15 mg per 24 hours)

STORAGE
Nitroglycerin ointment and patches should be stored at room temperature in their original containers. The ointment container should always be tightly capped.

USES
Nitroglycerin is used to prevent angina (chest pain). It is a vasodilator that relaxes the muscles of the blood vessels, causing an increase in the oxygen supply to the heart. The ointment and patches do not act quickly—they should not

be used to treat chest pain that has already started.

TREATMENT

The ointment comes with an applicator with which the prescribed dosage can easily be measured and applied. Before a new dose is applied, the previous dose should be thoroughly removed. Each dose should be applied to a new site on the skin. Do not rub or massage the ointment into the skin. Just spread the ointment in a thin, even layer, covering an area of about the same size each time. Avoid contact of the ointment with other parts of the body, since it is absorbed wherever it touches the skin. Either use plastic or rubber gloves to apply the ointment, or wash your hands immediately after applying the medication. Cover the ointment only if directed to do so by your doctor.

The transdermal system (patches) allows controlled, continuous release of nitroglycerin. Patches are convenient and easy to use. For best results, apply the patch to a hairless or clean-shaven area of skin, avoiding scars and wounds. Choose a site (such as the chest or upper arm) that is not subject to excessive movement. It is all right to bathe or shower with a patch in place. In the event that a patch becomes dislodged, discard and replace it. Replace a patch by applying a new unit before removing the old one. This allows for uninterrupted drug therapy; and skin irritation is minimized since the site is changed each time. If redness or irritation develops at the application site, consult your physician. Some people are sensitive to the materials used to make the patches. Do not trim or cut the patches. This alters the dose of the medication.

If you miss an application of this medication, apply the missed dose as soon as possible, unless it is more than halfway through the interval between doses. In that case do not apply the missed dose at all; just return to your regular dosing schedule. Do not double the next dose.

SIDE EFFECTS

Minor. Dizziness; flushing of the face; headache; lightheadedness; nausea; vomiting; and weakness. These side effects should disappear in several days, as your body adjusts to the medication.

Acetaminophen may help to relieve headaches.

If you feel dizzy or light-headed, sit or lie down awhile; get up slowly, and be careful on stairs. To avoid dizziness or light-headedness when you stand, contract and relax the muscles of your legs for a few moments before rising. Do this by pushing one foot against the floor while raising the other foot slightly, alternating feet so that you are "pumping" your legs in a pedaling motion.

Major. Tell your doctor about any side effects that are persistent or particularly bothersome. IT IS ESPECIALLY IMPORTANT TO TELL YOUR DOCTOR about fainting; palpitations; rash; or sweating.

INTERACTIONS

The combination of alcohol and nitroglycerin can lead to dizziness and fainting. Nitroglycerin can increase the side effects of the tricyclic anti-depressants.

Before starting to take nitroglycerin, BE SURE TO TELL YOUR DOCTOR if you are already taking one of these medications.

WARNINGS

• Tell your doctor about unusual or allergic reactions you have had to any medications, especially to nitroglycerin or isosorbide dinitrate.

• Before starting to take this medication, be sure to tell your doctor if you now have, or if you have ever had, severe anemia, glaucoma, head injury, low blood pressure, a recent heart attack, or thyroid disease.

• If this drug makes you dizzy or light-headed, do not take part in any activity that requires alertness, such as driving a car or operating potentially dangerous equipment.

• Before having any surgery or other medical or dental treatment, be sure your doctor or dentist knows that you are taking this medication.

• Tolerance to this medication may develop within one to three months. If it seems to lose its effectiveness, contact your doctor.

• You should not discontinue use of nitroglycerin unless you first consult your doctor. Stopping the drug abruptly may lead to further chest pain. Your doctor may therefore

want to decrease your dosage gradually.
• While taking this medication, do not take any over-the-counter (non-prescription) asthma, allergy, sinus, cough, cold, or diet preparations without first checking with your doctor or pharmacist. Some of these drugs decrease the effectiveness of nitroglycerin.
• Nitroglycerin is highly flammable. Do not use it in places where it might be ignited.
• Be sure to tell your doctor if you are pregnant. Although this drug appears to be safe, extensive studies in pregnant women have not yet been completed. Also, tell your doctor if you are breastfeeding an infant. It is not known whether or not nitroglycerin passes into breast milk.

Nitroglyn—see nitroglycerin (systemic)

Nitrol—see nitroglycerin (topical)

Nitrolin—see nitroglycerin (systemic)

Nitro-Long—see nitroglycerin (systemic)

Nitronet—see nitroglycerin (systemic)

Nitrong—see nitroglycerin (systemic)

Nitrong—see nitroglycerin (topical)

Nitrospan—see nitroglycerin (systemic)

Nitrostat—see nitroglycerin (systemic)

Nitrostat—see nitroglycerin (topical)

Nizoral—see ketoconazole

Noctec—see chloral hydrate

Nolvadex—see tamoxifen

Noradryl—see diphenhydramine

Norcet—see acetaminophen and hydrocodone combination

Nordette—see oral contraceptives

Nordryl—see diphenhydramine

Norgesic—see orphenadrine, aspirin, and caffeine combination

Norgesic Forte—see orphenadrine, aspirin, and caffeine combination

Norinyl—see oral contraceptives

Norlestrin—see oral contraceptives

Normatane Expectorant—see phenylephrine, phenylpropanolamine, brompheniramine, and guaifenesin combination

Nor-Mil—see diphenoxylate and atropine

Noroxine—see levothyroxine

Norpace—see disopyramide

Norpace CR—see disopyramide

Norpanth—see propantheline

Norpramin—see desipramine

Nor-Tet—see tetracycline

---

nortriptyline

BRAND NAMES (Manufacturers)
Aventyl (Lilly)
Pamelor (Sandoz)

TYPE OF DRUG
Tricyclic anti-depressant (mood elevator)
INGREDIENT
nortriptyline as the hydrochloride salt
DOSAGE FORMS
Tablets (10 mg, 25 mg, and 75 mg)
Oral solution (10 mg per 5 ml teaspoonful)
STORAGE
This medication should be stored at room temperature in a tightly closed container.

USES

Nortriptyline is used to relieve the symptoms of mental depression. This medication belongs to a group of drugs referred to as the tricyclic anti-depressants. These medicines are thought to relieve depression by increasing the concentration of certain chemicals necessary for nerve transmission in the brain.

TREATMENT

This medication should be taken exactly as your doctor prescribes. It can be taken with water or with food to lessen the chance of stomach irritation, unless your doctor tells you to do otherwise.

If you miss a dose of this medication, take the missed dose as soon as possible, then return to your regular dosing schedule. However, if the dose you missed was a once-a-day bedtime dose, do not take that dose in the morning; check with your doctor instead. If the dose is taken in the morning, it may cause some unwanted side effects. Never double the dose.

The effects of therapy with this medication may not become apparent for two or three weeks.

SIDE EFFECTS

Minor. Agitation; anxiety; blurred vision; confusion; constipation; cramps; diarrhea; dizziness; drowsiness; dry mouth; fatigue; heartburn; insomnia; loss of appetite; nausea; peculiar tastes in the mouth; restlessness; sweating; vomiting; weakness; and weight gain or loss. As your body adjusts to the medication, these side effects should disappear.

Dry mouth can be relieved by chewing sugarless gum, or by sucking on ice chips or a piece of hard candy.

To relieve constipation, increase the amount of fiber (bran, salads, whole-grain breads, fresh vegetables and fruits) in your diet, and drink more water (unless your doctor directs you to do otherwise).

To avoid dizziness or light-headedness when you stand, contract and relax the muscles of your legs for a few moments before rising. Do this by pushing one foot against the floor while raising the other foot slightly, alternating feet so that you are "pumping" your legs in a pedaling motion.

This medication may cause increased sensitivity to sunlight. You should therefore avoid prolonged exposure to sunlight and sunlamps. Wear protective clothing, and use an effective sunscreen.

Major. Tell your doctor about any side effects that are persistent or particularly bothersome. IT IS ESPECIALLY IMPORTANT TO TELL YOUR DOCTOR about unusual bleeding or bruising; chest pain; convulsions; difficulty urinating; enlarged or painful breasts (in both sexes); fainting; fever; fluid retention; hair loss; hallucinations; headaches; impotence; mood changes; mouth sores; nervousness; nightmares; numbness in the fingers or toes; palpitations; ringing in the ears; seizures; skin rash; sleep disorders; sore throat; swelling; tremors; uncoordinated movements or balance problems; or yellowing of the eyes or skin.

INTERACTIONS

Nortriptyline interacts with a number of other types of medication.

1. Extreme drowsiness can occur when this medicine is taken with central nervous system depressants (medicines that slow the activity of the nervous system), including alcohol, antihistamines, barbiturates, benzodiazepine tranquilizers, muscle relaxants, narcotics, pain medications, phenothiazine tranquilizers, and sleeping medications.

2. Nortriptyline may decrease the effectiveness of anti-seizure medications and may block the blood-pressure-lowering effects of clonidine and guanethidine.

3. Oral contraceptives (estrogens) can increase the side effects and reduce the effectiveness of the tricyclic anti-depressants (including nortriptyline).

4. Tricyclic anti-depressants may increase the side effects of thyroid medication and over-the-counter (non-prescription) cough, cold, asthma, allergy, sinus, and diet medications.

5. The concurrent use of tricyclic anti-depressants and monoamine oxidase (MAO) inhibitors should be undertaken very carefully, because the combination may result in fever, convulsions, or high blood pressure.

Before starting to take nortriptyline, BE SURE TO TELL YOUR DOCTOR if you are already taking any of the medications listed above.

WARNINGS

• Tell your doctor if you have had unusual or allergic reactions to medications, especially to nortriptyline or any of the other tricyclic anti-depressants (amitriptyline, imipramine, doxepin, trimipramine, amoxapine, protriptyline, desipramine, maprotiline).

• Tell your doctor if you now have, or if you have ever had, asthma, high blood pressure, liver or kidney disease, heart disease, a recent heart attack, circulatory disease, stomach problems, intestinal problems, alcoholism, difficulty urinating, enlarged prostate gland, epilepsy, glaucoma, thyroid disease, mental illness, or electroshock therapy.

• If this drug makes you dizzy or drowsy, do not take part in any activity that requires alertness, such as driving a car or operating potentially dangerous equipment.

• Before having any surgery or other medical or dental treatment, be sure to tell your doctor or dentist that you are taking this medication.

• Do not stop taking this drug suddenly. Abruptly stopping it can cause nausea, headache, stomach upset, fatigue, or a worsening of your condition. Your doctor may want to reduce the dosage gradually.

• The effects of this medication may last as long as seven days after you have stopped taking it, so continue to observe all precautions during that period.

• Be sure to tell your doctor if you are pregnant. Problems in humans have not been reported; however, studies in animals have shown that this type of medication can cause side effects to the fetus when given to the mother in large doses during pregnancy. Also, tell your doctor if you are breastfeeding an infant. Small amounts of this drug can pass into the breast milk and may cause unwanted effects, such as irritability or sleeping problems, in the nursing infant.

Novafed A—see pseudoephedrine and chlorpheniramine combination

Nutracort—see hydrocortisone (topical)

Nydrazid—see isoniazid

Nysolone—see triamcinolone, neomycin, nystatin, and gramicidin combination (topical)

---

nystatin

BRAND NAMES (Manufacturers)
Candex (Miles)
Korostatin (Youngs Drug)
Mycostatin (Squibb)
Nilstat (Lederle)
nystatin (various manufacturers)
O-V Statin (Squibb)
TYPE OF DRUG
Anti-fungal
INGREDIENT
nystatin
DOSAGE FORMS
Oral tablets (100,000 units and 500,000 units)
Oral suspension (100,000 units per ml)
Vaginal tablets (100,000 units)
Topical cream, ointment, lotion, and powder (100,000 units per gram)
STORAGE
Nystatin should be stored at room temperature in a tightly closed, light-resistant container. This medication should never be frozen.

USES

Nystatin is used to treat fungal infections of the throat, gastrointestinal tract, skin, and vagina. This medication works by chemically binding to the cell membranes of the fungus organisms. It causes the cell contents to leak out, killing the fungus.

TREATMENT

You can take the oral tablet form of nystatin either on an empty stomach or with food or milk (as directed by your doctor).

The oral suspension and lotion should be shaken well, just before using each dose The contents tend to settle on the bottom of the bottle, so it is necessary to shake the container to evenly distribute the ingredients and equalize the doses.

Each dose of the oral suspension should then be measured carefully, with a specially designed, 5 ml measuring spoon. An ordinary kitchen teaspoon is not accurate enough. Place half of the dose in each side of your mouth. Try to hold the suspension in the mouth or swish it through the mouth for as long as possible.

The vaginal tablets are packaged with patient instructions and an applicator for inserting the tablets into the vagina. Read the instructions carefully before using this product.

Occasionally, the vaginal tablets are prescribed to be taken orally (to treat mouth or throat infections). The tablets are sucked on to increase contact time with the mouth and throat.

The region where you are to apply the topical cream, ointment, lotion, or powder should be washed carefully and patted dry. A sufficient amount of medication should then be applied to the affected area. An occlusive dressing should NOT be applied over the medication (unless your doctor directs you to do so).

If you are using the powder form of this drug to treat a foot infection, sprinkle the powder liberally into your shoes and socks.

Try not to miss any doses of this medication. If you do miss a dose, take/apply the missed dose as soon as possible, unless it is almost time for the next dose. In that case don't take/apply the missed dose at all; just return to your regular dosing schedule. Do not double the next dose.

It is important to continue to take this medication for the entire time prescribed by your doctor (usually seven to 14 days), even if the symptoms disappear before the end of that period. If you stop taking the drug too soon, resistant fungi are given a chance to continue growing, and your infection could recur.

SIDE EFFECTS

Minor. Oral forms: diarrhea; nausea; vomiting. Topical and vaginal forms: itching. These side effects should disappear in several days, as your body adjusts to the medication.

Major. Tell your doctor about any side effects that are persistent or particularly bothersome. IT IS ESPECIALLY IMPORTANT TO TELL YOUR DOCTOR about a rash.

INTERACTIONS

Nystatin does not interact with other medications, if it is used according to directions.

WARNINGS

• Tell your doctor about unusual or allergic reactions you have had to any medications, especially to nystatin.

• If you are using this drug to treat a vaginal infection, avoid sexual intercourse, or ask your partner to wear a condom, until treatment is completed. These measures help prevent reinfection. Use the vaginal tablets continuously, even during a menstrual period. Unless instructed otherwise by your doctor, do not douche during the treatment period or during the three weeks after you stop using the vaginal tablets. Wear cotton panties, rather than those made of nylon or other non-porous materials, especially while you are being treated for fungal infections of the vagina. You may wish to wear a panty liner while using the vaginal tablets, to prevent soiling of your underwear.

• Some of these products contain F.D. & C. Yellow Dye No. 5 (tartrazine), which can cause allergic-type symptoms (rash, shortness of breath, fainting) in certain susceptible individuals.

• This medication has been prescribed for your current

infection only. Another infection later on, or one that someone else has, may require a different medicine. You should not give your medicine to other people, or use it for other infections, unless your doctor specifically directs you to do so.

● If your symptoms of infection do not begin to improve two or three days after starting nystatin, CONTACT YOUR DOCTOR. This medication may not be effective against the organism causing your infection.

● Be sure to tell your doctor if you are pregnant. Although nystatin appears to be safe during pregnancy, extensive studies in humans have not yet been completed. Also, tell your doctor if you are breastfeeding an infant. It is not known whether or not nystatin passes into breast milk.

Obalan—see phendimetrazine

Obe-Nix—see phentermine

Obephen—see phentermine

Obermine—see phentermine

Obestin-30—see phentermine

Obeval—see phendimetrazine

Obezine—see phendimetrazine

Omnipen—see ampicillin

Onset—see isosorbide dinitrate

Ophthacet—see sodium sulfacetamide (ophthalmic)

Optimine—see azatadine

Oradrate—see chloral hydrate

Orahist—see phenylpropanolamine and chlorpheniramine combination

oral contraceptives

BRAND NAMES (Manufacturers)
Brevicon (Syntex)
Demulen (Searle)
Enovid-E (Searle)
Loestrin (Parke-Davis)
Lo-Ovral (Wyeth)
Modicon (Ortho)
Nordette (Wyeth)
Norinyl (Syntex)
Norlestrin (Parke-Davis)
Ortho-Novum (Ortho)
Ovral (Wyeth)
Ovcon (Mead Johnson)
Ovulen (Searle)

TYPE OF DRUG
Oral contraceptive (birth control pill)

INGREDIENTS
Estrogens and progestins (female sex hormones)

DOSAGE FORM
Tablets (in packages of 21 or 28 tablets; when 28 tablets are present, seven of the tablets are either placebos or contain iron)

STORAGE
Oral contraceptives should be stored at room temperature. They should be kept in their original container, which is designed to help you keep track of your dosing schedule.

USES
Oral contraceptives change the hormone balance of the body to prevent pregnancy.

TREATMENT
To avoid stomach irritation, you can take oral contraceptives with food or with a full glass of water or milk.

In order to become accustomed to taking this medication, try to take it at the same time every day.

Use a supplemental method of birth control for the first three weeks after you start taking oral contraceptives (the medication takes time to become fully effective).

Even if you do not start to menstruate on schedule at the

end of the pill cycle, begin the next cycle of pills at the prescribed time. Many women taking oral contraceptives have irregular menstruation.

If you miss a dose of this medication and you are on a 21-day schedule, take the missed dose as soon as you remember. If you don't remember until the next day, take the dose of that day plus the one you missed; then return to your regular dosing schedule. If you miss two days' doses, you should take two tablets a day for the next two days; then return to your regular dosing schedule. You should also use another form of birth control during those four days. If you miss your dose three days in a row, you should stop taking this drug and use a different method of birth control until your period begins or your doctor ascertains that you are not pregnant. If you are on the 28-day schedule, and you miss taking any one of the first 21 tablets, you should follow the instructions for the 21-day schedule. If you missed taking any of the last seven tablets, there is no danger of pregnancy, but you should take the first pill of the next month's cycle on the regularly scheduled day.

SIDE EFFECTS

Minor. Abdominal cramps; acne; backache; bloating; change in appetite; changes in sexual desire; diarrhea; dizziness; fatigue; headache; itching; nasal congestion; nausea; nervousness; vaginal irritation; and vomiting. These side effects should disappear in several weeks, as your body adjusts to the medication.

If you feel dizzy, sit or lie down awhile; get up slowly, and be careful on stairs.

This medication can increase your sensitivity to sunlight. Avoid prolonged exposure to sunlight and sunlamps. Wear protective clothing and sunglasses, and use an effective sunscreen.

Major. Tell your doctor about any side effects that are persistent or particularly bothersome. IT IS ESPECIALLY IMPORTANT TO TELL YOUR DOCTOR about abdominal pain; unusual bleeding or bruising; breakthrough vaginal bleeding (spotting); changes in menstrual flow; chest pain; pain in your calves; depression; difficult or painful urination; enlarged or tender breasts; hearing changes; increase or decrease in hair growth; migraine headaches; numbness or tingling; rash; skin color changes; swelling of the feet, ankles, or lower legs; vaginal itching; weight changes; or yellowing of the eyes or skin

INTERACTIONS

Oral contraceptives interact with several other types of medication.

1. Pain relievers, anti-migraine preparations, rifampin, barbiturates, phenylbutazone, phenytoin, primidone, carbamazepine, isoniazid, neomycin, penicillins, tetracycline, chloramphenicol, sulfonamide antibiotics, nitrofurantoin, and ampicillin can decrease the effectiveness of oral contraceptives.

2. Oral contraceptives can reduce the effectiveness of oral anti-coagulants (blood thinners, such as warfarin), anticonvulsants, tricyclic anti-depressants, anti-hypertensive agents, oral anti-diabetic agents, and vitamins.

3. Oral contraceptives can increase the blood levels of caffeine, diazepam, chlordiazepoxide, metoprolol, propranolol, adrenocorticosteroids (cortisone-like medications), imipramine, clomipramine, phenytoin, and phenylbutazone, which can lead to an increase in side effects.

4. Oral contraceptives can decrease the blood levels and effectiveness of lorazepam and oxazepam.

BE SURE TO TELL YOUR DOCTOR if you are already taking any of the medications listed above.

WARNINGS

• Tell your doctor about unusual or allergic reactions you have had to any medications, especially to estrogens, progestins, or progesterones.

• Before starting to take this medication, be sure to tell your doctor if you now have, or if you have ever had, asthma, bleeding problems, breast cancer, clotting disorders, diabetes mellitus (sugar diabetes), endometriosis, epilepsy, gallbladder disease, heart disease, kidney disease, liver disease, mental depression, migraine headaches, porphyria, strokes, uterine tumors, vaginal bleeding, vitamin deficiencies, or thyroid disease.

• Some women who have used an oral contraceptive have had difficulty becoming pregnant after discontinuing use of the drug. Most of these women had had scanty or irregular menstrual periods before starting to use an oral contraceptive. Possible subsequent difficulty in becoming pregnant is a matter that you should discuss with your doctor before using an oral contraceptive.

● Your pharmacist will give you a booklet with every prescription that explains birth control pills. Read this booklet carefully. It contains exact directions on how to use this medicine correctly and describes the risks involved.

● Women over 30 years of age and women who smoke while taking this medication have an increased risk of developing serious heart or blood vessel side effects.

● If this drug makes you dizzy, avoid taking part in any activity that requires alertness, such as driving a car or operating potentially dangerous equipment.

● Oral contraceptives can change the clotting properties of blood. Before having any surgery or other medical or dental treatment, be sure your doctor or dentist knows that you are taking this medication.

● This type of drug has been known or suspected to cause cancer. If you have a family history of cancer, you should consult your doctor before taking oral contraceptives.

● Be sure to tell your doctor if you are pregnant. Oral contraceptives have been associated with birth defects in animals and in humans. Because hormones have long-term effects on the body, oral contraceptives should be stopped at least three months prior to becoming pregnant. Another method of birth control should be used for those three months. Also, tell your doctor if you are breastfeeding an infant. This medication passes into breast milk.

Oramide—see tolbutamide

Oramine Spancaps—see phenylpropanolamine and chlorpheniramine combination

Orasone—see prednisone (systemic)

Oretic—see hydrochlorothiazide

Oreton Methyl—see methyltestosterone

Orinase—see tolbutamide

Ornade—see phenylpropanolamine and chlorpheniramine combination

---

orphenadrine, aspirin, and caffeine combination

BRAND NAMES (Manufacturers)
Norgesic (Riker)
Norgesic Forte (Riker)
TYPE OF DRUG
Muscle relaxant and analgesic (pain reliever)
INGREDIENTS
orphenadrine as the citrate salt, aspirin, and caffeine
DOSAGE FORM
Tablets (25 mg orphenadrine, 385 mg aspirin, and 30 mg caffeine—Norgesic); (50 mg orphenadrine, 770 mg aspirin, and 60 mg caffeine—Norgesic Forte)
STORAGE
This medication should be stored at room temperature in a tightly closed, light-resistant container.

USES
Orphenadrine, aspirin, and caffeine is used to relax muscles and to relieve the pain of sprains, strains, and other muscle injuries. Orphenadrine acts as a central nervous system (brain and spinal cord) depressant, which blocks reflexes involved in producing and maintaining muscle spasms. It does not act directly on tense muscles. Caffeine is a central nervous system stimulant that acts by constricting the blood vessels in the head. This may help relieve headaches.

TREATMENT
These tablets should be taken with a full glass of water. In order to avoid stomach irritation, you can also take this medication with food or milk (unless your doctor directs you to do otherwise).

If you miss a dose of this medication and remember within a hour, take the missed dose, then return to your regular dosing schedule. If it has been longer than an hour, don't take the missed dose at all; just return to your regular dosing schedule. Do not double the next dose.

SIDE EFFECTS

Minor. Blurred vision; confusion; constipation; diarrhea; dizziness; drowsiness; dry mouth; headache; indigestion; insomnia; nausea; nervousness; vomiting; and weakness. These side effects should disappear in several days, as your body adjusts to the medication.

If you are constipated, increase the amount of fiber in your diet (fresh fruits and vegetables, salads, bran, and whole-grain breads), and drink more water (unless your doctor directs you to do otherwise).

If you feel dizzy or light-headed, sit or lie down awhile; get up slowly, and be careful on stairs.

To relieve mouth dryness, suck on ice chips or a piece of hard candy, or chew sugarless gum.

Major. Tell your doctor about any side effects that are persistent or particularly bothersome. IT IS ESPECIALLY IMPORTANT TO TELL YOUR DOCTOR about severe abdominal pain; bloody or black, tarry stools; chest tightness; difficulty breathing; difficulty urinating; hearing loss; palpitations; rash; or ringing in the ears.

INTERACTIONS

This medication interacts with several other types of drugs.
1. Orphenadrine can cause extreme drowsiness when combined with other central nervous system depressants (drugs that slow the activity of the nervous system), such as alcohol, antihistamines, barbiturates, benzodiazepine tranquilizers, and sleeping medications, or with tricyclic anti-depressants. It can cause confusion, anxiety, and tremors when combined with propoxyphene.
2. Aspirin can increase the active blood levels of methotrexate, oral anti-diabetic agents, and oral anti-coagulants (blood thinners, such as warfarin), which can lead to an increase in side effects.

3. The anti-gout activity of probenecid and sulfinpyra-zone are decreased by aspirin.
4. The gastrointestinal side effects of anti-inflammation medications may be increased by aspirin.
Before starting to take this medication, BE SURE TO TELL YOUR DOCTOR if you are already taking any of the medications listed above.

WARNINGS

● Tell your doctor about unusual or allergic reactions you have had to medications, especially to orphenadrine, caffeine, aspirin, other salicylates, methyl salicylate, or to non-steroidal anti-inflammatory agents (such as diflunisal, fenoprofen, ibuprofen, indomethacin, meclofenamate, naproxen, oxyphenbutazone, phenylbutazone, piroxicam, sulindac, tolmetin, and zomepirac).
● Tell your doctor if you now have, or if you have ever had, anemia, bladder obstruction, glaucoma, gout, kidney disease, liver disease, myasthenia gravis, peptic ulcers, enlarged prostate gland, intestinal obstruction, or bleeding problems.
● This medication should not be taken as a substitute for rest, physical therapy, or other measures recommended by your doctor to treat your condition.
● If this medication makes you dizzy or drowsy, or blurs your vision, do not take part in any activity that requires alertness, such as driving a car or operating potentially dangerous equipment.
● Before having any surgery or other medical or dental treatment, be sure to tell your doctor or dentist that you are taking this medication. Treatment with aspirin-containing drugs is usually discontinued several days before any major surgery, to prevent bleeding complications.
● Because this product contains aspirin, additional medications that contain aspirin should not be taken without your doctor's approval. Check the labels on over-the-counter (non-prescription) pain, sinus, allergy, asthma, cough, and cold products to see if they contain aspirin.
● Small doses or occasional use of aspirin usually does not affect urine sugar tests. However, diabetic patients should know that if they are regularly taking six or more of

the regular tablets or three or more of the double-strength tablets of this medication each day, false-positive urine sugar tests could result.

● Be sure to tell your doctor if you are pregnant. Aspirin can prolong labor if it is taken by the mother close to term, and can cause heart problems in newborn infants. Also, tell your doctor if you are breastfeeding an infant. It is not known whether or not orphenadrine passes into breast milk, but small quantities of aspirin and caffeine are able to pass into breast milk.

Ortega-Otic M—see hydrocortisone, polymyxin B, and neomycin combination (otic)

Ortho-Novum—see oral contraceptives

Otobione Otic—see hydrocortisone, polymyxin B, and neomycin combination (otic)

Otocort—see hydrocortisone, polymyxin B, and neomycin combination (otic)

Otoreid-HC—see hydrocortisone, polymyxin B, and neomycin combination (otic)

Ovcon—see oral contraceptives

Ovral—see oral contraceptives

O-V Statin—see nystatin

Ovulen—see oral contraceptives

oxacillin

BRAND NAMES (Manufacturers)
Bactocill (Beecham)
Prostaphlin (Bristol)
TYPE OF DRUG
Antibiotic (infection fighter)

INGREDIENT
oxacillin
DOSAGE FORMS
Capsules (250 mg and 500 mg)
Oral solution (250 mg per 5 ml teaspoonful)
STORAGE
Oxacillin capsules should be stored at room temperature in a tightly closed container. The oral solution should be stored in the refrigerator in a tightly closed container. Any unused portion of the solution should be discarded after 14 days, because the drug loses its potency after that time. This medication should never be frozen.

USES
Oxacillin is used to treat a wide variety of bacterial infections, usually involving *Staphylococcus* bacteria. It acts by severely injuring the cell walls of the infecting bacteria, thereby preventing them from growing and multiplying.

Oxacillin kills susceptible bacteria, but is not effective against viruses, parasites, or fungi.

TREATMENT
Oxacillin should be taken on an empty stomach or with a glass of water, one hour before or two hours after a meal. This medication should never be taken with fruit juices or carbonated beverages, because the acidity of these drinks destroys the drug in the stomach.

The oral solution should be measured carefully, with a specially designed, 5 ml measuring spoon. An ordinary kitchen teaspoon is not accurate enough.

Oxacillin works best when the level of medicine in your bloodstream is kept constant. It is best therefore to take the doses at evenly spaced intervals, day and night. For example, if you are taking four doses a day, the doses should be spaced six hours apart.

If you miss a dose of this medication, take the missed dose immediately. However, if you do not remember to take the missed dose until it is almost time for your next dose, take it; then space the following dose about halfway through the regular interval between doses. Then return to your regular dosing schedule. Try not to skip any doses.

It is important to continue to take this medication for the

entire time prescribed by your doctor (usually seven to 14 days), even if the symptoms of infection disappear before the end of that period. If you stop taking the drug too soon, resistant bacteria are given a chance to continue growing, and the infection could recur.

SIDE EFFECTS

Minor. Diarrhea; heartburn; nausea; and vomiting. These side effects should disappear in several days, as your body adjusts to the medication.

Major. Tell your doctor about any side effects that are persistent or particularly bothersome. IT IS ESPECIALLY IMPORTANT TO TELL YOUR DOCTOR about bloating; chills; cough; difficulty breathing; fever; irritation of the mouth; muscle aches; rash; rectal or vaginal itching; severe diarrhea; sore throat; or darkened tongue. Also, if your symptoms of infection seem to be getting worse rather than improving, you should contact your doctor.

INTERACTIONS

Oxacillin interacts with several other types of medications.

1. Probenecid can increase the blood concentrations of this medication.

2. Oxacillin may decrease the effectiveness of oral contraceptives (birth control pills), and pregnancy could result. You should therefore use another form of birth control while taking this medication. Discuss this with your doctor.

TELL YOUR DOCTOR if you are currently taking any of the medications listed above.

WARNINGS

● Tell your doctor about unusual or allergic reactions you have had to any medications, especially to oxacillin, penicillins, or to cephalosporin antibiotics, penicillamine, or griseofulvin.

● Tell your doctor if you now have, or if you have ever had, kidney disease, asthma, or allergies.

● This medication has been prescribed for your current infection only. Another infection later on, or one that someone else has, may require a different medicine. You should not give your medicine to other people or use it for other infections, unless your doctor specifically directs you to do so.

• Diabetics taking oxacillin should know that this drug can cause a false-positive sugar reaction with a Clinitest urine glucose test. To avoid this problem, while taking oxacillin you should switch to Clinistix or Tes-Tape to test your urine sugar.

• Be sure to tell your doctor if you are pregnant. Although oxacillin appears to be safe during pregnancy, extensive studies in humans have not yet been completed. Also, tell your doctor if you are breastfeeding an infant. Small amounts of this medication pass into breast milk and may temporarily alter the bacteria in the intestinal tract of the nursing infant, resulting in diarrhea.

---

oxandrolone

BRAND NAME (Manufacturer)
Anavar (Searle)
TYPE OF DRUG
Anabolic hormone
INGREDIENT
oxandrolone
DOSAGE FORM
Tablets (2.5 mg)
STORAGE
Oxandrolone should be stored at room temperature in a tightly closed, light-resistant container.

USES
This medication is used to treat anemia and osteoporosis (bone loss). Oxandrolone belongs to a group of drugs known as anabolic hormones (steroids). It works by promoting the buildup of body tissues, including red blood cells and bone.

TREATMENT
You can take oxandrolone either on an empty stomach or, to reduce stomach irritation, with food or milk (as directed by your doctor).

If you miss a dose of this medication, take the missed

dose as soon as possible, unless it is almost time for your next dose. In that case, do not take the missed dose at all; just return to your regular dosing schedule. Do not double the next dose.

SIDE EFFECTS

Minor. Chills; decreased sexual ability; diarrhea; increase or decrease in sexual desire; stomach upset; or trouble sleeping. These side effects should disappear in several weeks, as your body adjusts to the medication.

Major. Tell your doctor about any side effects that are persistent or particularly bothersome. IT IS ESPECIALLY IMPORTANT TO TELL YOUR DOCTOR about acne or oily skin; bloody or black, tarry stools; unusual bleeding or bruising; breath odor; deepening of the voice (in women); depression; enlarged or painful breasts (in both sexes); increased or decreased hair growth; severe headaches; loss of appetite; menstrual irregularities; muscle cramps; sore throat or fever; swelling of the feet or legs; weakness; weight gain or loss; or yellowing of the eyes or skin.

INTERACTIONS

Oxandrolone interacts with several medications.

1. It can increase the effects of anti-coagulants (blood thinners, such as warfarin), which can lead to bleeding complications.

2. Diabetic patients should know that oxandrolone can decrease blood glucose levels. The dosage of oral anti-diabetic medications may therefore require adjustment when this medication is started.

BE SURE TO TELL YOUR DOCTOR if you are already taking either of these types of medications.

WARNINGS

• Tell your doctor about unusual or allergic reactions you have had to any medications, especially to oxandrolone or to other anabolic hormones (such as dromostanolone, ethylestrenol, nandrolone, oxymetholone, or stanozolol).

• Before starting to take this medication, be sure to tell your doctor if you now have, or if you have ever had, breast cancer; heart disease; hypercalcemia; kidney disease; liver disease; prostate cancer; or enlarged prostate gland.

• To obtain the maximum benefit from this medication, eat a well-balanced diet that provides adequate protein and calories.

• Athletes sometimes use anabolic steroids to increase performance. However, there is conflicting and inconclusive evidence as to whether or not these drugs increase muscle strength. There is also some question as to their safety.

• Be sure to tell your doctor if you are pregnant. Oxandrolone crosses the placenta and can cause masculine characteristics, such as increased body hair, in the developing fetus. (Note: this drug does NOT affect the sex of the fetus, which is determined at conception.) Also, tell your doctor if you are breastfeeding an infant. It is not known whether or not oxandrolone passes into breast milk.

---

oxazepam

BRAND NAME (Manufacturer)
Serax (Wyeth)
TYPE OF DRUG
Sedative/hypnotic (anti-anxiety medication)
INGREDIENT
oxazepam
DOSAGE FORMS
Capsules (10 mg, 15 mg, and 30 mg)
Tablets (15 mg)
STORAGE
This medication should be stored at room temperature in a tightly closed, light-resistant container.

USES

Oxazepam is prescribed to treat symptoms of anxiety, and sometimes to treat anxiety associated with depression or alcohol withdrawal. It is not clear exactly how this medicine works, but it may relieve anxiety by acting as a depressant of the central nervous system. Oxazepam is currently used by many people to relieve nervousness. It is effective for this purpose for short periods, but it is important to try to remove the cause of the anxiety as well.

TREATMENT

This medication should be taken exactly as directed by your doctor. It can be taken with food or a full glass of water if stomach upset occurs. Do not take oxazepam with a dose of antacids, since they may retard its absorption.

If you are taking this medication regularly and you miss a dose, take the missed dose immediately if you remember within an hour of the scheduled time. If more than an hour has passed, skip the dose you missed and wait for the next scheduled dose. Do not double the dose.

SIDE EFFECTS

Minor. Bitter taste in mouth; constipation; depression; diarrhea; dizziness; drowsiness (after a night's sleep); dry mouth; fatigue; flushing; headache; heartburn; excess saliva; loss of appetite; nausea; nervousness; sweating; and vomiting. These side effects should disappear, as your body adjusts to the medication.

Dry mouth can be relieved by chewing sugarless gum or by sucking on ice chips.

If you feel dizzy, sit or lie down awhile; get up slowly, and be careful on stairs.

Major. Tell your doctor about any side effects that are persistent or particularly bothersome. iT IS ESPECIALLY IMPORTANT TO TELL YOUR DOCTOR about blurred or double vision; chest pain; severe depression; difficulty urinating; fainting; falling; fever; joint pain; hallucinations; mouth sores; nightmares; palpitations; rash; shortness of breath; slurred speech; sore throat; uncoordinated movements; unusual excitement; unusual tiredness; or yellowing of the eyes or skin.

INTERACTIONS

Oxazepam interacts with several other types of medication.

1. To prevent over-sedation, this drug should not be taken with alcohol, other sedative drugs, or central nervous system depressants (such as antihistamines, barbiturates, muscle relaxants, pain medicines, narcotics, medicines for seizures, phenothiazine tranquilizers), or with anti-depressants.

2. This medication may decrease the effectiveness of carbamazepine, levodopa, and oral anti-coagulants (blood thinners), and may increase the effects of phenytoin.

3. Disulfiram and isoniazid can increase the blood levels of oxazepam, which can lead to toxic effects.

4. Concurrent use of rifampin may decrease the effectiveness of oxazepam.

If you are currently taking any of the medications listed above, CONSULT YOUR DOCTOR about their use.

WARNINGS

● Tell your doctor about unusual or allergic reactions you have had to any medications, especially to oxazepam or other benzodiazepine tranquilizers (such as alprazolam, chlordiazepoxide, clorazepate, diazepam, flurazepam, halazepam, lorazepam, prazepam, temazepam, or triazolam).

● Tell your doctor if you now have, or if you have ever had, liver disease, kidney disease, epilepsy, lung disease, myasthenia gravis, porphyria, mental depression, or mental illness.

● This medicine can cause drowsiness. Avoid tasks that require mental alertness, such as driving a car or using potentially dangerous machinery.

● Oxazepam has the potential for abuse and must be used with caution. Tolerance may develop quickly; do not increase the dosage without first consulting your doctor. It is also important not to stop taking this drug suddenly if you have been taking it in large amounts, or if you have used it for several weeks. Your doctor may want to reduce the dosage gradually.

● This is a safe drug when used properly. When it is combined with other sedative drugs or alcohol, however, serious side effects can develop.

● Oxazepam contains F.D. & C. Yellow Dye No. 5 (tartrazine), which can cause allergic-type reactions (shortness of breath, wheezing, rash, or fainting) in certain susceptible individuals.

● Be sure to tell your doctor if you are pregnant. This type of medicine may increase the chance of birth defects if it is taken during the first three months of pregnancy. In addition, too much use of this medicine during the last six months of pregnancy may cause the baby to become dependent on it. This may result in withdrawal side effects in the newborn. Also, use of this medicine during the last weeks of pregnancy may cause drowsiness, slowed heartbeat, and breathing difficulties in the infant. Tell your doctor if you are breastfeeding an infant. Oxazepam may pass into breast milk and cause drowsiness, slowed heartbeat, and breathing difficulties in the nursing infant.

Oxlopar—see oxytetracycline

oxtriphylline

BRAND NAMES (Manufacturers)
Choledyl (Parke-Davis)
Choledyl SA (Parke-Davis)
oxtriphylline (various manufacturers)
TYPE OF DRUG
Bronchodilator
INGREDIENT
oxtriphylline (theophylline as the choline salt)
DOSAGE FORMS
Tablets (100 mg and 200 mg)
Sustained-release tablets (400 mg and 600 mg)
Oral pediatric liquid (50 mg per 5 ml teaspoonful)
Oral elixir (100 mg per 5 ml teaspoonful)
STORAGE
Oxtriphylline tablets, liquid, and elixir should be stored at room temperature in tightly closed containers. This medication should never be frozen.

USES
This medication is used to treat breathing problems (wheezing and shortness of breath) caused by asthma, bronchitis, or emphysema. It relaxes the smooth muscle of the bronchial airways (breathing tubes), which opens the air passages to the lungs, and allows air to move in and out more easily.

TREATMENT
Oxtriphylline should be taken on an empty stomach 30 to 60 minutes before, or two hours after, a meal. If this medi-

cation causes stomach irritation, however, you can take it with food or with a full glass of water or milk (unless your doctor directs you to do otherwise).

Anti-diarrhea medication prevents the absorption of oxtriphylline. Therefore, at least one hour should separate doses of these two types of medication.

The sustained-release tablets should be swallowed whole (if the tablet is scored for breaking, you can break it along these lines). Chewing, crushing, or crumbling the tablets destroys their sustained-release activity, and possibly increases the side effects.

Each dose of the oral liquid should be measured carefully, with a specially designed, 5 ml measuring spoon. An ordinary kitchen teaspoon is not accurate enough.

Oxtriphylline works best when the level of the medicine in your bloodstream is kept constant. It is best therefore to take it at evenly spaced intervals, day and night. For example, if you are to take four doses a day, the doses should be spaced six hours apart.

Try not to miss any doses of this medication. If you do miss a dose, take the missed dose as soon as possible, unless it is almost time for the next dose. In that case, do not take the missed dose at all; just return to your regular dosing schedule. Do not double the next dose.

SIDE EFFECTS

Minor. Diarrhea; dizziness; flushing; headache; heartburn; increased urination; insomnia; irritability; loss of appetite; nausea; nervousness; stomach pain; and vomiting. These side effects should disappear in several days, as your body adjusts to the medication.

If you feel dizzy or light-headed, sit or lie down awhile; get up slowly, and be careful on stairs.

Major. Tell your doctor about any side effects that are persistent or particularly bothersome. IT IS ESPECIALLY IMPORTANT TO TELL YOUR DOCTOR about bloody or black, tarry stools; confusion; convulsions; difficulty breathing; fainting; muscle twitches; palpitations; rash; severe abdominal pain; or unusual weakness.

INTERACTIONS

Oxtriphylline interacts with several other medications.

1. It can increase the effects (increased diuresis) of furo-semide.

2. Reserpine, in combination with oxtriphylline, can cause a rapid heart rate.

3. Beta-blockers (atenolol, metoprolol, nadolol, pindolol, propranolol, and timolol) can block the effectiveness of oxtriphylline.

4. Phenobarbital can increase the elimination of oxtriphylline from the body, decreasing its effectiveness.

5. Cimetidine, erythromycin, troleanodomycin, allopurinol, and thiabendazole can decrease the elimination of oxtriphylline from the body, increasing its side effects. BE SURE TO TELL YOUR DOCTOR if you are already taking any of the medications listed above.

WARNINGS

● Tell your doctor about any unusual or allergic reactions you have had to medications, especially to oxtriphylline, aminophylline, caffeine, dyphylline, theophylline, or theobromine.

● Tell your doctor if you now have, or if you have ever had, fibrocystic breast disease, heart disease, kidney disease, low or high blood pressure, liver disease, stomach ulcers, thyroid disease, or an enlarged prostate gland.

● Cigarette or marijuana smoking may affect this drug's action. BE SURE TO TELL YOUR DOCTOR if you smoke. Also, do not suddenly stop smoking without informing your doctor.

● High fever, diarrhea, the flu, and influenza vaccinations can also affect the actions of this drug. Therefore, tell your doctor about episodes of high fever or prolonged diarrhea. Before having any vaccinations, especially those to prevent the flu, be sure to tell your doctor that you are taking this medication.

● Avoid drinking large amounts of caffeine-containing beverages (coffee, cocoa, tea, and cola drinks) and avoid eating large amounts of chocolate. These products may increase the side effects of oxtriphylline.

● Do not change your diet without first consulting your doctor. Char-broiled foods or a high-protein, low-carbohydrate diet may affect the action of this drug.

● Before having any surgery or other medical or dental

treatment, be sure your doctor or dentist knows that you are taking this medication.

• Before taking any over-the-counter (non-prescription) asthma, allergy, cough, cold, sinus, or diet product, ask your doctor or pharmacist. These products may add to the side effects of oxtriphylline.

• Be sure to tell your doctor if you are pregnant. Although oxtriphylline appears to be safe during pregnancy, extensive studies in humans have not yet been completed. Birth defects have been observed in the offspring of animals who received large doses of this drug during pregnancy. Also, tell your doctor if you are breastfeeding an infant. Small amounts of oxtriphylline pass into breast milk and may cause irritability, fretfulness, or insomnia in nursing infants.

---

oxybutynin

BRAND NAME (Manufacturer)
Ditropan (Marion)
TYPE OF DRUG
Anti-spasmodic
INGREDIENT
oxybutynin as the chloride salt
DOSAGE FORMS
Tablets (5 mg)
Oral syrup (5 mg per 5 ml teaspoonful)
STORAGE
Oxybutynin tablets and syrup should be stored at room temperature in tightly closed containers.

USES

Oxybutynin is used to relieve the symptoms associated with urinary incontinence (inability to control the bladder) or urinary frequency. It works directly on the muscle of the bladder, increasing bladder capacity, thereby delaying the initial desire to urinate.

TREATMENT

Oxybutynin can be taken either on an empty stomach with water only or, to reduce stomach irritation, with food or milk (as directed by your doctor).

Each dose of the oral syrup should be measured carefully, with a specially designed, 5 ml measuring spoon. An ordinary kitchen teaspoon is not accurate enough.

If you miss a dose of this medication, take the missed dose as soon as possible, unless it is almost time for the next dose. In that case, do not take the missed dose at all; just return to your regular dosing schedule. Do not double the next dose.

SIDE EFFECTS

Minor. Bloating; blurred vision; constipation; decreased sweating; dizziness; dry mouth; drowsiness; insomnia; nausea; vomiting; and weakness. These side effects should disappear in several weeks, as your body adjusts to the medication.

To relieve constipation, increase the amount of fiber in your diet (bran, salads, fresh fruits and vegetables, and whole-grain breads), exercise, and drink more water (unless your doctor directs you to do otherwise).

If you feel dizzy, sit or lie down awhile; change positions slowly, and be careful on stairs.

To help relieve mouth dryness, chew sugarless gum, or suck on ice chips or a piece of hard candy.

This medication can also cause increased sensitivity of your eyes to sunlight. Sunglasses may help relieve the discomfort caused by bright lights.

Major. Tell your doctor about any side effects that are persistent or particularly bothersome. IT IS ESPECIALLY IMPORTANT TO TELL YOUR DOCTOR about difficult or painful urination; decreased sexual ability; eye pain; itching; palpitations; or skin rash.

INTERACTIONS

Oxybutynin does not interact with other medications, if it is used according to directions.

WARNINGS

● Tell your doctor about unusual or allergic reactions you have had to any medications, especially to oxybutynin.

● Before starting to take this medication, be sure to tell your doctor if you now have, or if you have ever had, severe bleeding; glaucoma; heart disease; hiatal hernia; high blood pressure; intestinal blockage; kidney disease; liver disease; myasthenia gravis; enlarged prostate gland; thyroid disease; toxemia of pregnancy; ulcerative colitis; or urinary retention.

• If this drug makes you dizzy or blurs your vision, avoid taking part in activities that require alertness, such as driving a car or operating potentially dangerous equipment.

• This medication can decrease sweating and heat release from the body. You should therefore avoid getting overheated (strenuous exercise in hot weather; hot baths, showers, and saunas).

• Be sure to tell your doctor if you are pregnant. Although oxybutynin appears to be safe during pregnancy, extensive studies in humans have not yet been completed. Also, tell your doctor if you are breastfeeding an infant. This medication may decrease milk production. It is not known whether or not oxybutynin passes into breast milk.

oxycodone hydrochloride, oxycodone terephthalate, and aspirin—see aspirin and oxycodone combination

oxycodone hydrochloride with acetaminophen—see acetaminophen and oxycodone combination

Oxydess II—see dextroamphetamine

oxymetholone

BRAND NAME (Manufacturer)
Anadrol-50 (Syntex)
TYPE OF DRUG
Anabolic hormone
INGREDIENT
oxymetholone
DOSAGE FORM
Tablets (50 mg)
STORAGE
Oxymetholone should be stored at room temperature in a tightly closed container.

USES

This medication is used to treat anemia and osteoporosis (bone loss). Oxymetholone belongs to a group of drugs known as anabolic hormones (steroids). It works by promoting the buildup of body tissues, including red blood cells and bone.

TREATMENT

You can take oxymetholone either on an empty stomach or, to reduce stomach irritation, with food or milk (as directed by your doctor).

If you miss a dose of this medication, take the missed dose as soon as possible, unless it is almost time for your next dose. In that case, do not take the missed dose at all; just return to your regular dosing schedule. Do not double the next dose.

SIDE EFFECTS

Minor. Chills; decreased sexual ability; diarrhea; increased or decreased sexual desire; stomach upset; or trouble sleeping. These side effects should disappear in several weeks, as your body adjusts to the medication.

Major. Tell your doctor about any side effects that are persistent or particularly bothersome. IT IS ESPECIALLY IMPORTANT TO TELL YOUR DOCTOR about acne or oily skin; bloody or black, tarry stools; unusual bleeding or bruising; breath odor; deepening of the voice (in women); depression; enlarged or painful breasts (in both sexes); increased or decreased hair growth; severe headaches; loss of appetite; menstrual irregularities; muscle cramps; sore throat or fever; swelling of the feet or legs; weakness; weight gain or loss; or yellowing of the eyes or skin.

INTERACTIONS

Oxymetholone interacts with several medications.

1. It can increase the effects of oral anti-coagulants (blood thinners, such as warfarin), which can lead to bleeding complications.

2. Diabetic patients should know that oxymetholone can decrease blood glucose levels. The dosage of oral anti-diabetic medications or insulin may therefore need to be ad-

justed when this medication is started.
BE SURE TO TELL YOUR DOCTOR if you are already taking either of these types of medication.

WARNINGS

● Tell your doctor about unusual or allergic reactions you have had to any medications, especially to oxymetholone or to other anabolic hormones (such as dromostanolone, nandrolone, oxandrolone, or stanozolol).

● Before starting to take this medication, be sure to tell your doctor if you now have, or if you have ever had, breast cancer, heart disease, hypercalcemia (high blood calcium levels), kidney disease, liver disease, prostate cancer, or an enlarged prostate gland.

● To obtain maximum benefit from this medication, eat a well-balanced diet that provides adequate protein and calories.

● Athletes sometimes use anabolic steroids to increase performance. However, there is conflicting and inconclusive evidence as to whether or not these drugs increase muscle strength. There is also some question as to their safety.

● Be sure to tell your doctor if you are pregnant. Oxymetholone crosses the placenta and can cause masculine characteristics, such as increased body hair, in the developing fetus. (Note: this drug does NOT affect the sex of the fetus, which is determined at conception.) Also, tell your doctor if you are breastfeeding an infant. It is not known whether or not oxymetholone passes into breast milk.

---

oxytetracycline

BRAND NAMES (Manufacturers)
E.P. Mycin (Edwards)
Oxlopar (Parke-Davis)
oxytetracycline hydrochloride (various manufacturers)
Terramycin (Pfipharmecs)
Tetramine (Tutag)
Uri-Tet (American Urologicals)
TYPE OF DRUG
Antibiotic (infection fighter)

INGREDIENT
oxytetracycline as the hydrochloride salt
DOSAGE FORMS
Tablets (125 mg)
Capsules (125 mg and 250 mg)
Oral syrup (125 mg per 5 ml teaspoonful)
STORAGE
Oxytetracycline tablets, capsules, and oral syrup should be stored at room temperature in tightly closed light-resistant containers. Any unused portion of the oral syrup should be discarded after 14 days, because the drug loses its potency after that period. This medication should never be frozen.

USES
Oxytetracycline is used to treat acne and a wide variety of bacterial infections. It acts by inhibiting the growth of bacteria. Bacteria may be partly responsible for the development of acne lesions. Oxytetracycline kills susceptible bacteria, but is not effective against viruses or fungi.

TREATMENT
Ideally, this medication should be taken on an empty stomach, one hour before or two hours after a meal. It should be taken with a full glass of water in order to avoid throat or esophagus (swallowing tube) irritation. If this drug causes stomach upset, however, you can take it with food or water (unless your doctor directs you to do otherwise).

Avoid consuming any dairy products, including milk and cheese, within two hours of any dose of this drug. Avoid taking antacids or laxatives containing aluminum, calcium, or magnesium within an hour or two of a dose. Avoid taking any medication containing iron within three hours of a dose. These products chemically bind oxytetracycline in the stomach and gastrointestinal tract, and prevent the drug from being absorbed into the body.

The oral syrup form of this medication should be measured carefully with a specially designed, 5 ml measuring teaspoon. An ordinary kitchen teaspoon is not accurate enough. The oral syrup should not be mixed with any other substance, unless your doctor directs you to do so.

Oxytetracycline works best when the level of medicine in your bloodstream is kept constant. Therefore, it is best to take each dose at evenly spaced times, day and night. For example, if you are to take four doses a day, the doses should be spaced six hours apart.

If you miss a dose of this medication, take the missed dose immediately. However, if you do not remember to take the missed dose until it is almost time for your next dose, take it; then space the next dose about halfway through the regular interval between doses. Then return to your regular dosing schedule. Try not to skip any doses.

It is important to continue to take this medication for the entire time prescribed by your doctor, even if the symptoms disappear before the end of that period. If you stop taking the drug too soon, resistant bacteria are given a chance to continue growing, and the infection could recur.

SIDE EFFECTS

Minor. Diarrhea; dizziness; loss of appetite; nausea; stomach cramps and upset; vomiting; and discoloration of the nails. These side effects should disappear in several days, as your body adjusts to the medication.

Oxytetracycline can increase your sensitivity to sunlight. In order to avoid this side effect, limit your exposure to sunlight and sunlamps. Wear protective clothing and sunglasses, and use an effective sunscreen.

Major. Tell your doctor about any side effects that are persistent or particularly bothersome. IT IS ESPECIALLY IMPORTANT TO TELL YOUR DOCTOR about unusual bleeding or bruising; darkened tongue; difficulty breathing; joint pain; mouth irritation; rash; rectal or vaginal itching; sore throat and fever; or yellowing of the eyes or skin. Also, if your symptoms of infection seem to be getting worse rather than improving, you should contact your doctor.

INTERACTIONS

Oxytetracycline interacts with other types of medication.

1. It can increase the absorption of digoxin, which may lead to digoxin toxicity.

2. The gastrointestinal side effects (nausea, vomiting,

stomach upset) of theophylline may be increased by oxytetracycline.

3. The dosage of oral anti-coagulants (blood thinners, such as warfarin) may need to be adjusted when this medication is started.

4. Oxytetracycline may decrease the effectiveness of oral contraceptives (birth control pills), and pregnancy could result. You should therefore use another form of birth control while taking tetracycline. Discuss this with your doctor.

TELL YOUR DOCTOR if you are currently taking any of the medications listed above.

WARNINGS

- Tell your doctor about unusual or allergic reactions you have had to any medications, especially to oxytetracycline or to tetracycline, doxycline, or minocycline.
- Tell your doctor if you now have, or if you have ever had, kidney or liver disease.
- Oxytetracycline can affect tests for syphilis; tell your doctor you are taking this medication if you are also being treated for this disease.
- Make sure that your prescription for oxytetracycline is marked with the drug's expiration date. The drug should be discarded after the expiration date. If the medication is used after it has expired, serious side effects (especially to the kidneys) could result.
- This medication has been prescribed for your current infection only. Another infection later on, or one that someone else has, may require a different medicine. You should not give your medicine to other people, or use it for other infections, unless your doctor specifically directs you to do so.
- Be sure to tell your doctor if you are pregnant or if you are breastfeeding an infant. Oxytetracycline crosses the placenta and passes into breast milk. If used during their development, this drug can cause permanent discoloration of the teeth and can inhibit tooth and bone growth. In addition, it should not be used for infants or for children less than eight years of age.

oxytetracycline hydrochloride—see oxytetracycline

Palbar—see atropine, scopolamine, hyoscyamine, and phenobarbital combination

Palmiron—see iron supplements

Pamelor—see nortriptyline

Panadol with Codeine—see acetaminophen and codeine combination

Panasol—see prednisone (systemic)

Pancrease—see pancrelipase

---

pancreatin

BRAND NAMES (Manufacturers)
Pancreatin* (Lilly)
Pancreatin Enseals* (Lilly)
Viokase (Viobin)
*Note that pancreatin is also available over-the-counter (non-prescription).
TYPE OF DRUG
Digestive enzymes
INGREDIENTS
lipase, protease, and amylase
DOSAGE FORMS
Tablets (6,500 U [units] lipase, 32,000 U protease, and 48,000 U amylase)
Powder (15,000 U lipase, 7,500 U protease, and 112,500 U amylase per 0.75 grams of powder)
STORAGE
Pancreatin tablets and powder should be stored at room temperature, in tightly closed containers.

USES
This medication is a combination of digestive (pancreatic) enzymes obtained from pigs or cows. These enzymes aid in the digestion and absorption of fats and starch. Pancreatin is used to treat pancreatic enzyme deficiencies result-

ing from conditions such as pancreatitis, cystic fibrosis, or gastrointestinal bypass surgery.

TREATMENT

In order to obtain the maximum benefit, you should take pancreatin just before or with meals or snacks. The powder can be added to food; the tablets can also be crushed and mixed with food.

If you miss a dose of this medication, do not take the missed dose at all; just return to your regular dosing schedule. Do not double the next dose.

SIDE EFFECTS

Minor. Diarrhea; nausea; and stomach cramps. These side effects should disappear in several weeks, as your body adjusts to the medication.

Major. Tell your doctor about any side effects that are persistent or particularly bothersome. IT IS ESPECIALLY IMPORTANT TO TELL YOUR DOCTOR about bloody urine, hives, joint pain, skin rash, or swelling of the feet or legs.

INTERACTIONS

Pancreatin can decrease the absorption of iron from the gastrointestinal tract, which may lead to nutritional deficiency. Your doctor may want to prescribe iron supplements if this becomes a problem. Cimetidine or antacids are often prescribed concurrently with pancreatin in order to maximize its effectiveness. However, calcium- or magnesium containing antacids should be avoided—they decrease this medication's effectiveness. You should discuss these effects with your doctor.

WARNINGS

• Tell your doctor about unusual or allergic reactions you have had to medications, especially to pancreatin, pancrelipase, or any other digestive enzymes.

• Patients who have allergies to pork or beef products may also be allergic to pancreatin, since it is obtained from pigs and cows.

• The powder form of this medication can be very irritating to the nose and throat. Therefore, try to avoid inhaling the particles

• Be sure to tell your doctor if you are pregnant. Although pancreatin appears to be safe during pregnancy, extensive studies have not yet been completed. Also, tell your doctor if you are breastfeeding an infant. It is not known whether or not pancreatin passes into breast milk.

pancrelipase

BRAND NAMES (Manufacturers)
Cotazym (Organon)
Cotazym-S (Organon)
Ilozyme (Adria)
Ku-Zyme HP (Kremers-Urban)
Pancrease (McNeil)
TYPE OF DRUG
Digestive enzymes
INGREDIENTS
lipase, protease, and amylase
DOSAGE FORMS
Tablets (11,000 U [units] lipase, 30,000 U protease, and 30,000 U amylase)
Capsules (8,000 U lipase, 30,000 U protease, and 30,000 U amylase; 5,000 U lipase, 20,000 U protease, and 20,000 U amylase; 4,000 U lipase, 25,000 U protease, and 20,000 U amylase)
Powder packets (16,000 U lipase, 60,000 U protease, and 60,000 U amylase; 40,000 U lipase, 150,000 U protease, and 150,000 U amylase)
STORAGE
Pancrelipase tablets, capsules, and powder should be stored at room temperature, in tightly closed containers.

USES
This medication is a combination of digestive (pancreatic) enzymes obtained from pigs. These enzymes aid in the digestion and absorption of starch and fats. Pancrelipase is used to treat pancreatic enzyme deficiencies resulting from conditions such as pancreatitis, cystic fibrosis, or gastrointestinal bypass surgery.

TREATMENT

In order to obtain the maximum benefit, you should take pancrelipase just before or with meals or snacks. The powder can be added to food; the tablets can also be crushed and mixed with food.

If you are taking the capsules containing the enteric-coated microspheres, swallow the capsule whole. Chewing, crushing, or breaking the capsules decreases their effectiveness, and increases the side effects. However, if you have difficulty swallowing the capsules, you can open them and sprinkle the contents on a small amount of liquid or soft food, which you should then swallow without chewing. DO NOT mix this medication with alkaline foods (such as dairy products)—they can reduce its effectiveness.

If you miss a dose of this medication, do not take the missed dose at all; just return to your regular dosing schedule. Do not double the next dose.

SIDE EFFECTS

Minor. Diarrhea; nausea; and stomach cramps. These side effects should disappear in several weeks, as your body adjusts to the medication.

Major. Tell your doctor about any side effects that are persistent or particularly bothersome. IT IS ESPECIALLY IMPORTANT TO TELL YOUR DOCTOR about bloody urine, hives, joint pain, skin rash, or swelling of the feet or legs.

INTERACTIONS

Pancrelipase can decrease the absorption of iron from the gastrointestinal tract, which may lead to nutritional deficiency. Your doctor may want to prescribe iron supplements if this becomes a problem. Cimetidine or antacids are often prescribed concurrently with pancrelipase, in order to maximize its effectiveness. However, calcium or magnesium-containing antacids should be avoided—they decrease this medication's effectiveness. You should discuss these effects with your doctor.

WARNINGS

• Tell your doctor about unusual or allergic reactions you have had to medications, especially to pancrelipase, pan-

creatin, or any other digestive enzymes.
● Patients who have allergies to pork products may also be allergic to pancrelipase, since it is obtained from pigs.
● The powder form of this medication can be very irritating to the nose and throat. Therefore, try to avoid inhaling the particles.
● Be sure to tell your doctor if you are pregnant. Although pancrelipase appears to be safe during pregnancy, extensive studies have not yet been completed. Also, tell your doctor if you are breastfeeding an infant. It is not known whether or not pancrelipase passes into breast milk.

Panheprin—see heparin

Panmycin—see tetracycline

Panwarfin—see warfarin

Papacon—see papaverine

---

papaverine

BRAND NAMES (Manufacturers)
Cerespan (USV)
Delapav (Dunhall)
Dilart (Trimen)
Myobid (Laser)
Papacon (CMC)
papaverine hydrochloride (various manufacturers)
Pavabid Plateau (Marion)
Pavacap Unicelles (Reid-Provident)
Pavacen Cenules (Central)
Pavadur (Century)
Pavadyl (Bock)
Pavagen (Rugby)
Pava-Par (Paramed)
Pava-RX (Blaine)
Pavased (Mallard)
Pavasule (Misemer)
Pavatine (Major)

Pavatym (Everett)
Paverine Spancaps (Vortech)
Paverolan Lanacaps (Lanneth)
Vasal Granucaps (Reid-Provident)
Vasocap (Keene)
Vasospan (Ulmer)

TYPE OF DRUG
Vasodilator

INGREDIENT
papaverine as the hydrochloride salt

DOSAGE FORMS
Tablets (30 mg, 60 mg, 100 mg, 200 mg, and 300 mg)
Sustained-release tablets (200 mg)
Sustained-release capsules (150 mg and 300 mg)

STORAGE
Papaverine should be stored at room temperature, in tightly closed containers.

USES
Papaverine is used to treat circulation disorders. It is a vasodilator that acts directly on the muscles of the blood vessels to increase the blood supply to various parts of the body.

TREATMENT
In order to avoid stomach irritation, you can take papaverine with food or with a full glass of water or milk. Ask your doctor if you can take it with an antacid.

The sustained-release tablets and capsules should be swallowed whole. Breaking, crushing, or chewing these tablets or capsules destroys their sustained-release activity, and possibly increases the side effects.

If you miss a dose of this medication, take the missed dose as soon as possible, unless it is almost time for the next dose. In that case, do not take the missed dose at all; just return to your regular dosing schedule. Do not double the next dose.

SIDE EFFECTS
Minor. Abdominal distress; blurred vision; constipation; diarrhea; dizziness; drowsiness; fatigue; flushing; headache; loss of appetite; nausea; and sweating. These side ef-

fects should disappear in several days, as your body adjusts to the medication.

If you feel dizzy, sit or lie down awhile; get up slowly, and be careful on stairs.

To relieve constipation, increase the amount of fiber in your diet (bran, salads, fresh fruits and vegetables, and whole-grain breads), exercise, and drink more water (unless your doctor directs you to do otherwise).

Major. Tell your doctor about any side effects that are persistent or particularly bothersome. IT IS ESPECIALLY IMPORTANT TO TELL YOUR DOCTOR about depression; difficulty breathing; palpitations; rash; unusual bleeding or bruising; or yellowing of the eyes or skin.

INTERACTIONS

Concurrent use of papaverine and levodopa can lead to decreased effectiveness of levodopa. Before starting to take papaverine, BE SURE TO TELL YOUR DOCTOR if you are already taking levodopa.

WARNINGS

• Tell your doctor about unusual or allergic reactions you have had to any medications, especially to papaverine.

• Before starting to take this medication, be sure to tell your doctor if you now have, or if you have ever had, angina (chest pain), glaucoma, heart block, liver disease, low or high blood pressure, a recent heart attack, or Parkinson's disease.

• A government panel has recently reviewed the effectiveness of this medication in the treatment of hardening of the arteries, leg cramps, and in the prevention of stroke. This drug may not be as effective as once thought. Discuss this with your doctor.

• Before taking any over-the-counter (non-prescription) cough, cold, allergy, asthma, sinus, or diet medication, check with your doctor or pharmacist. Some of these products can decrease the effectiveness of papaverine.

• If this drug makes you dizzy or drowsy, do not take part in any activity that requires alertness, such as driving a car or operating potentially dangerous equipment.

• The beneficial effects of this medication may be decreased by the nicotine in cigarettes. Try to stop smoking.

● To prevent dizziness and fainting while taking this medication, avoid drinking large quantities of alcohol, and avoid getting overheated (strenuous exercise in hot weather; hot baths, showers, and saunas).

● Be sure to tell your doctor if you are pregnant. Although papaverine appears to be safe, extensive studies in pregnant women have not yet been completed. Also, tell your doctor if you are breastfeeding an infant. It is not known whether or not papaverine passes into breast milk.

papaverine hydrochloride—see papaverine

Paracet Forte—see chlorzoxazone and acetaminophen combination

Parafon Forte—see chlorzoxazone and acetaminophen combination

Pargesic—see propoxyphene

---

pargyline

BRAND NAME (Manufacturer)
Eutonyl (Abbott)
TYPE OF DRUG
Monoamine oxidase (MAO) inhibitor and anti-hypertensive
INGREDIENT
pargyline as the hydrochloride salt
DOSAGE FORM
Tablets (10 mg, 25 mg, and 50 mg)
STORAGE
Pargyline should be stored at room temperature, in a tightly closed container.

USES

Pargyline belongs to a group of drugs known as monoamine oxidase (MAO) inhibitors. It is used to treat high blood pressure. It is not exactly clear how this medication works, but it is thought to decrease the activity of the chemicals responsible for increasing blood pressure.

TREATMENT

Pargyline can be taken either on an empty stomach or, to avoid stomach irritation, with food or milk (unless your doctor directs you to do otherwise).

In order to become accustomed to taking this medication, try to take the dose(s) at the same time(s) each day. If you are taking a single daily dose, it is best to take the dose in the morning (to avoid sleeping difficulties).

Pargyline does not cure high blood pressure, but it will help to control the condition, as long as you continue to take it.

If you miss a dose of this medication and remember within two hours of the scheduled time, take the missed dose immediately. If more than two hours have passed, do not take the missed dose at all; just return to your regular dosing schedule. Do not double the next dose.

SIDE EFFECTS

Minor. Constipation; dizziness; drowsiness; dry mouth; hallucinations; headache; increased appetite and weight gain; insomnia; nausea; restlessness; and sweating. These side effects should disappear in several weeks, as your body adjusts to the medication.

To relieve constipation, increase the amount of fiber in your diet (bran, salads, fresh fruits and vegetables, and whole-grain breads), and drink more water (unless your doctor directs you to do otherwise).

If you feel dizzy, sit or lie down awhile. Change positions slowly, and be careful on stairs.

To help relieve mouth dryness, chew sugarless gum, or suck on ice chips or a piece of hard candy.

Pargyline can increase your sensitivity to sunlight. You should therefore avoid prolonged exposure to sunlight and sunlamps. Wear protective clothing and sunglasses, and use an effective sunscreen.

Major. Tell your doctor about any side effects that are persistent or particularly bothersome. IT IS ESPECIALLY IMPORTANT TO TELL YOUR DOCTOR about blurred vision; chest pain; difficulty urinating; fainting; fever; muscle aches or twitching; palpitations; swelling of the feet or legs; or yellowing of the eyes or skin.

If you experience a severe headache, stiff neck, chest

pain, palpitations, or vomiting while taking this medication, CONTACT YOUR DOCTOR OR AN EMERGENCY ROOM IMMEDIATELY. These symptoms may be the result of a food or drug interaction.

INTERACTIONS

Pargyline interacts with a number of drugs and foods.

1. Concurrent use of pargyline with central nervous system depressants (drugs that slow the activity of the brain and spinal cord), such as alcohol, barbiturates, benzodiazepine tranquilizers, muscle relaxants, narcotics, pain medications, phenothiazine tranquilizers, and sleeping medications, or with tricyclic anti-depressants can lead to extreme drowsiness.

2. The dosage of anti-convulsion medication may need to be adjusted when pargyline is started.

3. Use of pargyline within 14 days of tricyclic anti-depressants, carbamazepine, cyclobenzaprine, other monoamine oxidase inhibitors, methyldopa, guanethidine, reserpine, levodopa, meperidine or other narcotics, amphetamines, ephedrine, methylphenidate, phenylpropanolamine, or pseudoephedrine can lead to serious, and sometimes fatal, side effects.

4. Tyramine-containing foods and beverages (aged cheeses, sour cream, yogurt, pickled herring, chicken livers, canned figs, raisins, bananas, avocados, soy sauce, broad bean pods, yeast extracts, beer, and certain wines); excessive amounts of caffeine-containing beverages (coffee, tea, cola); or chocolate can also cause serious reactions in patients on pargyline therapy.

5. Pargyline can increase the blood-sugar-lowering effects of insulin and oral anti-diabetic medications.

Before starting to take pargyline, BE SURE TO TELL YOUR DOCTOR if you are already taking any of the medications listed above. Be sure you are aware of the foods that interact with this medication.

WARNINGS

- Tell your doctor about unusual or allergic reactions you have had to any medications, especially to pargyline.
- Before starting to take this medication, be sure to tell your doctor if you now have, or if you have ever had,

asthma, bronchitis, diabetes mellitus (sugar diabetes), epilepsy, glaucoma, severe headaches, heart or blood vessel disease, kidney disease, liver disease, mental disorders, Parkinson's disease, pheochromocytoma, or thyroid disease.

• If this drug makes you dizzy or drowsy, do not take part in any activities that require alertness, such as driving a car or operating potentially dangerous equipment.

• Before having any surgery or other medical or dental treatment, be sure your doctor or dentist knows that you are taking this medication.

• Check with your doctor or pharmacist before taking any over-the-counter (non-prescription) asthma, allergy, cough, cold, diet, or sinus preparation. Concurrent use of some of these products with pargyline can lead to serious side effects.

• Pargyline 25 mg tablets contain F.D. & C. Yellow Dye No. 5 (tartrazine), which can cause allergic-type symptoms (fainting, shortness of breath, rash) in certain susceptible individuals.

• If you have angina, do not increase your amount of physical activity unless you check with your doctor. Pargyline can decrease the symptoms of angina without decreasing the risks of strenuous exercise.

• Be sure to tell your doctor if you are pregnant. Although pargyline appears to be safe during pregnancy, extensive studies have not yet been completed. Also, tell your doctor if you are breastfeeding an infant. It is not known whether or not pargyline passes into breast milk.

Parlodel—see bromocriptine

Parmine—see phentermine

Pathocil—see dicloxacillin

Pavabid Plateau—see papaverine

Pavacap Unicelles—see papaverine

Pavacen Cenules—see papaverine

Pavadur—see papaverine

Pavadyl—see papaverine

Pavagen—see papaverine

Pava-Par—see papaverine

Pava-RX—see papaverine

Pavased—see papaverine

Pavasule—see papaverine

Pavatine—see papaverine

Pavatym—see papaverine

Paverine Spancaps—see papaverine

Paverolan Lanacaps—see papaverine

Paxipam—see halazepam

PBR-12—see phenobarbital

PDM—see phendimetrazine

Pediaflor—see sodium fluoride

Pediamycin—see erythromycin

Pediazole—see erythromycin and sulfisoxazole combination

Pedi-Cort V—see hydrocortisone and iodochlorhydroxyquin combination (topical)

Pedi-Vit with Fluoride Drops—see vitamins, multiple, with fluoride

pemoline

BRAND NAME (Manufacturer)
Cylert (Abbott)
TYPE OF DRUG
Stimulant
INGREDIENT
pemoline
DOSAGE FORMS
Tablets (18.75 mg, 37.5 mg, and 75 mg)
Chewable tablets (37.5 mg)
STORAGE
Pemoline should be stored at room temperature in a tightly closed container.

USES

Pemoline is a central nervous system (brain) stimulant that is used to treat attention deficit disorders (hyperkinetic syndrome). It is not yet clear how pemoline works to improve behavioral effects in children, but it seems to decrease hyperactivity and to increase attention span.

TREATMENT

Pemoline can be taken either on an empty stomach or with food or milk (as directed by your doctor). The chewable tablets can be either chewed or swallowed whole.

If you miss a dose of this medication, take the missed dose as soon as possible, unless it is almost time for the next dose. In that case, do not take the missed dose at all; just return to your regular dosing schedule. Do not double the next dose.

You may not observe the full therapeutic benefits of this medication for three to four weeks after it is started.

SIDE EFFECTS

Minor. Dizziness; drowsiness; headache; insomnia; irritability; loss of appetite; nausea; stomach ache; or weight loss. These side effects should disappear in several days, as your body adjusts to the medication.

If you feel dizzy, sit or lie down awhile; get up slowly, and be careful on stairs.

Major. Tell your doctor about any side effects that are per-

sistent or particularly bothersome. IT IS ESPECIALLY IM-
PORTANT TO TELL YOUR DOCTOR about convulsions;
depression; hallucinations; palpitations; skin rash; unusual
movements of the tongue, lips, face, hands, or feet; or yellowing of the eyes or skin.

INTERACTIONS
Pemoline should not interact with other medications, if it
is used according to directions.

WARNINGS
● Tell your doctor about unusual or allergic reactions you
have had to any medications, especially to pemoline.
● Before starting to take this medication, be sure to tell
your doctor if you now have, or if you have ever had, kidney disease, liver disease, or mental disorders.
● If this drug makes you dizzy or drowsy, do not take part
in any activities that require alertness, such as driving a car
or operating potentially dangerous equipment. Children
should also be cautious while climbing trees or playing.
● This medication has the potential for abuse, and must
be used with caution. It should therefore not be taken in
larger doses, or for longer periods, than prescribed by your
doctor. In addition, you should not stop taking pemoline
unless you first check with your doctor. Stopping the drug
abruptly can lead to a withdrawal reaction. Your doctor
may therefore want to reduce the dosage gradually.
● Your doctor may want to interrupt pemoline therapy
("drug holiday") for short periods occasionally, to see if
the symptoms of the attention deficit disorder have disap-
peared.
● Be sure to tell your doctor if you are pregnant. Although pemoline appears to be safe, extensive studies in
humans during pregnancy have not yet been completed.
Also, tell your doctor if you are breastfeeding an infant. It
is not known whether or not pemoline passes into breast
milk.

Penapar-VK—see penicillin VK

Penbritin—see ampicillin

penicillamine

BRAND NAMES (Manufacturers)
Cuprimine (Merck Sharp & Dohme)
Depen Titratabs (Wallace)
TYPE OF DRUG
Chelator and anti-rheumatic
INGREDIENT
penicillamine
DOSAGE FORMS
Tablets (250 mg)
Capsules (125 mg and 250 mg)
STORAGE
Penicillamine tablets and capsules should be stored at room temperature, in tightly closed containers.

USES

This medication is used to treat Wilson's disease (high blood copper levels), severe rheumatoid arthritis, and cystinuria (high urine levels of cystine). Penicillamine binds to copper and cystine, which prevents their harmful effects on the body. It is not clearly understood how penicillamine works to relieve rheumatoid arthritis.

TREATMENT

In order to obtain maximum benefit from penicillamine, you should take it on an empty stomach, one hour before or two hours after a meal. To ensure maximum absorption of this drug, each dose should be separated from doses of other medications, or from food and milk, by at least an hour.

If you miss a dose of this medication, take the missed dose as soon as possible, unless it is almost time for the next dose. In that case, do not take the missed dose at all; just return to your regular dosing schedule. Do not double the next dose.

The full benefits of this medication may not become apparent for as long as three months after beginning therapy.

SIDE EFFECTS

Minor. Altered taste sensations; diarrhea; loss of appetite; nausea; stomach upset; and vomiting. These side effects should disappear in several days, as your body adjusts to the medication.

Major. Tell your doctor about any side effects that are persistent or particularly bothersome. IT IS ESPECIALLY IMPORTANT TO TELL YOUR DOCTOR about breast enlargement (in both sexes); difficult or painful urination; difficulty breathing; joint pain; loss of hair; mouth sores; ringing in the ears; skin rash; sore throat; tingling sensations in the fingers or toes; unusual bleeding or bruising; or wheezing.

INTERACTIONS

Penicillamine interacts with several other types of medication.

1. The absorption of penicillamine from the gastrointestinal tract can be decreased by iron or antacids.

2. Penicillamine can decrease the blood levels and beneficial effects of digoxin.

3. Concurrent use of penicillamine and gold salts, hydroxychloroquine, phenylbutazone, oxyphenbutazone, or anti-cancer drugs can lead to increased side effects to the blood and kidneys.

BE SURE TO TELL YOUR DOCTOR if you are already taking any of the medications listed above.

WARNINGS

● Tell your doctor about unusual or allergic reactions you have had to any medications, especially to penicillamine or penicillins.

● Before starting to take this medication, be sure to tell your doctor if you now have, or if you have ever had, blood disorders or kidney disease.

● Do not stop taking this drug unless you first check with your doctor. Stopping the drug and restarting it at a later time can lead to increased side effects.

● Penicillamine can decrease the body's ability to repair wounds, so be careful to avoid injuring yourself while you are taking this medication. This warning is especially important for diabetic patients.

● Before having any surgery or other medical or dental treatment, be sure to tell your doctor or dentist that you are taking this drug.

• Your doctor may want you to take pyridoxine (vitamin B$_6$) to prevent some of the side effects (tingling sensations) of penicillamine.

• Be sure to tell your doctor if you are pregnant. Penicillamine has been reported to cause birth defects in both animals and humans. Also, tell your doctor if you are breastfeeding an infant. It is not known whether or not penicillamine passes into breast milk.

---

penicillin G

BRAND NAMES (Manufacturers)
M-Cillin B (Misemer)
penicillin G potassium (various manufacturers)
Pentids (Squibb)
Pfizerpen G (Pfipharmecs)
SK-Penicillin G (Smith Kline & French)

TYPE OF DRUG
Antibiotic (infection fighter)

INGREDIENT
penicillin G potassium

DOSAGE FORMS
Tablets (125 mg, 250 mg, and 500 mg; 250,000 and 500,000 units)
Oral solution (125 mg and 250 mg; and 250,000 units per 5 ml teaspoonful)

STORAGE
Penicillin G tablets should be stored at room temperature in a tightly closed container. The oral solution should be stored in the refrigerator in a tightly closed container. Any unused portion of the solution should be discarded after 14 days, because the drug loses its potency after that time. This medication should never be frozen.

USES

Penicillin G is used to treat a wide variety of bacterial infections, including infections in the middle ear, upper and lower respiratory tracts, and the urinary tract. It acts by severely injuring the cell walls of the infecting bacteria, thereby preventing them from growing and multiplying.

Penicillin G kills susceptible bacteria, but is not effective against viruses, parasites, or fungi.

TREATMENT

Penicillin G should be taken on an empty stomach or with a glass of water, one hour before or two hours after a meal. This medication should never be taken with fruit juices or carbonated beverages, because the acidity of these drinks destroys the drug in the stomach.

The oral solution should be measured carefully, with a specially designed, 5 ml measuring spoon. An ordinary kitchen teaspoon is not accurate enough.

Penicillin G works best when the level of medicine in your bloodstream is kept constant. It is best therefore to take the doses at evenly spaced intervals, day and night. For example, if you are taking four doses a day, the doses should be spaced six hours apart.

If you miss a dose of this medication, take the missed dose immediately. However, if you do not remember to take the missed dose until it is almost time for your next dose, take it; then space the following dose about halfway through the regular interval between doses. Then return to your regular dosing schedule. Try not to skip any doses.

It is important to continue to take this medication for the entire time prescribed by your doctor (usually seven to 14 days), even if the symptoms of infection disappear before the end of that period. If you stop taking the drug too soon, resistant bacteria are given a chance to continue growing, and the infection could recur.

SIDE EFFECTS

Minor. Diarrhea; heartburn; nausea; and vomiting. These side effects should disappear in several days, as your body adjusts to the medication.

Major. Tell your doctor about any side effects that are persistent or particularly bothersome. IT IS ESPECIALLY IMPORTANT TO TELL YOUR DOCTOR about bloating; chills; cough; darkened tongue; difficulty breathing; fever; irritation of the mouth; muscle aches; rash; rectal or vaginal itching; severe diarrhea; or sore throat. Also, if your symptoms of infection seem to be getting worse rather than improving, you should contact your doctor.

INTERACTIONS

Penicillin G interacts with several other types of medication.

1. Probenecid can increase the blood concentrations of this medication.

2. Oral neomycin may decrease the absorption of penicillin from the gastrointestinal tract.

3. Penicillin G may decrease the effectiveness of oral contraceptives (birth control pills), and pregnancy could result. You should therefore use another form of birth control while taking this medication. Discuss this with your doctor.

TELL YOUR DOCTOR if you are already taking any of the medications listed above.

WARNINGS

• Tell your doctor about unusual or allergic reactions you have had to any medications, especially to penicillins, ampicillin, amoxicillin, cephalosporin antibiotics, penicillamine, or griseofulvin.

• Tell your doctor if you now have, or if you have ever had, kidney disease, asthma, or allergies.

• This medication has been prescribed for your current infection only. Another infection later on, or one that someone else has, may require a different medicine. You should not give your medicine to other people or use it for other infections, unless your doctor specifically directs you to do so.

• Diabetics taking penicillin should know that this drug can cause a false-positive sugar reaction with a Clinitest urine glucose test. To avoid this problem, while taking penicillin you should switch to Clinistix or Tes-Tape to test your urine sugar.

• Some of these products contain F.D. & C. Yellow Dye No. 5 (tartrazine), which can cause allergic-type reactions (shortness of breath, wheezing, rash, or fainting) in certain susceptible individuals.

• Be sure to tell your doctor if you are pregnant. Although penicillin appears to be safe during pregnancy, extensive studies in humans have not yet been completed. Also, tell your doctor if you are breastfeeding an infant. Small amounts of this medication pass into breast milk and may temporarily alter the bacteria in the intestinal tract of the nursing infant, resulting in diarrhea.

penicillin G potassium—see penicillin G

---

penicillin VK

BRAND NAMES (Manufacturers)
Beepen-VK (Beecham)
Betapen-VK (Bristol)
Deltapen-VK (Trimen)
Ledercillin VK (Lederle)
Penapar-VK (Parke-Davis)
penicillin VK (various manufacturers)
Pen-Vee K (Wyeth)
Pfizerpen VK (Pfipharmecs)
Repen-VK (Reid-Provident)
Robicillin VK (Robins)
SK-Penicillin (Smith Kline & French)
Uticillin VK (Upjohn)
V-Cillin K (Lilly)
Veetids (Squibb)

TYPE OF DRUG
Antibiotic (infection fighter)

INGREDIENT
penicillin potassium phenoxymethyl

DOSAGE FORMS
Tablets (125 mg, 250 mg, and 500 mg)
Oral solution (125 mg and 250 mg per 5 ml teaspoonful)

STORAGE
Penicillin VK tablets should be stored at room temperature in a tightly closed container. The oral solution should be stored in the refrigerator in a tightly closed container. Any unused portion of the solution should be discarded after 14 days, because the drug loses its potency after that time. This medication should never be frozen.

USES
Penicillin VK is used to treat a wide variety of bacterial infections, including infections in the middle ear, upper and

lower respiratory tracts, and the urinary tract. It acts by severely injuring the cell walls of the infecting bacteria, thereby preventing them from growing and multiplying. Penicillin VK kills susceptible bacteria, but is not effective against viruses, parasites, or fungi.

TREATMENT

Penicillin VK should be taken on an empty stomach or with a glass of water, one hour before or two hours after a meal. This medication should never be taken with fruit juices or carbonated beverages, because the acidity of these drinks destroys the drug in the stomach.

The oral solution should be measured carefully, with a specially designed, 5 ml measuring spoon. An ordinary kitchen teaspoon is not accurate enough.

Penicillin VK works best when the level of the medicine in your bloodstream is kept constant. It is best therefore to take the doses at evenly spaced intervals, day and night. For example, if you are taking four doses a day, the doses should be spaced six hours apart.

If you miss a dose of this medication, take the missed dose immediately. However, if you do not remember to take the missed dose until it is almost time for your next dose, take it; then space the following dose about halfway through the regular interval between doses. Then return to your regular dosing schedule. Try not to skip any doses.

It is important to continue to take this medication for the entire time prescribed by your doctor (usually seven to 14 days), even if the symptoms of infection disappear before the end of that period. If you stop taking the drug too soon, resistant bacteria are given a chance to continue growing, and the infection could recur.

SIDE EFFECTS

Minor. Diarrhea; heartburn; nausea; and vomiting. These side effects should disappear in several days, as your body adjusts to the medication.

Major. Tell your doctor about any side effects that are persistent or particularly bothersome. IT IS ESPECIALLY IMPORTANT TO TELL YOUR DOCTOR about bloating; chills; cough; darkened tongue; difficulty breathing; fever; irritation of the mouth; muscle aches; rash; rectal or vaginal itching; severe diarrhea; or sore throat. Also, if your symptoms of infection seem to be getting worse rather than improving, you should contact your doctor.

INTERACTIONS

Penicillin VK interacts with several other types of medications.

1. Probenecid can increase the blood concentrations of this medication.

2. Oral neomycin may decrease the absorption of penicillin from the gastrointestinal tract.

3. Penicillin VK may decrease the effectiveness of oral contraceptives (birth control pills), and pregnancy could result. You should therefore use another form of birth control while taking this medication. Discuss this with your doctor.

TELL YOUR DOCTOR if you are already taking any of the medications listed above.

WARNINGS

● Tell your doctor about unusual or allergic reactions you have had to any medications, especially to penicillins, ampicillin, amoxicillin, cephalosporin antibiotics, penicillamine, or griseofulvin.

● Tell your doctor if you now have, or if you have ever had, kidney disease, asthma, or allergies.

● This medication has been prescribed for your current infection only. Another infection later on, or one that someone else has, may require a different medicine. You should not give your medicine to other people or use it for other infections, unless your doctor specifically directs you to do so.

● Diabetics taking penicillin should know that this drug can cause a false-positive sugar reaction with a Clinitest urine glucose test. To avoid this problem, while taking penicillin you should switch to Clinistix or Tes-Tape to test your urine sugar.

● Be sure to tell your doctor if you are pregnant. Although penicillin appears to be safe during pregnancy, extensive studies in humans have not yet been completed. Also, tell your doctor if you are breastfeeding an infant. Small amounts of this medication pass into breast milk and may temporarily alter the bacteria in the intestinal tract of the nursing infant, resulting in diarrhea.

Pensyn—see ampicillin

---

pentaerythritol tetranitrate

BRAND NAMES (Manufacturers)
Duotrate Plateau Caps (Marion)
Naptrate (Vortech)
Pentol (Major)
Pentraspan SR (Vitarine)
Pentritol Tempules (USV)
Pentylan (Lannett)
Peritrate (Parke-Davis)
P.E.T.N. (various manufacturers)
Vaso-80 Unicelles (Reid-Provident)
TYPE OF DRUG
Anti-anginal
INGREDIENT
pentaerythritol tetranitrate
DOSAGE FORMS
Tablets (10 mg, 20 mg, 40 mg, and 80 mg)
Sustained-release tablets (80 mg)
Sustained-release capsules (30 mg, 45 mg, 60 mg, and 80 mg)
STORAGE
Pentaerythritol tetranitrate should be stored at room temperature in tightly closed containers. This medication loses its potency if exposed to heat or moisture.

USES

Pentaerythritol tetranitrate is used to prevent angina (chest pain). It dilates blood vessels, which increases the oxygen supply to the heart, thereby preventing chest pain. It does not relieve pain once an angina attack has begun.

TREATMENT

To ensure that the maximum amount of medication is absorbed into the bloodstream, you should take pentaerythritol tetranitrate on an empty stomach (at least 30 minutes before or one hour after a meal), with a glass of water (unless your doctor directs you to do otherwise).

The sustained-release tablets or capsules should be swallowed whole. Chewing, crushing, or breaking these tablets or capsules destroys their sustained-release activity, and possibly increases the side effects.

If you miss a dose of this medication and remember within two hours (six hours for the sustained-release tablets or capsules) of the scheduled time, take the missed dose immediately. Then return to your regular dosing schedule. Never double the dose (unless your doctor specifically directs you to do so).

SIDE EFFECTS

Minor. Dizziness; flushing or redness of the face and neck; headache; light-headedness; nausea; and vomiting. These side effects should disappear in several days, as your body adjusts to the medication.

If you feel dizzy or light-headed, sit or lie down awhile; change positions slowly, and be careful on stairs.

Acetaminophen may help relieve mild headaches.

Major. Tell your doctor about any side effects that are persistent or particularly bothersome. IT IS ESPECIALLY IMPORTANT TO TELL YOUR DOCTOR about fainting; palpitations; or skin rash.

INTERACTIONS

Alcohol can increase the blood-pressure-lowering effects of pentaerythritol tetranitrate, which can lead to serious side effects. You should therefore avoid drinking alcoholic beverages while taking this medication.

WARNINGS

● Tell your doctor about unusual or allergic reactions you have had to medications, especially to pentaerythritol tetranitrate or to any other nitrate product (such as erythrityl tetranitrate, isosorbide dinitrate, or nitroglycerin).

● Before starting to take this medication, be sure to tell your doctor if you now have, or if you have ever had, anemia, a recent heart attack, or thyroid disease.

● If this medication makes you dizzy or light-headed, avoid taking part in activities that require alertness, such as driving a car or operating potentially dangerous equipment.

● Tolerance to this medication can develop after prolonged use. If you begin to notice a decrease in effectiveness, contact your doctor. Do not increase the dose of this medication without first checking with your doctor. Stopping the drug abruptly can lead to a worsening in your condition. Your doctor may therefore want to reduce your dosage gradually.

● Before taking any over-the-counter (non-prescription) cough, cold, allergy, asthma, sinus, or diet preparation, check with your doctor. Some of these products can reduce the effectiveness of pentaerythritol tetranitrate.

● If you find whole or partially dissolved sustained-release tablets or capsules in your stool, contact your doctor. This indicates that you are not digesting and absorbing the tablets or capsules completely.

● Be sure to tell your doctor if you are pregnant. Although pentaerythritol tetranitrate appears to be safe during pregnancy, extensive studies in humans have not yet been completed. Also, tell your doctor if you are breast-feeding an infant. It is not known whether or not pentaerythritol tetranitrate passes into breast milk.

Pentazine Expectorant with Codeine—see
promethazine, potassium guaiacolsulfonate, and
codeine combination

Pentazine VC Expectorant with Codeine—see
phenylephrine, potassium guaiacolsulfonate,
promethazine, and codeine combination

---

pentazocine

BRAND NAME (Manufacturer)
Talwin NX (Winthrop)
TYPE OF DRUG
Analgesic (pain reliever)
INGREDIENTS
pentazocine as the hydrochloride salt; naloxone as the hydrochloride salt

DOSAGE FORM
Tablets (50 mg pentazocine and 0.5 mg naloxone)
STORAGE
Pentazocine tablets should be stored at room temperature in a tightly closed, light-resistant container.

USES
Pentazocine is a narcotic analgesic that acts directly on the central nervous system (brain and spinal cord) to relieve moderate to severe pain. Naloxone is added to this compound to prevent abuse. It is not absorbed from the gastrointestinal tract, but does block the action of pentazocine if the drug is injected into the body.

TREATMENT
In order to avoid stomach upset, you can take pentazocine with food or with a full glass of milk or water.

This medication works most effectively if you take it at the onset of pain, rather than waiting until the pain becomes intense.

If you are taking this medication on a regular schedule and you miss a dose, take the missed dose as soon as possible, unless it is almost time for your next dose. In that case, don't take the missed dose at all; just return to your regular dosing schedule. Do not double the next dose.

SIDE EFFECTS
Minor. Constipation; dizziness; drowsiness; dry mouth; false sense of well-being; flushing; light-headedness; loss of appetite; nausea; rash; sweating; and painful or difficult urination. These side effects should disappear in several days, as your body adjusts to the medication.

If you are constipated, increase the amount of fiber in your diet (raw vegetables, fruits, salads, bran, and whole-grain breads), and drink more water (unless your doctor directs you to do otherwise).

Chew sugarless gum, or suck on ice chips or a piece of hard candy, to reduce mouth dryness.

If you feel dizzy, light-headed, or nauseated, sit or lie down awhile; get up from a sitting or lying position slowly, and be careful on stairs.

Major. Tell your doctor about any side effects that are per-

sistent or particularly bothersome. IT IS ESPECIALLY IM-
PORTANT TO TELL YOUR DOCTOR about anxiety;
difficulty breathing; excitation; fatigue; pounding heartbeat; restlessness; sore throat and fever; tremors; or weakness.

INTERACTIONS

Pentazocine interacts with several other types of drugs.

1. Concurrent use of it with other central nervous system
depressants (drugs that slow the activity of the nervous system), such as antihistamines, barbiturates, benzodiazepine tranquilizers, muscle relaxants, phenothiazine
tranquilizers, and alcohol, or with tricyclic anti-depressants can cause extreme drowsiness.

2. A monoamine oxidase (MAO) inhibitor taken within
14 days of this medication can lead to unpredictable and
severe side effects.

3. Cimetidine, combined with this medication, can cause
confusion, disorientation, seizures, and shortness of
breath.

TELL YOUR DOCTOR if you are already taking any of the
medications listed above.

WARNINGS

• Tell your doctor about unusual or allergic reactions you
have had to any medications, especially to pentazocine or
to other narcotic analgesics (such as codeine, hydrocodone, hydromorphone, meperidine, methadone, morphine, oxycodone, and propoxyphene).

• Tell your doctor if you now have, or if you have ever
had, acute abdominal conditions, asthma, brain disease,
colitis, epilepsy, gallstones or gallbladder disease, head injuries, heart disease, kidney disease, liver disease, lung
disease, mental illness, emotional disorders, enlarged
prostate gland, thyroid disease, or urethral stricture.

• If this drug makes you dizzy or drowsy, do not take part
in any activity that requires alertness, such as driving a car
or operating potentially dangerous equipment.

• Before having any surgery or other medical or dental
treatment, be sure to tell your doctor or dentist that you are
taking this medication.

• Because this product contains pentazocine, it has the

potential for abuse, and must be used with caution. Usually, it should not be taken on a regular schedule for longer than ten days, unless your doctor directs you to do so. Tolerance develops quickly; do not increase the dosage or stop taking the drug abruptly, unless you first consult your doctor. If you have been taking large amounts of this medication, or have been taking it for long periods, you may experience a withdrawal reaction (muscle aches, diarrhea, gooseflesh, runny nose, nausea, vomiting, shivering, trembling, stomach cramps, sleep disorders, irritability, weakness, yawning, and sweating) when you stop taking it. Your doctor may therefore want to reduce the dosage gradually.

● Be sure to tell your doctor if you are pregnant. The effects of this medication during the early stages of pregnancy have not yet been thoroughly studied in humans. However, pentazocine, used regularly in large doses during the later stages of pregnancy, may result in addiction of the fetus—leading to withdrawal symptoms (irritability, excessive crying, tremors, fever, vomiting, diarrhea, sneezing, and yawning) at birth. Also, tell your doctor if you are breastfeeding an infant. Small amounts of this medication may pass into breast milk and cause excessive drowsiness in the nursing infant.

Pentids—see penicillin G

---

pentobarbital

BRAND NAMES (Manufacturers)
Nembutal (Abbott)
pentobarbital sodium (various manufacturers)
TYPE OF DRUG
Sedative/hypnotic (sleeping aid)
INGREDIENT
pentobarbital as the sodium salt
DOSAGE FORMS
Capsules (30 mg, 50 mg, and 100 mg)
Oral elixir (18.2 mg per 5 ml teaspoonful)
Suppositories (30 mg, 60 mg, 120 mg, and 200 mg)

STORAGE

Pentobarbital capsules and oral elixir should be stored at room temperature in tightly closed containers. The suppositories should be stored in the refrigerator. Pentobarbital should never be frozen.

USES

This medication belongs to a group of drugs known as barbiturates, which are central nervous system depressants (drugs that slow the activity of the brain and spinal cord). It is used as a sleeping aid in the treatment of insomnia.

TREATMENT

You can take pentobarbital at bedtime. The capsules or oral elixir can be taken with water, food, or milk.

Each dose of the oral elixir should be measured carefully, with a specially designed, 5 ml measuring spoon. An ordinary kitchen teaspoon is not accurate enough. The elixir can be taken straight or mixed with water, milk, or fruit juice.

To insert the suppository form of this medication, first unwrap it and moisten it slightly with water (if the suppository is too soft, run cold water over it or refrigerate it for 30 minutes before you unwrap it). Lie down on your left side, with your right knee bent. Push the suppository well into the rectum with your finger. Try to avoid having a bowel movement for at least an hour.

You should not use this drug as a sleeping aid for more than two weeks. With prolonged use, pentobarbital loses its ability to produce or maintain sleep.

SIDE EFFECTS

Minor. Constipation; diarrhea; dizziness; drowsiness; headache; a "hangover" feeling; muscle or joint pain; nausea; stomach upset; and vomiting. These side effects should disappear in several days, as your body adjusts to the medication.

If you feel dizzy or light-headed, sit or lie down awhile; get up slowly, and be careful on stairs.

To relieve constipation, increase the amount of fiber in your diet (bran, salads, fresh fruits and vegetables, and whole-grain breads), exercise, and drink more water (unless your doctor directs you to do otherwise).

Major. Tell your doctor about any side effects that are persistent or particularly bothersome. IT IS ESPECIALLY IMPORTANT TO TELL YOUR DOCTOR about chest tightness; confusion; depression; difficulty breathing; excitation; fatigue; feeling faint; hives or itching; loss of coordination; skin rash; slurred speech; sore throat; unusual bleeding or bruising; unusual weakness; or yellowing of the eyes or skin.

INTERACTIONS

Pentobarbital interacts with several other types of medication.

1. Concurrent use of it with other central nervous system depressants (such as antihistamines, benzodiazepine tranquilizers, muscle relaxants, narcotics, pain medications, phenothiazine tranquilizers, and alcohol) or with tricyclic anti-depressants can cause extreme drowsiness.

2. Valproic acid, chloramphenicol, and monoamine oxidase (MAO) inhibitors can prolong the effects of pentobarbital.

3. Pentobarbital can decrease the blood levels and effectiveness of oral anti-coagulants (blood thinners, such as warfarin), digoxin, tricyclic anti-depressants, cortisone-like medicines, doxycycline, quinidine, estrogens, birth control pills, phenytoin, acetaminophen, and carbamazepine.

4. The combination of pentobarbital and furosemide can cause low blood pressure and fainting.

5. Pentobarbital can increase the side effects of cyclophosphamide or large doses of acetaminophen.

Before starting to take pentobarbital, BE SURE TO TELL YOUR DOCTOR if you are already taking any of the medications listed above.

WARNINGS

● Tell your doctor about unusual or allergic reactions you have had to any medications, especially to pentobarbital or to other barbiturates (such as amobarbital, butabarbital, mephobarbital, metharbital, phenobarbital, primidone, or secobarbital).

● Before starting to take this medication, be sure to tell your doctor if you now have, or if you have ever had, acute or chronic (long-term) pain; Addison's disease (an under-active adrenal gland); diabetes mellitus (sugar diabetes); kidney disease; liver disease; lung disease; mental depression; porphyria; or thyroid disease.

● Since this medication makes you drowsy, do not take part in any activity that requires alertness, such as driving a car or operating potentially dangerous equipment.

● This drug has the potential for abuse and must be used with caution. Tolerance develops quickly; do not increase the dosage or stop taking this drug unless you first consult your doctor. If you have been taking pentobarbital for a long time or have been taking large doses, you may experience anxiety, muscle twitching, tremors, weakness, dizziness, nausea, vomiting, insomnia, or blurred vision when you stop taking it. To avoid this reaction, your doctor may want to reduce your dosage gradually.

● Be sure to tell your doctor if you are pregnant. Barbiturates cross the placenta, and there has been an association between birth defects and the use of this class of drugs during pregnancy. Such drugs may also lead to an increase in bleeding complications in the newborn. The risks should be discussed with your doctor. In addition, if pentobarbital is used for prolonged periods during the last three months of pregnancy, there is a chance that the infant will be born addicted to the medication, and will experience a withdrawal reaction (convulsions and irritability) at birth. Also, tell your doctor if you are breast-feeding an infant. Small amounts of pentobarbital pass into breast milk and may cause excessive drowsiness or breathing problems in nursing infants.

pentobarbital sodium—see pentobarbital

Pentol—see pentaerythritol tetranitrate

Pentraspan SR—see pentaerythritol tetranitrate

Pentritol Tempules—see pentaerythritol tetranitrate

Pentylan—see pentaerythritol tetranitrate

Pen-Vee K—see penicillin VK

Percocet-5—see acetaminophen and oxycodone combination

Percodan—see aspirin and oxycodone combination

Percodan-Demi—see aspirin and oxycodone combination

Periactin—see cyproheptadine

Peritrate—see pentraerythritol tetranitrate

Permitil—see fluphenazine

Permitil Chronotabs—see fluphenazine

---

perphenazine

BRAND NAMES (Manufacturers)
Trilafon (Schering)
Trilafon Repetabs (Schering)
TYPE OF DRUG
Phenothiazine tranquilizer
INGREDIENT
perphenazine
DOSAGE FORMS
Tablets (2 mg, 4 mg, 8 mg, and 16 mg)
Oral concentrate (16 mg per 5 ml teaspoonful)
Sustained-release tablets (8 mg)
STORAGE
The tablet forms of this medication should be stored at room temperature in tightly closed, light-resistant containers. The oral concentrate form of this medication should be stored in the refrigerator in a tightly closed, light-resistant container. If the oral concentrate turns to a slight yellow color, the medicine is still effective and can be used. However, if it changes color markedly, or has particles floating in it, it should not be used, but discarded down the sink. This medication should never be frozen.

USES

Perphenazine is prescribed to treat the symptoms of certain types of mental illness, such as emotional symptoms of psychosis, the manic phase of manic-depressive illness, and severe behavioral problems in children. This medication is thought to relieve the symptoms of mental illness by blocking certain chemicals involved with nerve transmission in the brain.

TREATMENT

To avoid stomach irritation, you can take the tablet form of this medication with a meal or with a glass of water or milk (unless your doctor directs you to do otherwise).

The sustained-release tablets should be taken whole; do not crush or break them prior to swallowing. This would release the medication all at once—defeating the purpose of the sustained-release tablets.

The oral concentrate form of this medication should be measured carefully with the dropper provided, then added to 4 ounces ($1/2$ cup) or more of water, milk, juice, or a carbonated beverage, or to applesauce or pudding, immediately prior to administration. To prevent possible loss of effectiveness, the medication should not be diluted in tea, coffee, or apple juice.

Antacids and anti-diarrhea medicine may decrease the absorption of this medication from the gastrointestinal tract. Therefore, at least an hour should separate doses of one of these medicines and perphenazine.

If you miss a dose of this medication, take the missed dose as soon as possible and return to your regular dosing schedule. If it is almost time for the next dose, however, skip the one you missed and return to your regular schedule. Do not double the next dose (unless your doctor directs you to do so).

The full effects of this medication for the control of emotional or mental symptoms may not become apparent for two weeks after you start to take it.

SIDE EFFECTS

Minor. Blurred vision; constipation; decreased sweating; diarrhea; discoloration of the urine to red, pink, or red-brown; dizziness; drooling; drowsiness; dry mouth; fatigue; jitteriness; menstrual irregularities; nasal congestion; restlessness; tremors; vomiting; and weight gain. As your body adjusts to the medication, these side effect should disappear.

If you are constipated, increase the amount of fiber in your diet (raw vegetables, fruits, salads, bran, and whole-grain breads), and drink more water (unless your doctor directs you to do otherwise).

Chew sugarless gum, or suck on ice chips or a piece of hard candy, to reduce mouth dryness.

This medication can cause increased sensitivity to sunlight. It is therefore important to avoid prolonged exposure to sunlight and sunlamps. Wear protective clothing, and use an effective sunscreen.

To avoid dizziness or light-headedness when you stand, contract and relax the muscles of your legs for a few moments before rising. Do this by pushing one foot against the floor while raising the other foot slightly, alternating feet so that you are "pumping" your legs in a pedaling motion.

Major. Tell your doctor about any side effects that are persistent or particularly bothersome. IT IS ESPECIALLY IMPORTANT TO TELL YOUR DOCTOR about breast enlargement (in both sexes); chest pain; convulsions; darkened skin; difficulty swallowing or breathing; fainting; fever; impotence; involuntary movements of the face, mouth, jaw, or tongue; palpitations; rash; sleep disorders; sore throat; uncoordinated movements; unusual bleeding or bruising; visual disturbances; weakness; or yellowing of the eyes or skin.

INTERACTIONS

Perphenazine interacts with other types of medication.

1. It can cause extreme drowsiness when combined with alcohol or other central nervous system depressants (drugs that slow the activity of the nervous system), such as barbiturates, benzodiazepine tranquilizers, muscle relaxants, narcotics, and pain medications, or with tricyclic anti-depressants.

2. Perphenazine can decrease the effectiveness of amphetamines, guanethidine, anti-convulsants, and levodopa.

3. The side effects of epinephrine, monoamine oxidase (MAO) inhibitors, propranolol, phenytoin, and tricyclic anti-depressants may be increased when combined with this medication.

4. Lithium may increase the side effects and decrease the effectiveness of this medication.

Before starting to take perphenazine, BE SURE TO TELL YOUR DOCTOR if you are already taking any of the medications listed above.

WARNINGS

• Tell your doctor about unusual or allergic reactions you have had to any medications, especially to perphenazine or other phenothiazine tranquilizers (such as acetophenazine, carphenazine, chlorpromazine, fluphenazine, mesoridazine, piperacetazine, prochlorperazine, promazine, thioridazine, trifluoperazine, and triflupromazine), or to loxapine.

• Tell your doctor if you now have, or if you have ever had, any blood disease, bone marrow disease, brain disease, breast cancer, blockage in the urinary or digestive tracts, alcoholism, drug-induced depression, epilepsy, severe high or low blood pressure, diabetes mellitus (sugar diabetes), glaucoma, heart or circulatory disease, liver disease, lung disease, Parkinson's disease, peptic ulcers, or an enlarged prostate gland.

• Tell your doctor about any recent exposure to a pesticide or an insecticide. Perphenazine may increase the side effects from the exposure.

• To prevent over-sedation, avoid drinking alcoholic beverages while taking this medication.

• If this medication makes you dizzy or drowsy, do not take part in any activity that requires alertness, such as driving a car or operating potentially dangerous equipment. Be careful on stairs and avoid getting up suddenly from a lying or sitting position.

• Before having any surgery or other medical or dental treatment, be sure your doctor or dentist knows that you are taking this medication.

• Some of the side effects caused by this drug can be prevented by taking an anti-parkinson drug. Discuss this with your doctor.

- Perphenazine has been reported to cause certain tumors in rats. This effect has not been shown to occur in humans.
- This medication can decrease sweating and heat release from the body. You should therefore avoid getting overheated (strenuous exercise in hot weather; hot baths, showers, and saunas).
- Do not stop taking this medication suddenly. If the drug is stopped abruptly, you may experience nausea, vomiting, stomach upset, headache, increased heart rate, insomnia, tremulousness, or a worsening of your condition. Your doctor may want to reduce the dosage gradually.
- If you are planning to have a myelogram, or any procedure in which dye will be injected into your spinal cord, tell your doctor that you are taking this medication.
- Avoid spilling the oral concentrate form of this medication on your skin or clothing; it may cause redness and irritation of the skin.
- While taking this medication, do not take any over-the-counter (non-prescription) medication for weight control, or for cough, cold, allergy, asthma, or sinus problems, unless you first check with your doctor. The combination of these medications may cause high blood pressure.
- Be sure to tell your doctor if you are pregnant. Small amounts of this medication cross the placenta. Although there are reports of safe use of this drug during pregnancy, there are also reports of liver disease and tremors in newborn infants whose mothers received this type of medication close to term. Also, tell your doctor if you are breastfeeding an infant. Small amounts of this medication pass into breast milk and may cause unwanted effects in the nursing infant.

---

perphenazine and amitriptyline combination

BRAND NAMES (Manufacturers)
Etrafon (Schering)
Triavil (Merck Sharp & Dohme)

TYPE OF DRUG
Phenothiazine tranquilizer and tricyclic anti-depressant (mood elevator)

INGREDIENTS
perphenazine, and amitriptyline as the hydrochloride salt

DOSAGE FORM
Tablets (2 mg perphenazine and 10 mg amitriptyline; 2 mg perphenazine and 25 mg amitriptyline; 4 mg perphenazine and 10 mg amitriptyline; 4 mg perphenazine and 25 mg amitriptyline; and 4 mg perphenazine and 50 mg amitriptyline)

STORAGE
Perphenazine and amitriptyline tablets should be stored at room temperature in a tightly closed, light-resistant container.

USES
Perphenazine and amitriptyline combination is used to relieve anxiety or depression. Amitriptyline belongs to a group of drugs referred to as tricyclic anti-depressants. These medicines are thought to relieve depression by decreasing the concentration of certain chemicals in the brain. Perphenazine is a phenothiazine tranquilizer. It is thought to relieve the symptoms of mental illness by blocking certain chemicals involved with nerve transmission in the brain.

TREATMENT
This medication should be taken exactly as your doctor prescribes. In order to avoid stomach irritation, you can take the tablets with food or with a full glass of water or milk (unless your doctor directs you to do otherwise).

Antacids and anti-diarrhea medicines may decrease the absorption of this medication from the gastrointestinal tract. Therefore, at least one hour should separate doses of perphenazine and amitriptyline and one of these medicines.

If you miss a dose of this medication, take the missed dose as soon as possible, then return to your regular dosing schedule. If it is within two hours of your next dose, however, do not take the missed dose at all; just return to your regular schedule. Do not double the next dose.

The full benefits of this medication for the control of emotional or mental symptoms may not become apparent for two weeks after you start to take it.

SIDE EFFECTS

Minor. Agitation; bloating; blurred vision; confusion; constipation; cramps; diarrhea; dizziness; drowsiness; dry mouth; fatigue; headache; heartburn; insomnia; loss of appetite; nasal congestion; nausea; numbness in the fingers or toes; peculiar tastes in the mouth; restlessness; stomach upset; sweating; vomiting; weakness; and weight gain or loss. These side effects should disappear in several days, as your body adjusts to the medication.

Dry mouth can be relieved by chewing sugarless gum, or by sucking on ice chips or a piece of hard candy.

To relieve constipation, increase the amount of fiber in your diet (bran, fresh fruits and vegetables, salads, and whole-grain breads), exercise, and drink more water (unless your doctor directs you to do otherwise).

To avoid dizziness and light-headedness when you stand, contract and relax the muscles of your legs for a few moments before rising. Do this by pushing one foot against the floor while raising the other foot slightly, alternating feet so that you are "pumping" your legs in a pedaling motion.

This medication can increase your sensitivity to sunlight. You should therefore avoid prolonged exposure to sunlight and sunlamps. Wear protective clothing and sunglasses; and use an effective sunscreen.

Amitriptyline can cause the urine to turn blue-green in color—this is a harmless effect.

Major. Tell your doctor about any side effects that are persistent or particularly bothersome. IT IS ESPECIALLY IMPORTANT TO TELL YOUR DOCTOR about convulsions; difficult or painful urination; enlarged or painful breasts (in both sexes); fainting; fever; hair loss; hallucinations; chest tightness; impotence; menstrual irregularities; mood changes; mouth sores; nervousness; nightmares; palpitations; rash; ringing in the ears; sore throat; tremors; uncoordinated movements or balance problems; unusual bleeding or bruising; or yellowing of the eyes or skin.

INTERACTIONS

Perphenazine and amitriptyline combination interacts with several other types of medication.

1. Extreme drowsiness can occur if this medication is taken with central nervous system depressants (drugs that slow the activity of the nervous system), including alcohol, antihistamines, barbiturates, benzodiazepine tranquilizers, muscle relaxants, narcotics, pain medications, and sleeping medications, or with other anti-depressants.

2. Amitriptyline may decrease the effectiveness of anti-seizure medications and block the blood-pressure-lowering effects of clonidine and guanethidine.

3. Estrogens and oral contraceptives can increase the side effects and reduce the effectiveness of amitriptyline.

4. Amitriptyline may increase the side effects of thyroid medication and of over-the-counter (non-prescription) cough, cold, allergy, asthma, sinus, and diet medications.

5. The concurrent use of this medication with mono-amine oxidase (MAO) inhibitors should be undertaken very carefully, because the combination may result in fever, convulsions, or high blood pressure.

6. Perphenazine can decrease the effectiveness of amphetamines, guanethidine, and levodopa.

7. The side effects of epinephrine and propranolol may be increased by perphenazine.

Before starting to take this medication, BE SURE TO TELL YOUR DOCTOR if you are already taking any of the medications listed above.

WARNINGS

• Tell your doctor about any unusual or allergic reactions you have had to medications, especially to perphenazine or other phenothiazine tranquilizers (such as chlorpromazine, mesoridazine, fluphenazine, promazine, thioridazine, or prochlorperazine), or to amitriptyline or other tricyclic anti-depressants (such as desipramine, doxepin, imipramine, or nortriptyline).

• Tell your doctor if you now have, or if you have ever had, asthma, breast cancer, brain disease, diabetes mellitus (sugar diabetes), electroshock therapy, epilepsy, glaucoma, heart disease, a recent heart attack, liver disease, lung disease, kidney disease, thyroid disease, intestinal or urinary tract blockage, low or high blood pressure, Parkinson's disease, peptic ulcers, or an enlarged prostate gland.

• The effects of this medication may last as long as seven days after you've stopped taking it, so continue to observe all precautions during that period.

• To prevent over-sedation, avoid drinking alcoholic beverages while taking this medication.

• If this medication makes you dizzy or drowsy, do not take part in any activity that requires alertness, such as driving a car or operating potentially dangerous equipment. Be careful on stairs, and avoid getting up suddenly from a lying or sitting position.

• Prior to having surgery or any other medical or dental treatment, be sure your doctor or dentist knows that you are taking this medication.

• Perphenazine has been reported to cause certain tumors in rats. This effect has not been shown to occur in humans.

• This medication can decrease sweating and heat release from the body. You should therefore avoid getting overheated (strenuous exercise in hot weather; hot baths, showers, and saunas).

• Do not stop taking this medication suddenly. If the drug is stopped abruptly you may experience nausea, vomiting, stomach upset, headache, increased heart rate, insomnia, tremulousness, or a worsening of your condition. Your doctor may therefore want to reduce the dosage gradually.

• If you are planning to have a myelogram, or any procedure in which dye will be injected into your spinal cord, tell your doctor that you are taking this medication.

• While taking this medication, do not take any over-the-counter (non-prescription) medication for weight control, or for cough, cold, asthma, allergy, or sinus problems, unless you first check with your doctor. The combination of these medications with perphenazine and amitriptyline may cause high blood pressure.

• Be sure to tell your doctor if you are pregnant. Small amounts of this medication cross the placenta. Although there are reports of safe use of this drug during pregnancy, there are also reports of liver disease and tremors in newborn infants whose mothers received this type of medication close to term. Also, tell your doctor if you are breastfeeding an infant. Small amounts of this medication pass into breast milk and may cause unwanted effects in the nursing infant.

Persantine—see dipyridamole

Pertofrane—see desipramine

Pethadol—see meperidine

P.E.T.N.—see pentaerythritol tetranitrate

Pfizer-E—see erythromycin

Pfizerpen A—see ampicillin

Pfizerpen G—see penicillin G

Pfizerpen VK—see penicillin VK

Phen-Amin—see diphenhydramine

Phenaphen with Codeine—see acetaminophen and codeine combination

Phenazodine—see phenazopyridine

---

phenazopyridine

BRAND NAMES (Manufacturers)
Azodine (Vortech)
Azo-Standard* (Webcon)
Baridium* (Pfeiffer)
Di-Azo* (Kay)
Phenazodine (Lannett)
phenazopyridine hydrochloride (various manufacturers)
Pyridiate (various manufacturers)
Pyridium (Parke-Davis)
*Phenazopyridine 100 mg tablets are also available over-the-counter (non-prescription) under several brand names.

Tablet/Capsule Identification Guide

On the following pages, you will find color photos of hundreds of the most commonly prescribed drugs in tablet and capsule form. These photos will help you to identify your prescription medications, and will help you to make sure that the prescription your doctor wrote refers to the same medication you received from your pharmacist. If you note any discrepancy, call your pharmacist immediately.

HOW TO USE THIS SECTION

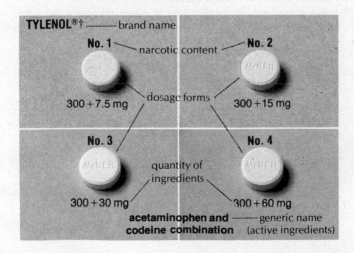

†Drug contains multiple ingredients; quantities and ingredients are listed respectively.

Tablet/Capsule Identification Guide

Prescription drugs are displayed in alphabetical order by brand name. Included are one or more dosage forms of the particular medication. The generic name is listed below the photograph(s) of each prescription medication. A generic name is generally a shortened form of the chemical name of a drug (or, in the case of a combination medication, a list of its active ingredients). This is the name under which you will be able to read more about your medications (in the Drug Profiles section of this book). If, for example, you have been prescribed Tylenol No. 2, you will find your medication discussed in detail within the "acetaminophen and codeine combination" profile.

Some medications are composed of more than one active ingredient. The quantities of each ingredient are listed under each photo, in the order in which they appear in the generic name. For example, Tylenol No. 2 contains 300 mg of acetaminophen and 15 mg of codeine. The terms No. 1 and No. 2 refer to a designation used by many manufacturers to denote the codeine (or other narcotic) content of certain medications. This type of term does not appear in all photographs—only those photographs of medications that have a narcotic component. In our example, the term No. 1 refers to the 7.5 mg codeine content; No. 2 is 15 mg, etc. (This is described in more detail within the appropriate Drug Profiles.)

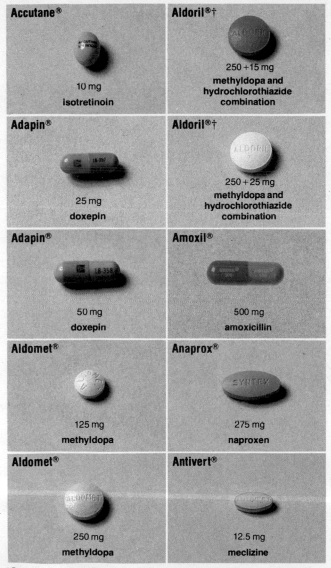

Accutane®

10 mg

isotretinoin

Aldoril®†

250 + 15 mg

methyldopa and
hydrochlorothiazide
combination

Adapin®

25 mg

doxepin

Aldoril®†

250 + 25 mg

methyldopa and
hydrochlorothiazide
combination

Adapin®

50 mg

doxepin

Amoxil®

500 mg

amoxicillin

Aldomet®

125 mg

methyldopa

Anaprox®

275 mg

naproxen

Aldomet®

250 mg

methyldopa

Antivert®

12.5 mg

meclizine

† Drug contains multiple ingredients; quantities and ingredients are listed respectively.

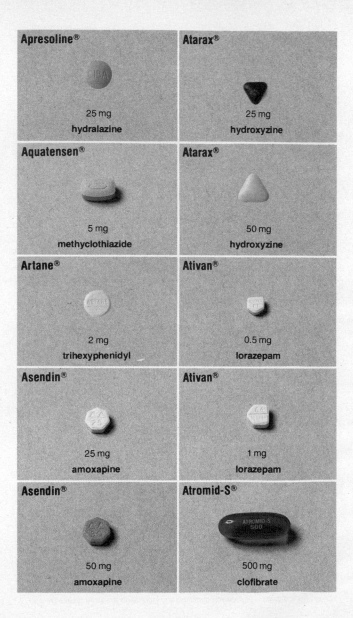

Apresoline®	**Atarax®**
25 mg	25 mg
hydralazine	hydroxyzine
Aquatensen®	**Atarax®**
5 mg	50 mg
methyclothiazide	hydroxyzine
Artane®	**Ativan®**
2 mg	0.5 mg
trihexyphenidyl	lorazepam
Asendin®	**Ativan®**
25 mg	1 mg
amoxapine	lorazepam
Asendin®	**Atromid-S®**
50 mg	500 mg
amoxapine	clofibrate

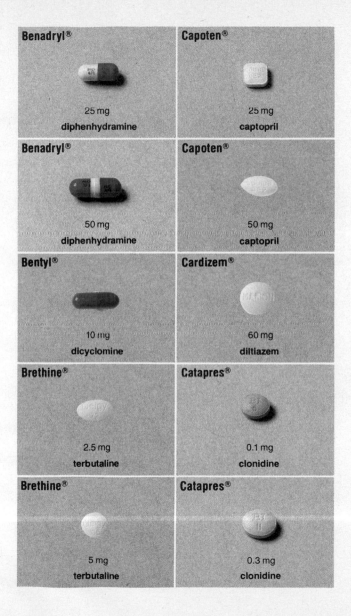

Benadryl® 25 mg diphenhydramine	**Capoten®** 25 mg captopril
Benadryl® 50 mg diphenhydramine	**Capoten®** 50 mg captopril
Bentyl® 10 mg dicyclomine	**Cardizem®** 60 mg diltiazem
Brethine® 2.5 mg terbutaline	**Catapres®** 0.1 mg clonidine
Brethine® 5 mg terbutaline	**Catapres®** 0.3 mg clonidine

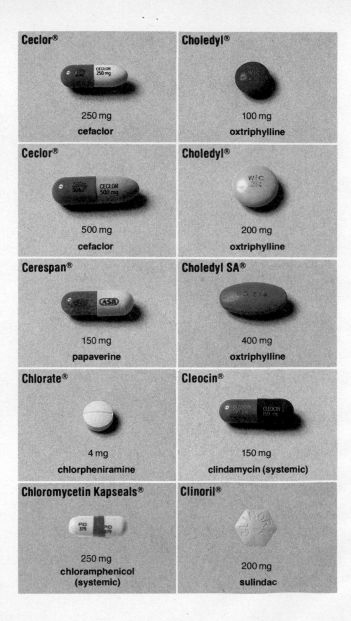

Ceclor®

250 mg

cefaclor

Choledyl®

100 mg

oxtriphylline

Ceclor®

500 mg

cefaclor

Choledyl®

200 mg

oxtriphylline

Cerespan®

150 mg

papaverine

Choledyl SA®

400 mg

oxtriphylline

Chlorate®

4 mg

chlorpheniramine

Cleocin®

150 mg

clindamycin (systemic)

Chloromycetin Kapseals®

250 mg

chloramphenicol
(systemic)

Clinoril®

200 mg

sulindac

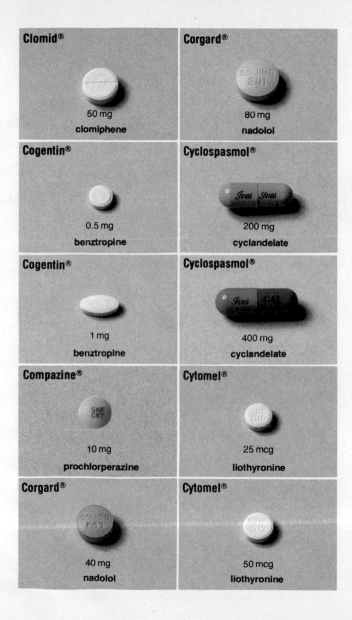

Clomid®

50 mg

clomiphene

Corgard®

80 mg

nadolol

Cogentin®

0.5 mg

benztropine

Cyclospasmol®

200 mg

cyclandelate

Cogentin®

1 mg

benztropine

Cyclospasmol®

400 mg

cyclandelate

Compazine®

10 mg

prochlorperazine

Cytomel®

25 mcg

liothyronine

Corgard®

40 mg

nadolol

Cytomel®

50 mcg

liothyronine

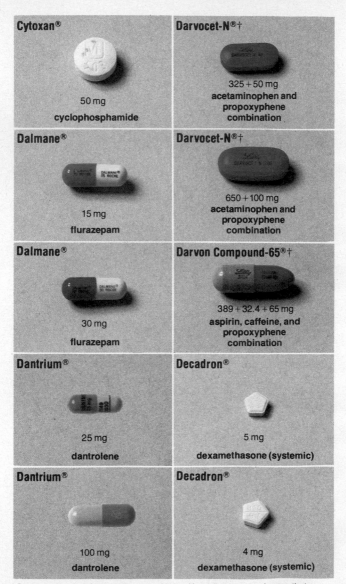

Cytoxan®

50 mg

cyclophosphamide

Dalmane®

15 mg

flurazepam

Dalmane®

30 mg

flurazepam

Dantrium®

25 mg

dantrolene

Dantrium®

100 mg

dantrolene

Darvocet-N®†

325 + 50 mg

acetaminophen and
propoxyphene
combination

Darvocet-N®†

650 + 100 mg

acetaminophen and
propoxyphene
combination

Darvon Compound-65®†

389 + 32.4 + 65 mg

aspirin, caffeine, and
propoxyphene
combination

Decadron®

5 mg

dexamethasone (systemic)

Decadron®

4 mg

dexamethasone (systemic)

† Drug contains multiple ingredients; quantities and ingredients are listed respectively.

Desyrel®	**Dilantin®**
50 mg	30 mg
trazodone	phenytoin
Desyrel®	**Dilantin®**
100 mg	100 mg
trazodone	phenytoin
Diabeta®	**Ditropan®**
5 mg	5 mg
glyburide	oxybutynin
Diabinese®	**Diulo®**
100 mg	2.5 mg
chlorpropamide	metolazone
Diabinese®	**Diulo®**
250 mg	5 mg
chlorpropamide	metolazone

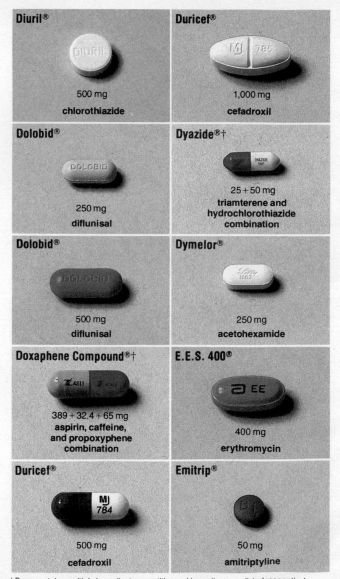

Diuril®

500 mg

chlorothiazide

Duricef®

1,000 mg

cefadroxil

Dolobid®

250 mg

diflunisal

Dyazide®†

25 + 50 mg

triamterene and
hydrochlorothiazide
combination

Dolobid®

500 mg

diflunisal

Dymelor®

250 mg

acetohexamide

Doxaphene Compound®†

389 + 32.4 + 65 mg
aspirin, caffeine,
and propoxyphene
combination

E.E.S. 400®

400 mg

erythromycin

Duricef®

500 mg

cefadroxil

Emitrip®

50 mg

amitriptyline

†Drug contains multiple ingredients; quantities and ingredients are listed respectively.

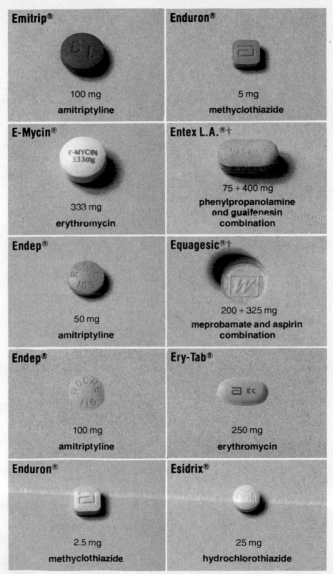

Emitrip®	**Enduron®**
100 mg	5 mg
amitriptyline	methyclothiazide
E-Mycin®	**Entex L.A.®†**
E-MYCIN 333mg	ENTEX L.A.
333 mg	75 + 400 mg
erythromycin	phenylpropanolamine and guaifenesin combination
Endep®	**Equagesic®†**
ROCHE 103	W
50 mg	200 + 325 mg
amitriptyline	meprobamate and aspirin combination
Endep®	**Ery-Tab®**
ROCHE 116	EC
100 mg	250 mg
amitriptyline	erythromycin
Enduron®	**Esidrix®**
2.5 mg	25 mg
methyclothiazide	hydrochlorothiazide

†Drug contains multiple ingredients; quantities and ingredients are listed respectively.

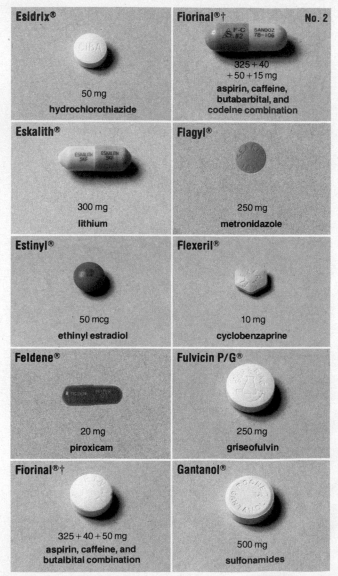

Esidrix®

50 mg

hydrochlorothiazide

Fiorinal®† No. 2

325 + 40
+ 50 + 15 mg

aspirin, caffeine,
butabarbital, and
codeine combination

Eskalith®

300 mg

lithium

Flagyl®

250 mg

metronidazole

Estinyl®

50 mcg

ethinyl estradiol

Flexeril®

10 mg

cyclobenzaprine

Feldene®

20 mg

piroxicam

Fulvicin P/G®

250 mg

griseofulvin

Fiorinal®†

325 + 40 + 50 mg

aspirin, caffeine, and
butalbital combination

Gantanol®

500 mg

sulfonamides

† Drug contains multiple ingredients; quantities and ingredients are listed respectively.

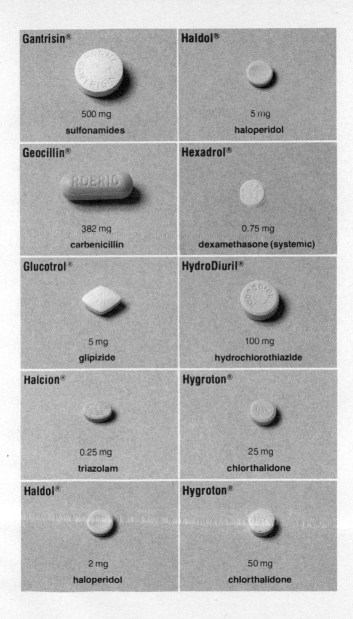

Gantrisin®	**Haldol®**
500 mg	5 mg
sulfonamides	haloperidol
Geocillin®	**Hexadrol®**
382 mg	0.75 mg
carbenicillin	dexamethasone (systemic)
Glucotrol®	**HydroDiuril®**
5 mg	100 mg
glipizide	hydrochlorothiazide
Halcion®	**Hygroton®**
0.25 mg	25 mg
triazolam	chlorthalidone
Haldol®	**Hygroton®**
2 mg	50 mg
haloperidol	chlorthalidone

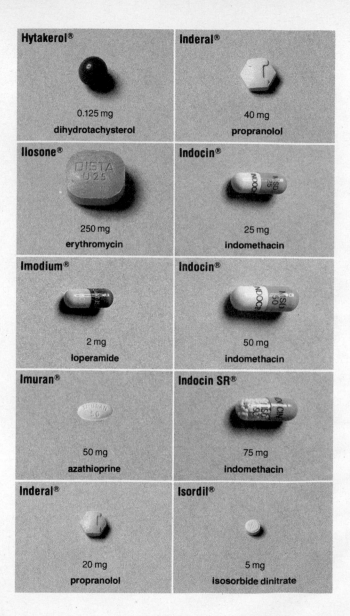

Hytakerol®

0.125 mg

dihydrotachysterol

Inderal®

40 mg

propranolol

Ilosone®

DISTA
U25

250 mg

erythromycin

Indocin®

ISD
INDOCIN 25

25 mg

indomethacin

Imodium®

2 mg

loperamide

Indocin®

INDOCIN MSD 50

50 mg

indomethacin

Imuran®

IMURAN 50

50 mg

azathioprine

Indocin SR®

INDOCIN MSD 693

75 mg

indomethacin

Inderal®

20 mg

propranolol

Isordil®

5 mg

isosorbide dinitrate

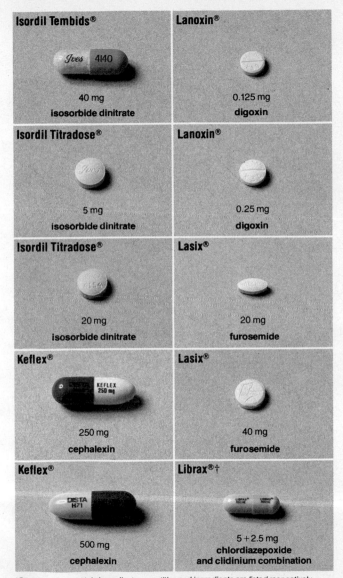

Isordil Tembids®

40 mg

isosorbide dinitrate

Isordil Titradose®

5 mg

isosorbide dinitrate

Isordil Titradose®

20 mg

isosorbide dinitrate

Keflex®

250 mg

cephalexin

Keflex®

500 mg

cephalexin

Lanoxin®

0.125 mg

digoxin

Lanoxin®

0.25 mg

digoxin

Lasix®

20 mg

furosemide

Lasix®

40 mg

furosemide

Librax®†

5 + 2.5 mg

chlordiazepoxide
and clidinium combination

†*Drug contains multiple ingredients; quantities and ingredients are listed respectively.*

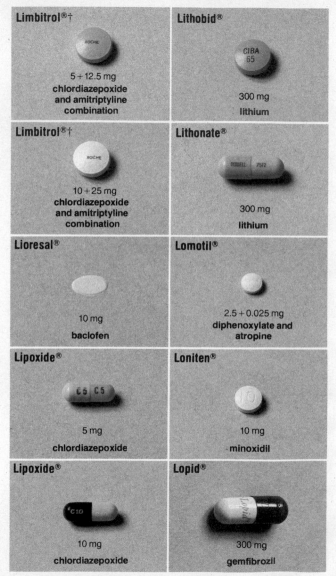

Limbitrol®†

5 + 12.5 mg
**chlordiazepoxide
and amitriptyline
combination**

Lithobid®

300 mg
lithium

Limbitrol®†

10 + 25 mg
**chlordiazepoxide
and amitriptyline
combination**

Lithonate®

300 mg
lithium

Lioresal®

10 mg
baclofen

Lomotil®

2.5 + 0.025 mg
**diphenoxylate and
atropine**

Lipoxide®

5 mg
chlordiazepoxide

Loniten®

10 mg
minoxidil

Lipoxide®

10 mg
chlordiazepoxide

Lopid®

300 mg
gemfibrozil

† Drug contains multiple ingredients; quantities and ingredients are listed respectively.

Lopressor® 50 mg metoprolol	**Ludiomil®** 50 mg maprotiline
Lopressor® 100 mg metoprolol	**Macrodantin®** 100 mg nitrofurantoin
Loxitane® 10 mg loxapine	**Mandelamine®** 1,000 mg methenamine
Loxitane® 25 mg loxapine	**Meclomen®** 50 mg meclofenamate
Ludiomil® 25 mg maprotiline	**Meclomen®** 100 mg meclofenamate

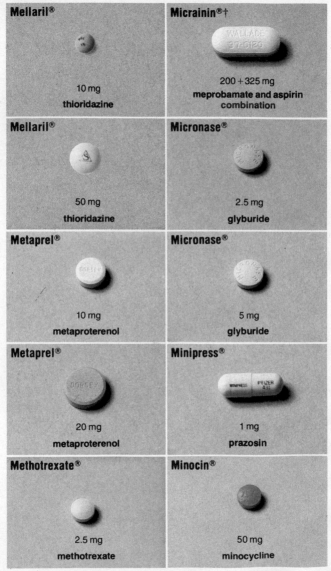

Mellaril®	**Micrainin®†**
10 mg	200 + 325 mg
thioridazine	meprobamate and aspirin combination

Mellaril®	**Micronase®**
50 mg	2.5 mg
thioridazine	glyburide

Metaprel®	**Micronase®**
10 mg	5 mg
metaproterenol	glyburide

Metaprel®	**Minipress®**
20 mg	1 mg
metaproterenol	prazosin

Methotrexate®	**Minocin®**
2.5 mg	50 mg
methotrexate	minocycline

† *Drug contains multiple ingredients; quantities and ingredients are listed respectively.*

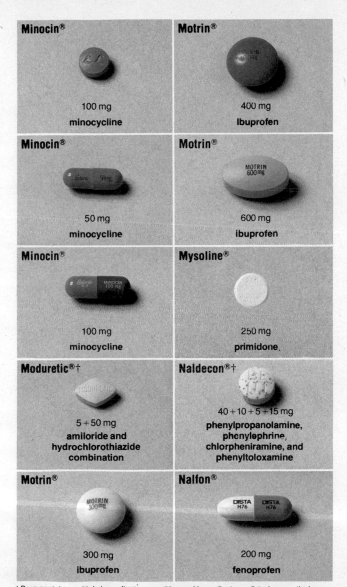

Minocin®	**Motrin®**
100 mg	400 mg
minocycline	Ibuprofen
Minocin®	**Motrin®**
50 mg	600 mg
minocycline	ibuprofen
Minocin®	**Mysoline®**
100 mg	250 mg
minocycline	primidone
Moduretic®†	**Naldecon®†**
5 + 50 mg	40 + 10 + 5 + 15 mg
amiloride and hydrochlorothiazide combination	phenylpropanolamine, phenylephrine, chlorpheniramine, and phenyltoloxamine
Motrin®	**Nalfon®**
300 mg	200 mg
ibuprofen	fenoprofen

†Drug contains multiple ingredients; quantities and ingredients are listed respectively.

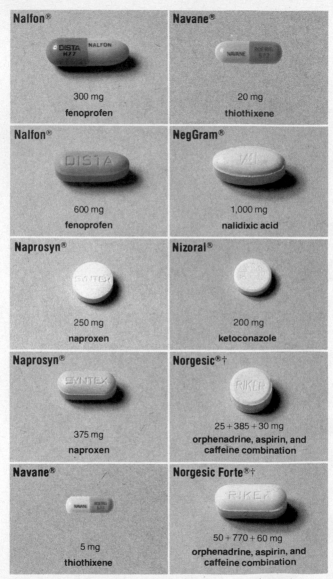

Nalfon®

300 mg

fenoprofen

Navane®

20 mg

thiothixene

Nalfon®

600 mg

fenoprofen

NegGram®

1,000 mg

nalidixic acid

Naprosyn®

250 mg

naproxen

Nizoral®

200 mg

ketoconazole

Naprosyn®

375 mg

naproxen

Norgesic®†

25 + 385 + 30 mg

orphenadrine, aspirin, and
caffeine combination

Navane®

5 mg

thiothixene

Norgesic Forte®†

50 + 770 + 60 mg

orphenadrine, aspirin, and
caffeine combination

† *Drug contains multiple ingredients; quantities and ingredients are listed respectively.*

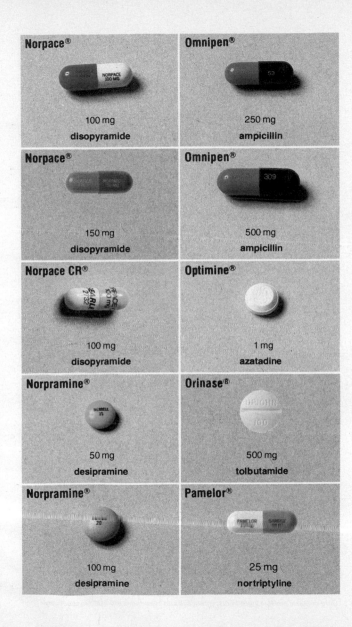

Norpace® 100 mg disopyramide	**Omnipen®** 250 mg ampicillin
Norpace® 150 mg disopyramide	**Omnipen®** 500 mg ampicillin
Norpace CR® 100 mg disopyramide	**Optimine®** 1 mg azatadine
Norpramine® 50 mg desipramine	**Orinase®** 500 mg tolbutamide
Norpramine® 100 mg desipramine	**Pamelor®** 25 mg nortriptyline

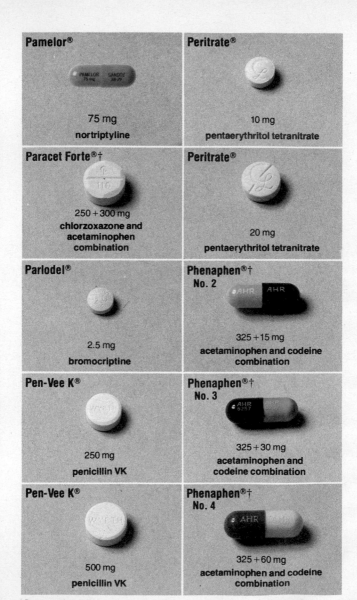

Pamelor®

75 mg

nortriptyline

Paracet Forte®†

250 + 300 mg

chlorzoxazone and
acetaminophen
combination

Parlodel®

2.5 mg

bromocriptine

Pen-Vee K®

250 mg

penicillin VK

Pen-Vee K®

500 mg

penicillin VK

Peritrate®

10 mg

pentaerythritol tetranitrate

Peritrate®

20 mg

pentaerythritol tetranitrate

**Phenaphen®†
No. 2**

325 + 15 mg

acetaminophen and codeine
combination

**Phenaphen®†
No. 3**

325 + 30 mg

acetaminophen and
codeine combination

**Phenaphen®†
No. 4**

325 + 60 mg

acetaminophen and codeine
combination

†Drug contains multiple ingredients; quantities and ingredients are listed respectively.

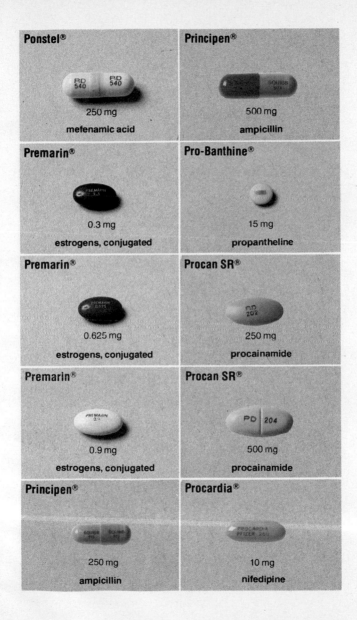

Ponstel®

250 mg

mefenamic acid

Principen®

500 mg

ampicillin

Premarin®

0.3 mg

estrogens, conjugated

Pro-Banthine®

15 mg

propantheline

Premarin®

0.625 mg

estrogens, conjugated

Procan SR®

250 mg

procainamide

Premarin®

0.9 mg

estrogens, conjugated

Procan SR®

500 mg

procainamide

Principen®

250 mg

ampicillin

Procardia®

10 mg

nifedipine

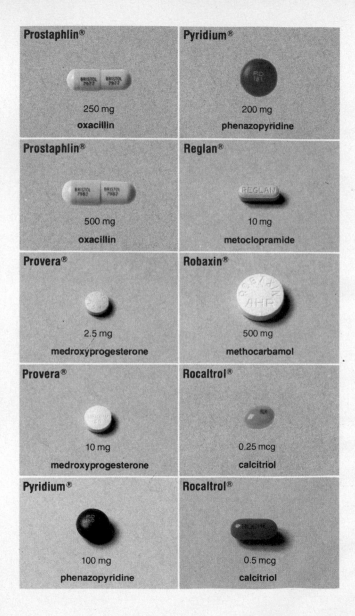

Prostaphlin®

250 mg

oxacillin

Prostaphlin®

500 mg

oxacillin

Provera®

2.5 mg

medroxyprogesterone

Provera®

10 mg

medroxyprogesterone

Pyridium®

100 mg

phenazopyridine

Pyridium®

200 mg

phenazopyridine

Reglan®

10 mg

metoclopramide

Robaxin®

500 mg

methocarbamol

Rocaltrol®

0.25 mcg

calcitriol

Rocaltrol®

0.5 mcg

calcitriol

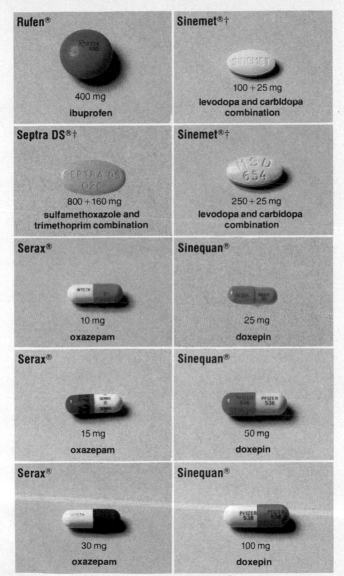

Rufen®

400 mg

ibuprofen

Sinemet®†

100 + 25 mg

levodopa and carbidopa
combination

Septra DS®†

800 + 160 mg

sulfamethoxazole and
trimethoprim combination

Sinemet®†

250 + 25 mg

levodopa and carbidopa
combination

Serax®

10 mg

oxazepam

Sinequan®

25 mg

doxepin

Serax®

15 mg

oxazepam

Sinequan®

50 mg

doxepin

Serax®

30 mg

oxazepam

Sinequan®

100 mg

doxepin

†Drug contains multiple ingredients; quantities and ingredients are listed respectively.

Slow-K®

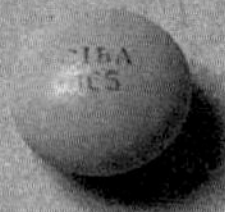

8 mEq

potassium chloride

Sumycin®

250 mg

tetracycline

Soma®

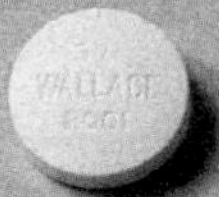

350 mg

carisoprodol

Symmetrel®

100 mg

amantadine

Sorbitrate®

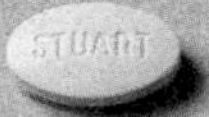

5 mg

isosorbide dinitrate

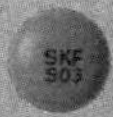

Synthroid®

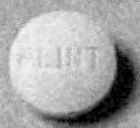

0.05 mg

levothyroxine

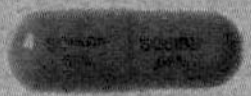

Sorbitrate®

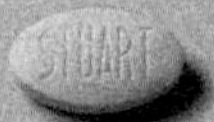

10 mg

isosorbide dinitrate

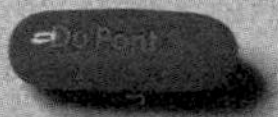

Synthroid®

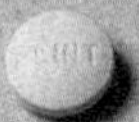

0.1 mg

levothyroxine

Stelazine®

1 mg

trifluoperazine

Synthroid®

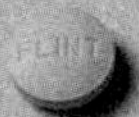

0.15 mg

levothyroxine

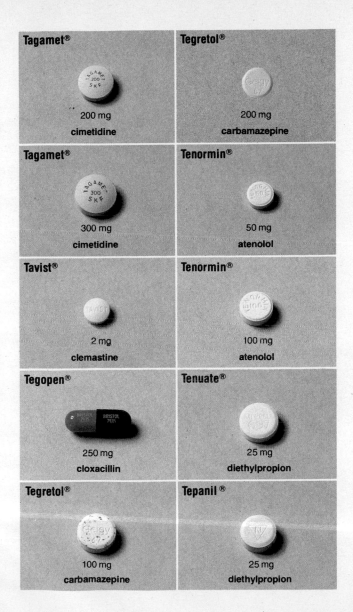

Tagamet®	Tegretol®
200 mg	200 mg
cimetidine	carbamazepine
Tagamet®	Tenormin®
300 mg	50 mg
cimetidine	atenolol
Tavist®	Tenormin®
2 mg	100 mg
clemastine	atenolol
Tegopen®	Tenuate®
250 mg	25 mg
cloxacillin	diethylpropion
Tegretol®	Tepanil®
100 mg	25 mg
carbamazepine	diethylpropion

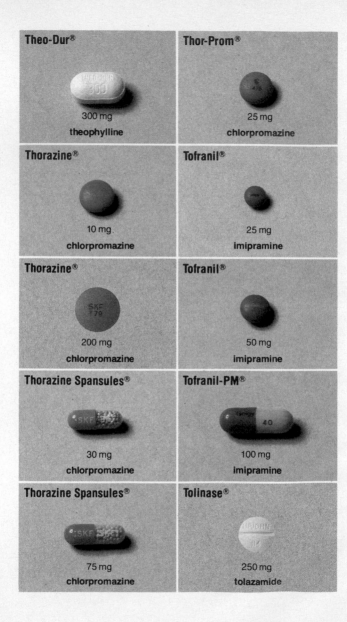

Theo-Dur®
300 mg
theophylline

Thor-Prom®
25 mg
chlorpromazine

Thorazine®
10 mg
chlorpromazine

Tofranil®
25 mg
imipramine

Thorazine®
200 mg
chlorpromazine

Tofranil®
50 mg
imipramine

Thorazine Spansules®
30 mg
chlorpromazine

Tofranil-PM®
100 mg
imipramine

Thorazine Spansules®
75 mg
chlorpromazine

Tolinase®
250 mg
tolazamide

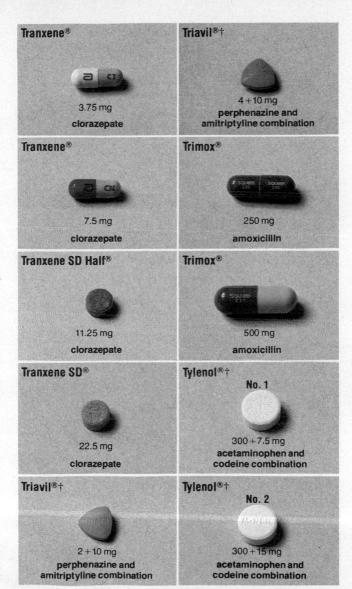

Tranxene®

3.75 mg

clorazepate

Tranxene®

7.5 mg

clorazepate

Tranxene SD Half®

11.25 mg

clorazepate

Tranxene SD®

22.5 mg

clorazepate

Triavil®†

2 + 10 mg

perphenazine and
amitriptyline combination

Triavil®†

4 + 10 mg

perphenazine and
amitriptyline combination

Trimox®

250 mg

amoxicillin

Trimox®

500 mg

amoxicillin

Tylenol®†

No. 1

300 + 7.5 mg

acetaminophen and
codeine combination

Tylenol®†

No. 2

300 + 15 mg

acetaminophen and
codeine combination

†Drug contains multiple ingredients; quantities and ingredients are listed respectively.

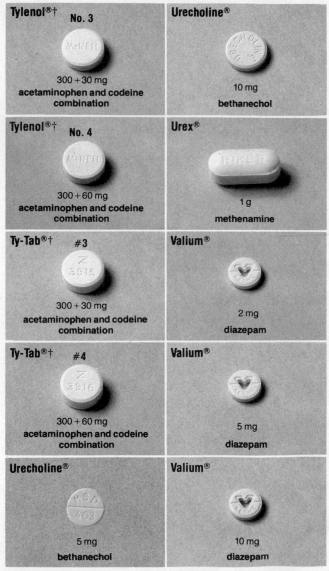

Tylenol®† No. 3
300 + 30 mg
acetaminophen and codeine combination

Urecholine®
10 mg
bethanechol

Tylenol®† No. 4
300 + 60 mg
acetaminophen and codeine combination

Urex®
1 g
methenamine

Ty-Tab®† #3
300 + 30 mg
acetaminophen and codeine combination

Valium®
2 mg
diazepam

Ty-Tab®† #4
300 + 60 mg
acetaminophen and codeine combination

Valium®
5 mg
diazepam

Urecholine®
5 mg
bethanechol

Valium®
10 mg
diazepam

† Drug contains multiple ingredients; quantities and ingredients are listed respectively.

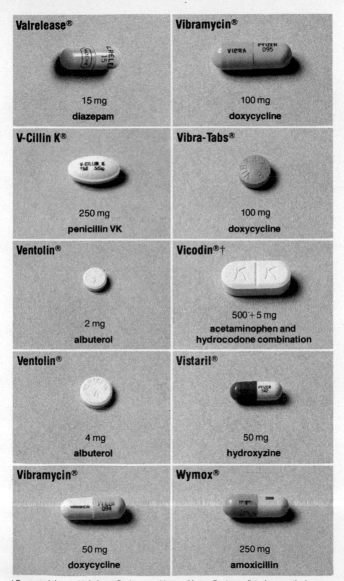

Valrelease®

15 mg

diazepam

Vibramycin®

100 mg

doxycycline

V-Cillin K®

250 mg

penicillin VK

Vibra-Tabs®

100 mg

doxycycline

Ventolin®

2 mg

albuterol

Vicodin®†

500 + 5 mg

acetaminophen and
hydrocodone combination

Ventolin®

4 mg

albuterol

Vistaril®

50 mg

hydroxyzine

Vibramycin®

50 mg

doxycycline

Wymox®

250 mg

amoxicillin

† *Drug contains multiple ingredients; quantities and ingredients are listed respectively.*

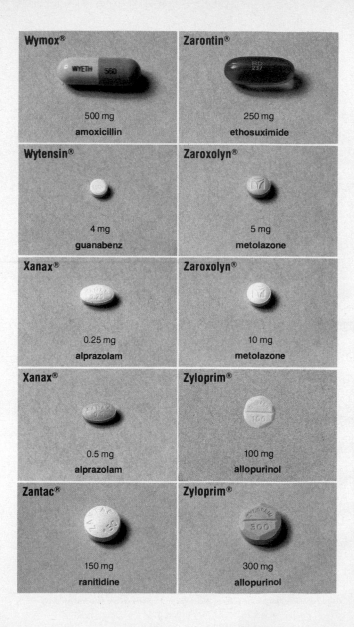

Wymox®

500 mg

amoxicillin

Zarontin®

250 mg

ethosuximide

Wytensin®

4 mg

guanabenz

Zaroxolyn®

5 mg

metolazone

Xanax®

0.25 mg

alprazolam

Zaroxolyn®

10 mg

metolazone

Xanax®

0.5 mg

alprazolam

Zyloprim®

100 mg

allopurinol

Zantac®

150 mg

ranitidine

Zyloprim®

300 mg

allopurinol

TYPE OF DRUG
Urinary tract analgesic (pain reliever)
INGREDIENT
phenazopyridine as the hydrochloride salt
DOSAGE FORM
Tablets (100 mg and 200 mg)
STORAGE
Phenazopyridine tablets should be stored at room temperature in a tightly closed, light-resistant container.

USES
Phenazopyridine is used for the symptomatic relief of the burning, pain, and discomfort caused by urinary tract infections or irritations. It is excreted in the urine, where it exerts a topical analgesic effect on the urinary tract. This medication is not useful for other types of pain.

TREATMENT
Phenazopyridine tablets should be taken with a full glass of water, either with meals or immediately after a meal.

If you miss a dose of this medication, take the missed dose as soon as possible, unless it is almost time for the next dose. In that case, do not take the missed dose at all; just return to your regular dosing schedule. Do not double the next dose.

SIDE EFFECTS
Minor. Dizziness; headache; indigestion; nausea; stomach cramps; and vomiting. These side effects should disappear in several days, as your body adjusts to the medication.

If you feel dizzy, sit or lie down awhile; get up slowly, and be careful on stairs.

Phenazopyridine causes your urine to become orange-red in color. This is not harmful; however, it may stain your clothing. The urine will return to its normal color soon after the drug is discontinued.

Major. Tell your doctor about any side effects that are persistent or particularly bothersome. IT IS ESPECIALLY IMPORTANT TO TELL YOUR DOCTOR about a bluish color of the skin or fingernails; skin rash; unusual fatigue; or yellowing of the eyes or skin.

INTERACTIONS

Phenazopyridine does not interact with other medications, as long as it is used according to directions.

WARNINGS

• Tell your doctor about unusual or allergic reactions you have had to any medications, especially to phenazopyridine.

• Tell your doctor if you now have, or if you have ever had, kidney disease.

• If this drug makes you dizzy, do not take part in any activity that requires alertness, such as driving a car or operating potentially dangerous equipment.

• Diabetic patients using this medication may get delayed reactions or false-positive readings for sugar or ketones with urine tests. Clinitest is not affected by this medication, but the other urine sugar tests are.

• Be sure to tell your doctor if you are pregnant. Although there are no reports of any problems with this drug during pregnancy in either humans or animals, extensive studies have not yet been completed. Also, tell your doctor if you are breastfeeding an infant. Small amounts of phenazopyridine may pass into breast milk.

phenazopyridine hydrochloride—see phenazopyridine

---

phendimetrazine

BRAND NAMES (Manufacturers)

Adipost (Ascher)
Adphen (Ferndale)
Anorex (Dunhall)
Bacarate (Reid-Provident)
Bontril PDM (Carnrick)
Di-Ap-Trol (Foy)
Dyrexan-OD (Trimen)
Hyrex 105 (Hyrex)
Limit (Bock)
Melfiat (Reid-Provident)
Metra (O'Neal)
Obalan (Lannett)

Obeval (Vale)
Obezine (Western Research)
PDM (Century)
phendimetrazine tartrate (various manufacturers)
Phenzine (Mallard)
Plegine (Ayerst)
Prelu-2 (Boehringer Ingelheim)
Slyn-LL (Edwards)
Sprx-1 (Reid-Provident)
Statobex (Lemmon)
Trimcaps (Maynard)
Trimstat (Laser)
Trimtabs (Maynard)
Weh-less (Hauck)
Weightrol (Vortech)

TYPE OF DRUG
Anorectic (appetite suppressant)

INGREDIENT
phendimetrazine as the hydrochloride salt

DOSAGE FORMS
Tablets (35 mg)
Capsules (35 mg)
Sustained-release capsules (105 mg)

STORAGE
Phendimetrazine should be stored at room temperature in tightly closed, light-resistant containers.

USES
Phendimetrazine is used as an appetite suppressant during the first few weeks of dieting, to help establish new eating habits. This medication is thought to relieve hunger by altering nerve impulses to the appetite control center in the brain. Its effectiveness lasts only for short periods (three to 12 weeks), however.

TREATMENT
You can take phendimetrazine with a full glass of water, one hour before meals (unless your doctor directs you to do otherwise).

The sustained-release form of this medication should be swallowed whole. Breaking, chewing, or crushing these capsules destroys their sustained-release activity, and may increase the side effects.

In order to avoid difficulty falling asleep, the last dose of this medication each day should be taken four to six hours (regular tablets) or ten to 14 hours (sustained-release capsules) before bedtime.

If you miss a dose of this medication, take the missed dose as soon as possible, unless it is almost time for your next dose. In this case, don't take the missed dose at all; just return to your regular dosing schedule. Do not double the next dose.

SIDE EFFECTS

Minor. Blurred vision; constipation; diarrhea; dizziness; dry mouth; false sense of well-being; fatigue; insomnia; irritability; nausea; nervousness; restlessness; stomach pain; sweating; tremors; unpleasant taste in the mouth; and vomiting. These side effects should disappear in several days, as your body adjusts to the medication.

Dry mouth can be relieved by sucking on ice chips or a piece of hard candy, or by chewing sugarless gum.

In order to prevent constipation, increase the amount of fiber in your diet (raw vegetables, fruits, salads, bran, and whole-grain breads), and drink more water (unless your doctor tells you not to do so).

Major. Tell your doctor about any side effects that are persistent or particularly bothersome. IT IS ESPECIALLY IMPORTANT TO TELL YOUR DOCTOR about changes in sexual desire; chest pain; difficulty urinating; enlarged breasts (in either sex); fever; hair loss; headaches; impotence; menstrual irregularities; mental depression; mood changes; mouth sores; muscle pains; palpitations; rash; sore throat; or unusual bleeding or bruising.

INTERACTIONS

Phendimetrazine interacts with several other types of medication.

1. Use of it within 14 days of a monoamine oxidase (MAO) inhibitor (isocarboxazid, pargyline, phenelzine, tranylcypromine) can result in high blood pressure and other side effects.

2. Barbiturate medications and phenothiazine tranquil-

izers (especially chlorpromazine) can antagonize (act against) the appetite suppressant activity of this medication.
3. Phendimetrazine can decrease the blood-pressure-lowering effects of antihypertensive medications (especially guanethidine), and may alter insulin and oral antidiabetic medication dosage requirements in diabetic patients.
4. The side effects of other central nervous system stimulants, such as caffeine, over-the-counter (non-prescription) appetite suppressants, or cough, allergy, asthma, sinus, or cold preparations, may be increased by this medication.
Before starting to take phendimetrazine, TELL YOUR DOCTOR if you are already taking any of the medications listed above.

WARNINGS

• Tell your doctor about unusual or allergic reactions you have had to any medications, especially to phendimetrazine or other appetite suppressants (such as benzphetamine, phenmetrazine, diethylpropion, fenfluramine, mazindol, or phentermine), or to epinephrine, norepinephrine, ephedrine, amphetamines, dextroamphetamine, phenylephrine, phenylpropanolamine, pseudoephedrine, albuterol, metaproterenol, or terbutaline.
• Tell your doctor if you now have, or if you have ever had, angina (chest pain); diabetes mellitus (sugar diabetes); emotional disturbances; glaucoma; heart or cardiovascular disease; high blood pressure; thyroid disease; or a history of drug abuse.
• Phendimetrazine can mask the symptoms of extreme fatigue, and can cause dizziness or light-headedness. Your ability to perform tasks that require alertness, such as driving a car or operating potentially dangerous machinery, may be decreased. Appropriate caution should therefore be taken.
• Before having any surgery or other medical or dental treatment, be sure to tell your doctor or dentist that you are taking this medication.
• Phendimetrazine is related to amphetamine and may be habit-forming when taken for long periods of time (both physical and psychological dependence can occur).

You should not increase the dosage of this medication or take it for longer than 12 weeks, unless you first consult your doctor. It is also important that you not stop taking this medication abruptly—fatigue, sleep disorders, mental depression, nausea, vomiting, or stomach cramps or pain could occur. Your doctor may therefore want to decrease your dosage gradually.

● Be sure to tell your doctor if you are pregnant. Although studies of phendimetrazine in humans have not yet been completed, some of the appetite suppressants have been shown to cause side effects in the fetuses of animals who received large doses during pregnancy. Also, tell your doctor if you are breastfeeding an infant. It is not known whether or not this medication passes into breast milk.

phendimetrazine tartrate—see phendimetrazine

---

phenelzine

BRAND NAME (Manufacturer)
Nardil (Parke-Davis)
TYPE OF DRUG
Monoamine oxidase inhibitor (anti-depressant)
INGREDIENT
phenelzine as the sulfate salt
DOSAGE FORM
Tablets (15 mg)
STORAGE
Phenelzine should be stored at room temperature, in a tightly closed, light-resistant container.

USES
This medication is used to treat depression. Phenelzine belongs to a group of drugs known as monoamine oxidase (MAO) inhibitors. It is not clearly understood how phenelzine works, but it is thought to increase the amounts of certain chemicals in the brain that act to relieve depression.

TREATMENT
You can take phenelzine either on an empty stomach or,

to avoid stomach irritation, with food or milk (as directed by your doctor).

If you are taking a single daily dose, it is best to take the dose in the morning, in order to avoid sleeping difficulties.

If you miss a dose of this medication and remember within two hours of the scheduled time, take the missed dose immediately. If more than two hours have passed, do not take the missed dose at all; just return to your regular dosing schedule. Do not double the next dose.

The full therapeutic benefits of this medication may not be observed for up to four weeks after you start to take it.

SIDE EFFECTS

Minor. Constipation; diarrhea; dizziness; drowsiness; dry mouth; fatigue; headache; insomnia; nausea; restlessness; stomach upset; sweating; and weakness. These side effects should disappear in several weeks, as your body adjusts to the medication.

If you feel dizzy, sit or lie down awhile; get up slowly, and be careful on stairs.

To relieve constipation, increase the amount of fiber in your diet (bran, salads, fresh fruits and vegetables, and whole-grain breads), exercise, and drink more water (unless your doctor directs you to do otherwise).

To relieve mouth dryness, chew sugarless gum, or suck on ice chips or a piece of hard candy.

Phenelzine can increase your sensitivity to sunlight. You should therefore avoid prolonged exposure to sunlight and sunlamps. Wear protective clothing and sunglasses, and use an effective sunscreen.

Major. Tell your doctor about any side effects that are persistent or particularly bothersome. IT IS ESPECIALLY IMPORTANT TO TELL YOUR DOCTOR about anxiety; blurred vision; chills; confusion; convulsions; darkened tongue; difficult or painful urination; fainting; false sense of well-being; hallucinations; jitteriness; mental disorders; palpitations; rapid weight gain (three to five pounds within a week); ringing in the ears; changes in sexual ability; uncoordination; or yellowing of the eyes or skin.

If you experience a severe headache, stiff neck, chest pains, palpitations, or vomiting while taking this medication, CONTACT YOUR DOCTOR OR AN EMERGENCY

ROOM IMMEDIATELY. These symptoms may be the result of a food or drug interaction.

INTERACTIONS

Phenelzine interacts with a number of drugs and foods.

1. Concurrent use of phenelzine with central nervous system depressants (drugs that slow the activity of the brain and spinal cord), such as alcohol, barbiturates, benzodiazepine tranquilizers, muscle relaxants, narcotics, pain medications, phenothiazine tranquilizers, and sleeping medications, or with tricyclic anti-depressants can lead to extreme drowsiness.

2. The dosage of anti-convulsion medication may need to be adjusted when phenelzine is started.

3. The use of phenelzine within 14 days of tricyclic anti-depressants, carbamazepine, cyclobenzaprine, other monoamine oxidase inhibitors, methyldopa, guanethidine, reserpine, levodopa, meperidine or other narcotics, amphetamines, ephedrine, methylphenidate, phenylpropanolamine, or pseudoephedrine can lead to serious, and sometimes fatal, side effects.

4. Tyramine-containing foods and beverages (aged cheeses, sour cream, yogurt, pickled herring, chicken livers, canned figs, raisins, bananas, avocados, soy sauce, broad bean pods, yeast extracts, beer, and certain wines); excessive amounts of caffeine-containing beverages (coffee, tea, cola); or chocolate can also cause serious reactions in patients on phenelzine therapy.

5. Phenelzine can increase the blood-sugar-lowering effects of insulin and oral anti-diabetic medications.

Before starting to take this medication, BE SURE TO TELL YOUR DOCTOR if you are already taking any of the medications listed above. Be sure you are aware of the foods that interact with phenelzine.

WARNINGS

• Tell your doctor about unusual or allergic reactions you have had to any medications, especially to phenelzine.

• Before starting to take this medication, be sure to tell your doctor if you now have, or if you have ever had, asthma, bronchitis, diabetes mellitus (sugar diabetes), epilepsy, glaucoma, severe headaches, heart or blood vessel disease, kidney disease, liver disease, mental disorders, Parkinson's disease, pheochromocytoma, or thyroid disease.

● If this drug makes you dizzy or drowsy, do not take part in any activities that require alertness, such as driving a car or operating potentially dangerous equipment.

● Before having any surgery or other medical or dental treatment, be sure your doctor or dentist knows that you are taking this medication.

● Check with your doctor or pharmacist before taking any over-the-counter (non-prescription) asthma, allergy, cough, cold, diet, or sinus preparations. Concurrent use of some of these products with phenelzine can lead to serious side effects.

● If you also have angina, do not increase your amount of physical activity unless you first check with your doctor. Phenelzine can decrease the symptoms of angina without decreasing the risks of strenuous exercise.

● Be sure to tell your doctor if you are pregnant. Studies in animals have shown that phenelzine can cause birth defects if it is taken in high doses during pregnancy. Studies in humans have not yet been completed. Also, tell your doctor if you are breastfeeding an infant. Small amounts of phenelzine may pass into breast milk.

Phenergan Expectorant with Codeine—see promethazine, potassium guaiacolsulfonate, and codeine combination

Phenergan VC with Codeine—see phenylephrine, potassium guaiacolsulfonate, promethazine, and codeine combination

Phenetron—see chlorpheniramine

---

phenmetrazine

BRAND NAME (Manufacturer)
Preludin (Boehringer Ingelheim)
TYPE OF DRUG
Anorectic (appetite suppressant)

INGREDIENT
phenmetrazine as the hydrochloride salt
DOSAGE FORMS
Tablets (25 mg)
Sustained-release tablets (50 mg and 75 mg)
STORAGE
Phenmetrazine should be stored at room temperature in tightly closed, light-resistant containers.

USES
Phenmetrazine is used as an appetite suppressant during the first few weeks of dieting, to help establish new eating habits. This medication is thought to relieve hunger by altering nerve impulses to the appetite control center in the brain. Its effectiveness lasts only for short periods (three to 12 weeks), however.

TREATMENT
You can take phenmetrazine with a full glass of water one hour before meals (unless your doctor directs you to do otherwise).

The sustained-release form of this medication should be swallowed whole. Breaking, chewing, or crushing these tablets destroys their sustained-release activity, and may increase the side effects.

In order to avoid difficulty falling asleep, the last dose of this medication each day should be taken four to six hours (regular tablets) or ten to 14 hours (sustained-release tablets) before bedtime.

If you miss a dose of this medication, take the missed dose as soon as possible, unless it is almost time for your next dose. In that case, don't take the missed dose at all; just return to your regular dosing schedule. Do not double the next dose.

SIDE EFFECTS
Minor. Blurred vision; constipation; diarrhea; dizziness; dry mouth; false sense of well-being; fatigue; insomnia; irritability; nausea; nervousness; restlessness; stomach pain; sweating; tremors; unpleasant taste in the mouth; and vomiting. These side effects should disappear in several days, as your body adjusts to the medication.

Dry mouth can be relieved by sucking on ice chips or a piece of hard candy, or by chewing sugarless gum.

In order to prevent constipation, increase the amount of fiber in your diet (raw vegetables, fruits, salads, bran, and whole-grain breads), and drink more water (unless your doctor tells you not to do so)

Major. Tell your doctor about any side effects that are persistent or particularly bothersome. IT IS ESPECIALLY IMPORTANT TO TELL YOUR DOCTOR about changes in sexual desire; chest pain; difficulty urinating; enlarged breasts (in either sex); fever; hair loss; headaches; impotence; menstrual irregularities; mental depression; mood changes; mouth sores; muscle pains; palpitations; rash; sore throat; or unusual bleeding or bruising.

INTERACTIONS

Phenmetrazine interacts with several other medications.

1. Use of it within 14 days of a monoamine oxidase (MAO) inhibitor (isocarboxazid, pargyline, phenelzine, tranylcypromine) can result in high blood pressure and other side effects.

2. Barbiturate medications and phenothiazine tranquilizers (especially chlorpromazine) can antagonize (act against) the appetite suppressant activity of this medication.

3. Phenmetrazine can decrease the blood-pressure-lowering effects of anti-hypertensive medications (especially guanethidine), and may alter insulin and oral anti-diabetic medication dosage requirements in diabetic patients.

4. The side effects of other central nervous system stimulants, such as caffeine, over-the-counter (non-prescription) appetite suppressants, or cough, cold, sinus, asthma, or allergy preparations, may be increased by this medication.

TELL YOUR DOCTOR if you are already taking any of the medications listed above.

WARNINGS

● Tell your doctor about unusual or allergic reactions you have had to any medications, especially to phenmetrazine or other appetite suppressants (such as benzphetamine, phendimetrazine, diethylpropion, fenfluramine, mazindol, or phentermine), or to epinephrine, norepinephrine, ephedrine, amphetamines, dextroamphetamine, phenylephrine, phenylpropanolamine, pseudoephedrine, albuterol, metaproterenol, or terbutaline.

● Tell your doctor if you now have, or if you have ever had, angina (chest pain); diabetes mellitus (sugar diabetes); emotional disturbances; glaucoma; heart or cardiovascular disease; high blood pressure; thyroid disease; or a history of drug abuse.

● Phenmetrazine can mask the symptoms of extreme fatigue, and can cause dizziness or light-headedness. Your ability to perform tasks that require alertness, such as driving a car or operating potentially dangerous machinery, may be decreased. Appropriate caution should therefore be taken.

● Before having any surgery or other medical or dental treatment, be sure to tell your doctor or dentist that you are taking this medication.

● Phenmetrazine is related to amphetamine and may be habit-forming when taken for long periods of time (both physical and psychological dependence can occur). Therefore, you should not increase your dosage of this medication or take it for longer than 12 weeks, unless you first consult your doctor. It is also important that you not stop taking this medication abruptly—fatigue, sleep disorders, mental depression, nausea or vomiting, or stomach cramps or pain could occur. Your doctor may want to decrease the dosage gradually in order to prevent these side effects.

● Be sure to tell your doctor if you are pregnant. Although studies of phenmetrazine in humans have not yet been completed, some of the appetite suppressants have been shown to cause side effects in the fetuses of animals who received large doses during pregnancy. Also, tell your doctor if you are breastfeeding an infant. It is not known whether or not this medication passes into breast milk.

phenobarbital

BRAND NAMES (Manufacturers)
Barbita (Vortech)

Luminal Ovoids (Winthrop)
PBR-12 (Scott-Alison)
phenobarbital (various manufacturers)
Sedadrops (Merrell Dow)
SK-Phenobarbital (Smith Kline & French)
Solfoton (Poythress)

TYPE OF DRUG

Sedative and anti-convulsant

INGREDIENT

phenobarbital

DOSAGE FORMS

Tablets (8 mg, 15 mg, 16 mg, 30 mg, 32 mg, 65 mg, and
  100 mg)
Capsules (16 mg)
Sustained-release capsules (65 mg)
Oral liquid (15 mg and 20 mg per 5 ml teaspoonful)
Pediatric drops (16 mg per ml)

STORAGE

Phenobarbital tablets and capsules should be stored at
room temperature in tightly closed containers. The oral
liquid and pediatric drops should be stored at room temperature in tightly closed, light-resistant containers. Phenobarbital liquid should not be used if the solution
becomes cloudy—it is no longer effective. This medication should never be frozen.

USES

Phenobarbital is used to control convulsions, to relieve
anxiety or tension, and as a sleeping aid. Phenobarbital
belongs to a group of drugs known as barbiturates. The
barbiturates are central nervous system (brain and spinal
cord) depressants (drugs that slow the activity of the nervous system).

TREATMENT

In order to avoid stomach irritation, you should take phenobarbital with food or with a full glass of water or milk.
  The pediatric drops and oral liquid should be measured
carefully, with the dropper provided or with a specially designed, 5 ml measuring spoon. An ordinary kitchen teaspoon is not accurate enough. The liquid dose can be
taken straight, or diluted with water, milk, or fruit juice.

The sustained-release capsules should be swallowed whole. Chewing, crushing, or breaking these capsules destroys their sustained-release activity, and may increase the side effects.

If phenobarbital is being taken as a sleeping aid, take it 30 to 60 minutes before you want to go to sleep.

If you are taking this medication for the treatment of seizures, phenobarbital works best when the level of medicine in your bloodstream is kept constant. It is best therefore to take it at evenly spaced intervals, day and night. For example, if you are to take three doses a day, the doses should be spaced eight hours apart.

If you are taking this medication on a regular basis and you miss a dose, take the missed dose as soon as possible (if you remember within an hour). Then return to your regular dosing schedule. If more than an hour has passed, do not take the missed dose at all; just return to your regular dosing schedule. Do not double the next dose. If you are taking this medication to control seizures and you miss more than two doses, contact your doctor.

SIDE EFFECTS

Minor. Constipation; diarrhea; dizziness, drowsiness, headache; a "hangover" feeling; muscle or joint pain; nausea; stomach upset; and vomiting. These side effects should disappear in several days, as your body adjusts to the medication.

If you feel dizzy or light-headed, sit or lie down awhile; get up slowly, and be careful on stairs.

To relieve constipation, increase the amount of fiber in your diet (fresh fruits and vegetables, bran, salads, and whole-grain breads), exercise, and drink more water (unless your doctor directs you to do otherwise).

Major. Tell your doctor about any side effects that are persistent or particularly bothersome. IT IS ESPECIALLY IMPORTANT TO TELL YOUR DOCTOR about chest tightness; confusion; depression; difficulty breathing; excitation; fatigue; feeling faint; hives or itching; loss of coordination; skin rash; slurred speech; sore throat; unusual bleeding or bruising; unusual weakness; or yellowing of the eyes or skin.

INTERACTIONS

Phenobarbital interacts with several other types of medication.

1. Concurrent use of it with other central nervous system depressants (such as antihistamines, benzodiazepine tranquilizers, muscle relaxants, narcotics, pain medications, phenothiazine tranquilizers, sleeping medications, and alcohol) or with tricyclic anti-depressants can cause extreme drowsiness.

2. Valproic acid, chloramphenicol, and monoamine oxidase (MAO) inhibitors can prolong the effects of the barbiturates.

3. Phenobarbital can increase the elimination from the body, and decrease the effectiveness, of oral anti-coagulants (blood thinners, such as warfarin), digoxin, tricyclic anti-depressants, cortisone-like medications, doxycycline, quinidine, estrogens, birth control pills, phenytoin, acetaminophen, and carbamazepine.

4. Phenobarbital can decrease the absorption of griseofulvin from the gastrointestinal tract.

5. The combination of phenobarbital and furosemide can cause low blood pressure and fainting.

6. Phenobarbital can increase the side effects of cyclophosphamide or large doses of acetaminophen.

BE SURE TO TELL YOUR DOCTOR if you are already taking any of the medications listed above.

WARNINGS

● Tell your doctor about unusual or allergic reactions you have had to any medications, especially to phenobarbital or other barbiturates (such as amobarbital, butabarbital, mephobarbital, pentobarbital, primidone, and secobarbital).

● Tell your doctor if you now have, or if you have ever had, acute or chronic (long-term) pain; Addison's disease (an underactive adrenal gland); diabetes mellitus (sugar diabetes); kidney disease; liver disease; lung disease; mental depression; porphyria; or thyroid disease.

● Before having any surgery or other medical or dental treatment, be sure to tell your doctor or dentist that you are taking this medication.

● If this medication makes you dizzy or drowsy, do not

take part in any activity that requires alertness, such as driving a car or operating potentially dangerous equipment.

● This drug has the potential for abuse, and must be used with caution. Tolerance develops quickly; do not increase the dosage or stop taking this drug unless you first consult your doctor. If you have been taking this drug for a long time or have been taking large doses, you may experience anxiety; muscle twitching; tremors; weakness; dizziness; nausea; vomiting; insomnia; or blurred vision when you stop taking it. Your doctor may therefore want to reduce your dosage gradually.

● Some of these products contain F.D. & C. Yellow Dye No. 5 (tartrazine), which can cause allergic-type reactions (difficulty breathing, rash, or fainting) in certain susceptible individuals.

● Be sure to tell your doctor if you are pregnant. Phenobarbital crosses the placenta, and birth defects have been associated with the use of this medication during pregnancy. If phenobarbital is used during the last three months of the pregnancy, there is a chance that the infant will be born addicted to the medication and will experience a withdrawal reaction (seizures and irritability) at birth. The infant could also be born with bleeding problems. The risks and benefits of treatment should be discussed with your doctor. Also, tell your doctor if you are breastfeeding an infant. Small amounts of phenobarbital pass into breast milk and may cause excessive drowsiness in the nursing infant.

Phentamine——see phentermine

phentermine

BRAND NAMES (Manufacturers)
Adipex-P (Lemmon)
Fastin (Beecham)
Ionamin (Pennwalt)
Obe-Nix (Holloway)
Obephen (Mallard)
Obermine (O'Neal)

Obestin-30 (Ferndale)
Parmine (Parmed)
Phentamine (Major)
phentermine hydrochloride (various manufacturers)
Phentrol (Vortech)
Unifast Unicelles (Reid-Provident)
Wilpowr (Foy)

TYPE OF DRUG

Anorectic (appetite suppressant)

INGREDIENT

phentermine as the hydrochloride salt or resin complex

DOSAGE FORMS

Tablets (8 mg, 15 mg, 30 mg, and 37.5 mg)
Capsules (8 mg, 15 mg, 30 mg, and 37.5 mg)

STORAGE

Phentermine should be stored at room temperature in tightly closed, light-resistant containers.

USES

Phentermine is used as an appetite suppressant during the first few weeks of dieting, to help establish new eating habits. This medication is thought to relieve hunger by altering nerve impulses to the appetite control center in the brain. Its effectiveness lasts only for short periods (three to 12 weeks), however.

TREATMENT

You can take phentermine with a full glass of water one hour before meals (unless your doctor directs you to do otherwise).

In order to avoid difficulty falling asleep, the last dose of this medication each day should be taken four to six hours before bedtime.

If you miss a dose of this medication, take the missed dose as soon as possible, unless it is almost time for your next dose. In that case, don't take the missed dose at all; just return to your regular dosing schedule. Do not double the next dose.

SIDE EFFECTS

Minor. Blurred vision; constipation; diarrhea; dizziness; dry mouth; false sense of well-being; fatigue; insomnia; ir ritability; nausea; nervousness; restlessness; stomach pain; sweating; tremors; unpleasant taste in the mouth; and vomiting. These side effects should disappear in several days, as your body adjusts to the medication.

Dry mouth can be relieved by sucking on ice chips or a piece of hard candy, or by chewing sugarless gum.

In order to prevent constipation, increase the amount of fiber in your diet (raw vegetables, fruits, salads, bran, and whole-grain breads) and drink more water (unless your doctor tells you not to do so).

Major. Tell your doctor about any side effects that are persistent or particularly bothersome. IT IS ESPECIALLY IMPORTANT TO TELL YOUR DOCTOR about changes in sexual desire; chest pain; difficulty urinating; enlarged breasts (in both sexes); fever; hair loss; headaches; impotence; menstrual irregularities; mental depression; mood changes; mouth sores; muscle pains; palpitations; rash; or sore throat.

INTERACTIONS

Phentermine interacts with other types of medication.

1. Use of it within 14 days of a monoamine oxidase (MAO) inhibitor (isocarboxazid, pargyline, phenelzine, tranylcypromine) can result in high blood pressure and other side effects.

2. Barbiturate medications and phenothiazine tranquilizers (especially chlorpromazine) can antagonize (act against) the appetite suppressant activity of this medication.

3. Phentermine can decrease the blood-pressure-lowering effects of anti-hypertensive medications (especially guanethidine), and may alter insulin and oral anti-diabetic medication dosage requirements in diabetic patients.

4. The side effects of other central nervous system stimulants, such as caffeine, over-the-counter (non-prescription) appetite suppressants, or cough, cold, sinus, asthma, or allergy preparations, may be increased by this medication. TELL YOUR DOCTOR if you are already taking any of the medications listed above.

WARNINGS

• Tell your doctor about unusual or allergic reactions you

have had to any medications, especially to phentermine or other appetite suppressants (such as benzphetamine, phendimetrazine, diethylpropion, fenfluramine, mazindol, or phenmetrazine), or to epinephrine, norepinephrine, ephedrine, amphetamines, dextroamphetamine, phenylephrine, phenylpropanolamine, pseudoephedrine, albuterol, metaproterenol, or terbutaline.

● Tell your doctor if you now have, or if you have ever had, angina (chest pain); diabetes mellitus (sugar diabetes); emotional disturbances; glaucoma; heart or cardiovascular disease; high blood pressure; thyroid disease; or a history of drug abuse.

● Phentermine can mask the symptoms of extreme fatigue, and can cause dizziness or light-headedness. Your ability to perform tasks that require alertness, such as driving a car or operating potentially dangerous machinery, may be decreased. Appropriate caution should therefore be taken.

● Before having any surgery or other medical or dental treatment, be sure to tell your doctor or dentist that you are taking this medication.

● Phentermine is related to amphetamine and may be habit-forming when taken for long periods of time (both physical and psychological dependence can occur). You should therefore not increase the dosage of this medication or take it for longer than 12 weeks, unless you first consult your doctor. It is also important that you not stop taking this medication abruptly—fatigue, sleep disorders, mental depression, nausea, vomiting, or stomach cramps or pain could occur. Your doctor may therefore want to decrease your dosage gradually.

● Be sure to tell your doctor if you are pregnant. Although studies of phentermine in humans have not yet been completed, some of the appetite suppressants have been shown to cause side effects in the fetuses of animals who received large doses during pregnancy. Also, tell your doctor if you are breastfeeding an infant. It is not known whether or not this medication passes into breast milk.

phentermine hydrochloride—see phentermine

Phentrol—see phentermine

phenylbutazone

BRAND NAMES (Manufacturers)
Azolid (USV)
Butazolidin (Geigy)
phenylbutazone (various manufacturers)
TYPE OF DRUG
Non-steroidal anti-inflammatory analgesic (pain reliever)
INGREDIENT
phenylbutazone
DOSAGE FORMS
Tablets (100 mg)
Capsules (100 mg)
STORAGE
Phenylbutazone tablets and capsules should be stored at
room temperature in tightly closed containers.

USES

Phenylbutazone is used to reduce pain, redness, and
swelling due to arthritis or thrombophlebitis. It is not
clearly understood how phenylbutazone works, but it is
thought to relieve pain and inflammation by blocking the
production of substances that sensitize pain receptors or
of substances responsible for an inflammatory response.

TREATMENT

In order to avoid stomach upset, you can take phenylbutazone with food or with a full glass of water or milk. Ask
your doctor if you can take phenylbutazone with an antacid.

If you miss a dose of this medication, and you are taking
it once or twice a day, take the missed dose as soon as possible, unless it is almost time for the next dose. In that
case, don't take the missed dose at all; just return to your
regular dosing schedule. Do not double the next dose.

If you are taking phenylbutazone three or more times
per day, and you miss a dose, take the missed dose right
away (if you remember within an hour of the correct time);
then take the next dose as scheduled. If more than an hour
has passed, however, don't take the missed dose at all; just
return to your regular schedule. Do not double the next
dose.

SIDE EFFECTS

Minor. Abdominal pain; bloating; constipation; diarrhea; drowsiness; gas; headache; heartburn; indigestion; irritability; nausea; numbness; vomiting; and weakness These side effects should disappear in several days, as your body adjusts to the medication.

Acetaminophen may be helpful in relieving headaches.

To relieve constipation, increase the amount of fiber in your diet (fresh fruits and vegetables, bran, salads, and whole-grain breads), exercise, and drink more water (unless your doctor directs you to do otherwise).

Major. Tell your doctor about any side effects that are persistent or particularly bothersome. IT IS ESPECIALLY IMPORTANT TO TELL YOUR DOCTOR about bloody or black, tarry stools; blurred vision; confusion; depression; difficulty breathing; difficulty hearing; difficult or painful urination; fatigue; fever; itching; mouth sores; rash; ringing in the ears; severe abdominal pain; sore throat; swelling of the ankles; tremors; unusual bleeding or bruising; weight gain of more than three pounds within a week; or yellowing of the eyes or skin.

INTERACTIONS

Phenylbutazone interacts with several other types of medication.

1. It can increase the kidney side effects of penicillamine; increase the skin reactions of chloroquine, gold compounds, and hydroxychloroquine, and increase the effects on the blood of anti-neoplastics (anti-cancer medicines), chloramphenicol, colchicine, gold compounds, pyrimethamine, and trimethoprim.

2. Alcohol and anti-inflammatory medicines can increase the gastrointestinal side effects of phenylbutazone.

3. Phenylbutazone can decrease the blood levels and effectiveness of digitoxin.

4. The active blood levels and side effects of oral anti-coagulants (blood thinners, such as warfarin), oral anti-diabetic medicines, methotrexate, and phenytoin can be increased by phenylbutazone.

Before starting to take this medication, BE SURE TO TELL YOUR DOCTOR if you are already taking any of the medications listed above.

WARNINGS

- Tell your doctor about unusual or allergic reactions you have had to any medications, especially to phenylbutazone or other non-steroidal, anti-inflammatory medications (such as aspirin, diflunisal, fenoprofen, ibuprofen, indomethacin, meclofenamate, mefenamic acid, naproxen, oxyphenbutazone, sulfinpyrazone, sulindac, tolmetin, and zomepirac).
- Tell your doctor if you now have, or if you have ever had, anemia, blood disorders, heart disease, hypertension, inflamed salivary glands, kidney disease, liver disease, mouth sores, pancreatitis, peptic ulcers, polymyalgia rheumatica, stomach problems, temporal arteritis, or thyroid disease.
- Use of this drug has been associated with leukemia, although there is no definite proof that the drug causes the disease.
- If phenylbutazone makes you dizzy or drowsy, avoid activities that require alertness, such as driving a car or operating potentially dangerous equipment.
- Because phenylbutazone can prolong your bleeding time, it is important to tell your doctor or dentist that you are taking this drug, before having any surgery or other medical or dental treatment.
- This medication can cause serious blood disorders. Therefore, it should never be used for trivial aches or pains.
- This drug should be used for a short time only. Follow your doctor's directions exactly, and never exceed the recommended dosage.
- Some of these products contain F.D. & C. Yellow Dye No. 5 (tartrazine), which can cause allergic-type symptoms (shortness of breath, rash, fainting) in certain susceptible individuals.
- Be sure to tell your doctor if you are pregnant. Although studies in humans have not yet been completed, unwanted effects have been reported in the offspring of animals that received large doses of this drug during pregnancy. If taken late in pregnancy, phenylbutazone can also prolong labor. Also, tell your doctor if you are breastfeeding an infant. Small doses of phenylbutazone pass into breast milk.

phenylephrine, phenylpropanolamine, brompheniramine, and guaifenesin combination

BRAND NAMES (Manufacturers)
Bromphen Expectorant (Rugby)
Dimetane Expectorant (Robins)
Midatane Expectorant (Vangard)
Normatane Expectorant (Vortech)
Puretane Expectorant (Purepac)
Rotane Expectorant (Three P Products)
Tamine Expectorant (Geneva Generics)
Triphen Expectorant (Bay)

TYPE OF DRUG
Adrenergic (decongestant), antihistamine, and expectorant

INGREDIENTS
phenylephrine as the hydrochloride salt, phenylpropanolamine as the hydrochloride salt, brompheniramine as
the maleate salt, guaifenesin, and alcohol

DOSAGE FORM
Oral expectorant (5 mg phenylephrine, 5 mg phenylpropanolamine, 2 mg brompheniramine, 100 mg
guaifenesin, and 3.5% alcohol per 5 ml teaspoonful)

STORAGE
Phenylephrine, phenylpropanolamine, brompheniramine,
and guaifenesin combination expectorant should be
stored at room temperature in a tightly closed container.
This medication should never be frozen.

USES
This drug combination is used to relieve the coughing and
congestion of allergy and the common cold.

Phenylephrine and phenylpropanolamine belong to a
group of drugs known as adrenergic agents (decongestants). They act by constricting blood vessels in the nasal
passages, thereby reducing swelling and congestion.

Brompheniramine belongs to a group of drugs known as
antihistamines, which are used to relieve or prevent symptoms of allergy. Antihistamines block the actions of hista-

mine, a chemical released by the body during an allergic reaction.

Guaifenesin is an expectorant, a drug that loosens bronchial secretions.

TREATMENT

In order to avoid stomach upset, you can take phenylephrine, phenylpropanolamine, brompheniramine, and guaifenesin combination with food or with a full glass of milk or water (unless your doctor directs you to do otherwise).

The expectorant should be measured carefully, with a specially designed, 5 ml measuring spoon. An ordinary kitchen teaspoon is not accurate enough.

If you miss a dose of this medication, take the missed dose as soon as possible, unless it is almost time for your next dose. In that case, don't take the missed dose at all; just return to your regular dosing schedule. Do not double the next dose.

SIDE EFFECTS

Minor. Anxiety; blurred vision; constipation; diarrhea; dizziness; drowsiness; dry mouth, nose, and throat; heartburn; insomnia; irritability; loss of appetite; nasal congestion; nausea; restlessness; reduced sweating; vomiting; and weakness. These side effects should disappear in several days, as your body adjusts to the medication.

If you are constipated, increase the amount of fiber in your diet (raw vegetables, fruits, salads, bran, and whole-grain breads), and drink more water (unless your doctor tells you not to do so).

Chew sugarless gum, or suck on ice chips or a piece of hard candy, to reduce mouth dryness.

This medication can increase your sensitivity to sunlight. It is therefore important to avoid prolonged exposure to sunlight and sunlamps. Wear protective clothing, and use an effective sunscreen.

If you feel dizzy or light-headed, sit or lie down awhile; get up from a sitting or lying position slowly, and be careful on stairs.

In order to avoid difficulty falling asleep, take the last

dose of this medication several hours before bedtime.

Major. Tell your doctor about any side effects that are persistent or particularly bothersome. IT IS ESPECIALLY IMPORTANT TO TELL YOUR DOCTOR about chest pain; convulsions; difficult or painful urination; difficulty breathing; fainting; hallucinations; headaches; loss of coordination; confusion; mood changes; nosebleeds; palpitations; rash; severe abdominal pain; sore throat; or unusual bleeding or bruising.

INTERACTIONS

This drug combination interacts with several other types of medications.

1. Concurrent use of this medication with central nervous system depressants (drugs that slow the activity of the nervous system), such as barbiturates, benzodiazepine tranquilizers, muscle relaxants, narcotics, pain medications, phenothiazine tranquilizers, and alcohol, or with tricyclic anti-depressants can cause extreme drowsiness.

2. Monoamine oxidase (MAO) inhibitors (isocarboxazid, pargyline, phenelzine, tranylcypromine) and tricyclic anti-depressants can increase the side effects of this medication.

3. The side effects of the antihistamine part of this medication may be increased by quinidine, procainamide, haloperidol, and phenothiazine tranquilizers, and the side effects of the decongestant component can be increased by digoxin or over-the-counter (non-prescription) diet aids, or by allergy, asthma, cough, cold, or sinus preparations.

4. The blood-pressure-lowering effects of guanethidine may be decreased by this medication.

TELL YOUR DOCTOR if you are already taking any of the medications listed above.

WARNINGS

● Tell your doctor about unusual or allergic reactions you have had to any medications, especially to brompheniramine or other antihistamines (such as azatadine, chlorpheniramine, carbinoxamine, clemastine, cyproheptadine, dexchlorpheniramine, dimenhydrinate, dimethindene, diphenhydramine, diphenylpyraline, doxylamine,

hydroxyzine, promethazine, pyrilamine, trimeprazine, tripelennamine, tripolidine); to phenylpropanolamine,
phenylephrine, or other adrenergic agents (such as albuterol, amphetamines, ephedrine, epinephrine, isoproterenol, métaproterenol, norepinephrine, pseudoephedrine,
or terbutaline); or to guaifenesin.
- Tell your doctor if you now have, or if you have ever
had, diabetes mellitus (sugar diabetes), epilepsy, glaucoma, heart or blood vessel disease, hiatal hernia, high
blood pressure, myasthenia gravis, obstructed bladder or
intestinal tract, peptic ulcers, enlarged prostate gland, or
thyroid disease.
- Because this drug can reduce sweating and heat release
from the body, you should avoid excessive work or exercising in hot weather.
- While you are taking this medication, drink at least
eight glasses of water a day, to help loosen bronchial secretions.
- This medication can cause drowsiness. Your ability to
perform tasks that require alertness, such as driving a car
or operating potentially dangerous machinery, may be decreased. Appropriate caution should therefore be taken.
- Be sure to tell your doctor if you are pregnant. The effects of this medication during pregnancy have not yet
been thoroughly studied in humans. Also, tell your doctor
if you are breastfeeding an infant. Small amounts of this
medication pass into breast milk and may cause unusual
excitement or irritability in nursing infants.

---

phenylephrine, potassium guaiacolsulfonate, promethazine, and codeine combination

BRAND NAMES (Manufacturers)
Mallergan-VC Expectorant with Codeine (Mallard)
Pentazine VC Expectorant with Codeine (Century)

Phenergan VC with Codeine (Wyeth)
Promethazine Hydrochloride VC Expectorant with Codeine (various manufacturers)

TYPE OF DRUG

Adrenergic (decongestant), antihistamine, expectorant, and cough suppressant combination

INGREDIENTS

phenylephrine as the hydrochloride salt, potassium guaiacolsulfonate, promethazine as the hydrochloride salt, and codeine as the phosphate salt

DOSAGE FORM

Oral syrup (5 mg phenylephrine, 44 mg potassium guaiacolsulfonate, 5 mg promethazine, 10 mg codeine, and 7% alcohol per 5 ml teaspoonful)

STORAGE

This medication should be stored at room temperature in a tightly closed, light-resistant container. This medication should never be frozen.

USES

This combination medication is used to provide symptomatic relief of coughs due to colds, minor upper respiratory infections, and allergy.

Phenylephrine belongs to a group of drugs known as adrenergic agents (decongestants), which constrict blood vessels in the nasal passages to reduce swelling and congestion.

Promethazine belongs to a group of drugs known as antihistamines (antihistamines block the actions of histamine, a chemical released by the body during an allergic reaction). It is used to relieve or prevent symptoms of allergy.

Potassium guaiacolsulfonate is an expectorant; it loosens bronchial secretions.

TREATMENT

To avoid stomach upset, you can take this medication with food or with a full glass of milk or water (unless your doctor directs you to do otherwise).

The oral syrup should be shaken well, just before measuring each dose. The contents tend to settle on the bottom of the bottle, so it is necessary to shake the container to evenly distribute the ingredients and equalize the doses. Each dose should then be measured carefully, with a specially designed, 5 ml measuring spoon. An ordinary kitchen teaspoon is not accurate enough.

If you miss a dose of this medication, take the missed dose as soon as possible, unless it is almost time for your next dose. In that case, don't take the missed dose at all; just return to your regular dosing schedule. Do not double the next dose.

SIDE EFFECTS

Minor. Blurred vision; constipation; diarrhea; dizziness; dry mouth; heartburn; insomnia; loss of appetite; confusion; nasal congestion; nausea; nervousness; rash; restlessness; sweating; vomiting; and weakness. These side effects should disappear in several days, as your body adjusts to the medication.

If you are constipated, increase the amount of fiber in your diet (raw vegetables, fruits, salads, bran, and whole-grain breads), and drink more water (unless your doctor tells you not to do so).

Chew sugarless gum, or suck on ice chips or a piece of hard candy, to reduce mouth dryness.

This medication can cause increased sensitivity to sunlight. It is therefore important to avoid prolonged exposure to sunlight and sunlamps. Wear protective clothing, and use an effective sunscreen.

If you feel dizzy or light-headed, sit or lie down awhile; get up from a sitting or lying position slowly, and be careful on stairs.

In order to avoid difficulty falling asleep, check with your doctor to see if you can take the last dose of this medication several hours before bedtime each day.

Major. Tell your doctor about any side effects that are persistent or particularly bothersome. IT IS ESPECIALLY IMPORTANT TO TELL YOUR DOCTOR about convulsions; difficult or painful urination; difficulty breathing; disturbed coordination; excitation; fainting; headaches; muscle spasms; nightmares; nosebleeds; severe abdominal pain; sore throat or fever; or yellowing of the eyes or skin.

INTERACTIONS

This drug combination interacts with several other types of medication.

1. Concurrent use of this medication with central nervous system depressants (drugs that slow the activity of the nervous system), such as barbiturates, benzodiazepine tranquilizers, muscle relaxants, narcotics, pain medications, phenothiazine tranquilizers, and alcohol, or with tricyclic anti-depressants can cause extreme drowsiness.

2. This medication can decrease the effectiveness of amphetamines, guanethidine, anti-convulsants, and levodopa.

3. The side effects of monoamine oxidase (MAO) inhibitors (isocarboxazid, pargyline, phenelzine, tranylcypromine) and tricyclic anti-depressants may also be increased.

TELL YOUR DOCTOR if you are already taking any of the medications listed above.

WARNINGS

• Tell your doctor about unusual or allergic reactions you have had to medications, especially to promethazine or other antihistamines (such as azatadine, brompheniramine, carbinoxamine, clemastine, cyproheptadine, chlorpheniramine, dexbrompheniramine, dimenhydrinate, dimethindene, diphenhydramine, diphenylpyraline, doxylamine, hydroxyzine, pyrilamine, trimeprazine, tripelennamine, or tripolidine); to phenothiazine tranquilizers; potassium guaiacolsulfonate; phenylephrine or other adrenergic agents (such as albuterol, amphetamines, ephedrine, epinephrine, isoproterenol, metaproterenol, norepinephrine, pseudoephedrine, phenylpropanolamine, or terbutaline), or to codeine or any other narcotic cough suppressant or pain medication.

• Tell your doctor if you now have, or if you have ever had, asthma, brain disease, blockage of the urinary or digestive tract, diabetes mellitus (sugar diabetes), colitis, gallbladder disease, glaucoma, heart or blood vessel disease, high blood pressure, kidney disease, liver disease, lung disease, peptic ulcers, enlarged prostate gland, or thyroid disease.

- This medication can cause drowsiness. Your ability to perform tasks that require alertness, such as driving a car or operating potentially dangerous machinery, may be decreased. Appropriate caution should therefore be taken.
- While you are taking this medication, drink at least eight glasses of water a day to help loosen bronchial secretions.
- Because this product contains codeine, there is potential for abuse, so it must be used with caution. It usually should not be taken for longer than ten days at a time. Tolerance may develop quickly; do not increase the dosage unless you first consult your doctor.
- Before having surgery or any other medical or dental treatment, be sure to tell your doctor or dentist that you are taking this medication.
- Be sure to tell your doctor if you are pregnant. The effects of this medication during the early stages of pregnancy have not yet been thoroughly studied in humans. However, codeine, used regularly during the later stages of pregnancy, may lead to addiction of the fetus, resulting in withdrawal symptoms (irritability, excessive crying, tremors, fever, vomiting, diarrhea, sneezing, and yawning) in the newborn infant. Also, tell your doctor if you are breast-feeding an infant. Small amounts of this medication pass into breast milk and may cause unusual excitement or irritability in nursing infants.

---

phenylpropanolamine and caramiphen combination

BRAND NAMES (Manufacturers)
Bay-Ornade (Bay)
Caramiphen Edisylate and Phenylpropanolamine Hydrochloride (Lederle)
Tuss-Ade (Henry Schein)
Tuss-Allergine Modified T.D. (Rugby)
Tuss-Ornade (Smith Kline & French)
TYPE OF DRUG
Adrenergic (decongestant) and cough suppressant

INGREDIENTS

phenylpropanolamine as the hydrochloride salt; caramiphen as the edisylate salt

DOSAGE FORMS

Sustained-release capsules (75 mg phenylpropanolamine and 40 mg caramiphen)

Oral liquid (12.5 mg phenylpropanolamine, 6.7 mg caramiphen, and 5% alcohol per 5 ml teaspoonful)

STORAGE

Phenylpropanolamine and caramiphen capsules or oral liquid should be stored at room temperature in tightly closed containers. This medication should never be frozen.

USES

This drug combination is used to relieve the coughing and congestion associated with the common cold.

Phenylpropanolamine belongs to a group of drugs known as adrenergic agents (decongestants). They act by constricting blood vessels in the nasal passages, thereby reducing swelling and congestion.

Caramiphen is a non-narcotic cough suppressant that acts at the cough center in the brain.

TREATMENT

In order to avoid stomach upset, you can take this medication with food or with a full glass of milk or water (unless your doctor directs you to do otherwise).

The sustained-release capsules should be swallowed whole. Breaking, chewing, or crushing these capsules destroys their sustained-release activity, and may increase the side effects.

The oral liquid form of this medication should be measured carefully with a specially designed, 5 ml measuring spoon. An ordinary kitchen teaspoon is not accurate enough.

If you miss a dose of this medication, take the missed dose as soon as possible, unless it is almost time for your next dose. In that case, don't take the missed dose at all; just return to your regular dosing schedule. Do not double the next dose.

SIDE EFFECTS

Minor. Blurred vision; constipation; diarrhea; dizziness; drowsiness; heartburn; insomnia; irritability; loss of appetite; nasal congestion; nausea; nervousness; restlessness; upset stomach; and vomiting. These side effects should disappear in several days, as your body adjusts to the medication.

If you are constipated, increase the amount of fiber in your diet (raw vegetables, fruits, salads, bran, and whole-grain breads), and drink more water (unless your doctor directs you to do otherwise).

If you feel dizzy or light-headed, sit or lie down awhile; get up from a sitting or lying position slowly, and be careful on stairs.

In order to avoid difficulty falling asleep, take the last dose of this medication several hours before bedtime.

Major. Tell your doctor about any side effects that are persistent or particularly bothersome. IT IS ESPECIALLY IMPORTANT TO TELL YOUR DOCTOR about chest pain; difficult or painful urination; fainting; headaches; nosebleeds; palpitations; or uncoordinated body movements.

INTERACTIONS

Phenylpropanolamine and caramiphen combination interacts with several other types of medications.

1. Monoamine oxidase (MAO) inhibitors (isocarboxazid, pargyline, phenelzine, tranylcypromine) can increase the side effects of this medication.

2. The blood-pressure-lowering effects of guanethidine may be decreased by this medication.

3. The side effects of phenylpropanolamine may be increased by digoxin, over-the-counter (non-prescription) diet aids, or by allergy, asthma, cough, cold, or sinus preparations.

TELL YOUR DOCTOR if you are already taking any of the medications listed above.

WARNINGS

● Tell your doctor about unusual or allergic reactions you have had to any medications, especially to caramiphen or phenylpropanolamine, or to other adrenergic agents (such

as albuterol, amphetamines, ephedrine, epinephrine, isoproterenol, metaproterenol, norepinephrine, pseudoephedrine, or terbutaline).
● Tell your doctor if you now have, or if you have ever
had, asthma, diabetes mellitus (sugar diabetes), glaucoma,
heart or blood vessel disease, high blood pressure, an enlarged prostate gland, or thyroid disease.
● This medication can cause drowsiness. Your ability to
perform tasks that require alertness, such as driving a car
or operating potentially dangerous machinery, may be decreased. Appropriate caution should therefore be taken.
● Be sure to tell your doctor if you are pregnant. The effects of this medication during pregnancy have not yet
been thoroughly studied in humans. Also, tell your doctor
if you are breastfeeding an infant. Small amounts of this
medication may pass into breast milk.

phenylpropanolamine and chlorpheniramine combination

BRAND NAMES (Manufacturers)
Allergine Modified (Rugby)
Condrin-LA (Mallard)
Deconade (H.L. Moore)
Drize (Ascher)
Orahist (Vangard)
Oraminic Spancaps (Vortech)
Ornade (Smith Kline & French)
Phenylpropanolamine HCl and Chlorpheniramine Male-
    ate (Lederle)
Resaid T.D. (Geneva Generics)
Rhinolar-Ex 12 (McGregor)
Triaminic-12* (Dorsey)
*Phenylpropanolamine and chlorpheniramine combina-
    tion is also available over-the-counter (non-prescrip-
    tion), under the brand name of Triaminic-12.
TYPE OF DRUG
Adrenergic (decongestant) and antihistamine

INGREDIENTS
phenylpropanolamine as the hydrochloride salt; chlorpheniramine as the maleate salt

DOSAGE FORMS
Sustained-release capsules (75 mg phenylpropanolamine and 12 mg chlorpheniramine)

Oral syrup (12.5 mg phenylpropanolamine and 2 mg chlorpheniramine per 5 ml teaspoonful)

STORAGE
Phenylpropanolamine and chlorpheniramine capsules and oral syrup should be stored at room temperature in tightly closed containers. This medication should never be frozen.

USES
This drug combination is used to relieve the symptoms of upper respiratory tract infections, hay fever and other allergies, and sinusitis (inflammation of the sinuses).

Phenylpropanolamine belongs to a group of drugs known as adrenergic agents (decongestants). They act by constricting blood vessels in the nasal passages, thereby reducing swelling and congestion.

Chlorpheniramine belongs to a group of drugs known as antihistamines (antihistamines block the action of histamine, a chemical released by the body during an allergic reaction). It is therefore used to relieve or prevent symptoms of allergy.

TREATMENT
In order to avoid stomach upset, you can take phenylpropanolamine and chlorpheniramine combination with food or with a full glass of milk or water (unless your doctor directs you to do otherwise).

The oral syrup form of this medication should be measured carefully, with a specially designed, 5 ml measuring spoon. An ordinary kitchen teaspoon is not accurate enough.

The sustained-release capsules should be swallowed whole. Breaking, chewing, or crushing these capsules destroys their sustained-release activity, and may increase the side effects.

If you miss a dose of this medication, take the missed dose as soon as possible, unless it is almost time for your next dose. In that case, don't take the missed dose at all; just return to your regular dosing schedule. Do not double the next dose.

SIDE EFFECTS

Minor. Anxiety; blurred vision; constipation; diarrhea; dizziness; drowsiness; dry mouth, nose, and throat; heartburn; insomnia; irritability; loss of appetite; nasal congestion; nausea; restlessness; reduced sweating; vomiting; and weakness. These side effects should disappear in several days, as your body adjusts to the medication.

If you are constipated, increase the amount of fiber in your diet (raw vegetables, fruits, salads, bran and whole-grain breads), and drink more water (unless your doctor directs you to do otherwise).

This medication can increase your sensitivity to sunlight. It is therefore important to avoid prolonged exposure to sunlight and sunlamps. Wear protective clothing, and use an effective sunscreen.

If you feel dizzy or light-headed, sit or lie down awhile; get up from a sitting or lying position slowly, and be careful on stairs.

In order to avoid difficulty falling asleep, take the last dose of this medication several hours before bedtime.

Major. Tell your doctor about any side effects that are persistent or particularly bothersome. IT IS ESPECIALLY IMPORTANT TO TELL YOUR DOCTOR about chest pain; convulsions; difficult or painful urination; difficulty breathing; fainting; hallucinations; headaches; loss of coordination; confusion; mood changes; nosebleeds; palpitations; rash; severe abdominal pain; sore throat; or unusual bleeding or bruising.

INTERACTIONS

Phenylpropanolamine and chlorpheniramine combination interacts with several other types of medication.

1. Concurrent use of this medication with central nervous system depressants (drugs that slow the activity of the nervous system), such as barbiturates, benzodiazepine tranquilizers, muscle relaxants, narcotics, pain medication, phenothiazine tranquilizers, and alcohol, or with tricyclic anti-depressants can cause extreme drowsiness.

2. Monoamine oxidase (MAO) inhibitors (isocarboxazid, pargyline, phenelzine, tranylcypromine) and tricyclic anti-depressants can increase the side effects of this medication.

3. The side effects of the antihistamine part of this medication may be increased by quinidine, procainamide, haloperidol, and phenothiazine tranquilizers; and the side effects of the decongestant component may be increased by digoxin, over-the-counter (non-prescription) diet aids, or by allergy, asthma, cough, cold, or sinus preparations.

4. The blood-pressure-lowering effects of guanethidine may be decreased by this medication.

TELL YOUR DOCTOR if you are already taking any of the medications listed above.

WARNINGS

• Tell your doctor about unusual or allergic reactions you have had to any medications, especially to chlorpheniramine or other antihistamines (such as azatadine, bromodiphenhydramine, brompheniramine, carbinoxamine, clemastine, cyproheptadine, dexchlorpheniramine, dimenhydrinate, dimethindene, diphenhydramine, diphenylpyraline, doxylamine, hydroxyzine, promethazine, pyrilamine, trimeprazine, tripelennamine, and tripolidine); or to phenylpropanolamine or other adrenergic agents (such as albuterol, amphetamines, ephedrine, epinephrine, isoproterenol, metaproterenol, norepinephrine, pseudoephedrine, and terbutaline).

• Tell your doctor if you now have, or if you have ever had, diabetes mellitus (sugar diabetes), epilepsy, glaucoma, heart or blood vessel disease, hiatal hernia, high blood pressure, myasthenia gravis, obstructed bladder or intestinal tract, peptic ulcers, enlarged prostate gland, or thyroid disease.

• Because this drug can reduce sweating and heat release from the body, you should avoid excessive work or exercising in hot weather.

• This medication can cause drowsiness. Your ability to

perform tasks that require alertness, such as driving a car or operating potentially dangerous machinery, may be decreased. Appropriate caution should therefore be taken.

● Be sure to tell your doctor if you are pregnant. The effects of this medication during pregnancy have not yet been thoroughly studied in humans. Also, tell your doctor if you are breastfeeding an infant. Small amounts of this medication pass into breast milk and may cause unusual excitement or irritability in nursing infants.

phenylpropanolamine and guaifenesin combination

BRAND NAMES (Manufacturers)
Entex L.A. (Norwich-Eaton)
Voxin-PG (Norwich-Eaton)
TYPE OF DRUG
Adrenergic (decongestant) and expectorant
INGREDIENTS
phenylpropanolamine as the hydrochloride salt;
  guaifenesin
DOSAGE FORM
Sustained-release tablets (75 mg phenylpropanolamine and 400 mg guaifenesin)
STORAGE
Phenylpropanolamine and guaifenesin combination tablets should be stored at room temperature in a tightly closed container.

USES
This drug combination is used to relieve the coughing and congestion associated with colds, sinusitis (inflammation of the sinuses), sore throat, bronchitis, and asthma.

Phenylpropanolamine belongs to a group of drugs known as adrenergic agents (decongestants). They act by constricting blood vessels in the nasal passages, thereby reducing swelling and congestion.

Guaifenesin is an expectorant, a drug that loosens bronchial secretions.

TREATMENT

In order to avoid stomach upset, you can take phenylpropanolamine and guaifenesin combination with food or
with a full glass of milk or water (unless your doctor directs
you to do otherwise).

These sustained-release tablets should be swallowed
whole. Breaking, chewing, or crushing these tablets destroys their sustained-release activity, and may increase the
side effects.

If you miss a dose of this medication, take the missed
dose as soon as possible, unless it is almost time for your
next dose. In that case, don't take the missed dose at all;
just return to your regular dosing schedule. Do not double
the next dose.

SIDE EFFECTS

Minor. Insomnia; nervousness; and restlessness. These
side effects should disappear in several days, as your body
adjusts to the medication.

In order to avoid difficulty falling asleep, take the last
dose of this medication several hours before bedtime.

Major. Tell your doctor about any side effects that are persistent or particularly bothersome. IT IS ESPECIALLY IM-
PORTANT TO TELL YOUR DOCTOR about fainting;
headaches; nosebleeds; or palpitations.

INTERACTIONS

Phenylpropanolamine and guaifenesin combination interacts with several other types of medication.

1. Monoamine oxidase (MAO) inhibitors (isocarboxazid,
pargyline, phenelzine, tranylcypromine) can increase the
side effects of this medicaiton.

2. The blood-pressure-lowering effects of guanethidine
may be decreased by this medication.

3. The side effects of the decongestant component of this
medication can be increased by digoxin, or by over-the-
counter (non-prescription) allergy, asthma, cough, cold,
diet, or sinus preparations.

Before starting to take this medication, BE SURE TO TELL
YOUR DOCTOR if you are already taking any of the drugs
listed above.

WARNINGS

- Tell your doctor about unusual or allergic reactions you have had to any medications, especially to guaifenesin or phenylpropanolamine, or to other adrenergic agents (such as albuterol, amphetamines, ephedrine, epinephrine, iso-proterenol, metaproterenol, norepinephrine, pseudoeph-edrine, or terbutaline).
- Tell your doctor if you now have, or if you have ever had, diabetes mellitus (sugar diabetes), glaucoma, heart or blood vessel disease, high blood pressure, enlarged prostate gland, or thyroid disease.
- While you are taking this medication, drink at least eight glasses of water a day, to help loosen bronchial secretions.
- Be sure to tell your doctor if you are pregnant. The effects of this medication during pregnancy have not yet been thoroughly studied in humans. Also, tell your doctor if you are breastfeeding an infant. Small amounts of this medication may pass into breast milk.

---

phenylpropanolamine, phenylephrine, and brompheniramine combination

BRAND NAMES (Manufacturers)
Bromophen T.D. (Rugby)
Bromphen Compound T.D. (Henry Schein)
Brompheniramine, Phenylephrine, and Phenylpropanol-
amine (Lederle)
Cordamine-PA (Cord)
Dimetapp Extentabs (Robins)
Histatapp TD (Upsher-Smith)
Midatap (Vangard)
Purebrom Compound T.D. (Purepac)
Tagatap (Reid-Provident)
Tamine SR (Geneva Generics)
TYPE OF DRUG
Adrenergic (decongestant) and antihistamine

INGREDIENTS
phenylpropanolamine as the hydrochloride salt, phenylephrine as the hydrochloride salt, and brompheniramine as the maleate salt

DOSAGE FORMS
Sustained-release tablets (15 mg phenylpropanolamine, 15 mg phenylephrine, and 12 mg brompheniramine)
Oral elixir (5 mg phenylpropanolamine, 5 mg phenylephrine, 4 mg brompheniramine, and 2.3% alcohol per 5 ml teaspoonful)

STORAGE
Phenylpropanolamine, phenylephrine, and brompheniramine combination tablets and oral elixir should be stored at room temperature in tightly closed, light-resistant containers. This medication should never be frozen.

USES
This drug combination is used to relieve the symptoms of upper respiratory tract infections, hay fever and other allergies, and sinusitis (inflammation of the sinuses).

Phenylpropanolamine and phenylephrine belong to a group of drugs known as adrenergic agents (decongestants). They act by constricting blood vessels in the nasal passages, thereby reducing swelling and congestion.

Brompheniramine belongs to a group of drugs known as antihistamines (antihistamines block the actions of histamine, a chemical released by the body during an allergic reaction). It is therefore used to relieve or prevent symptoms of allergy.

TREATMENT
In order to avoid stomach upset, you can take phenylpropanolamine, phenylephrine, and brompheniramine combination with food or with a full glass of milk or water (unless your doctor directs you to do otherwise).

The oral elixir form of this medication should be measured carefully, with a specially designed, 5 ml measuring spoon. An ordinary kitchen teaspoon is not accurate enough.

The sustained-release tablets should be swallowed whole. Breaking, chewing, or crushing these tablets destroys their sustained-release activity, and may increase the side effects.

If you miss a dose of this medication, take the missed dose as soon as possible, unless it is almost time for your next dose. In that case, don't take the missed dose at all; just return to your regular dosing schedule. Do not double the next dose.

SIDE EFFECTS

Minor. Anxiety; blurred vision; constipation; diarrhea; dizziness; drowsiness; dry mouth, nose, and throat; heartburn; insomnia; irritability; loss of appetite; nasal congestion; nausea; restlessness; reduced sweating; vomiting; and weakness. These side effects should disappear in several days, as your body adjusts to the medication.

If you are constipated, increase the amount of fiber in your diet (raw vegetables, fruits, salads, bran, and whole-grain breads), and drink more water (unless your doctor directs you to do otherwise).

Chew sugarless gum, or suck on ice chips or a piece of hard candy, to reduce mouth dryness.

This medication can increase your sensitivity to sunlight. It is therefore important to avoid prolonged exposure to sunlight and sunlamps. Wear protective clothing, and use an effective sunscreen.

If you feel dizzy or light-headed, sit or lie down awhile; get up from a sitting or lying position slowly, and be careful on stairs.

In order to avoid difficulty falling asleep, take the last dose of this medication several hours before bedtime.

Major. Tell your doctor about any side effects that are persistent or particularly bothersome. IT IS ESPECIALLY IMPORTANT TO TELL YOUR DOCTOR about chest pain; confusion; convulsions; difficult or painful urination; difficulty breathing; fainting; hallucinations; headaches; loss of coordination; mood changes; nosebleeds; palpitations; rash; severe abdominal pain; sore throat; or unusual bleeding or bruising.

INTERACTIONS

Phenylpropanolamine, phenylephrine, and bromphenir-

amine combination interacts with several other types of
medication.

1. Concurrent use of this medication with central nervous
system depressants (drugs that slow the activity of the nervous system), such as barbiturates, benzodiazepine tranquilizers, muscle relaxants, narcotics, pain medications,
phenothiazine tranquilizers, and alcohol, or with tricyclic
anti-depressants can cause extreme drowsiness.

2. Monoamine oxidase (MAO) inhibitors (isocarboxazid,
pargyline, phenelzine, tranylcypromine) and tricyclic anti-
depressants can increase the side effects of this medication.

3. The side effects of the antihistamine part of this medication may be increased by quinidine, procainamide, haloperidol, and phenothiazine tranquilizers; and the side effects of the decongestant component may be increased by
digoxin, or by over-the-counter (non-prescription) allergy,
asthma, cough, cold, diet, or sinus preparations.

4. The blood-pressure-lowering effects of guanethidine
may be decreased by this medication.

TELL YOUR DOCTOR if you are already taking any of the
medications listed above.

WARNINGS

● Tell your doctor about unusual or allergic reactions you
have had to any medications, especially to brompheniramine or to other antihistamines (such as azatadine,
chlorpheniramine, carbinoxamine, clemastine, cyproheptadine, dexchlorpheniramine, dimenhydrinate, dimethindene, diphenhydramine, diphenylpyraline, doxylamine,
hydroxyzine, promethazine, pyrilamine, trimeprazine, tripelennamine, and tripolidine); or to phenylpropanolamine, phenylephrine, or other adrenergic agents (such as
albuterol, amphetamines, ephedrine, epinephrine, isoproterenol, metaproterenol, norepinephrine, pseudoephedrine, and terbutaline).

● Tell your doctor if you now have, or if you have ever
had, diabetes mellitus (sugar diabetes), epilepsy, glaucoma, heart or blood vessel disease, hiatal hernia, high
blood pressure, myasthenia gravis, obstructed bladder or

intestinal tract, peptic ulcers, enlarged prostate gland, or
thyroid disease.
● Because this drug can reduce sweating and heat release
from the body, you should avoid excessive work or exercising in hot weather.
● This medication can cause drowsiness. Your ability to
perform tasks that require alertness, such as driving a car
or operating potentially dangerous machinery may be decreased. Appropriate caution should therefore be taken.
● Be sure to tell your doctor if you are pregnant. The effects of this medication during pregnancy have not yet
been thoroughly studied in humans. Also, tell your doctor
if you are breastfeeding an infant. Small amounts of this
medication pass into breast milk and may cause unusual
excitement or irritability in nursing infants.

---

phenylpropanolamine, phenylephrine, chlorpheniramine, and phenyltoloxamine combination

BRAND NAMES (Manufacturers)
Amaril D Spantab (Vortech)
Condecal (Geneva Generics)
Decongestabs (H.L. Moore)
Naldecon (Bristol)
QuadraHist (Henry Schein)
Sinocon (Vangard)
Tri-Phen-Chlor (Rugby)
Tudencon (Reid-Provident)
TYPE OF DRUG
Adrenergic (decongestant) and antihistamine
INGREDIENTS
phenylpropanolamine as the hydrochloride salt, phenyl-
ephrine as the hydrochloride salt, chlorpheniramine as
the maleate salt, and phenyltoloxamine as the citrate salt

DOSAGE FORMS

Sustained-release tablets (40 mg phenylpropanolamine, 10 mg phenylephrine, 5 mg chlorpheniramine, and 15 mg phenyltoloxamine)

Oral syrup (20 mg phenylpropanolamine, 5 mg phenylephrine, 2.5 mg chlorpheniramine, and 7.5 mg phenyltoloxamine per 5 ml teaspoonful)

Oral pediatric drops (5 mg phenylpropanolamine, 1.25 mg phenylephrine, 0.5 mg chlorpheniramine, and 2 mg phenyltoloxamine per ml)

STORAGE

Phenylpropanolamine, phenylephrine, chlorpheniramine, and phenyltoloxamine combination tablets, oral syrup, and oral pediatric drops should be stored at room temperature, in tightly closed containers. This medication should never be frozen.

USES

This drug combination is used to relieve symptoms of upper respiratory tract infections, hay fever and other allergies, and sinusitis (inflammation of the sinuses).

Phenylpropanolamine and phenylephrine belong to a group of drugs known as adrenergic agents (decongestants). They act by constricting blood vessels in the nasal passages, thereby reducing swelling and congestion.

Chlorpheniramine and phenyltoloxamine belong to a group of drugs known as antihistamines (antihistamines block the actions of histamine, a chemical released by the body during an allergic reaction). They are therefore used to relieve or prevent the symptoms of allergy.

TREATMENT

In order to avoid stomach upset, you can take phenylpropanolamine, phenylephrine, chlorpheniramine, and phenyltoloxamine combination with food or with a full glass of milk or water (unless your doctor directs you to do otherwise).

The oral pediatric drops should be measured carefully with the dropper provided.

The oral syrup form of this medication should be measured carefully, with a specially designed, 5 ml measuring spoon. An ordinary teaspoon isn't accurate enough.

The sustained-release tablets should be swallowed whole. Breaking, chewing, or crushing these tablets destroys their sustained-release activity, and may increase the side effects.

If you miss a dose of this medication, take the missed dose as soon as possible, unless it is almost time for your next dose. In that case, don't take the missed dose at all; just return to your regular dosing schedule. Do not double the next dose.

SIDE EFFECTS

Minor. Anxiety; blurred vision; constipation; diarrhea; dizziness; drowsiness; dry mouth, nose, and throat; heartburn; insomnia; irritability; loss of appetite; nasal congestion; reduced sweating; restlessness; vomiting; and weakness. These side effects should disappear in several days, as your body adjusts to the medication.

If you are constipated, increase the amount of fiber in your diet (raw vegetables, fruits, salads, bran, and whole-grain breads), and drink more water (unless your doctor directs you to do otherwise).

Chew sugarless gum, or suck on ice chips or a piece of hard candy, to reduce mouth dryness.

This medication can increase your sensitivity to sunlight. It is therefore important to avoid prolonged exposure to sunlight and sunlamps. Wear protective clothing, and use an effective sunscreen.

If you feel dizzy or light-headed, sit or lie down awhile; get up from a sitting or lying position slowly, and be careful on stairs.

In order to avoid difficulty falling asleep, take the last dose of this medication several hours before bedtime.

Major. Tell your doctor about any side effects that are persistent or particularly bothersome. IT IS ESPECIALLY IMPORTANT TO TELL YOUR DOCTOR about chest pain; convulsions; difficult or painful urination; difficulty breathing; fainting; hallucinations; headaches; loss of coordination; confusion; mood changes; nosebleeds; palpitations; rash; severe abdominal pain; sore throat; or unusual bleeding or bruising.

INTERACTIONS

Phenylpropanolamine, phenylephrine, chlorpheniramine, and phenyltoloxamine combination interacts with several other types of medication.

1. Concurrent use of this medication with central nervous system depressants (drugs that slow the activity of the nervous system), such as barbiturates, benzodiazepine tranquilizers, muscle relaxants, narcotics, pain medications, phenothiazine tranquilizers, and alcohol, or with tricyclic anti-depressants can cause extreme drowsiness.

2. Monoamine oxidase (MAO) inhibitors (isocarboxazid, pargyline, phenelzine, tranylcypromine) and tricyclic anti-depressants can increase the side effects of this medication.

3. The side effects of the antihistamine part of this medication may be increased by quinidine, procainamide, haloperidol, and phenothiazine tranquilizers; and the side effects of the decongestant component may be increased by digoxin or by over-the-counter (non-prescription) allergy, asthma, cough, cold, diet, or sinus preparations.

4. The blood-pressure-lowering effects of guanethidine may be decreased by this medication.

TELL YOUR DOCTOR if you are already taking any of the medications listed above.

WARNINGS

• Tell your doctor about unusual or allergic reactions you have had to medications, especially to chlorpheniramine, phenyltoloxamine, or any other antihistamine (such as azatadine, bromodiphenhydramine, brompheniramine, carbinoxamine, clemastine, cyproheptadine, dexchlorpheniramine, dimenhydrinate, dimethindene, diphenhydramine, diphenylpyraline, doxylamine, hydroxyzine, promethazine, pyrilamine, trimeprazine, tripelennamine, or tripolidine); or to phenylpropanolamine, phenylephrine, or any other adrenergic agent (such as albuterol, amphetamines, ephedrine, epinephrine, isoproterenol, meta-

proterenol, norepinephrine, or terbutaline).
● Tell your doctor if you now have, or if you have ever had, diabetes mellitus (sugar diabetes), epilepsy, glaucoma, heart or blood vessel disease, hiatal hernia, high blood pressure, myasthenia gravis, obstructed bladder or intestinal tract, peptic ulcers, enlarged prostate gland, or thyroid disease.
● Because this drug can reduce sweating and heat release from the body, you should avoid excessive work or exercising in hot weather.
● This medication can cause drowsiness. Your ability to perform tasks that require alertness, such as driving a car or operating potentially dangerous machinery, may be decreased. Appropriate caution should therefore be taken.
● Be sure to tell your doctor if you are pregnant. The effects of this medication during pregnancy have not yet been thoroughly studied in humans. Also, tell your doctor if you are breastfeeding an infant. Small amounts of this medication pass into breast milk and may cause unusual excitement or irritability in nursing infants.

Phenylpropanolamine HCl and Chlorpheniramine Maleate—see phenylpropanolamine and chlorpheniramine combination

---

phenyltoloxamine and hydrocodone combination

BRAND NAME (Manufacturer)
Tussionex (Pennwalt)
TYPE OF DRUG
Antihistamine and cough suppressant combination
INGREDIENTS
phenyltoloxamine and hydrocodone
DOSAGE FORMS
Tablets (10 mg phenyltoloxamine and 5 mg hydrocodone)
Capsules (10 mg phenyltoloxamine and 5 mg hydrocodone)

Oral suspension (10 mg phenyltoloxamine and 5 mg hy-
    drocodone per 5 ml teaspoonful)
STORAGE
The tablets, capsules, and oral suspension should be
stored at room temperature in tightly closed containers.
This medication should never be frozen

USES
This combination medication is used to provide symptomatic relief of coughs due to colds, minor upper respiratory
infections, and allergy.

Phenyltoloxamine belongs to a group of drugs known as
antihistamines (antihistamines block the action of histamine, a chemical released by the body during an allergic
reaction). It is therefore used to relieve or prevent symptoms of allergy.

Hydrocodone is a narcotic cough suppressant, which
acts at the cough reflex center in the brain.

TREATMENT
To avoid stomach upset, you can take this medication with
food or with a full glass of milk or water (unless your doctor directs you to do otherwise).

The suspension form of this medication should be
shaken well just before measuring each dose. The contents tend to settle on the bottom of the bottle, so it is necessary to shake the container to evenly distribute the
ingredients and equalize the doses. Each dose should then
be measured carefully, with a specially designed, 5 ml
measuring spoon. An ordinary kitchen teaspoon is not accurate enough.

If you miss a dose of this medication, take the missed
dose as soon as possible, unless it is almost time for your
next dose. In that case, don't take the missed dose at all;
just return to your regular dosing schedule. Do not double
the next dose.

SIDE EFFECTS
Minor. Blurred vision; constipation; diarrhea; difficult or
painful urination; dizziness; dry mouth, throat, or nose; irritability; loss of appetite; confusion; nausea; restlessness;
ringing or buzzing in the ears; rash; stomach upset; and

unusual increase in sweating. These side effects should disappear in several days, as your body adjusts to the medication.

If you are constipated, increase the amount of fiber in your diet (raw vegetables, fruits, salads, bran, and whole-grain breads), and drink more water (unless your doctor tells you not to do so).

Chew sugarless gum, or suck on ice chips or a piece of hard candy, to reduce mouth dryness.

This medication can cause increased sensitivity to sunlight. It is therefore important to avoid prolonged exposure to sunlight and sunlamps. Wear protective clothing, and use an effective sunscreen.

If you feel dizzy or light-headed, sit or lie down awhile; get up from a sitting or lying position slowly, and be careful on stairs.

Major. Tell your doctor about any side effects that are persistent or particularly bothersome. IT IS ESPECIALLY IMPORTANT TO TELL YOUR DOCTOR about chest pain; feeling faint; headaches; nosebleeds; palpitations; severe abdominal pain; sore throat; or unusual bleeding or bruising.

INTERACTIONS

This drug combination interacts with several other types of medication.

1. Concurrent use of this medication with central nervous system depressants (drugs that slow the activity of the nervous system), such as barbiturates, benzodiazepine tranquilizers, muscle relaxants, narcotics, pain medications, phenothiazine tranquilizers, and alcohol, or with tricyclic anti-depressants can cause extreme drowsiness.

2. Monoamine oxidase (MAO) inhibitors (isocarboxazid, pargyline, phenelzine, tranylcypromine) and tricyclic anti-depressants can increase the side effects of this medication.

TELL YOUR DOCTOR if you are already taking any of the medications listed above.

WARNINGS

• Tell your doctor about unusual or allergic reactions you have had to any medications, especially to phenyltoloxamine or other antihistamines (such as azatadine, brompheniramine, bromodiphenhydramine, carbinoxamine, clemastine, cyproheptadine, chlorpheniramine, dexbrompheniramine, dimenhydrinate, dimethindene, diphenhydramine, diphenylpyraline, doxylamine, hydroxyzine, promethazine, pyrilamine, trimeprazine, tripelennamine, or tripolidine); or to hydrocodone or any other narcotic cough suppressant or pain medication.

• Tell your doctor if you now have, or if you have ever had, asthma, brain disease, blockage of the urinary or digestive tract, diabetes mellitus (sugar diabetes), colitis, gallbladder disease, glaucoma, heart or blood vessel disease, high blood pressure, kidney disease, liver disease, lung disease, peptic ulcers, enlarged prostate gland, or thyroid disease.

• This medication can cause drowsiness. Your ability to perform tasks that require alertness, such as driving a car or operating potentially dangerous machinery, may be decreased. Appropriate caution should therefore be taken.

• While you are taking this medication, drink at least eight glasses of water a day to help loosen bronchial secretions.

• Because this product contains hydrocodone, there is potential for abuse, so it must be used with caution. Usually, you should not take it for longer than ten days at a time (unless your doctor directs you to do so) Tolerance may develop quickly; do not increase the dosage unless you first consult your doctor

• Before having surgery or any other medical or dental treatment, be sure to tell your doctor or dentist that you are taking this medication.

• Be sure to tell your doctor if you are pregnant. The effects of this medication during the early stages of pregnancy have not yet been thoroughly studied in humans. However, hydrocodone, used regularly during the later stages of pregnancy, may lead to addiction of the fetus, resulting in withdrawal symptoms (irritability, excessive crying, tremors, fever, vomiting, diarrhea, sneezing, and yawning) in the newborn infant. Also, tell your doctor if you are breastfeeding an infant. Small amounts of this medication pass into breast milk and may cause unusual excitement or irritability in nursing infants.

phenytoin

BRAND NAMES (Manufacturers)
Dilantin (Parke-Davis)
Dilantin Infatab (Parke-Davis)
Diphenylan (Lannett)
Ditan (Mallard)
phenytoin (various manufacturers)
TYPE OF DRUG
Anti-convulsant
INGREDIENT
phenytoin
DOSAGE FORMS
Capsules (30 mg and 100 mg)
Chewable tablets (50 mg)
Oral suspension (30 mg and 125 mg per 5 ml teaspoonful)
STORAGE
Phenytoin capsules, tablets, and oral suspension should be stored at room temperature in tightly closed, light-resistant containers. This medication should never be frozen.

USES
Phenytoin is used to control epilepsy. It is not clear exactly how phenytoin works to control convulsions, but it appears to prevent the spread of seizure activity in the brain.

TREATMENT
In order to avoid stomach irritation, and to increase this drug's absorption, you can take phenytoin with food or with a full glass of water or milk (unless your doctor directs you to do otherwise).

The tablets should be chewed before swallowing.

The suspension form of this medication should be shaken well just before measuring each dose. The contents tend to settle on the bottom of the bottle, so it is necessary to shake the container to evenly distribute the ingredients and equalize the doses. Each dose should then be measured carefully, with a specially designed, 5 ml measuring spoon. An ordinary kitchen teaspoon is not accurate enough.

Phenytoin works best when the level of medicine in

your bloodstream is kept constant. It is best therefore to take the doses at evenly spaced intervals, day and night. For example, if you are taking three doses a day, the doses should be spaced eight hours apart.

If you miss a dose of this medication, take the missed dose as soon as possible, unless it is almost time for the next dose. In that case, do not take the missed dose at all; just return to your regular dosing schedule. Do not double the next dose. If you miss two or more doses in a row, contact your doctor.

SIDE EFFECTS

Minor. Blurred vision; constipation; drowsiness; headache; insomnia; muscle twitching; nausea; and vomiting. These side effects should disappear in several days, as your body adjusts to the medication.

To relieve constipation, increase the amount of fiber in your diet (bran, salads, fresh fruits and vegetables, and whole-grain breads), exercise, and drink more water (unless your doctor directs you to do otherwise).

Phenytoin may cause your urine to change to a pink, red, or red-brown color. This is a harmless effect.

Major. Tell your doctor about any side effects that are persistent or particularly bothersome. IT IS ESPECIALLY IMPORTANT TO TELL YOUR DOCTOR about a change in facial features; chest pain; confusion; dizziness; gum enlargement; hairiness; joint pain; nervousness; numbness; rash; slurred speech; sore throat; swollen glands; uncoordinated movements; unusual bleeding or bruising; or yellowing of the eyes or skin.

INTERACTIONS

Phenytoin interacts with a number of other medications.
1. The effectiveness of phenytoin can be decreased by alcohol, barbiturates, folic acid, tricyclic anti-depressants, reserpine, molindone, phenothiazine tranquilizers, and haloperidol.
2. Phenytoin can decrease the effectiveness of calcifediol, warfarin, quinidine, disopyramide, dexamethasone, doxycycline, levodopa, and oral contraceptives.
3. The side effects of chloramphenicol, cimetidine, warfarin, disulfiram, isoniazid, oxyphenbutazone, phenylbu-

tazone, sulfonamide antibiotics, tolbutamide, chlordiaz-epoxide, chlorpromazine, diazepam, estrogens, ethosux-imide, methylphenidate, and prochlorperazine can be increased by phenytoin.

4. Valproic acid can either increase or decrease the effects of phenytoin.

5. The dosage of oral anti-diabetic medications may need to be adjusted when phenytoin is started.

6. Phenytoin may decrease the absorption of furosemide from the gastrointestinal tract, decreasing its effectiveness.

7. Antacids, calcium, oxacillin, and anti-neoplastics (anti-cancer drugs) may decrease the gastrointestinal absorption and effectiveness of phenytoin.

Before starting to take phenytoin, BE SURE TO TELL YOUR DOCTOR if you are already taking any of the medications listed above.

WARNINGS

• Tell your doctor about unusual or allergic reactions you have had to any medications, especially to phenytoin, ethotoin, or mephenytoin.

• Before starting to take this medication, be sure to tell your doctor if you now have, or if you have ever had, blood disorders, diabetes mellitus (sugar diabetes), or liver disease.

• If this drug makes you dizzy or drowsy, do not take part in any activities that require alertness, such as driving a car or operating potentially dangerous equipment. Children should be careful while playing or climbing trees.

• Before having any surgery or other medical or dental treatment, be sure your doctor or dentist knows that you are taking phenytoin.

• Do not stop taking this medication unless you first consult your doctor. If this drug is stopped abruptly, you may experience uncontrollable seizures. Your doctor may therefore want to reduce your dosage gradually. Be sure you have enough medication on hand for holidays and vacations.

• Although several generic versions of this drug are available, you should not switch from one brand to another without your doctor's careful assessment and complete approval.

• Therapy with phenytoin may cause your gums to enlarge enough to cover your teeth. Gum enlargement can be minimized, at least partially, by good dental care—frequent brushing, and massaging of the gums with the rubber tip of a good toothbrush.

• Be sure to tell your doctor if you are pregnant. Birth defects have been reported more often in infants whose mothers have seizure disorders. It is unclear if the increased risk of birth defects is associated with the disorder or with the anti-convulsion medications, such as phenytoin, that are used to treat them. The risks and benefits of treatment should be discussed with your doctor. Also, tell your doctor if you are breastfeeding an infant. Phenytoin passes into breast milk and can cause extreme drowsiness in the nursing infant.

Phenzine—see phendimetrazine

Phos-Flur—see sodium fluoride

Phyllocontin—see aminophylline

Pilocar—see pilocarpine (ophthalmic)

---

pilocarpine (ophthalmic)

BRAND NAMES (Manufacturers)
Adsorbocarpine (Alcon)
Akarpine (Akorn)
Almocarpine (Ayerst)
Isopto Carpine (Alcon)
Pilocar (CooperVision)
pilocarpine hydrochloride (various manufacturers)
Pilocel (BioProducts)
Pilomiotin (CooperVision)
Piloptic (Muro)
TYPE OF DRUG
Anti-glaucoma ophthalmic solution
INGREDIENT
pilocarpine as the hydrochloride salt

DOSAGE FORMS

Ophthalmic drops (0.25%, 0.5%, 1%, 1.5%, 2%, 3%, 4%, 5%, 6%, 8%, and 10%)

Ocular therapeutic system (oval ring of plastic that contains pilocarpine. The ring is placed in the eye and the drug is released gradually, over a period of seven days.)

STORAGE

Pilocarpine eye drops should be stored at room temperature in a tightly closed container. This medication should never be frozen. If this medication discolors or turns brown, it should be discarded. A color change demonstrates a loss of potency.

The ocular therapeutic system form of this medication should be stored in the refrigerator, in its original container.

USES

Pilocarpine ophthalmic is used to reduce the increased pressure in the eye caused by glaucoma or other eye conditions. When pilocarpine is applied to the eye, it constricts the pupil and increases the flow of fluid (aqueous humor) out of the eye, thereby reducing the pressure.

TREATMENT

Wash your hands with soap and water before applying this medication. In order to avoid contamination of the eye drops, be careful not to touch the dropper or let it touch your eye; and DO NOT wipe off or rinse the dropper after use.

To apply the eye drops, tilt your head back and pull down your lower eyelid with one hand to make a pouch below the eye. Drop the prescribed amount of medicine into this pouch and slowly close your eyes. Try not to blink. Keep your eyes closed for a minute or two, and place one finger at the corner of the eye, next to your nose, applying a slight pressure (this is done to prevent loss of the medication into the nose and throat canal). Then wipe away any excess with a clean tissue. If you don't think the medicine got into the eye, repeat the process once. Since the drops are somewhat difficult to apply, you may want to have someone else apply them for you.

If you have been prescribed more than one type of eye

drop, after instilling pilocarpine, wait at least five minutes before using any other eye medication (to give the pilocarpine a chance to work).

The ocular therapeutic system comes packaged with detailed instructions for insertion and removal. Follow these directions carefully. Damaged or deformed ocular therapeutic systems should not be placed or retained in the eye. Use a new system instead.

If you miss a dose of this medication, apply the missed dose as soon as possible, then return to your regular dosing schedule. However, if it is almost time for the next dose, skip the one you missed. Do not double the next dose.

SIDE EFFECTS

Minor. Blurred vision; brow ache; headache; and twitching of the eyelids. These side effects should disappear in several days, as your body adjusts to the medication.

Major Tell your doctor about any side effects that are persistent or particularly bothersome. IT IS ESPECIALLY IMPORTANT TO TELL YOUR DOCTOR about diarrhea; difficult or painful urination; flushing; muscle tremors; nausea; nearsightedness; palpitations; shortness of breath; stomach cramps; or sweating.

INTERACTIONS

This medication does not interact with other drugs, as long as it is applied according to directions.

WARNINGS

• Tell your doctor about any unusual or allergic reactions you have had to medications, especially to pilocarpine.
• Tell your doctor if you now have, or if you have ever had, asthma, epilepsy, heart disease, peptic ulcers, thyroid disease, or blockage of the urinary tract.
• This medication can cause difficulty in adjusting to low light levels. Caution should therefore be exercised during night driving, and while performing hazardous tasks in poor lighting.
• Be sure to tell your doctor if you are pregnant. The effects of this drug during pregnancy have not yet been thoroughly studied in humans, but small amounts of pilocar-

pine may be absorbed into the bloodstream. Also, tell your doctor if you are breastfeeding an infant. Small amounts of pilocarpine may pass into breast milk.

pilocarpine hydrochloride—see pilocarpine (ophthalmic)

Pilocel—see pilocarpine (ophthalmic)

Pilomiotin—see pilocarpine (ophthalmic)

Piloptic—see pilocarpine (ophthalmic)

---

pindolol

BRAND NAME (Manufacturer)
Visken (Sandoz)
TYPE OF DRUG
Beta-adrenergic blocking agent
INGREDIENT
pindolol
DOSAGE FORM
Tablets (5 mg and 10 mg)
STORAGE
Pindolol should be stored at room temperature in a tightly closed, light-resistant container.

USES
Pindolol is used to treat high blood pressure. It belongs to a group of medicines known as beta-adrenergic blocking agents or, more commonly, beta-blockers. These drugs work by controlling nerve impulses along certain nerve pathways.

TREATMENT
This medicine can be taken with a glass of water, with meals, immediately following meals, or on an empty stomach (depending on your doctor's instructions). Try to take the medication at the same time(s) each day.

Try not to miss any doses of this medicine. If you do miss a dose, take the missed dose as soon as possible. However, if the next scheduled dose is within eight hours (if you are taking this medicine once a day) or within four hours (if you are taking this medicine more than once a day), do not take the missed dose at all; just return to your regular dosing schedule. Do not double the next dose.

It is important to remember that pindolol does not cure high blood pressure, but it will help to control the condition, as long as you continue to take it.

SIDE EFFECTS

Minor. Anxiety; cold hands or feet (due to decreased blood circulation to skin, fingers, and toes); constipation; decreased sexual ability; diarrhea; drowsiness; dryness of the eyes, mouth, and skin; difficulty sleeping; headache; nausea; numbness or tingling of the fingers or toes; tiredness; or weakness. These side effects should disappear during treatment, as your body adjusts to the medicine.

If you are extra-sensitive to the cold, be sure to dress warmly during cold weather.

Plain, non-medicated eye drops (artificial tears) may help to relieve eye dryness.

Sucking on ice chips or chewing sugarless gum helps to relieve mouth or throat dryness.

Major. Tell your doctor about any side effects that are persistent or particularly bothersome. IT IS ESPECIALLY IMPORTANT TO TELL YOUR DOCTOR about confusion; difficulty breathing, or wheezing; dizziness; fever and sore throat; hair loss; hallucinations; light-headedness; mental depression; nightmares; rapid weight gain (three to five pounds within a week); reduced alertness; skin rash; swelling; or unusual bleeding or bruising.

INTERACTIONS

Pindolol interacts with a number of other medications.
1. Indomethacin, aspirin, or other salicylates may decrease the blood-pressure-lowering effects of the beta-blockers.
2. Concurrent use of beta-blockers and calcium channel blockers (diltiazem, nifedipine, and verapamil) can lead to heart failure or very low blood pressure.
3. Cimetidine can increase the blood concentrations of pindolol, which can result in greater side effects.

4. Side effects may also be increased when beta-blockers are taken with clonidine, digoxin, epinephrine, phenylephrine, phenylpropanolamine, phenothiazine tranquilizers, reserpine, or monoamine oxidase (MAO) inhibitors. At least 14 days should separate the use of a beta-blocker and an MAO inhibitor.

5. Beta-blockers may antagonize (work against) the effects of theophylline, aminophylline, albuterol, metaproterenol, and terbutaline.

6. Beta-blockers can also interact with insulin or oral antidiabetic agents—raising or lowering blood sugar levels or masking the symptoms of low blood sugar.

BE SURE TO TELL YOUR DOCTOR if you are already taking any of the medicines listed above.

WARNINGS

● Before starting to take this medication, it is important to tell your doctor if you have ever had unusual or allergic reactions to any beta-blocking medication (atenolol, metoprolol, nadolol, pindolol, propranolol, or timolol).

● Tell your doctor if you now have, or if you have ever had, allergies, asthma, hay fever, eczema, slow heartbeat, bronchitis, diabetes mellitus (sugar diabetes), emphysema, heart or blood vessel disease, kidney disease, liver disease, thyroid disease, or poor circulation in the fingers or toes.

● You may want to check your pulse while taking this medication. If your pulse is much slower than your usual rate (or if it is less than 50 beats per minute), check with your doctor. A pulse rate that is too slow may cause circulation problems.

● This medicine may affect your body's response to exercise. Make sure you discuss with your doctor a safe amount of exercise for your medical condition.

● It is important that you do not stop taking this medicine without first checking with your doctor. Some conditions may become worse when the medicine is stopped suddenly, and the danger of a heart attack is increased in some patients. Your doctor may want you to gradually reduce the amount of medicine you take, before stopping completely. Make sure that you have enough medicine on hand to last through vacations, holidays, and weekends.

- Before having any kind of surgery or other medical or dental treatment, tell your physician or dentist that you are taking pindolol. Often, this medication will be discontinued 48 hours prior to any major surgery.
- Pindolol can cause dizziness, drowsiness, light-headedness, or decreased alertness. You should therefore exercise caution while driving a car or using potentially dangerous machinery.
- While taking this medicine, do not use any over-the-counter (non-prescription) allergy, asthma, cough, cold, sinus, or diet preparations, unless you first check with your pharmacist or doctor. Some of these medicines can result in high blood pressure and slow heartbeat if taken in conjunction with a beta-blocker.
- Be sure to tell your doctor if you are pregnant. Animal studies have shown that some beta-blockers can cause problems in pregnancy when used at very high doses. Adequate studies have not been completed in humans, but there has been some association between beta-blockers used during pregnancy and low birth rate, as well as breathing problems and slow heart rate in newborn infants. However, other reports have shown no effects on newborn infants. Also, tell your doctor if you are breast-feeding an infant. Although this medicine has not been shown to cause problems in breast-fed infants, some of the medicine may pass into breast milk.

---

piroxicam

BRAND NAME (Manufacturer)
Feldene (Pfizer)
TYPE OF DRUG
Non-steroidal anti-inflammatory analgesic (pain reliever)
INGREDIENT
piroxicam
DOSAGE FORM
Capsules (10 mg and 20 mg)
STORAGE
This medication should be stored in a tightly closed container at room temperature, away from heat and direct sunlight.

USES

Piroxicam is used to treat the inflammation (pain, swelling, and stiffness) of certain types of arthritis, gout, bursitis, and tendinitis.

TREATMENT

You should take this medication on an empty stomach, 30 to 60 minutes before meals, or two hours after meals, so that it gets into your bloodstream quickly. To decrease stomach irritation, your doctor may want you to take the medicine with food or antacids.

It is important to take piroxicam on schedule and not to miss any doses. If you do miss a dose, take the missed dose as soon as possible. However, if you are taking this drug once a day and are six hours late, OR if you take this drug twice a day and are two hours late, don't take the missed dose at all; just return to your regular dosing schedule. Do not double the next dose.

If you are taking piroxicam to relieve arthritis, you must take it regularly, as directed by your doctor. It may take up to three months before you feel the full benefits of this medication. Piroxicam does not cure arthritis, but it will help to control the condition, as long as you continue to take it.

SIDE EFFECTS

Minor. Bloating; constipation; difficulty sleeping; dizziness; drowsiness; headache; heartburn; indigestion; lightheadedness; loss of appetite; nausea; nervousness; soreness of the mouth; unusual sweating; or vomiting. As your body adjusts to the drug, these side effects should disappear.

If you become dizzy, sit or lie down awhile; get up slowly from a sitting or lying position, and be careful on stairs.

Acetaminophen may be helpful in relieving any headaches.

Major. Tell your doctor about any side effects that are persistent or particularly bothersome. IT IS ESPECIALLY IMPORTANT TO TELL YOUR DOCTOR about bloody or black, tarry stools; blurred vision; depression; difficult or painful urination; difficulty breathing, or wheezing; confusion; a problem with hearing; ringing or buzzing in the ears; skin rash, hives, or itching; stomach pain; swelling of the feet; tightness in the chest; pounding heartbeat; unexplained sore throat and fever; unusual bleeding or bruising; unusual fatigue or weakness; unusual weight gain; or yellowing of the eyes or skin.

INTERACTIONS
Piroxicam interacts with several types of medication.
1. Anti-coagulants (blood thinners, such as warfarin) can lead to an increase in bleeding complications.
2. Aspirin, salicylates, or other anti-inflammation medications can increase stomach irritation.
BE SURE TO TELL YOUR DOCTOR if you are already taking any of these medications.

WARNINGS
• Before you take this medication, it is important to tell your doctor if you have ever had unusual or allergic reactions to piroxicam or any of the other chemically related drugs (including aspirin or other salicylates, diflunisal, fenoprofen, ibuprofen, meclofenamate, mefanamic acid, naproxen, oxyphenbutazone, phenylbutazone, indomethacin, sulindac, tolmetin, and zomepirac).
• Tell your doctor if you now have, or if you have ever had, bleeding problems; colitis, stomach ulcers, or other stomach problems; epilepsy; heart disease; high blood pressure; asthma; kidney disease; liver disease; mental illness; or Parkinson's disease.
• If this drug makes you dizzy or drowsy, do not take part in any activity that requires alertness, such as driving a car or operating potentially dangerous equipment.
• Because this drug can prolong bleeding time, it is important to tell your doctor or dentist that you are taking this drug, before having any surgery or other medical or dental treatment.
• Stomach problems are more likely to occur if you take aspirin regularly or drink alcohol while being treated with this medication. These should therefore be avoided (unless your doctor directs you to do otherwise).

• Be sure to tell your doctor if you are pregnant. Although studies in humans have not yet been completed, unwanted side effects (on the heart) have been reported in the offspring of animals who received this type of drug during pregnancy. If taken late in pregnancy, it can also prolong labor. Also, tell your doctor if you are breastfeeding an infant. Small amounts of piroxicam can pass into breast milk.

Plegine—see phendimetrazine

Point-Two—see sodium fluoride

Poladex T.D.—see dexchlorpheniramine

Polaramine—see dexchlorpheniramine

Polycillin—see ampicillin

Polyflex—see chlorzoxazone and acetaminophen combination

Polymox—see amoxicillin

Poly-Vi-Flor—see vitamins, multiple, with fluoride

Polyvite with Fluoride Drops—see vitamins, multiple, with fluoride

Pondimin—see fenfluramine

Ponstel—see mefenamic acid

Potachlor—see potassium chloride

Potasalan—see potassium chloride

Potage—see potassium chloride

Potassine—see potassium chloride

potassium chloride

BRAND NAMES (Manufacturers)

Cena K (Century)
Kaochlor (Adria)
Kaon (Adria)
Kato (Syntex)
Kay Ciel (Berlex)
KEFF (Lemmon)
K-Lor (Abbott)
Klor-Con (Upsher-Smith)
Klorvess (Dorsey)
Klotrix (Mead Johnson)
K-Lyte-Cl (Mead Johnson)
K-Tab (Abbott)
Micro-K (Robbins)
Potachlor (Ray)
Potasalan (Lannett)
Potage (Lemmon)
Potassine (Recsei)
potassium chloride (various manufacturers)
Rum-K (Fleming)
SK-Potassium Chloride (Smith Kline & French)
Slow-K (Ciba)

TYPE OF DRUG

Potassium replacement

INGREDIENT

potassium as the chloride salt

DOSAGE FORMS

Effervescent tablets (20 mEq, 25 mEq, and 50 mEq)
Sustained-release tablets (6.7 mEq, 8 mEq, and 10 mEq)
Enteric-coated tablets (4 mEq and 13 mEq)
Sustained-release capsules (8 mEq)
Oral liquid (10 mEq, 20 mEq, 30 mEq, and 40 mEq per 15 ml tablespoonful)
Oral powder (15 mEq, 20 mEq, and 25 mEq per packet)

STORAGE

Potassium chloride should be stored at room temperature in tightly closed containers.

USES

This medication is used to prevent or treat potassium deficiency, especially that caused by diuretics (water pills).

TREATMENT

In order to avoid stomach irritation, you should take potassium chloride with food or immediately after a meal. In order to become accustomed to taking this medication, try to take it at the same time(s) each day.

Each dose of the liquid form of this medication should be measured carefully, with a specially designed measuring spoon. An ordinary kitchen spoon is not accurate enough.

If you are taking the liquid, powder, or effervescent tablet form of this medication, you should dilute each dose in at least four ounces (1/2 glass) of cold water or juice. Be sure the medication has dissolved completely and has stopped fizzing before you drink it. Then sip it slowly. DO NOT use tomato juice to dissolve this medication (unless your doctor directs you to do so). Tomato juice contains a great deal of sodium.

The sustained-release tablets and capsules should be swallowed whole. Chewing, crushing, or breaking these tablets or capsules destroys their sustained-release activity, and possibly increases the side effects.

If you miss a dose of this medication, take the missed dose as soon as possible, unless it is within two hours of the next scheduled dose. In that case, do not take the missed dose at all; just return to your regular dosing schedule. Do not double the next dose.

SIDE EFFECTS

Minor. Diarrhea; nausea; stomach pains; and vomiting. These side effects should disappear in several days, as your body adjusts to the medication.

Major. Tell your doctor about any side effects that are persistent or particularly bothersome. IT IS ESPECIALLY IMPORTANT TO TELL YOUR DOCTOR about anxiety; bloody or black, tarry stools; confusion; difficulty breathing; numbness or tingling in the arms, legs, or feet; palpitations; severe abdominal pain; or unusual weakness.

INTERACTIONS

Potassium chloride interacts with other medication.

1. The combination of potassium chloride with amiloride, spironolactone, or triamterene can lead to hyperkalemia (high levels of potassium in the bloodstream).
2. The combination of digoxin and high doses of potassium chloride can lead to heart problems.
Before starting to take potassium chloride, BE SURE TO TELL YOUR DOCTOR if you are already taking any of the medications listed above.

WARNINGS
● Tell your doctor about unusual or allergic reactions you have had to any medications, especially to potassium.
● Before starting to take this medication, be sure to tell your doctor if you now have, or if you have ever had, Addison's disease, acute dehydration, heart disease, heat cramps, hyperkalemia, intestinal blockage, kidney disease, myotonia congenita, or peptic ulcers.
● Ask your doctor about using a salt substitute instead of potassium chloride; salt substitutes are similar, but less expensive and more convenient. However, salt substitutes should only be used with your doctor's approval. Too much potassium can be dangerous.
● If you are taking the tablets and you find the wax matrix tablet in your stool, there is no reason for concern; the potassium chloride has been absorbed from the matrix.
● Some of these products contain F.D. & C. Yellow Dye No. 5 (tartrazine), which can cause allergic-type symptoms (rash, shortness of breath, fainting) in certain susceptible individuals.
● Be sure to tell your doctor if you are pregnant. Although this drug appears to be safe, extensive studies in pregnant women have not yet been completed. Also, tell your doctor if you are breastfeeding an infant. Small amounts of potassium pass into breast milk.

prazepam

BRAND NAME (Manufacturer)
Centrax (Parke-Davis)
TYPE OF DRUG
Sedative/hypnotic (anti-anxiety medication)

INGREDIENT
prazepam
DOSAGE FORMS
Capsules (5 mg, 10 mg, and 20 mg)
Tablets (10 mg)
STORAGE
This medication should be stored at room temperature in tightly closed, light-resistant containers.

USES
Prazepam is prescribed to treat symptoms of anxiety. It is not clear exactly how this medicine works, but it may relieve anxiety by acting as a depressant of the central nervous system. This drug is currently used by many people to relieve nervousness. It is effective for this purpose for short periods, but it is important to try to remove the cause of the anxiety as well.

TREATMENT
Prazepam should be taken exactly as directed by your doctor. It can be taken with food or a full glass of water if stomach upset occurs. Do not take this medication with a dose of antacids, since they may retard its absorption.

If you are taking this medication regularly and you miss a dose, and remember within an hour of the scheduled time, take the missed dose immediately. If more than an hour has passed, skip the dose you missed and wait for the next scheduled dose. Do not double the next dose.

SIDE EFFECTS
Minor. Bitter taste in mouth; constipation; depression; diarrhea; dizziness; drowsiness (after a night's sleep); dry mouth; fatigue; flushing; headache; heartburn; excess saliva; loss of appetite; nausea; nervousness; sweating; and vomiting. As your body adjusts to the medicine, these side effects should disappear.

Dry mouth can be relieved by chewing sugarless gum or by sucking on ice chips.

If you feel dizzy, sit or lie down awhile; get up slowly, and be careful on stairs.

Major. Tell your doctor about any side effects that are persistent or particularly bothersome. IT IS ESPECIALLY IM-

PORTANT TO TELL YOUR DOCTOR about blurred or double vision; chest pain; difficulty urinating; fainting; falling; fever; joint pain; hallucinations; mouth sores; nightmares; palpitations; rash; severe depression; shortness of breath; slurred speech; sore throat; uncoordinated movements; unusual excitement; unusual tiredness; or yellowing of the eyes or skin.

INTERACTIONS

Prazepam interacts with a number of other medications.
1. To prevent over-sedation, this drug should not be taken with alcohol, other sedative drugs, central nervous system depressants (such as antihistamines, barbiturates, muscle relaxants, pain medicines, narcotics, medicines for seizures, or phenothiazine tranquilizers), or with anti-depressants.
2. This medication may decrease the effectiveness of carbamazepine, levodopa, and oral anti-coagulants (blood thinners).
3. It may increase the effects of phenytoin.
4. Disulfiram, isoniazid, and cimetidine can increase the blood levels of prazepam, which can lead to toxic effects.
5. Concurrent use of rifampin may decrease the effectiveness of prazepam.
If you are already taking any of the medications listed above, CONSULT YOUR DOCTOR about their use.

WARNINGS

• Tell your doctor about unusual or allergic reactions you have had to any medications, especially to prazepam or to other benzodiazepine tranquilizers (such as alprazolam, chlordiazepoxide, clorazepate, diazepam, flurazepam, halazepam, lorazepam, oxazepam, temazepam, or triazolam).
• Tell your doctor if you now have, or if you have ever had, liver disease, kidney disease, epilepsy, lung disease, myasthenia gravis, porphyria, mental depression, or mental illness.
• This medicine can cause drowsiness. Avoid tasks that require alertness, such as driving a car or using potentially dangerous machinery.
• Prazepam has the potential for abuse and must be used

with caution. Tolerance may develop quickly; do not increase the dosage without first consulting your doctor. It is also important not to stop this drug suddenly if you have been taking it in large amounts or if you have used it for several weeks. Your doctor may want to reduce the dosage gradually.

• This is a safe drug when used properly. When it is combined with other sedative drugs or alcohol, however, serious side effects can develop.

• Be sure to tell your doctor if you are pregnant. This type of medicine may increase the chance of birth defects if it is taken during the first three months of pregnancy. In addition, too much use of this medicine during the last six months of pregnancy may result in addiction of the fetus, leading to withdrawal side effects in the newborn. Also, use of this medicine during the last weeks of pregnancy may cause drowsiness, slowed heartbeat, and breathing difficulties in the infant. Tell your doctor if you are breast feeding an infant. This medicine can pass into the breastmilk and cause drowsiness, slowed heartbeat, and breathing difficulties in nursing infants.

---

prazosin

BRAND NAME (Manufacturer)
Minipress (Pfizer)
TYPE OF DRUG
Anti-hypertensive
INGREDIENT
prazosin as the hydrochloride salt
DOSAGE FORM
Capsules (1 mg, 2 mg, and 5 mg)
STORAGE
Prazosin capsules should be stored at room temperature in a tightly closed, light-resistant container.

USES

Prazosin is used to treat high blood pressure. It is a vasodilator that relaxes the muscles of the blood vessels, which in turn lowers blood pressure.

TREATMENT

To avoid stomach irritation, you can take prazosin with food or with a full glass of water or milk. In order to become accustomed to taking this medication, try to take it at the same time(s) each day.

The first dose of this medication can cause fainting. Therefore, it is often recommended that this dose be taken at bedtime.

If you miss a dose of this medication, take the missed dose as soon as possible, unless it is almost time for the next dose. In that case, do not take the missed dose at all; just return to your regular dosing schedule. Do not double the next dose.

Prazosin does not cure high blood pressure, but it will help to control the condition, as long as you continue to take it.

The effects of this medication may not become apparent for two weeks.

SIDE EFFECTS

Minor. Abdominal pain; constipation; diarrhea; dizziness; drowsiness; dry mouth; frequent urination; headache; impotence; itching; loss of appetite; nasal congestion; nausea; nervousness; sweating; tiredness; vivid dreams; vomiting; and weakness. These side effects should disappear in several weeks, as your body adjusts to the medication.

If you are constipated, increase the amount of fiber in your diet (raw vegetables, fruits, salads, bran, and whole-grained breads), and drink more water (unless your doctor directs you to do otherwise).

To relieve mouth dryness, chew sugarless gum, or suck on ice chips or a piece of hard candy.

If you feel dizzy or light-headed, sit or lie down awhile; get up slowly, and be careful on stairs. To avoid dizziness or light-headedness when you stand, contract and relax the muscles of your legs for a few moments before rising. Do this by pushing one foot against the floor while raising the other foot slightly, alternating feet so that you are "pumping" your legs in a pedaling motion.

Major. Tell your doctor about any side effects that are persistent or particularly bothersome. IT IS ESPECIALLY IM-

PORTANT TO TELL YOUR DOCTOR about blurred vision; chest pain; constant erection; depression; difficulty breathing; difficulty urinating; fainting; hallucinations; loss of hair; nosebleeds; palpitations; rapid weight gain (three to five pounds within a week); rash; ringing in the ears; swelling of the feet, legs, or ankles; or tingling of the fingers or toes.

INTERACTIONS

The combination of prazosin and alcohol can lead to a severe drop in blood pressure, and fainting.

WARNINGS

- Tell your doctor about unusual or allergic reactions you have had to any medications, especially to prazosin.
- Before starting to take this medication, be sure to tell your doctor if you now have, or if you have ever had, angina (chest pain) or kidney disease.
- Because initial therapy with this drug may cause dizziness or fainting, your doctor will probably start you on a low dose and increase the dosage gradually.
- If this drug makes you dizzy or drowsy or blurs your vision, do not take part in any activity that requires alertness, such as driving a car or operating potentially dangerous equipment.
- In order to avoid dizziness or fainting while taking this medication, try not to stand for long periods of time, avoid drinking excessive amounts of alcohol, and avoid getting overheated (strenuous exercise in hot weather; hot baths, showers, and saunas).
- Before taking any over-the-counter (non-prescription) sinus, allergy, asthma, cough, cold, or diet product, check with your doctor or pharmacist. Some of these products can cause an increase in blood pressure.
- Do not stop taking this medication unless you first check with your doctor. If you stop taking this drug abruptly, you may experience a sudden rise in blood pressure. Your doctor may therefore want to decrease your dosage gradually.
- Be sure to tell your doctor if you are pregnant. Although this drug appears to be safe, extensive studies in pregnant women have not yet been completed. Also, tell

your doctor if you are breastfeeding an infant. It is not known whether or not prazosin passes into breast milk.

Prednicen-M—see prednisone (systemic)

---

prednisolone (systemic)

BRAND NAMES (Manufacturers)
Cortalone (Halsey)
Delta-Cortef (Upjohn)
Fernisolone-P (Ferndale)
prednisolone (various manufacturers)
Predoxine-5 (Mallard)
Sterane (Pfipharmecs)
TYPE OF DRUG
Adrenocorticosteroid hormone
INGREDIENT
prednisolone
DOSAGE FORM
Tablets (1 mg and 5 mg)
STORAGE
Prednisolone tablets should be stored at room temperature in a tightly closed container.

USES
Your adrenal glands naturally produce certain cortisone-like chemicals. These chemicals are involved in various regulatory processes in the body (such as maintenance of fluid balance, temperature, and reactions to inflammation). Prednisolone belongs to a group of drugs known as adrenocorticosteroids (or cortisone-like medications). It is used to treat a variety of disorders, including endocrine and rheumatic disorders; asthma; blood diseases; certain cancers; eye disorders; gastrointestinal disturbances such as ulcerative colitis; respiratory diseases; and inflammations such as arthritis, dermatitis, and poison ivy. How this drug acts to relieve these disorders is not completely understood.

TREATMENT
In order to prevent stomach irritation, you can take pred-

nisolone with food or milk.

If you are taking only one dose of this medication each day, try to take it before 9:00 A.M. This will mimic the body's normal production of this type of chemical.

It is important to try not to miss any doses of prednisolone. However, if you do miss a dose of this medication:

1. If you are taking it more than once a day, take the missed dose as soon as possible and return to your regular dosing schedule. If it is already time for the next dose, double the dose.

2. If you are taking this medication once a day, take the dose you missed as soon as possible, unless you don't remember until the next day. In that case do not take the missed dose at all; just follow your regular dosing schedule. Do not double the next dose.

3. If you are taking this drug every other day, take it as soon as you remember. If you missed the scheduled time by a whole day, take it when you remember, then skip a day before you take the next dose. Do not double the next dose.

If you miss more than one dose, CONTACT YOUR DOCTOR.

SIDE EFFECTS

Minor. Dizziness; false sense of well-being; increased appetite; increased sweating; indigestion; menstrual irregularities; muscle weakness; nausea; reddening of the skin on the face; restlessness; sleep disorders; thinning of the skin; and weight gain. These side effects should disappear in several weeks, as your body adjusts to the medication.

To help avoid potassium loss while using this drug, take your dose with a glass of fresh or frozen orange juice, or eat a banana each day. The use of a salt substitute also helps prevent potassium loss. Check with your doctor.

Major. Tell your doctor about any side effects that are persistent or particularly bothersome. IT IS ESPECIALLY IMPORTANT TO TELL YOUR DOCTOR about abdominal enlargement; abdominal pain; acne or other skin problems; back or rib pain; bloody or black, tarry stools; blurred vision; convulsions; eye pain; fever and sore throat; growth impairment (in children); headaches; impaired healing of wounds; increased thirst and urination;

mental depression; mood changes; muscle wasting; night-mares; nosebleeds; rapid weight gain (three to five pounds within a week); rash; shortness of breath; unusual bruising or bleeding; or unusual weakness.

INTERACTIONS

Prednisolone interacts with other types of medication.

1. Alcohol, aspirin, and anti-inflammation medications (such as diflunisal, ibuprofen, indomethacin, mefenamic acid, meclofenamate, naproxen, piroxicam, sulindac, and tolmetin) aggravate the stomach problems that are common with use of this medication.

2. A change in the dosage requirements of oral anti-coagulants (blood thinners, such as warfarin), oral anti-diabetic drugs, or insulin may be necessary when this medication is started or stopped.

3. The loss of potassium caused by prednisolone can lead to serious side effects in individuals taking digoxin.

4. Thiazide diuretics (water pills) can increase the potassium loss caused by this medication.

5. Phenobarbital, phenytoin, rifampin, and ephedrine can increase the elimination of prednisolone from the body, thereby decreasing its effectiveness.

6. Oral contraceptives and estrogen-containing drugs may decrease the elimination of this drug from the body, which can lead to an increase in side effects.

7. Prednisolone can increase the elimination of aspirin and isoniazid, thereby decreasing the effectiveness of these two medications.

8. Cholestyramine and colestipol can chemically bind this medication in the stomach and gastrointestinal tract and prevent its absorption.

TELL YOUR DOCTOR if you are currently taking any of the medications listed above.

WARNINGS

● Tell your doctor about unusual or allergic reactions you have had to any medications, especially to prednisolone or other adrenocorticosteroids (such as betamethasone, cortisone, dexamethasone, fluprednisolone, hydrocortisone, methylprednisolone, paramethasone, prednisone, or triamcinolone).

• Tell your doctor if you now have, or if you have ever had, bone disease; diabetes mellitus (sugar diabetes); emotional instability; glaucoma; fungal infections; heart disease; high blood pressure; high cholesterol levels; myasthenia gravis; peptic ulcers; osteoporosis; thyroid disease; tuberculosis; severe ulcerative colitis; kidney disease; or liver disease.

• If you are using this medication for longer than a week, you may need to have your dosage adjusted if you are subjected to stress, such as serious infections, injury, or surgery. Discuss this with your doctor.

• If you have been taking this drug for more than a week, do not stop taking it suddenly. If it is stopped abruptly, you may experience abdominal or back pain, dizziness, fainting, fever, muscle or joint pain, nausea, vomiting, shortness of breath, or extreme weakness. Your doctor may therefore want to reduce the dosage gradually. Never increase the dosage or take the drug for longer than the prescribed time, unless you first consult your doctor.

• While you are taking this drug, you should not be vaccinated or immunized. Prednisolone decreases the effectiveness of vaccines and can lead to overwhelming infection if a live virus is administered.

• Before having any surgery or other medical or dental treatment, be sure your doctor or dentist knows that you are taking this medication.

• Because this drug can cause glaucoma and cataracts with long-term use, your doctor may want you to have your eyes examined by an ophthalmologist periodically during treatment.

• If you are taking prednisolone for prolonged periods, you should wear or carry an identification card or notice stating that you are taking an adrenocorticosteroid.

• This medication can raise blood sugar levels in diabetic patients. Blood sugar should therefore be monitored carefully with blood or urine tests when this medication is started.

• Some of these products contain F.D. & C. Yellow Dye No. 5 (tartrazine), which can cause allergic-type reactions (shortness of breath, wheezing, rash, or fainting) in certain susceptible individuals.

• Be sure to tell your doctor if you are pregnant. This

drug crosses the placenta. Although studies in humans have not yet been completed, birth defects have been observed in the fetuses of animals who were given large doses of this type of drug during pregnancy. Also, tell your doctor if you are breastfeeding an infant. Small amounts of this drug pass into breast milk and may cause growth suppression or a decrease in natural adrenocorticosteroid production in the nursing infant.

---

prednisone (systemic)

BRAND NAMES (Manufacturers)
Cortan (Halsey)
Deltasone (Upjohn)
Fernisone (Ferndale)
Liquid Pred (Muro)
Meticorten (Schering)
Orasone (Rowell)
Panasol (Seatrace)
Prednicen-M (Central)
prednisone (various manufacturers)
SK-Prednisone (Smith Kline & French)
Sterapred (Maynard)

TYPE OF DRUG
Adrenocorticosteroid hormone

INGREDIENT
prednisone

DOSAGE FORMS
Tablets (1 mg, 2.5 mg, 5 mg, 10 mg, 20 mg, 25 mg, and 50 mg)
Oral syrup (5 mg per 5 ml teaspoonful with 5% alcohol)

STORAGE
Prednisone tablets and oral syrup should be stored at room temperature in tightly closed containers.

USES
Your adrenal glands naturally produce certain cortisone-like chemicals. These chemicals are involved in various regulatory processes in the body (such as maintenance of fluid balance, temperature, and reactions to inflammation). Prednisone belongs to a group of drugs known as

adrenocorticosteroids (or cortisone-like medications). It is used to treat a variety of disorders, including endocrine and rheumatic disorders; asthma; blood diseases; certain cancers; eye disorders; gastrointestinal disturbances such as ulcerative colitis; respiratory diseases; and inflammations such as arthritis, dermatitis, and poison ivy. How this drug acts to relieve these disorders is not completely understood.

TREATMENT

In order to prevent stomach irritation, you can take prednisone with food or milk.

If you are taking only one dose of this medication each day, try to take it before 9:00 A.M. This will mimic the body's normal production of this type of chemical.

The oral syrup form of this medication should be measured carefully, with a specially designed, 5 ml measuring spoon. A kitchen teaspoon is not accurate enough.

It is important to try not to miss any doses of prednisone. However, if you do miss a dose of this medication:

1. If you are taking it more than once a day, take the missed dose as soon as possible and return to your regular dosing schedule. If it is already time for the next dose, double the dose.

2. If you are taking this medication once a day, take the dose you missed as soon as possible, unless you don't remember until the next day. In that case do not take the missed dose at all; just follow your regular dosing schedule. Do not double the next dose.

3. If you are taking this drug every other day, take it when you remember, then skip a day before you take the next dose. Do not double the dose.

If you miss more than one dose, CONTACT YOUR DOCTOR.

SIDE EFFECTS

Minor. Dizziness; false sense of well-being; increased appetite; increased sweating; indigestion; menstrual irregularities; muscle weakness; nausea; reddening of the skin on the face; restlessness; sleep disorders; thinning of the skin; and weight gain. These side effects should disappear in several weeks, as your body adjusts to the medication.

To help avoid potassium loss while using this drug, take your dose with a glass of fresh or frozen orange juice, or eat a banana each day. The use of a salt substitute also helps prevent potassium loss. Check with your doctor.

Major. Tell your doctor about any side effects that are persistent or particularly bothersome. IT IS ESPECIALLY IMPORTANT TO TELL YOUR DOCTOR about abdominal enlargement; abdominal pain; acne or other skin problems; back or rib pain; bloody or black, tarry stools; blurred vision; convulsions; eye pain; fever and sore throat; growth impairment (in children); headaches; impaired healing of wounds; increased thirst and urination; mental depression; mood changes; muscle wasting; nightmares; nosebleeds; rapid weight gain (three to five pounds within a week); rash; shortness of breath; unusual bruising or bleeding; or unusual weakness.

INTERACTIONS

Prednisone interacts with other types of medication.

1. Alcohol, aspirin, and anti-inflammation medications (diflunisal, ibuprofen, indomethacin, mefenamic acid, meclofenamate, naproxen, piroxicam, sulindac, and tolmetin) aggravate the stomach problems that are common with use of this medication.

2. A change in the dosage requirements of oral anti-coagulants (blood thinners, such as warfarin), oral anti-diabetic drugs, or insulin may be necessary when this medication is started or stopped.

3. The loss of potassium caused by prednisone can lead to serious side effects in individuals taking digoxin.

4. Thiazide diuretics (water pills) can increase the potassium loss caused by this medication.

5. Phenobarbital, phenytoin, rifampin, and ephedrine can increase the elimination of prednisone from the body, thereby decreasing its effectiveness.

6. Oral contraceptives and estrogen-containing drugs may decrease the elimination of this drug from the body, which can lead to an increase in side effects.

7. Prednisone can increase the elimination of aspirin and isoniazid, thereby decreasing the effectiveness of these two medications.

8. Cholestyramine and colestipol can chemically bind

this medication in the stomach and gastrointestinal tract and prevent its absorption.
TELL YOUR DOCTOR if you are currently taking any of the medications listed above.

WARNINGS

● Tell your doctor about unusual or allergic reactions you have had to any medications, especially to prednisone or other adrenocorticosteroids (such as betamethasone, cortisone, dexamethasone, fluprednisolone, hydrocortisone, methylprednisolone, paramethasone, prednisolone, or triamcinolone).

● Tell your doctor if you now have, or if you have ever had, bone disease; diabetes mellitus (sugar diabetes); emotional instability; glaucoma; fungal infections; heart disease; high blood pressure; high cholesterol levels; myasthenia gravis; peptic ulcers; osteoporosis; thyroid disease; tuberculosis; severe ulcerative colitis; kidney disease; or liver disease.

● If you are using this medication for longer than a week, you may need to have your dosage adjusted if you are subjected to stress, such as serious infections, injury, or surgery. Discuss this with your doctor.

● If you have been taking this drug for more than a week, do not stop taking it suddenly. If it is stopped abruptly, you may experience abdominal or back pain, dizziness, fainting, fever, muscle or joint pain, nausea, vomiting, shortness of breath, or extreme weakness. Your doctor may therefore want to reduce the dosage gradually. Never increase the dosage or take the drug for longer than the prescribed time, unless you first consult your doctor.

● While you are taking this drug, you should not be vaccinated or immunized. This medication decreases the effectiveness of vaccines and can lead to overwhelming infection if a live virus is administered.

● Before having any surgery or other medical or dental treatment, be sure your doctor or dentist knows that you are taking this medication.

● Because this drug can cause glaucoma and cataracts with long-term use, your doctor may want you to have your eyes examined by an ophthalmologist periodically during treatment.

● If you are taking this medication for prolonged periods, you should wear or carry an identification card or notice stating that you are taking an adrenocorticosteroid.

● This medication can raise blood sugar levels in diabetic patients. Blood sugar should therefore be monitored carefully with blood or urine tests when this medication is started.

● Be sure to tell your doctor if you are pregnant. Prednisone crosses the placenta. Although studies in humans have not yet been completed, birth defects have been observed in the fetuses of animals who were given large doses of this drug during pregnancy. Also, tell your doctor if you are breastfeeding an infant. Small amounts of this drug pass into breast milk and may cause growth suppression or a decrease in natural adrenocorticosteroid production in the nursing infant.

Predoxine-5—see prednisolone (systemic)

Prelu-2—see phendimetrazine

Preludin—see phenmetrazine

Premarin—see estrogens, conjugated

---

primidone

BRAND NAMES (Manufacturers)
Myidone (Major)
Mysoline (Ayerst)
primidone (various manufacturers)
Primoline (Rugby)
TYPE OF DRUG
Anti-convulsant
INGREDIENT
primidone
DOSAGE FORMS
Tablets (50 mg and 250 mg)
Oral suspension (250 mg per 5 ml teaspoonful)
STORAGE
Primidone tablets and oral suspension should be stored at

room temperature in tightly closed containers. This medication should never be frozen.

USES

Primidone is used to treat various seizure disorders. This drug is converted in the body to phenobarbital. It is not clear exactly how primidone or phenobarbital acts to decrease the number of seizures, but both drugs are central nervous system depressants (drugs that slow the activity of the brain and spinal cord).

TREATMENT

In order to avoid stomach irritation, you can take primidone with food or with a full glass of water or milk (unless your doctor directs you to do otherwise).

The oral suspension form of this medication should be shaken well, just before measuring each dose. The contents tend to settle on the bottom of the bottle, so it is necessary to shake the container to evenly distribute the ingredients and equalize the doses. Each dose should then be measured carefully, with a specially designed, 5 ml measuring spoon. An ordinary kitchen teaspoon is not accurate enough.

Primidone works best when the level of medicine in your bloodstream is kept constant. It is best therefore to take the doses at evenly spaced intervals, day and night. For example, if you are to take three doses a day, the doses should be spaced eight hours apart.

It is important to try not to miss any doses of this medication. If you do miss a dose, and remember within two hours of your scheduled time, take it immediately. If more than two hours have passed, do not take the missed dose; just return to your regular dosing schedule. Do not double the next dose. If you miss two or more consecutive doses, contact your doctor as soon as possible.

SIDE EFFECTS

Minor. Dizziness; drowsiness; fatigue; loss of appetite; nausea; and vomiting. These side effects should disappear in several days, as your body adjusts to the medication.

If you feel dizzy, sit or lie down awhile; get up slowly, and be careful on stairs.

Major. Tell your doctor about any side effects that are persistent or particularly bothersome. IT IS ESPECIALLY IMPORTANT TO TELL YOUR DOCTOR about blurred vision; emotional disturbances; irritability; loss of coordination; or skin rash.

INTERACTIONS

Primidone interacts with other types of medication.

1. Concurrent use of primidone with other central nervous system depressants (such as alcohol, antihistamines, barbiturates, benzodiazepine tranquilizers, muscle relaxants, narcotics, pain medications, phenothiazine tranquilizers, and sleeping medications) or with tricyclic antidepressants can lead to extreme drowsiness.

2. The blood levels and therapeutic effects of oral anticoagulants (blood thinners, such as warfarin), adrenocorticosteroids (cortisone-like medications), digitoxin, phenytoin, doxycycline, and tricyclic anti-depressants can be decreased by primidone.

3. Primidone can decrease the absorption of griseofulvin from the gastrointestinal tract, decreasing its effectiveness. Before starting to take primidone, BE SURE TO TELL YOUR DOCTOR if you are already taking any of the medications listed above.

WARNINGS

● Tell your doctor about unusual or allergic reactions you nave had to any medications, especially to primidone, phenobarbital, or other barbiturates (such as amobarbital, butabarbital, mephobarbital, pentobarbital, and secobarbital).

● Before starting to take primidone, be sure to tell your doctor if you now have, or if you have ever had, asthma, kidney disease, liver disease, or porphyria.

● If this drug makes you dizzy or drowsy, do not take part in any activities that require alertness, such as driving a car or operating potentially dangerous equipment.

● Before having any surgery or other medical or dental treatment, be sure your doctor or dentist knows that you are taking primidone.

● Do not stop taking this medication unless you first check with your doctor. Stopping the drug abruptly can lead to a worsening of your condition. Your doctor may therefore want to reduce your dosage gradually, or start you on another drug when primidone is stopped.

● Be sure to tell your doctor if you are pregnant. Birth defects have been reported more often in infants whose mothers have seizure disorders. It is unclear if the increased risk of birth defects is associated with the disorders or with the anti-convulsion medications, such as primidone, that are used to treat the condition. Such drugs may also lead to bleeding complications in the newborn. The risks and benefits of treatment should be discussed with your doctor. Also, tell your doctor if you are breast-feeding an infant. Primidone passes into breast milk and can cause extreme drowsiness in nursing infants.

Primoline—see primidone

Principen—see ampicillin

Proaqua—see benzthiazide

Probalan—see probenecid

Pro-Banthine—see propantheline

---

probenecid

BRAND NAMES (Manufacturers)
Benemid (Merck Sharp & Dohme)
Probalan (Lannett)
probenecid (various manufacturers)
SK-Probenecid (Smith Kline & French)
TYPE OF DRUG
Uricosuric (anti-gout preparation)
INGREDIENT
probenecid
DOSAGE FORM
Tablets (500 mg)
STORAGE
Probenecid should be stored at room temperature in a tightly closed container.

USES

Probenecid is used to prevent gout attacks. It increases the elimination through the kidneys of uric acid (the chemical responsible for gout's symptoms). Probenecid is also occasionally used in combination with penicillin or ampicillin, to increase the length of time that the antibiotics remain in the bloodstream.

TREATMENT

In order to avoid stomach irritation, you should take probenecid with a full glass of water or milk. You should also drink at least ten to 12 full eight-ounce glasses of liquids (not alcoholic beverages) each day to prevent formation of uric acid kidney stones.

If you miss a dose of this medication, take the missed dose as soon as possible, unless it is almost time for the next dose. In that case, do not take the missed dose at all; just return to your regular dosing schedule. Do not double the next dose.

SIDE EFFECTS

Minor. Dizziness; frequent urination; headache; loss of appetite; nausea; rash; sore gums; and vomiting. These side effects should disappear in several days, as your body adjusts to the medication.

If you feel dizzy, sit or lie down awhile; get up slowly, and be careful on stairs.

Major. Tell your doctor about any side effects that are persistent or particularly bothersome. IT IS ESPECIALLY IMPORTANT TO TELL YOUR DOCTOR about fatigue; fever; flushing; lower back pain; painful or difficult urination; sore throat; unusual bleeding or bruising; or yellowing of the eyes or skin.

INTERACTIONS

Probenecid interacts with several other types of medication.

1. Aspirin and pyrazinamide antagonize (act against) the anti-gout effects of probenecid.

2. The blood levels of methotrexate, sulfonamide antibiotics, cinoxacin, nitrofurantoin, oral anti-diabetic medicines, naproxen, indomethacin, rifampin, sulindac, dapsone, and clofibrate can be increased by probenicid, which can lead to an increase in side effects.

3. Alcohol, chlorthalidone, ethacrynic acid, furosemide, and thiazide diuretics (water pills) can increase blood uric acid levels, which can decrease the effectiveness of probenecid.

Before starting to take probenecid, BE SURE TO TELL YOUR DOCTOR if you are already taking any of the medications listed above.

WARNINGS

● Tell your doctor about unusual or allergic reactions you have had to any medications, especially to probenecid.

● Before starting to take probenecid, be sure to tell your doctor if you now have, or if you have ever had, blood diseases; diabetes mellitus; glucose-6-phosphate dehydrogenase (G6PD) deficiency; kidney stones; peptic ulcers; or porphyria.

● Diabetics using Clinitest urine glucose tests may get erroneously high readings of blood sugar levels while they are taking this drug. Temporarily changing to Clinistix or Tes-Tape urine tests will avoid this problem.

● If probenecid makes you dizzy, avoid tasks that require alertness, such as driving a car or operating potentially dangerous equipment.

● Avoid taking large amounts of vitamin C while on probenecid. Vitamin C can increase the risk of kidney stone formation.

● Probenecid is not effective for an attack of gout. It is used to prevent attacks.

● Be sure to tell your doctor if you are pregnant. Although probenecid appears to be safe, it does cross the placenta. Extensive studies in pregnant women have not yet been completed. Also, tell your doctor if you are breastfeeding an infant. It is not known whether or not probenecid passes into breast milk.

---

probucol

BRAND NAME (Manufacturer)
Lorelco (Merrell Dow)

TYPE OF DRUG
Anti-hyperlipidemic (lipid-lowering drug)
INGREDIENT
probucol
DOSAGE FORM
Tablets (250 mg)
STORAGE
Probucol should be stored at room temperature in a tightly closed, light-resistant container.

USES

This medication is used to treat hypercholesterolemia (high blood cholesterol levels) in patients who have not responded to diet, weight reduction, exercise, and control of blood sugar. It is not clear how probucol lowers blood cholesterol levels, but it is thought to decrease the body's own production of cholesterol.

TREATMENT

Probucol should be taken with meals, in order to maximize its effectiveness.

If you miss a dose of this medication, take the missed dose as soon as possible, unless it is almost time for the next dose. In that case, don't take the missed dose at all; just return to your regular dosing schedule. Do not double the next dose.

The therapeutic benefits of this medication may not become apparent for up to three months after it is started.

SIDE EFFECTS

Minor. Diarrhea; dizziness; gas; headache; insomnia; nausea; stomach upset; and vomiting. These side effects should disappear in several days, as your body adjusts to the medication.

If you feel dizzy, sit or lie down awhile; get up slowly, and be careful on stairs.

Major. Tell your doctor about any side effects that are persistent or particularly bothersome. IT IS ESPECIALLY IMPORTANT TO TELL YOUR DOCTOR about blurred vision; bloody or black, tarry stools; chest pain; impotence, palpitations; rash; ringing in the ears; sweating; tingling sensations; or unusual bleeding or bruising.

INTERACTIONS

Probucol does not interact with other medications, if it is used according to directions.

WARNINGS

● Tell your doctor about unusual or allergic reactions you have had to any medications, especially to probucol.

● Before starting to take this medication, be sure to tell your doctor if you now have, or if you have ever had, biliary tract disorders, gallstones or gallbladder disease, heart disease, or liver disease.

● Do not stop taking this medication unless you first check with your doctor. Stopping the drug abruptly may lead to a rapid increase in blood lipid (fats) and cholesterol levels. Your doctor may therefore want to start you on a special diet or another medication when probucol treatment is stopped.

● Be sure to tell your doctor if you are pregnant. Although probucol appears to be safe during pregnancy, extensive studies in humans have not yet been completed. If you and your doctor decide that you should stop the drug for a planned pregnancy, some form of birth control should be used for at least six months after probucol therapy is stopped, to assure that the drug has been completely eliminated from the body. Also, tell your doctor if you are breastfeeding an infant. It is not known whether or not probucol passes into breast milk.

---

procainamide

BRAND NAMES (Manufacturers)
procainamide hydrochloride (various manufacturers)
Procan (Parke-Davis)
Pronestyl (Squibb)
Sub-Quin (Scrip)
TYPE OF DRUG
Anti-arrhythmic
INGREDIENT
procainamide as the hydrochloride salt
DOSAGE FORMS
Tablets (250 mg, 375 mg, and 500 mg)

Sustained-release tablets (250 mg, 500 mg, and 750 mg)
Capsules (250 mg, 375 mg, and 500 mg)

STORAGE

Procainamide tablets and capsules should be stored in
tightly closed containers in a cool, dry place. Exposure to
moisture causes deterioration of this medication.

USES

Procainamide is used to treat heart arrhythmias. It corrects
irregular heartbeats and helps to achieve a more normal
rhythm.

TREATMENT

To increase absorption, take procainamide with a full glass
of water on an empty stomach, one hour before or two
hours after a meal. However, if it upsets your stomach, ask
your doctor if you can take it with food or milk.

Try to take it at the same time(s) each day. Procainamide
works best when the amount of drug in your bloodstream
is kept at a constant level. This medication should therefore be taken at evenly spaced intervals, day and night. For
example, if you are to take this medication four times per
day, the doses should be spaced six hours apart.

The sustained-release tablets should be swallowed
whole. Breaking, chewing, or crushing these tablets destroys their sustained-release activity, and possibly increases the side effects.

If you miss a dose of this medication, take the missed
dose immediately—if you remember within an hour or so.
If more than one hour has passed (or four hours for the
sustained-release tablets), do not take the missed dose;
just return to your regular dosing schedule. Do not double
the next dose.

SIDE EFFECTS

Minor. Bitter taste in the mouth; diarrhea; dizziness; dry
mouth; headache; itching; loss of appetite; nausea; stomach upset; and vomiting. These side effects should disappear in several days, as your body adjusts to the
medication.

If you feel dizzy, sit or lie down awhile; get up slowly,
and be careful on stairs.

To relieve mouth dryness, chew sugarless gum, or suck on ice chips or a piece of hard candy.

Major. Tell your doctor about any side effects that are persistent or particularly bothersome. IT IS ESPECIALLY IMPORTANT TO TELL YOUR DOCTOR about chest pain; chills; confusion; depression; fainting; fatigue; fever; giddiness; hallucinations; joint pain; palpitations; rash; sore throat; unusual bleeding or bruising; or weakness.

INTERACTIONS

Procainamide interacts with several other types of medication.

1. The combination of digoxin and procainamide can lead to an increase in side effects to the heart.

2. Procainamide can block the effectiveness of neostigmine, pyridostigmine, and prostigmine.

3. Cimetidine can increase the blood levels of procainamide, which can lead to an increase in side effects. Before starting to take procainamide, BE SURE TO TELL YOUR DOCTOR if you are already taking any of the medications listed above.

WARNINGS

• Tell your doctor about unusual or allergic reactions you have had to any medications, especially to procainamide, procaine, lidocaine, benzocaine, or tetracaine.

• Before starting this medication, be sure to tell your doctor if you now have, or if you have ever had, asthma, heart block, kidney disease, liver disease, myasthenia gravis, or systemic lupus erythematosus (SLE).

• If this drug makes you dizzy, do not take part in any activity that requires alertness, such as driving a car or operating potentially dangerous equipment.

• Before having any surgery or other medical or dental treatment, be sure your doctor or dentist knows that you are taking this medication.

• Do not stop taking this drug without first consulting your doctor. Stopping procainamide abruptly may cause a serious change in the activity of your heart. Your doctor may therefore want to reduce your dosage gradually.

• Some of these products contain F.D. & C. Yellow Dye No. 5 (tartrazine), which can cause allergic-type symptoms (rash, shortness of breath, fainting) in certain susceptible individuals.

● Be sure to tell your doctor if you are pregnant. Although this drug appears to be safe, extensive studies in pregnant women have not yet been completed. Also, tell your doctor if you are breastfeeding an infant. It is not known whether or not procainamide passes into breast milk.

procainamide hydrochloride—see procainamide

Procan—see procainamide

---

procarbazine

BRAND NAME (Manufacturer)
Matulane (Roche)
TYPE OF DRUG
Anti-neoplastic (anti-cancer drug)
INGREDIENT
procarbazine
DOSAGE FORM
Capsules (50 mg)
STORAGE
Procarbazine capsules should be stored at room temperature in a tightly closed, light-resistant container.

USES

This medication belongs to a group of drugs known as alkylating agents. It is used to treat a variety of cancers. Procarbazine is thought to work by binding to the rapidly growing cancer cells, thereby preventing their multiplication and growth.

TREATMENT

In order to prevent stomach irritation, you can take procarbazine with food or milk (unless your doctor directs you to do otherwise).

The timing of the dose of this medication is important. Be sure you completely understand your doctor's instructions on how and when this medication should be taken.

If you miss a dose of this medication and remember within a short period of time, take the missed dose immediately. If more than several hours have passed, check with your doctor to find out when the dose should be taken.

SIDE EFFECTS

Minor. Constipation; diarrhea; dizziness; drowsiness; dry mouth; headache; insomnia; loss of appetite; nausea; and vomiting. These side effects may disappear as your body adjusts to the medication. However, it is important to continue taking this medication, despite any nausea and vomiting that occur.

Procarbazine can also cause hair loss (which is reversible when the medication is stopped).

To relieve constipation, increase the amount of fiber in your diet (bran, salads, fresh fruits and vegetables, and whole-grain breads), exercise, and drink more water (unless your doctor directs you to do otherwise).

If you feel dizzy, sit or lie down awhile; get up slowly, and be careful on stairs.

To help relieve mouth dryness, chew sugarless gum, or suck on ice chips or a piece of hard candy.

This medication can increase your sensitivity to sunlight. You should therefore avoid prolonged exposure to sunlight and sunlamps. Wear protective clothing and sunglasses, and use an effective sunscreen.

Major. Tell your doctor about any side effects that are persistent or particularly bothersome. IT IS ESPECIALLY IMPORTANT TO TELL YOUR DOCTOR about unusual bleeding or bruising; bloody or black, tarry stools; blurred vision; chest pain; chills; confusion; convulsions; darkening of the skin; depression; difficulty swallowing; fainting; flushing; fever; hallucinations; altered hearing; itching; joint pain; lethargy; loss of coordination; menstrual irregularities; mouth sores; muscle pains; nervousness; nightmares; skin rash; slurred speech; sore throat; sweating; tingling sensations; tremors; weakness; or yellowing of the eyes or skin.

INTERACTIONS

Procarbazine interacts with other types of medication.

1. Concurrent use of it with central nervous system depressants (drugs that slow the activity of the brain and spinal cord), including alcohol, antihistamines, barbiturates, benzodiazepine tranquilizers, muscle relaxants, narcotics, pain medications, and phenothiazine tranquilizers, or with tricyclic anti-depressants can lead to extreme drowsiness.

2. Diabetic patients should know that procarbazine can increase the blood-sugar-lowering effects of insulin and oral anti-diabetic medications. Dosages of these medications may need to be adjusted when procarbazine is started.

3. The combination of procarbazine with guanethidine, levodopa, methyldopa, or reserpine can result in excitation and high blood pressure.

4. Concurrent use of procarbazine and tricyclic anti-depressants, monoamine oxidase (MAO) inhibitors, amphetamines, decongestants, or phenothiazine tranquilizers can lead to severe reactions. Tricyclic anti-depressants should be stopped seven days before starting procarbazine therapy, and MAO inhibitors should be stopped 14 days prior to starting therapy.

5. Ingestion of alcohol while taking procarbazine can result in fainting, flushing, headache, nausea, vomiting, and weakness.

Before starting to take procarbazine, BE SURE TO TELL YOUR DOCTOR if you are already taking any of the medications listed above.

WARNINGS

• Tell your doctor about unusual or allergic reactions you have had to any medications, especially to procarbazine.

• Before starting to take this medication, be sure to tell your doctor if you now have, or if you have ever had, blood disorders; chronic or recurrent infections; diabetes mellitus (sugar diabetes); kidney disease; or liver disease.

• If this drug makes you dizzy or drowsy, or blurs your vision, avoid taking part in any activity that requires alertness, such as driving a car or operating potentially dangerous equipment.

• Before having any surgery or other medical or dental treatment, be sure your doctor or dentist knows that you are taking this medication.

- You should not receive any immunizations or vaccinations while taking this medication. Procarbazine blocks the effectiveness of vaccines, and may result in an overwhelming infection if a live vaccine is administered.
- Procarbazine can lower your platelet count, thereby decreasing your body's ability to form blood clots. You should therefore be especially careful while brushing your teeth, flossing, or using toothpicks, razors, or fingernail scissors. Try to avoid falls and other injuries.
- While you are taking procarbazine , avoid eating foods containing tyramine (certain cheeses, soy sauce, fava beans, chicken liver, avocados, bananas, canned figs, raisins, beers, and certain wines). The combination can lead to severe hypertensive (high blood pressure) reactions.
- Procarbazine can decrease fertility in both men and women.
- Be sure to tell your doctor if you are pregnant. Birth defects have been reported in both humans and animals whose mothers received procarbazine during pregnancy. The risks should be discussed with your doctor. Also, tell your doctor if you are breastfeeding an infant. It is not known whether or not procarbazine passes into breast milk.

Procardia—see nifedipine

Prochlor-Iso—see prochlorperazine and isopropamide combination

---

prochlorperazine

BRAND NAMES (Manufacturers)
Chlorazine (Major)
Compazine (Smith Kline & French)
prochlorperazine maleate (various manufacturers)
TYPE OF DRUG
Phenothiazine tranquilizer and anti-emetic
INGREDIENT
prochlorperazine as the maleate salt
DOSAGE FORMS
Tablets (5 mg, 10 mg, and 25 mg)

Sustained-release capsules (10 mg, 15 mg, 30 mg, and 75 mg)
Suppositories (2.5 mg, 5 mg, and 25 mg)
Oral concentrate (10 mg per ml)
Oral syrup (5 mg per 5 ml teaspoonful)

STORAGE

The tablet and capsule forms of this medication should be stored at room temperature in tightly closed, light-resistant containers. The oral concentrate, oral syrup, and suppository forms should be stored in the refrigerator in tightly closed, light-resistant containers. If the oral concentrate or oral syrup turns to a slight yellow color, the medicine is still effective and can be used. However, if they change color markedly, or have particles floating in them, they should not be used, but discarded down the sink. Prochlorperazine should never be frozen.

USES

Prochlorperazine is prescribed to treat the symptoms of certain types of mental illness, such as emotional symptoms of psychosis, the manic phase of manic-depressive illness, and severe behavioral problems in children. This medication is thought to relieve the symptoms of mental illness by blocking certain chemicals involved with nerve transmission in the brain. Prochlorperazine is also frequently used to treat nausea and vomiting (this medication works at the vomiting center in the brain to relieve nausea and vomiting).

TREATMENT

To avoid stomach irritation, you can take the tablet or capsule form of this medication with a meal or with a glass of water or milk (unless your doctor directs you to do otherwise).

Antacids and anti-diarrhea medicine may decrease the absorption of this medication from the gastrointestinal tract. Therefore, at least one hour should separate doses of one of these medicines and prochlorperazine.

The sustained-release capsules should be swallowed whole; do not crush, break, or open them. Breaking the capsule releases the medication all at once—defeating the purpose of the sustained-release capsules.

Measure the oral syrup carefully, with a specially designed, 5 ml measuring spoon. An ordinary kitchen teaspoon is not accurate enough.

The oral concentrate form of this medication should be measured carefully with the dropper provided, then added to 4 ounces (½ cup) or more of water, milk, juice, or a carbonated beverage, or to applesauce or pudding, immediately prior to administration. To prevent possible loss of effectiveness, the medication should not be diluted in tea, coffee, or apple juice.

To use the suppository form of this medication, remove the foil wrapper (if the suppository is too soft to insert, refrigerate it for half an hour or run cold water over it before removing the wrapper), and moisten the suppository with water. Lie on your left side with your right knee bent. Push the suppository into the rectum, pointed end first. Lie still for a few minutes. Try to avoid having a bowel movement for at least an hour (to give the medication time to be absorbed).

If you miss a dose of this medication, take the missed dose as soon as possible and return to your regular dosing schedule. If it is almost time for the next dose, however, skip the one you missed and return to your regular schedule. Do not double the dose (unless your doctor directs you to do so).

The full effects of this medication for the control of emotional or mental symptoms may not become apparent for two weeks after you start to take it.

SIDE EFFECTS

Minor. Blurred vision; constipation; decreased sweating; diarrhea; discoloration of the urine to red, pink, or red-brown; dizziness; drooling; drowsiness; dry mouth; fatigue; jitteriness; menstrual irregularities; nasal congestion; restlessness; tremors; vomiting; and weight gain. As your body adjusts to the medication, these side effects should disappear.

If you are constipated, increase the amount of fiber in your diet (raw vegetables, fruits, salads, bran, and whole-grain breads), and drink more water (unless your doctor directs you to do otherwise).

Chew sugarless gum, or suck on ice chips or a piece of

hard candy, to reduce mouth dryness.

This medication can cause increased sensitivity to sunlight. It is therefore important to avoid prolonged exposure to sunlight and sunlamps. Wear protective clothing, and use an effective sunscreen.

To avoid dizziness or light-headedness when you stand, contract and relax the muscles of your legs for a few moments before rising. Do this by pushing one foot against the floor while raising the other foot slightly, alternating feet so that you are "pumping" your legs in a pedaling motion.

Major. Tell your doctor about any side effects that are persistent or particularly bothersome. IT IS ESPECIALLY IMPORTANT TO TELL YOUR DOCTOR about unusual bleeding or bruising; breast enlargement (in both sexes); chest pain; convulsions; darkened skin; difficulty swallowing or breathing; fainting; fever; impotence; involuntary movements of the face, mouth, jaw, or tongue; palpitations; rash; sleep disorders; sore throat; uncoordinated movements; visual disturbances; or yellowing of the eyes or skin.

INTERACTIONS

Prochlorperazine interacts with other medication.

1. It can cause extreme drowsiness when combined with alcohol or other central nervous system depressants (drugs that slow the activity of the nervous system), such as barbiturates, benzodiazepine tranquilizers, muscle relaxants, narcotics, and pain medications, or with tricyclic anti-depressants.

2. Prochlorperazine can decrease the effectiveness of amphetamines, guanethidine, anti-convulsants, and levodopa.

3. The side effects of epinephrine, monoamine oxidase (MAO) inhibitors, propranolol, phenytoin, and tricyclic anti-depressants may be increased when combined with this medication.

4. Lithium may increase the side effects, and decrease the effectiveness, of this medication.

Before starting to take prochlorperazine, BE SURE TO TELL YOUR DOCTOR if you are already taking any of the medications listed above.

WARNINGS

- Tell your doctor about any unusual or allergic reactions you have had to medications, especially to prochlorperazine or other phenothiazine tranquilizers (such as acetophenazine, carphenazine, chlorpromazine, fluphenazine, mesoridazine, perphenazine, piperacetazine, promazine, thioridazine, trifluoperazine, triflupromazine) or to loxapine.

- Tell your doctor if you now have, or if you have ever had, any blood disease, bone marrow disease, brain disease, breast cancer, blockage in the urinary or digestive tracts, alcoholism, drug-induced depression, epilepsy, severe high or low blood pressure, diabetes mellitus (sugar diabetes), glaucoma, heart or circulatory disease, liver disease, lung disease, Parkinson's disease, peptic ulcers, or an enlarged prostate gland.

- Tell your doctor about any recent exposure to a pesticide or an insecticide. Prochlorperazine may increase the side effects from the exposure.

- To prevent over-sedation, avoid drinking alcoholic beverages while taking this medication.

- If this medication makes you dizzy or drowsy, do not take part in any activity that requires alertness, such as driving a car or operating potentially dangerous equipment. Be careful on stairs and avoid getting up suddenly from a lying or sitting position.

- Prior to having surgery or any other medical or dental treatment, be sure your doctor or dentist knows that you are taking this medication.

- Some of the side effects caused by this drug can be prevented by taking an anti-parkinson drug. Discuss this with your doctor.

- Prochlorperazine has been reported to cause certain tumors in rats. This effect has not been shown to occur in humans.

- This medication can decrease sweating and heat release from the body. You should therefore avoid getting overheated (strenuous exercise in hot weather; hot baths, showers, and saunas).

- Do not stop taking prochlorperazine suddenly if you have been taking it for a prolonged period. If the drug is stopped abruptly, you may experience nausea, vomiting, stomach upset, headache, increased heart rate, insomnia, tremulousness, or a worsening of your condition. Your doctor may want to reduce the dosage gradually.

• If you are planning to have a myelogram, or any procedure in which dye will be injected into your spinal cord, tell your doctor that you are taking this medication.

• Avoid spilling the oral concentrate or syrup forms of this medication on your skin or clothing; they may cause redness and irritation of the skin.

• While taking this medication, do not take any over-the-counter (non-prescription) medication for weight control, or for cough, cold, allergy, asthma, or sinus problems, unless you first check with your doctor. The combination of these medications with prochlorperazine may cause high blood pressure.

• Be sure to tell your doctor if you are pregnant. Small amounts of this medication cross the placenta. Although there are reports of safe use of this drug during pregnancy, there are also reports of liver disease and tremors in newborn infants whose mothers received this type of medication close to term. Also, tell your doctor if you are breastfeeding an infant. Small amounts of this medication pass into breast milk and may cause unwanted effects in the nursing infant.

prochlorperazine and isopropamide combination

BRAND NAMES (Manufacturers)
Combid (Smith Kline & French)
Isopro T.D. (Rugby)
Prochlor-Iso (Henry Schein)
Pro-Iso (various manufacturers)
TYPE OF DRUG
Phenothiazine tranquilizer and anti-cholinergic
INGREDIENTS
prochlorperazine as the maleate salt; isopropamide as the iodide salt
DOSAGE FORM
Capsules (10 mg prochlorperazine and 5 mg isopropamide)

STORAGE

Prochlorperazine and isopropamide capsules should be stored at room temperature in a tightly closed, light-resistant container.

USES

Prochlorperazine and isopropamide combination is used to treat intestinal and stomach disorders, such as peptic ulcers and irritable bowel syndrome. Prochlorperazine belongs to a group of drugs known as phenothiazine tranquilizers. It acts on the brain to relieve nausea and vomiting, and also relieves anxiety by acting as a central nervous system (brain and spinal cord) depressant. Isopropamide is an anti-cholinergic agent that slows down the gastrointestinal tract and reduces the production of stomach acid.

TREATMENT

Prochlorperazine and isopropamide capsules should be taken with a full glass of water 30 minutes before a meal.

Antacids and anti-diarrhea medicine may decrease the absorption of this medication from the gastrointestinal tract. Therefore, at least one hour should separate doses of these medicines and this combination drug.

The capsules should be swallowed whole. Breaking, crushing, or opening the capsules destroys their sustained-release activity, and possibly increases the side effects.

If you miss a dose of this medication, take the missed dose as soon as possible, unless it is within 10 hours of your next scheduled dose. In that case, do not take the missed dose at all; just return to your regular dosing schedule. Do not double the next dose (unless your doctor directs you to do so).

SIDE EFFECTS

Minor. Bloating; blurred vision; constipation; dizziness; drowsiness; dry mouth; flaking skin; fever; headache; insomnia; jitteriness; menstrual irregularities; nasal congestion; nausea; nervousness; reduced sweating; and restlessness. These side effects should disappear in several days, as your body adjusts to the medication.

Dry mouth can be relieved by chewing sugarless gum, or by sucking on ice chips or a piece of hard candy.

To avoid dizziness or light-headedness when you stand, contract and relax the muscles of your legs for a few moments before rising. Do this by pushing one foot against the floor while raising the other foot slightly, alternating feet so that you are "pumping" your legs in a pedaling motion.

This medication may cause increased sensitivity to sunlight. You should therefore avoid prolonged exposure to sunlight and sunlamps. Wear protective clothing and sunglasses, and use an effective sunscreen.

Major. Tell your doctor about any side effects that are persistent or particularly bothersome. IT IS ESPECIALLY IMPORTANT TO TELL YOUR DOCTOR about unusual bleeding or bruising; back pain; chest tightness; convulsions; difficulty breathing; difficulty swallowing; difficult or painful urination; drooling; enlarged breasts (in both sexes); impotence; involuntary movements of the face, tongue, mouth, or jaw; muscle stiffness; eye pain; palpitations; rapid weight gain (three to five pounds within a week); rash; sore throat; tremors; uncoordinated movements; or yellowing of the eyes or skin.

INTERACTIONS

Prochlorperazine and isopropamide combination interacts with several types of medication.

1. It can cause extreme drowsiness when combined with alcohol or other central nervous system depressants (drugs that slow the activity of the nervous system), such as barbiturates, antihistamines, benzodiazepine tranquilizers, muscle relaxants, narcotics, pain medications, and sleeping medications, or with tricyclic anti-depressants.

2. Prochlorperazine can decrease the effectiveness of amphetamines, guanethidine, anti-convulsants, and levodopa.

3. The side effects of epinephrine, monoamine oxidase (MAO) inhibitors, propranolol, phenytoin, tricyclic anti-depressants, amantadine, haloperidol, procainamide, and quinidine may be increased when combined with this medication.

Before starting to take this medication, BE SURE TO TELL

YOUR DOCTOR if you are already taking any of the medications listed above.

WARNINGS

● Tell your doctor about unusual or allergic reactions you have had to medications, especially to prochlorperazine or other phenothiazine tranquilizers (such as chlorpromazine, fluphenazine, mesoridazine, promazine, or thioridazine); to isopropamide; to loxapine; or to iodine.

● Tell your doctor if you now have, or if you have ever had, blood diseases, brain tumor, drug-induced depression, epilepsy, glaucoma, heart disease, liver disease, lung disease, kidney disease, myasthenia gravis, hiatal hernia, high blood pressure, obstructed intestine or bladder, Parkinson's disease, peptic ulcers, thyroid disease, or ulcerative colitis.

● Some of these products contain F.D. & C. Yellow Dye No. 5 (tartrazine), which can cause allergic-type reactions (shortness of breath, wheezing, rash, or fainting) in certain susceptible individuals.

● To prevent over-sedation, avoid drinking alcoholic beverages while taking this medication.

● If this medication makes you dizzy or drowsy, do not take part in any activity that requires alertness, such as driving a car or operating potentially dangerous equipment. Be careful on stairs; and avoid getting up suddenly from a lying or sitting position.

● Prior to having surgery or any other medical or dental treatment, be sure your doctor or dentist knows that you are taking this medication.

● Prochlorperazine has been reported to cause certain tumors in rats. This effect has not been shown to occur in humans.

● This medication can decrease sweating and heat release from the body. You should therefore avoid getting overheated (strenuous exercise in hot weather; hot baths, showers, and saunas).

● Do not stop taking this medication suddenly. If the drug is stopped abruptly, you may experience nausea, vomiting, stomach upset, headache, increased heart rate, insomnia, tremulousness, or a worsening of your condition. Your

doctor may therefore want to reduce the dosage gradually.
● If you are planning to have a myelogram, or any procedure in which dye will be injected into your spinal cord,
tell your doctor that you are taking this medication.
● While taking this medication, do not take any over-the-
counter (non-prescription) medication for weight control,
or for cough, cold, allergy, asthma, or sinus problems, unless you first check with your doctor. The combination of
these medications may cause high blood pressure.
● Be sure to tell your doctor if you are pregnant. Small
amounts of this medication cross the placenta. Although
there are reports of safe use of this drug during pregnancy,
there are also reports of liver disease and tremors in newborn infants whose mothers received this type of medication close to term. Also, tell your doctor if you are
breastfeeding an infant. Small amounts of this medication
pass into breast milk and may cause unwanted effects in
the nursing infant.

prochlorperazine maleate—see prochlorperazine

Profene-65—see propoxyphene

Pro-Iso—see prochlorperazine and isopropamide
    combination

Proklar—see sulfonamides

Prolixin—see fluphenazine

Proloprim—see trimethoprim

Promapar—see chlorpromazine

---

promazine

BRAND NAMES (Manufacturers)
promazine hydrochloride (various manufacturers)
Prozine (Hauck)
Sparine (Wyeth)

TYPE OF DRUG
Phenothiazine tranquilizer
INGREDIENT
promazine as the hydrochloride salt
DOSAGE FORMS
Tablets (10 mg, 25 mg, 50 mg, and 100 mg)
Oral syrup (10 mg per 5 ml teaspoonful)
Oral concentrate (30 mg per ml)
STORAGE
The tablet form of this medication should be stored at room temperature in a tightly closed, light-resistant container. The oral concentrate and the oral syrup forms of this medication should be stored in the refrigerator in tightly closed, light-resistant containers. If the oral concentrate or oral syrup turns to a slight yellow color, the medicine is still effective and can be used. However, if they change color markedly, or have particles floating in them, they should not be used, but discarded down the sink.

USES
Promazine is prescribed to treat the symptoms of certain types of mental illness, such as emotional symptoms of psychosis, the manic phase of manic-depressive illness, and severe behavioral problems in children. This medication is thought to relieve the symptoms of mental illness by blocking certain chemicals involved with nerve transmission in the brain.

TREATMENT
To avoid stomach irritation, you can take the tablet form of this medication with a meal or with a glass of water or milk (unless your doctor directs you to do otherwise).

Measure the oral syrup carefully, with a specially designed, 5 ml measuring spoon. An ordinary kitchen teaspoon is not accurate enough.

The oral concentrate form of this medication should be measured carefully with the dropper provided, then added to four ounces (1/2 cup) or more of water, milk, juice, or a carbonated beverage, or to applesauce or pudding, immediately prior to administration. To prevent possible loss of effectiveness, the medication should not be diluted in tea, coffee, or apple juice.

If you miss a dose of this medication, take the missed dose as soon as possible, then return to your regular dosing schedule. If it is almost time for the next dose, however, skip the one you missed and return to your regular dosing schedule. Do not double the dose (unless your doctor directs you to do so).

Antacids and anti-diarrhea medicine may decrease the absorption of this medication from the gastrointestinal tract. Therefore, at least one hour should separate doses of one of these medicines and promazine.

The full effects of this medication for the control of emotional or mental symptoms may not become apparent for two weeks after you start to take it.

SIDE EFFECTS

Minor. Blurred vision; constipation; decreased sweating; diarrhea; discoloration of the urine to red, pink, or red-brown; dizziness; drooling; drowsiness; dry mouth; fatigue; jitteriness; menstrual irregularities; nasal congestion; restlessness; tremors; vomiting; and weight gain. As your body adjusts to the medication, these side effects should disappear.

If you are constipated, increase the amount of fiber in your diet (raw vegetables, fruits, salads, bran, and whole-grain breads), and drink more water (unless your doctor directs you to do otherwise).

Chew sugarless gum, or suck on ice chips or a piece of hard candy, to reduce mouth dryness.

This medication can cause increased sensitivity to sunlight. It is therefore important to avoid prolonged exposure to sunlight and sunlamps. Wear protective clothing, and use an effective sunscreen.

To avoid dizziness or light-headedness when you stand, contract and relax the muscles of your legs for a few moments before rising. Do this by pushing one foot against the floor while raising the other foot slightly, alternating feet so that you are "pumping" your legs in a pedaling motion.

Major. Tell your doctor about any side effects that are persistent or particularly bothersome. IT IS ESPECIALLY IMPORTANT TO TELL YOUR DOCTOR about unusual bleeding or bruising; breast enlargement (in both sexes);

chest pain; convulsions; darkened skin; difficulty swallowing or breathing; fainting; fever; impotence; involuntary
movements of the face, mouth, jaw, or tongue; palpitations; rash; sleep disorders; sore throat; uncoordinated
movements; visual disturbances; or yellowing of the eyes
or skin.

INTERACTIONS

Promazine interacts with other types of medication.

1. It can cause extreme drowsiness when combined with
alcohol or other central nervous system depressants (drugs
that slow the activity of the nervous system), such as barbiturates, benzodiazepine tranquilizers, muscle relaxants,
narcotics, and pain medications, or with tricyclic anti-
depressants.

2. Promazine can decrease the effectiveness of amphetamines, guanethidine, anti-convulsants, and levodopa.

3. The side effects of epinephrine, monoamine-oxidase
(MAO) inhibitors, propranolol, phenytoin, and tricyclic
anti-depressants may be increased when combined with
this medication.

4. Lithium may increase the side effects and decrease the
effectiveness of this medication.

BE SURE TO TELL YOUR DOCTOR if you are already taking any of the medications listed above.

WARNINGS

● Tell your doctor about unusual or allergic reactions you
have had to any medications, especially to promazine or
other phenothiazine tranquilizers (such as acetophenazine, carphenazine, chlorpromazine, fluphenazine, mesoridazine, perphenazine, piperacetazine, prochlorperazine, thioridazine, trifluoperazine, triflupromazine), or to
loxapine.

● Tell your doctor if you now have, or if you have ever
had, any blood disease, bone marrow disease, brain disease, breast cancer, blockage in the urinary or digestive
tracts, alcoholism, drug-induced depression, epilepsy, severe high or low blood pressure, diabetes mellitus (sugar
diabetes), glaucoma, heart or circulatory disease, liver disease, lung disease, Parkinson's disease, peptic ulcers, or
an enlarged prostate gland.

• Tell your doctor about any recent exposure to a pesti cide or an insecticide. Promazine may increase the side effects from the exposure.

• To prevent over-sedation, avoid drinking alcoholic beverages while taking this medication.

• If this medication makes you dizzy or drowsy, do not take part in any activity that requires alertness, such as driving a car or operating potentially dangerous equipment. Be careful on stairs; and avoid getting up suddenly from a lying or sitting position.

• Prior to having surgery or any other medical or dental treatment, be sure your doctor or dentist knows that you are taking this medication.

• Some of the side effects caused by this drug can be prevented by taking an anti-parkinson drug. Discuss this with your doctor.

• Promazine has been reported to cause certain tumors in rats. This effect has not been shown to occur in humans.

• This medication can decrease sweating and heat release from the body. You should therefore avoid getting overheated (strenuous exercise in hot weather; hot baths, showers, and saunas).

• Do not stop taking this medication suddenly. If the drug is stopped abruptly, you may experience nausea, vomiting, stomach upset, headache, increased heart rate, insomnia, tremulousness, or a worsening of your condition. Your doctor may therefore want to reduce the dosage gradually.

• If you are planning to have a myelogram, or any procedure in which dye will be injected into your spinal cord, tell your doctor that you are taking this medication.

• Avoid spilling the oral concentrate or oral syrup forms of this medication on your skin or clothing; they may cause redness and irritation of the skin.

• While taking this medication, do not take any over-the-counter (non-prescription) medication for weight control, or for cough, cold, allergy, asthma, or sinus problems, unless you first check with your doctor. The combination of these medications may cause high blood pressure.

• Be sure to tell your doctor if you are pregnant. Small amounts of this medication cross the placenta. Although there are reports of safe use of this drug during pregnancy, there are also reports of liver disease and tremors in new-born infants whose mothers received this medication close to term. Also, tell your doctor if you are breastfeeding an infant. Small amounts of this medication pass into breast milk and may cause unwanted effects in nursing infants.

promazine hydrochloride—see promazine

Promethazine Hydrochloride with Codeine—see promethazine, potassium guaiacolsulfonate, and codeine combination

Promethazine Hydrochloride VC Expectorant with Codeine—see phenylephrine, potassium guaiacolsulfonate, promethazine, and codeine combination

---

promethazine, potassium guaiacolsulfonate, and codeine combination

BRAND NAMES (Manufacturers)
Pentazine Expectorant with Codeine (Century)
Phenergan Expectorant with Codeine (Wyeth)
Promethazine Hydrochloride with Codeine (various manufacturers)
Prothazine with Codeine Expectorant (Vortech)
TYPE OF DRUG
Antihistamine, expectorant, and cough suppressant
INGREDIENTS
promethazine as the hydrochloride salt, potassium guaiacolsulfonate, and codeine as the phosphate salt
DOSAGE FORM
Oral syrup (5 mg promethazine, 44 mg potassium guaiacolsulfonate, 10 mg codeine, and 7% alcohol per 5 ml teaspoonful)

STORAGE

This medication should be stored at room temperature in a tightly closed, light-resistant container. This medication should never be frozen.

USES

This drug combination is used to provide symptomatic relief of coughs due to colds, minor upper respiratory infections, or allergy.

Promethazine belongs to a group of drugs known as antihistamines (antihistamines block the actions of histamine, a chemical released by the body during an allergic reaction). It is used to relieve or prevent symptoms of allergy.

Potassium guaiacolsulfonate is an expectorant, which loosens bronchial secretions.

Codeine is a narcotic cough suppressant that acts at the cough reflex center in the brain.

TREATMENT

To avoid stomach upset, you can take this medication with food or with a full glass of milk or water (unless your doctor directs you to do otherwise).

The oral syrup should be shaken well just before measuring each dose. The contents tend to settle on the bottom of the bottle, so it is necessary to shake the container to evenly distribute the ingredients and equalize the doses. Each dose should then be measured carefully, with a specially designed, 5 ml measuring spoon. An ordinary kitchen teaspoon is not accurate enough.

If you miss a dose of this medication, take the missed dose as soon as possible, unless it is almost time for your next dose. In that case, don't take the missed dose at all; just return to your regular dosing schedule. Do not double the next dose.

SIDE EFFECTS

Minor.   Blurred vision; constipation; diarrhea; difficult or painful urination; dizziness; dry mouth, throat, or nose; irritability; loss of appetite; confusion; nausea; restlessness; ringing or buzzing in the ears; rash; stomach upset; and unusual increase in sweating. These side effects should disappear in several days, as your body adjusts to the medication.

If you are constipated, increase the amount of fiber in your diet (raw vegetables, fruits, salads, bran, and whole-grain breads), and drink more water (unless your doctor tells you not to do so).

Chew sugarless gum, or suck on ice chips or a piece of hard candy, to reduce mouth dryness.

This medication can cause increased sensitivity to sunlight. It is therefore important to avoid prolonged exposure to sunlight and sunlamps. Wear protective clothing, and use an effective sunscreen.

If you feel dizzy or light-headed, sit or lie down awhile; get up from a sitting or lying position slowly, and be careful on stairs.

Major. Tell your doctor about any side effects that are persistent or particularly bothersome. IT IS ESPECIALLY IMPORTANT TO TELL YOUR DOCTOR about convulsions; difficulty breathing; difficult or painful urination; disturbed coordination; excitation; fainting; headaches; muscle spasms; nightmares; nosebleeds; palpitations; severe abdominal pain; sore throat or fever; or yellowing of the eyes or skin.

INTERACTIONS

This drug combination interacts with several other types of medication.

1. Concurrent use of it with central nervous system depressants (drugs that slow the activity of the nervous system), such as barbiturates, benzodiazepine tranquilizers, muscle relaxants, narcotics, pain medications, phenothiazine tranquilizers, and alcohol, or with tricyclic anti-depressants can cause extreme drowsiness.

2. This medication can decrease the effectiveness of amphetamines, guanethidine, anti-convulsants, and levodopa.

3. This combination medication can increase the side effects of monoamine oxidase (MAO) inhibitors (isocarboxazid, pargyline, phenelzine, tranylcypromine) and tricyclic anti-depressants.

TELL YOUR DOCTOR if you are already taking any of the medications listed above

WARNINGS

• Tell your doctor about unusual or allergic reactions you have had to medications, especially to promethazine or other antihistamines; to phenothiazine tranquilizers; potassium guaiacolsulfonate; codeine; or any other narcotic cough suppressant or pain medication.

• Tell your doctor if you now have, or if you have ever had, asthma, brain disease, blockage of the urinary or digestive tract, diabetes mellitus (sugar diabetes), colitis, gallstones or gallbladder disease, glaucoma, heart or blood vessel disease, high blood pressure, kidney disease, liver disease, lung disease, peptic ulcers, enlarged prostate gland, or thyroid disease.

• This medication can cause drowsiness. Your ability to perform tasks that require alertness, such as driving a car or operating potentially dangerous machinery, may be decreased. Appropriate caution should therefore be taken.

• While you are taking this medication, drink at least eight glasses of water a day (to help loosen bronchial secretions).

• Before having surgery or any other medical or dental treatment, be sure to tell your doctor or dentist that you are taking this medication.

• Because this product contains codeine, it has the potential for abuse, and must be used with caution. Usually, it should not be taken on a regular schedule for longer than ten days at a time. Tolerance develops quickly; do not increase the dosage or stop taking the drug abruptly, unless you first consult your doctor. If you have been taking large amounts of this medication or have been taking it for a long period of time, you may experience a withdrawal reaction (muscle aches, diarrhea, gooseflesh, runny nose, nausea, vomiting, shivering, trembling, stomach cramps, sleep disorders, irritability, weakness, yawning, and sweating) when you stop taking it. Your doctor may therefore want to reduce the dosage gradually.

• Be sure to tell your doctor if you are pregnant. The effects of this medication during the early stages of pregnancy have not yet been thoroughly studied in humans. However, codeine, used regularly during the later stages of pregnancy, may lead to addiction of the fetus, resulting in withdrawal symptoms (irritability, excessive crying, tremors, fever, vomiting, diarrhea, sneezing, and yawning) in the newborn infant. Also, tell your doctor if you are breast-feeding an infant. Small amounts of this medication pass into breast milk and may cause unusual excitement or irritability in nursing infants.

Pronestyl—see procainamide

---

propantheline

BRAND NAMES (Manufacturers)
Norpanth (Vortech)
Pro-Banthine (Searle)
propantheline bromide (various manufacturers)
SK-Propantheline Bromide (Smith Kline & French)
TYPE OF DRUG
Anti-cholinergic (anti-ulcer drug)
INGREDIENT
propantheline as the bromide salt
DOSAGE FORM
Tablets (7.5 mg and 15 mg)
STORAGE
Propantheline should be stored at room temperature, in a tightly closed container.

USES

Propantheline is used to treat peptic ulcers. It is thought to reduce the amount of acid formed in the stomach. It also relieves cramping and spasms of the gastrointestinal tract and bladder.

TREATMENT

In order to obtain the maximum benefit, you should take propantheline 30 minutes before meals and at bedtime (unless your doctor directs you to do otherwise).

If you miss a dose of this medication, do not take the

missed dose at all; just return to your regular dosing schedule. Do not double the next dose.

SIDE EFFECTS

Minor. Bloating; blurred vision, constipation; decreased sweating; dizziness; drowsiness; dry mouth; headache; increased sensitivity of the eyes to sunlight; nausea; nervousness; taste disorders; and vomiting. These side effects should disappear in several weeks, as your body adjusts to the medication.

To relieve constipation, increase the amount of fiber in your diet (bran, salads, fresh fruits and vegetables, and whole-grain breads), exercise, and drink more water (unless your doctor directs you to do otherwise).

If you feel dizzy, sit or lie down awhile; change positions slowly, and be careful on stairs.

Sunglasses may help to relieve the sensitivity of your eyes to sunlight.

Major. Tell your doctor about any side effects that are persistent or particularly bothersome. IT IS ESPECIALLY IMPORTANT TO TELL YOUR DOCTOR about decreased sexual ability; difficulty urinating; eye pain; itching; palpitations; or skin rash.

INTERACTIONS

Propantheline interacts with several other types of drugs.
1. Amantadine, antihistamines, disopyramide, haloperidol, monoamine oxidase (MAO) inhibitors, phenothiazine tranquilizers, procainamide, quinidine, and tricyclic antidepressants can increase the side effects of propantheline.
2. Antacids and anti-diarrhea medications can reduce the absorption of propantheline from the gastrointestinal tract, which can decrease its effectiveness. At least two hours should therefore separate doses of one of these types of medications and propantheline.
BE SURE TO TELL YOUR DOCTOR if you are already taking any of the medications listed above.

WARNINGS

● Tell your doctor about unusual or allergic reactions you have had to any medications, especially to propantheline.

● Before starting this medication, be sure to tell your doctor if you now have, or if you have ever had, glaucoma, heart disease, hiatal hernia, high blood pressure, intestinal blockage, kidney disease, liver disease, lung disease, myasthenia gravis, enlarged prostate gland, thyroid disease, ulcerative colitis, or urinary retention.

● This medication can decrease sweating and heat release from the body. You should therefore avoid getting overheated (strenuous exercise in hot weather; hot baths, showers, and saunas).

● If this medication makes you dizzy or drowsy, or blurs your vision, avoid taking part in activities that require alertness, such as driving a car or operating potentially dangerous equipment.

● Be sure to tell your doctor if you are pregnant. Although propantheline appears to be safe during pregnancy, extensive studies in humans have not yet been completed. Also, tell your doctor if you are breastfeeding an infant. It is not known whether or not propantheline passes into breast milk.

propantheline bromide—see propantheline

propoxyphene

BRAND NAMES (Manufacturers)
Darvon (Lilly)
Darvon-N (Lilly)
Dolene (Lederle)
Doxaphene (Major)
Pargesic (Parmed)
Profene-65 (Halsey)
propoxyphene hydrochloride (various manufacturers)
SK-65 (Smith Kline & French)
TYPE OF DRUG
Analgesic (pain reliever)
INGREDIENT
propoxyphene as the hydrochloride or napsylate salt
DOSAGE FORMS
Capsules (32 mg and 65 mg)
Tablets (100 mg)

STORAGE

This medication should be stored at room temperature in tightly closed containers.

USES

Propoxyphene is a narcotic analgesic that acts on the central nervous system to relieve mild to moderate pain.

TREATMENT

In order to avoid stomach upset, you can take propoxyphene with food or milk.

This medication works best if taken at the first sign of pain—don't wait for the pain to become severe.

If your doctor has prescribed this medication to be taken on a regular schedule and you miss a dose, take the missed dose as soon as possible, unless it is almost time for your next dose. In that case, do not take the missed dose at all; just return to your regular dosing schedule. Do not double the next dose.

SIDE EFFECTS

Minor. Dizziness; drowsiness; blurred vision; light-headedness; constipation; indigestion; nausea; nervousness; restlessness; vomiting; and weakness. As your body adjusts to the medication, these side effects should disappear.

If you are constipated, increase the amount of fiber in your diet (raw vegetables, fruits, salads, bran, and whole-grain breads), and drink more water (unless your doctor directs you to do otherwise).

If you feel dizzy, light-headed, or nauseated, sit or lie down awhile; get up from a sitting or lying position slowly, and be careful on stairs.

Major. Tell your doctor about any side effects that are persistent or particularly bothersome. IT IS ESPECIALLY IMPORTANT TO TELL YOUR DOCTOR about confusion; convulsions; darkening of the urine; depression; difficulty breathing; hallucinations; irregular heartbeat; ringing in the ears; skin rash; yellow stools; or yellowing of the eyes or skin.

INTERACTIONS

Propoxyphene can interact with several types of drugs.

1. Concurrent use of it with other central nervous system depressants (drugs that slow the activity of the nervous system), such as antihistamines, barbiturates, tranquilizers, sleeping medications, muscle relaxants, and other pain medications, or with tricyclic anti-depressants can cause extreme drowsiness.

2. Propoxyphene can increase carbamazepine blood levels, which in turn can result in greater side effects.

3. A monoamine oxidase (MAO) inhibitor taken within 14 days of this medication can lead to unpredictable and severe side effects.

4. Propoxyphene also interacts with alcohol, increasing its intoxicating effects. You should therefore avoid drinking alcoholic beverages while taking this medicine.

TELL YOUR DOCTOR if you are already taking any of the medications listed above.

WARNINGS

● Tell your doctor about unusual or allergic reactions you have had to any medications, especially to propoxyphene or to other narcotic analgesics (such as codeine, hydrocodone, hydromorphone, meperidine, methadone, morphine, and oxycodone).

● Tell your doctor if you now have, or if you have ever had, acute abdominal conditions, asthma, brain disease, colitis, epilepsy, gallstones or gallbladder disease, head injuries, heart disease, kidney disease, liver disease, lung disease, mental illness, emotional disorders, enlarged prostate gland, thyroid disease, or urethral stricture.

● If this drug makes you dizzy or drowsy, do not take part in any activity that requires alertness, such as driving a car or operating potentially dangerous equipment.

● Before having any surgery or other medical or dental treatment, be sure to tell your doctor or dentist that you are taking this medication.

● Propoxyphene has the potential for abuse, and must be used with caution. Usually, you should not take it on a regular schedule for longer than ten days (unless your doctor directs you to do so). Tolerance develops quickly; do not increase the dosage or stop taking the drug abruptly, unless you first consult your doctor. If you have been taking large amounts of this medication or have been taking it for long periods of time, you may experience a withdrawal reaction (muscle aches, diarrhea, gooseflesh, runny nose, nausea, vomiting, shivering, trembling, stomach cramps, sleep disorders, irritability, weakness, yawning, and sweating) when you stop taking it. Your doctor may therefore want to reduce the dosage gradually.

• Be sure to tell your doctor if you are pregnant. The effects of this medication during the early stages of pregnancy have not yet been thoroughly studied in humans. However, propoxyphene, used regularly in large doses during the later stages of pregnancy, can result in addiction of the fetus, leading to withdrawal symptoms (irritability, excessive crying, tremors, fever, vomiting, diarrhea, sneezing, and yawning) at birth. Also, tell your doctor if you are breastfeeding an infant. Small amounts of this medication may pass into breast milk and cause excessive drowsiness in the nursing infant.

propoxyphene hydrochloride—see propoxyphene

propoxyphene hydrochloride compound—see aspirin, caffeine, and propoxyphene combination

propoxyphene hydrochloride with acetaminophen—see acetaminophen and propoxyphene combination

---

propranolol

BRAND NAMES (Manufacturers)
Inderal (Ayerst)
Inderal LA (Ayerst)
TYPE OF DRUG
Beta-adrenergic blocking agent
INGREDIENT
propranolol
DOSAGE FORMS
Tablets (10 mg, 20 mg, 40 mg, 60 mg, 80 mg, and 90 mg)
Extended-release capsules (80 mg, 120 mg, and 160 mg)

STORAGE

Propranolol should be stored at room temperature in tightly closed, light-resistant containers.

USES

Propranolol is used to treat high blood pressure, angina pectoris (chest pain), and irregular heartbeats. It is also useful in preventing migraine headaches and preventing additional heart attacks in heart attack patients. Propranolol belongs to a group of medicines known as beta-adrenergic blocking agents or, more commonly, beta-blockers. These drugs work by controlling nerve impulses along certain nerve pathways.

TREATMENT

Propranolol can be taken with a glass of water, with meals, immediately following meals, or on an empty stomach—depending on your doctor's instructions. Try to take the medication at the same time(s) each day.

The extended-release capsules should be swallowed whole. Do not chew or crush them. Breaking the capsule releases the medication all at once—defeating the purpose of extended-release capsules.

It is important to remember that propranolol does not cure high blood pressure, but it will help to control the condition, as long as you continue to take it.

Try not to miss any doses of this medicine. If you do miss a dose, take the missed dose as soon as possible. However, if the next scheduled dose is within eight hours (if you are taking this medicine only once a day) or within four hours (if you are taking this medicine more than once a day), do not take the missed dose at all; just return to your regular dosing schedule. Do not double the next dose.

SIDE EFFECTS

Minor. Anxiety; cold hands or feet (due to decreased blood circulation to skin, fingers, and toes); constipation; decreased sexual ability; diarrhea; difficulty sleeping; drowsiness; dryness of the eyes, mouth, and skin; headache; nausea; nervousness; numbness or tingling of the fingers or toes; stomach discomfort; tiredness; or weakness. These side effects should disappear during treatment, as your body adjusts to the medicine.

If you are extra-sensitive to the cold, be sure to dress warmly during cold weather.

Plain, non-medicated eye drops (artificial tears) may help to relieve eye dryness.

Sucking on ice chips or chewing sugarless gum helps to relieve mouth and throat dryness.

Major. Tell your doctor about any side effects that are persistent or particularly bothersome. IT IS ESPECIALLY IMPORTANT TO TELL YOUR DOCTOR about breathing difficulty or wheezing; confusion; depression; dizziness; hair loss; hallucinations; light-headedness; nightmares; rapid weight gain (three to five pounds within a week); reduced alertness; swelling; sore throat and fever; skin rash; or unusual bleeding or bruising.

INTERACTIONS

Propranolol interacts with a number of other medications.
1. Indomethacin, aspirin, or other salicylates may decrease the blood-pressure-lowering effects of beta-blockers.
2. Concurrent use of beta-blockers and calcium channel blockers (diltiazem, nifedipine, and verapamil) can lead to heart failure or very low blood pressure.
3. Cimetidine can increase the blood concentrations of propranolol, which can result in greater side effects.
4. Side effects may also be increased when beta-blockers are taken with clonidine, digoxin, epinephrine, phenylephrine, phenylpropanolamine, phenothiazine tranquilizers, reserpine, or monoamine oxidase (MAO) inhibitors. At least 14 days should separate the use of a beta-blocker and an MAO inhibitor.
5. Beta-blockers may antagonize (work against) the effects of theophylline, aminophylline, albuterol, metaproterenol, and terbutaline.
6. Beta-blockers can also interact with insulin or oral anti-diabetic agents—raising or lowering blood sugar levels or masking the symptoms of low blood sugar.
BE SURE TO TELL YOUR DOCTOR if you are already taking any of the medications listed above.

WARNINGS

• Before starting to take this medication, it is important to tell your doctor if you have ever had unusual or allergic reactions to any beta-blocker (atenolol, metoprolol, nadolol, pindolol, propranolol, and timolol).

• Tell your doctor if you now have, or if you have ever had, allergies, asthma, hay fever, eczema, slow heartbeat, bronchitis, diabetes mellitus (sugar diabetes), emphysema, heart or blood vessel disease, kidney disease, liver disease, thyroid disease, or poor circulation in the fingers or toes.

• You may want to check your pulse while taking this medication. If your pulse is much slower than your usual rate (or if it is less than 50 beats per minute), check with your doctor. A pulse rate that is too slow may cause circulation problems.

• This medicine may affect your body's response to exercise. Make sure you ask your doctor what an appropriate amount of exercise would be for you, taking into account your medical condition.

• It is important that you do not stop taking this medicine without first checking with your doctor. Some conditions may become worse when the medicine is stopped suddenly, and the danger of a heart attack is increased in some patients. Your doctor may want you to gradually reduce the amount of medicine you take, before stopping completely. Make sure that you have enough medicine on hand to last through vacations, holidays, and weekends.

• Before having any surgery or other medical or dental treatment, tell your physician or dentist that you are taking this medicine. Often, this medication will be discontinued 48 hours prior to any major surgery.

• Propranolol can cause dizziness; drowsiness; lightheadedness; and decreased alertness. Therefore, exercise caution while driving a car or using any potentially dangerous machinery.

• While taking this medicine, do not use any over-the-counter (non-prescription) allergy, asthma, cough, cold, sinus, or diet preparation without first checking with your pharmacist or doctor. The combination of these medicines with a beta-blocker can result in high blood pressure and slow heartbeat.

• Be sure to tell your doctor if you are pregnant. Animal studies have shown that some beta-blockers can cause problems in pregnancy when used at very high doses. Adequate studies have not been done in humans, but there has been some association between beta-blockers used during pregnancy and low birth rate, as well as breathing problems and slow heart rate in the newborn infants. However, other reports have shown no effects on newborn infants. Also, tell your doctor if you are breastfeeding an infant. Although this medicine has not been shown to cause problems in breast-fed infants, some of the medicine may pass into breast milk.

propranolol and hydrochlorothiazide combination

BRAND NAME (Manufacturer)
Inderide (Ayerst)
TYPE OF DRUG
Beta-adrenergic blocking agent and diuretic (water pill)
INGREDIENTS
propranolol and hydrochlorothiazide
DOSAGE FORM
Tablets (40 mg propranolol and 25 mg hydrochlorothiazide; 80 mg propranolol and 25 mg hydrochlorothiazide)
STORAGE
Propranolol and hydrochlorothiazide should be stored at room temperature in a tightly closed, light-resistant container.

USES
Propranolol and hydrochlorothiazide is prescribed to treat high blood pressure. Hydrochlorothiazide is a diuretic (water pill), which reduces fluid accumulation in the body by increasing the elimination of sodium and water through the kidneys. Propranolol belongs to a group of medicines known as beta-adrenergic blocking agents or, more com-

monly, beta-blockers. They work by controlling nerve impulses along certain nerve pathways.

TREATMENT

This medication can be taken with a glass of water, with meals, immediately following meals, or on an empty stomach—depending on your doctor's instructions.

Try to take the medication at the same time(s) each day. Avoid taking a dose after 6:00 P.M.—this will prevent you from having to get up during the night to urinate.

If you miss a dose of this medication, take the missed dose as soon as possible, unless it is almost time for your next dose. In that case, do not take the missed dose at all; just wait until the next scheduled dose. Do not double the dose.

Propranolol and hydrochlorothiazide combination does not cure high blood pressure, but it will help to control the condition, as long as you continue to take it.

SIDE EFFECTS

Minor. Anxiety; constipation; cramps; decreased sexual ability; diarrhea; difficulty sleeping; drowsiness; dizziness; dryness of the eyes, mouth, and skin; headache; heartburn; itching; loss of appetite; nausea; nervousness; cold hands and feet (due to decreased blood circulation to skin, fingers, and toes); stomach discomfort; restlessness; tiredness; vomiting; and weakness. These side effects should disappear in several days, as your body adjusts to the medication.

If you become extra-sensitive to the cold, be sure to dress warmly during cold weather.

Plain, non-medicated eye drops (artificial tears) may help to relieve eye dryness.

Sucking on ice chips or chewing sugarless gum helps to relieve mouth and throat dryness.

To avoid dizziness or light-headedness when you stand, contract and relax the muscles of your legs for a few moments before rising. Do this by pushing one foot against the floor while raising the other foot slightly, alternating feet so that you are "pumping" your legs in a pedaling motion.

Hydrochlorothiazide can cause increased sensitivity to sunlight. It is therefore important to avoid prolonged exposure to sunlight and sunlamps. Wear protective clothing and sunglasses, and use an effective sunscreen.

Major. Tell your doctor about any side effects that are persistent or particularly bothersome. IT IS ESPECIALLY IMPORTANT TO TELL YOUR DOCTOR about blurred vision; confusion; depression; difficulty breathing; dry mouth; excessive thirst; excessive weakness; fever; hair loss; hallucinations; joint pain; mood changes; muscle spasms; nightmares; numbness or tingling in the fingers or toes; palpitations; rapid weight gain (three to five pounds within a week); reduced alertness; skin rash; sore throat; swelling; unusual bleeding or bruising; or yellowing of the eyes or skin.

INTERACTIONS

This medicine interacts with other medications.

1. Indomethacin, aspirin, and other salicylates have been shown to decrease the blood-pressure-lowering effects of beta-blockers.

2. Concurrent use of propranolol and calcium channel blockers (diltiazem, nifedipine, and verapamil) can lead to heart failure or very low blood pressure.

3. Cimetidine can increase the blood levels of propranolol, which can result in greater side effects. Side effects may also be increased when propranolol is taken with clonidine, digoxin, epinephrine, phenylephrine, phenylpropanolamine, phenothiazine tranquilizers, reserpine, or monoamine oxidase (MAO) inhibitors. At least 14 days should separate the use of propranolol and an MAO inhibitor.

4. Propranolol can antagonize (act against) the effects of theophylline, aminophylline, albuterol, metaproterenol, and terbutaline.

5. Propranolol can also interact with insulin and oral anti-diabetic agents—raising or lowering blood sugar levels and masking the symptoms of low blood sugar.

6. Hydrochlorothiazide can decrease the effectiveness of oral anti-coagulants (blood thinners, such as warfarin), anti-gout medications, and methenamine.

7. Fenfluramine may increase the blood-pressure-lowering effects of this drug, which can be dangerous.

8. Cholestyramine and colestipol can decrease the absorption of hydrochlorothiazide from the gastrointestinal tract—this medication should therefore be taken one hour before or four hours after cholestyramine or colestipol.

9. Hydrochlorothiazide may increase the side effects of amphotericin B; calcium; cortisone-like steroids (such as cortisone, dexamethasone, hydrocortisone, prednisone, prednisolone); digoxin; digitalis; lithium; quinidine; sulfonamide antibiotics; and vitamin D.

BE SURE TO TELL YOUR DOCTOR if you are already taking any of the medications listed above.

WARNINGS

● Tell your doctor about unusual or allergic reactions you have had to medications, especially to propranolol or any other beta-blocker (atenolol, metoprolol, nadolol, pindolol, or timolol); to hydrochlorothiazide or other diuretics (such as bendroflumethiazide, benzthiazide, chlorothiazide, chlorthalidone, cyclothiazide, hydroflumethiazide, methyclothiazide, metolozone, polythiazide, quinethazone, trichlormethiazide, or furosemide); or to any sulfa drug (oral anti-diabetic or sulfonamide antibiotic).

● Tell your doctor if you now have, or if you have ever had, asthma, diabetes mellitus (sugar diabetes), heart disease, gout, kidney disease or problems with urination, liver disease, pancreatitis, systemic lupus erythematosus, thyroid disease, or poor circulation in the fingers or toes.

● Hydrochlorothiazide can cause potassium loss. Signs of potassium loss include dry mouth, thirst, weakness, muscle pain or cramps, nausea, and vomiting. If you experience any of these symptoms, call your doctor. To help prevent this problem, your doctor may have blood tests performed periodically. To help avoid potassium loss, take this medication with a glass of fresh or frozen orange juice or cranberry juice, or eat a banana every day. The use of a salt substitute also helps to prevent potassium loss. Do not change your diet, however, until you discuss it with your doctor. Too much potassium may also be dangerous.

● While taking this medication, limit your intake of alco-

hol in order to prevent dizziness and light-headedness.
• Do not take any over-the-counter (non-prescription)
medication for weight control, or for allergy, asthma,
cough, cold, or sinus problems, unless you first check
with your doctor.
• To prevent severe water loss (dehydration) while taking
this medication, check with your doctor if you have any illness that causes severe nausea, vomiting, or diarrhea.
• This medication can raise blood sugar levels in diabetic
patients. Blood sugar should be monitored carefully with
blood or urine tests when this medication is started.
• You may want to check your pulse while taking this
medication. If your pulse is much slower than your usual
rate (or if it is less than 50 beats per minute), check with
your doctor. A pulse rate that slow may cause circulation
problems.
• Propranolol can affect your body's response to exercise.
Make sure you ask your doctor what an appropriate
amount of exercise would be for you, taking into account
your medical condition.
• Before having surgery or any other medical or dental
treatment, tell your doctor or dentist that you are taking
this medicine. Often, this medication will be discontinued
48 hours prior to any major surgery.
• This medication can cause dizziness, drowsiness, light-
headedness, or decreased alertness. Therefore, exercise
caution while driving a car or operating potentially dangerous machinery.
• It is important that you do not stop taking this medicine
unless you first check with your doctor. Some conditions
worsen when this medicine is stopped suddenly, and the
danger of a heart attack is increased in some patients. Your
doctor may therefore want you to gradually reduce the
amount of medicine you take, before stopping completely.
Make sure that you have enough medicine on hand to last
through vacations, holidays, and weekends.
• Be sure to tell your doctor if you are pregnant. Animal
studies have shown that some beta-blockers can cause
problems in pregnancy when used at very high doses. Adequate studies have not been completed in humans, but
there has been some association between beta-blockers

used during pregnancy and low birth rate, as well as breathing problems and slow heart rate in the newborn infants. However, other reports have shown no effects on newborn infants. Also, tell your doctor if you are breast-feeding an infant. Although problems in humans have not yet been reported, small amounts of propranolol and hydrochlorothiazide pass into breast milk.

Prostaphlin—see oxacillin

Protension—see aspirin, caffeine, and butalbital combination

Prothazine with Codeine Expectorant—see promethazine, potassium guaiacolsulfonate, and codeine combination

Protostat—see metronidazole

---

protriptyline

BRAND NAME (Manufacturer)
Vivactil (Merck Sharp & Dohme)
TYPE OF DRUG
Tricyclic anti-depressant (mood elevator)
INGREDIENT
protriptyline as the hydrochloride salt
DOSAGE FORM
Tablets (5 mg and 10 mg)
STORAGE
This medication should be stored at room temperature in a tightly closed container.

USES

Protriptyline is used to relieve the symptoms of mental depression. This medication belongs to a group of drugs referred to as the tricyclic anti-depressants. These medicines are thought to relieve depression by increasing the concentration of certain chemicals necessary for nerve transmission in the brain.

TREATMENT

This medication should be taken exactly as your doctor prescribes. You can take it with water or with food to lessen the chance of stomach irritation, unless your doctor tells you to do otherwise.

If you miss a dose of this medication, take the missed dose as soon as possible, then return to your regular dosing schedule. However, if the dose you missed was a once-a-day bedtime dose, do not take that dose in the morning; check with your doctor instead. If the dose is taken in the morning, it may cause some unwanted side effects. Never double the dose.

The effects of therapy with this medication may not become apparent for two or three weeks.

SIDE EFFECTS

Minor. Agitation; anxiety; blurred vision; confusion; constipation; cramps; diarrhea; dizziness; drowsiness; dry mouth; fatigue; headache; heartburn; insomnia; loss of appetite; nausea; peculiar tastes in the mouth; restlessness; sweating; vomiting; weakness; and weight gain or loss. As your body adjusts to the medication, these side effects should disappear.

Dry mouth can be relieved by chewing sugarless gum or by sucking on ice chips or a piece of hard candy.

To relieve constipation, increase the amount of fiber in your diet (bran, fresh fruits and vegetables, salads, and whole-grain breads), and drink more water (unless your doctor directs you to do otherwise).

To avoid dizziness or light-headedness when you stand, contract and relax the muscles of your legs for a few moments before rising. Do this by pushing one foot against the floor while raising the other foot slightly, alternating feet so that you are "pumping" your legs in a pedaling motion.

This medication may cause increased sensitivity to sunlight. You should therefore avoid prolonged exposure to sunlight and sunlamps. Wear protective clothing, and use an effective sunscreen.

Major. Tell your doctor about any side effects that are persistent or are particularly bothersome. IT IS ESPECIALLY IMPORTANT TO TELL YOUR DOCTOR about bleeding; chest pain; convulsions; difficulty urinating; enlarged or painful breasts (in both sexes); fainting; fever; fluid retention; hair loss; hallucinations; headaches; impotence; mood changes; mouth sores; nervousness; nightmares; nosebleeds; numbness in the fingers or toes; palpitations; ringing in the ears; seizures; skin rash; sleep disorders; sore throat; tremors; uncoordinated movements or balance problems; or yellowing of the eyes or skin.

INTERACTIONS

Protriptyline interacts with a number of other medications.
1. Extreme drowsiness can occur when this medicine is taken with central nervous system depressants (medicines that slow the activity of the nervous system), including alcohol, antihistamines, barbiturates, benzodiazepine tranquilizers, muscle relaxants, narcotics, pain medications, phenothiazine tranquilizers, and sleeping medications, or with other tricyclic anti-depressants.
2. Protriptyline may decrease the effectiveness of anti-seizure medications and may block the blood-pressure-lowering effects of clonidine and guanethidine.
3. Oral contraceptives (estrogens) can increase the side effects, and reduce the effectiveness, of tricyclic anti-depressants (including protriptyline).
4. Tricyclic anti-depressants may increase the side effects of thyroid medication and over-the-counter (non-prescription) cough, cold, allergy, asthma, sinus, and diet medications.
5. The concurrent use of tricyclic anti-depressants and monoamine oxidase (MAO) inhibitors should be undertaken very carefully, because the combination may result in fever, convulsions, or high blood pressure.
Before starting to take protriptyline, BE SURE TO TELL YOUR DOCTOR if you are already taking any of the medications listed above.

WARNINGS

• Tell your doctor if you have had unusual or allergic reactions to any medications, especially to protriptyline or other tricyclic anti-depressants (such as amitriptyline, imipramine, doxepin, trimipramine, amoxapine, desipramine, maprotiline, and nortriptyline).

• Tell your doctor if you now have, or if you have ever had, asthma, high blood pressure, liver or kidney disease, heart disease, a recent heart attack, circulatory disease, stomach problems, intestinal problems, alcoholism, difficulty urinating, enlarged prostate gland, epilepsy, glaucoma, thyroid disease, mental illness, or electroshock therapy.

• If this drug makes you dizzy or drowsy, do not take part in any activity that requires alertness, such as driving a car or operating potentially dangerous equipment.

• Before having any surgery or other medical or dental treatment, be sure to tell your doctor or dentist that you are taking this medication.

• Do not stop taking this drug suddenly. Stopping abruptly can cause nausea, headache, stomach upset, fatigue, or a worsening of your condition. Your doctor may want to reduce the dosage gradually.

• The effects of this medication may last as long as seven days after you have stopped taking it, so continue to observe all precautions during that period.

• Be sure to tell your doctor if you are pregnant. Problems in humans have not been reported; however, studies have shown side effects on the fetuses of animals who received this type of medication in large doses during pregnancy. Also, tell your doctor if you are breastfeeding an infant. Small amounts of this drug can pass into breast milk and may cause unwanted effects, such as irritability or sleeping problems, in nursing infants.

Proval—see acetaminophen and codeine combination

Proventil—see albuterol

Provera—see medroxyprogesterone

Prozine—see promazine

pseudoephedrine and azatadine combination

BRAND NAME (Manufacturer)
Trinalin Repetabs (Schering)
TYPE OF DRUG
Adrenergic (decongestant) and antihistamine
INGREDIENTS
pseudoephedrine as the sulfate salt; azatadine as the maleate salt
DOSAGE FORM
Sustained-release tablets (120 mg pseudoephedrine and 1 mg azatadine)
STORAGE
Pseudoephedrine and azatadine combination tablets should be stored at room temperature, in a tightly closed container.

USES

This drug combination is used to relieve the symptoms of upper respiratory tract infections, hay fever and other allergies, and sinusitis (inflammation of the sinuses).

Pseudoephedrine belongs to a group of drugs known as adrenergic agents (decongestants). They act by constricting blood vessels in the nasal passages to reduce swelling and congestion.

Azatadine belongs to a group of drugs known as antihistamines (antihistamines block the action of histamine, a chemical released by the body during an allergic reaction). It is therefore used to relieve or prevent symptoms of allergy.

TREATMENT

In order to avoid stomach upset, you can take pseudoephedrine and azatadine combination with food or with a full glass of milk or water (unless your doctor directs you to do otherwise).

The sustained-release tablets should be swallowed whole. Breaking, chewing, or crushing these tablets destroys their sustained-release activity, and may increase the side effects.

If you miss a dose of this medication, take the missed dose as soon as possible, unless it is almost time for your next dose. In that case, don't take the missed dose at all; just return to your regular dosing schedule. Do not double the next dose.

SIDE EFFECTS

Minor. Anxiety; blurred vision; constipation; diarrhea; dizziness; drowsiness; dry mouth, nose, and throat; heartburn; insomnia; irritability; loss of appetite; nasal congestion; nausea; restlessness; reduced sweating; vomiting; and weakness. These side effects should disappear in several days, as your body adjusts to the medication.

If you are constipated, increase the amount of fiber in your diet (raw vegetables, fruits, salads, bran, and whole-grain breads), and drink more water (unless your doctor directs you to do otherwise).

Chew sugarless gum, or suck on ice chips or a piece of hard candy, to reduce mouth dryness.

This medication can increase your sensitivity to sunlight. It is therefore important to avoid prolonged exposure to sunlight and sunlamps. Wear protective clothing, and use an effective sunscreen.

If you feel dizzy or light-headed, sit or lie down awhile; get up from a sitting or lying position slowly, and be careful on stairs.

In order to avoid difficulty falling asleep, take the last dose of this medication several hours before bedtime.

Major. Tell your doctor about any side effects that are persistent or particularly bothersome. IT IS ESPECIALLY IMPORTANT TO TELL YOUR DOCTOR about unusual bleeding or bruising; chest pain; difficulty breathing; confusion; convulsions; difficult or painful urination; fainting; hallucinations; headaches; loss of coordination; mood changes; nose bleeds; palpitations; rash; severe abdominal pain; or sore throat.

INTERACTIONS

Pseudoephedrine and azatadine combination can interact with several other medications.

1. Concurrent use of this medication with central nervous system depressants (drugs that slow the activity of the nervous system), such as barbiturates, benzodiazepine tranquilizers, muscle relaxants, narcotics, pain medications, phenothiazine tranquilizers, and alcohol, or with tricyclic anti-depressants can cause extreme drowsiness.

2. Monoamine oxidase (MAO) inhibitors (isocarboxazid, pargyline, phenelzine, tranylcypromine) and tricyclic anti-depressants can increase the side effects of this medication.

3. The side effects of the antihistamine part of this medication may be increased by quinidine, procainamide, haloperidol, and phenothiazine tranquilizers.

4. The side effects of the decongestant component may be increased by digoxin, over-the-counter (non-prescription) diet aids, or asthma, allergy, cough, cold, or sinus preparations.

5. The blood-pressure-lowering effects of guanethidine may be decreased by this medication.

TELL YOUR DOCTOR if you are currently taking any of the medications listed above.

WARNINGS

● Tell your doctor about unusual or allergic reactions you have had to any medications, especially to azatadine or other antihistamines (such as chlorpheniramine, brompheniramine, carbinoxamine, chlorpheniramine, clemastine, cyproheptadine, dexchlorpheniramine, dimenhydrinate, dimethindene, diphenhydramine, diphenylpyraline, doxylamine, hydroxyzine, promethazine, pyrilamine, trimeprazine, tripelennamine, and tripolidine); or to pseudoephedrine or other adrenergic agents (such as albuterol, amphetamines, ephedrine, epinephrine, isoproterenol, metaproterenol, norepinephrine, phenylpropanolamine, and terbutaline).

● Tell your doctor if you now have, or if you have ever had, diabetes mellitus (sugar diabetes), epilepsy, glaucoma, heart or blood vessel disease, hiatal hernia, high blood pressure, myasthenia gravis, obstructed bladder or intestinal tract, peptic ulcers, enlarged prostate gland, or thyroid disease.

● Because this drug can reduce sweating and heat release from the body, you should avoid excessive work and exercising in hot weather.

- This medication can cause drowsiness. Your ability to perform tasks that require alertness, such as driving a car or operating potentially dangerous machinery, may be decreased. Appropriate caution should therefore be taken.
- Be sure to tell your doctor if you are pregnant. The effects of this medication during pregnancy have not yet been thoroughly studied in humans. Also, tell your doctor if you are breastfeeding an infant. Small amounts of this medication pass into breast milk and may cause unusual excitement or irritability in nursing infants.

---

pseudoephedrine and carbinoxamine combination

BRAND NAME (Manufacturer)
Rondec (Ross)

TYPE OF DRUG
Adrenergic (decongestant) and antihistamine

INGREDIENTS
pseudoephedrine as the hydrochloride salt; carbinoxamine as the maleate salt

DOSAGE FORMS
Tablets (60 mg pseudoephedrine and 4 mg carbinoxamine)

Oral syrup (60 mg pseudoephedrine and 4 mg carbinoxamine per 5 ml teaspoonful)

Oral drops (25 mg pseudoephedrine and 2 mg carbinoxamine per ml)

STORAGE
Pseudoephedrine and carbinoxamine combination tablets, oral syrup, and oral drops should be stored at room temperature, in tightly closed containers. This medication should never be frozen.

USES
This drug combination is used to relieve symptoms of upper respiratory tract infections, hay fever and other allergies, and sinusitis (inflammation of the sinuses).

Pseudoephedrine belongs to a group of drugs known as

adrenergic agents (decongestants). They act by constricting blood vessels in the nasal passages to reduce swelling and congestion.

Carbinoxamine belongs to a group of drugs known as antihistamines (antihistamines block the actions of histamine, a chemical released by the body during an allergic reaction). It is therefore used to relieve or prevent symptoms of allergy.

TREATMENT

In order to avoid stomach upset, you can take pseudoephedrine and carbinoxamine combination with food or with a full glass of water (unless your doctor directs you to do otherwise).

The oral drops should be measured carefully, with the dropper provided.

The oral syrup form of this medication should be measured carefully, with a specially designed, 5 ml measuring spoon. An ordinary kitchen teaspoon is not accurate enough.

If you miss a dose of this medication, take the missed dose as soon as possible, unless it is almost time for your next dose. In that case, don't take the missed dose at all; just return to your regular dosing schedule. Do not double the next dose.

SIDE EFFECTS

Minor. Anxiety; blurred vision; constipation; diarrhea; dizziness; drowsiness; dry mouth, nose, and throat; heartburn; insomnia; irritability; loss of appetite; nasal congestion; nausea; restlessness; reduced sweating; vomiting; and weakness. These side effects should disappear in several days, as your body adjusts to the medication.

If you are constipated, increase the amount of fiber in your diet (raw vegetables, fruits, salads, bran, and whole-grain breads), and drink more water (unless your doctor directs you to do otherwise).

Chew sugarless gum, or suck on ice chips or a piece of hard candy, to reduce mouth dryness.

This medication can increase your sensitivity to sunlight. It is therefore important to avoid prolonged exposure to sunlight and sunlamps. Wear protective clothing, and use an effective sunscreen.

If you feel dizzy or light-headed, sit or lie down awhile; get up from a sitting or lying position slowly, and be careful on stairs.

In order to avoid difficulty falling asleep, take the last dose of this medication several hours before bedtime.

Major. Tell your doctor about any side effects that are persistent or particularly bothersome. IT IS ESPECIALLY IMPORTANT TO TELL YOUR DOCTOR about unusual bleeding or bruising; chest pain; difficulty breathing; confusion; convulsions; difficult or painful urination; fainting; hallucinations; headaches; loss of coordination; mood changes; nosebleeds; palpitations; rash; severe abdominal pain; or sore throat.

INTERACTIONS

Pseudoephedrine and carbinoxamine combination interacts with several other medications.

1. Concurrent use of it with central nervous system depressants (drugs that slow the activity of the nervous system), such as barbiturates, benzodiazepine tranquilizers, muscle relaxants, narcotics, pain medications, phenothiazine tranquilizers, and alcohol, or with tricyclic anti-depressants can cause extreme drowsiness.

2. Monoamine oxidase (MAO) inhibitors (isocarboxazid, pargyline, phenelzine, tranylcypromine) and tricyclic anti-depressants can increase the side effects of this medication.

3. The side effects of the antihistamine part of this medication may be increased by quinidine, procainamide, haloperidol, and phenothiazine tranquilizers.

4. The side effects of the decongestant component may be increased by digoxin, over-the-counter (non-prescription) diet aids, or asthma, allergy, cough, cold or sinus preparations.

5. The blood-pressure-lowering effects of guanethidine may be decreased by this medication.

TELL YOUR DOCTOR if you are currently taking any of the medications listed above.

WARNINGS

- Tell your doctor about unusual or allergic reactions you have had to any medications, especially to carbinoxamine or other antihistamines (such as azatadine, bromodiphenhydramine, chlorpheniramine, clemastine, cyproheptadine, dexchlorpheniramine, dimenhydrinate, dimethindene, diphenhydramine, diphenylpyraline, doxylamine, hydroxyzine, promethazine, pyrilamine, trimeprazine, tripelennamine, or tripolidine); or to pseudoephedrine or other adrenergic agent (such as albuterol, amphetamines, ephedrine, epinephrine, isoproterenol, metaproterenol, norepinephrine, phenylpropanolamine, and terbutaline).
- Tell your doctor if you now have, or if you have ever had, diabetes mellitus (sugar diabetes), epilepsy, glaucoma, heart or blood vessel disease, hiatal hernia, high blood pressure, myasthenia gravis, obstructed bladder or intestinal tract, peptic ulcers, enlarged prostate gland, or thyroid disease.
- Because this drug can reduce sweating and heat release from the body, you should avoid excessive work and exercising in hot weather.
- This medication can cause drowsiness. Your ability to perform tasks requiring alertness, such as driving a car or operating potentially dangerous machinery, may be decreased. Appropriate caution should therefore be taken.
- Be sure to tell your doctor if you are pregnant. The effects of this medication during pregnancy have not yet been thoroughly studied in humans. Also, tell your doctor if you are breastfeeding an infant. Small amounts of this medication pass into breast milk and may cause unusual excitement or irritability in nursing infants.

---

pseudoephedrine and chlorpheniramine combination

BRAND NAMES (Manufacturers)
Anafed (Everett)
Anamine T.D. (Maynard)

Brexin L.A. (Savage)
Chlorafed Adult Timecelles (Hauck)
Chlorafed (Half-Strength) (Hauck)
Chlor-Trimeton Decongestant* (Schering)
Chlor-Trimeton Decongestant Repetabs* (Schering)
Codimal-L.A. Cenules (Central)
Control-D (Beecham)
Deconamine (Berlex)
Deconamine SR (Berlex)
Duralex (American Urologicals)
Fedahist* (Rorer)
Hournaze (Delta)
Isoclor (American Critical Care)
Isoclor Timesules (American Critical Care)
Kronofed-A Jr. (Ferndale)
Kronofed-A Kronocaps (Ferndale)
ND Clear T.D. (Seatrace)
Novafed A (Merrell Dow)
Rhinafed-EX (McGregor)
Rinade-BID (EconoMed)
Sudafed Plus* (Burroughs Wellcome)
*Pseudoephedrine and chlorpheniramine combination is
    also available over-the-counter (non-prescription) under
    several brand names.

TYPE OF DRUG

Adrenergic (decongestant) and antihistamine

INGREDIENTS

Pseudoephedrine as the hydrochloride salt; chlor-
    pheniramine as the maleate salt

DOSAGE FORMS

Tablets (60 mg pseudoephedrine and 4 mg chlorpheni-
    amine)
Capsules (60 mg pseudoephedrine and 4 mg chlor-
    pheniramine)
Sustained-release capsules (120 mg pseudoephedrine and
    8 mg chlorpheniramine)
Oral elixir (30 mg pseudoephedrine and 2 mg chlorphen-
    iramine per 5 ml teaspoonful)
Oral syrup (30 mg pseudoephedrine and 2 mg chlorphen-
    iramine per 5 ml teaspoonful)

STORAGE
Pseudoephedrine and chlorpheniramine combination tablets, capsules, elixir, and syrup should be stored at room temperature in tightly closed containers. This medication should never be frozen.

USES
This drug combination is used to relieve the symptoms of upper respiratory tract infections, hay fever and other allergies, and sinusitis (inflammation of the sinuses).

Pseudoephedrine belongs to a group of drugs known as adrenergic agents (decongestants). They act by constricting blood vessels in the nasal passages to reduce swelling and congestion.

Chlorpheniramine belongs to a group of drugs known as antihistamines (antihistamines block the actions of histamine, a chemical released by the body during an allergic reaction). It is therefore used to relieve or prevent symptoms of allergy.

TREATMENT
In order to avoid stomach upset, you can take pseudoephedrine and chlorpheniramine combination with food or with a full glass of milk or water (unless your doctor directs you to do otherwise).

The oral syrup and elixir forms of this medication should be measured carefully, with a specially designed, 5 ml measuring spoon. An ordinary kitchen teaspoon is not accurate enough.

The sustained-release capsules should be swallowed whole. Breaking, chewing, or crushing these capsules destroys their sustained-release activity, and may increase the side effects.

If you miss a dose of this medication, take the missed dose as soon as possible, unless it is almost time for your next dose. In that case, don't take the missed dose at all; just return to your regular dosing schedule. Do not double the next dose.

SIDE EFFECTS
Minor. Anxiety; blurred vision; constipation; diarrhea;

dizziness; drowsiness; dry mouth, nose, and throat; heartburn; insomnia; irritability; loss of appetite; nasal congestion; nausea; restlessness; reduced sweating; vomiting; and weakness. These side effects should disappear in several days, as your body adjusts to this medication.

If you are constipated, increase the amount of fiber in your diet (raw vegetables, fruits, salads, bran, and whole-grain breads), and drink more water (unless your doctor directs you to do otherwise).

This medication can increase your sensitivity to sunlight. It is therefore important to avoid prolonged exposure to sunlight and sunlamps. Wear protective clothing, and use an effective sunscreen.

If you feel dizzy or light-headed, sit or lie down awhile; get up from a sitting or lying position slowly and be careful on stairs.

In order to avoid difficulty falling asleep, take the last dose of this medication several hours before bedtime.

Major. Tell your doctor about any side effects that are persistent or particularly bothersome. IT IS ESPECIALLY IMPORTANT TO TELL YOUR DOCTOR about unusual bleeding or bruising; chest pain; difficulty breathing; confusion; convulsions; difficult or painful urination; fainting; hallucinations; headaches; loss of coordination; mood changes; palpitations; rash; severe abdominal pain; or sore throat.

INTERACTIONS

This medication interacts with other medications.

1. Concurrent use of it with central nervous system depressants (drugs that slow the activity of the nervous system), such as barbiturates, benzodiazepine tranquilizers, muscle relaxants, narcotics, pain medication, phenothiazine tranquilizers, and alcohol, or with tricyclic antidepressants can cause extreme drowsiness.

2. Monoamine oxidase (MAO) inhibitors (isocarboxazid, pargyline, phenelzine, tranylcypromine) and tricyclic antidepressants can increase the side effects of this medication.

3. The side effects of the antihistamine part of this medication may be increased by quinidine, procainamide, haloperidol, and phenothiazine tranquilizers.

4. The side effects of the decongestant component may be increased by digoxin, over-the-counter (non-prescription) diet aids, or asthma, allergy, cough, cold, or sinus preparations.

5. The blood pressure-lowering-effects of guanethidine may be decreased by this medication.

TELL YOUR DOCTOR if you are currently taking any of the medications listed above.

WARNINGS

• Tell your doctor about unusual or allergic reactions you have had to any medications, especially to chlorpheniramine or to other antihistamines (such as azatadine, brompheniramine, carbinoxamine, clemastine, cyproheptadine, dexchlorpheniramine, dimenhydrinate, dimethindene, diphenhydramine, diphenylpyraline, doxylamine, hydroxyzine, promethazine, pyrilamine, trimeprazine, tripelennamine, or tripolidine); or to pseudoephedrine or other adrenergic agents (such as albuterol, amphetamines, ephedrine, epinephrine, isoproterenol, metaproterenol, norepinephrine, phenylpropanolamine, and terbutaline).

• Tell your doctor if you now have, or if you have ever had, diabetes mellitus (sugar diabetes), epilepsy, glaucoma, heart or blood vessel disease, hiatal hernia, high blood pressure, myasthenia gravis, obstructed bladder or intestinal tract, peptic ulcers, enlarged prostate gland, or thyroid disease.

• Because this drug can reduce sweating and heat release from the body, you should avoid excessive work or exercising in hot weather.

• This medication can cause drowsiness. Your ability to perform tasks that require alertness, such as driving a car or operating potentially dangerous machinery, may be decreased. Appropriate caution should therefore be taken.

• Be sure to tell your doctor if you are pregnant. The effects of this medication during pregnancy have not yet been thoroughly studied in humans. Also, tell your doctor if you are breastfeeding an infant. Small amounts of this medication pass into breast milk and may cause unusual excitement or irritability in nursing infants.

pseudoephedrine and dexbrompheniramine combination

BRAND NAMES (Manufacturers)
Dexbrompheniramine and Pseudoephedrine (Lederle)
Disophrol Chronotabs (Schering)
Drixoral* (Schering)
Duo-Hist (Henry Schein)
Efedra P.A. (Cord)
Histarall (H.L. Moore)
Pseudo-Mal (Rugby)
*Pseudoephedrine and dexbrompheniramine combination is also available over-the-counter (non-prescription).

TYPE OF DRUG
Adrenergic (decongestant) and antihistamine

INGREDIENTS
pseudoephedrine as the sulfate salt and dexbrompheniramine as the maleate salt

DOSAGE FORM
Sustained-release tablets (120 mg pseudoephedrine and 6 mg dexbrompheniramine)

STORAGE
Pseudoephedrine and dexbrompheniramine combination tablets should be stored at room temperature, in a tightly closed container.

USES
This drug combination is used to relieve the symptoms of upper respiratory tract infections, hay fever and other allergies, and sinusitis (inflammation of the sinuses).

Pseudoephedrine belongs to a group of drugs known as adrenergic agents (decongestants). They act by constricting blood vessels in the nasal passages to reduce swelling and congestion.

Dexbrompheniramine belongs to a group of drugs known as antihistamines (antihistamines block the actions of histamine, a chemical released by the body during an allergic reaction). It is therefore used to relieve or prevent symptoms of allergy.

TREATMENT

In order to avoid stomach upset, you can take pseudoephedrine and dexbromphiramine combination with food or with a full glass of milk or water (unless your doctor directs you to do otherwise).

The sustained-release tablets should be swallowed whole. Breaking, chewing, or crushing these tablets destroys their sustained-release activity and may increase the side effects.

If you miss a dose of this medication, take the missed dose as soon as possible, unless it is almost time for your next dose. In that case, don't take the missed dose at all; just return to your regular dosing schedule. Do not double the next dose.

SIDE EFFECTS

Minor. Anxiety; blurred vision; constipation; diarrhea; dizziness; drowsiness; dry mouth, nose, and throat; heartburn; insomnia; irritability; loss of appetite; nasal congestion; nausea; restlessness; reduced sweating; vomiting; and weakness. These side effects should disappear in several days, as your body adjusts to the medication.

If you are constipated, increase the amount of fiber in your diet (raw vegetables, fruits, salads, bran, and whole-grain breads), and drink more water (unless your doctor directs you to do otherwise).

Chew sugarless gum, or suck on ice chips or a piece of hard candy, to reduce mouth dryness.

This medication can increase your sensitivity to sunlight. It is therefore important to avoid prolonged exposure to sunlight and sunlamps. Wear protective clothing, and use an effective sunscreen.

If you feel dizzy or light-headed, sit or lie down awhile; get up from a sitting or lying position slowly, and be careful on stairs.

In order to avoid difficulty falling asleep, take the last dose of this medication several hours before bedtime.

Major. Tell your doctor about any side effects that are persistent or particularly bothersome. IT IS ESPECIALLY IMPORTANT TO TELL YOUR DOCTOR about unusual bleeding or bruising; chest pain; difficulty breathing; confusion; convulsions; difficult or painful urination; fainting; hallucinations; headaches; loss of coordination; mood changes; nosebleeds; palpitations; rash; severe abdominal pain; or sore throat.

INTERACTIONS

Pseudoephedrine and dexbrompheniramine combination interacts with several other medications.
1. Concurrent use of it with central nervous system depressants (drugs that slow the activity of the nervous system), such as barbiturates, benzodiazepine tranquilizers, muscle relaxants, narcotics, pain medications, phenothiazine tranquilizers, and alcohol, or with tricyclic anti-depressants can cause extreme drowsiness.
2. Monoamine oxidase (MAO) inhibitors (isocarboxazid, pargyline, phenelzine, tranylcypromine) and tricyclic anti-depressants can increase the side effects of this medication.
3. The side effects of the antihistamine part of this medication may be increased by quinidine, procainamide, haloperidol, and phenothiazine tranquilizers.
4. The side effects of the decongestant component may be increased by digoxin, over-the-counter (non-prescription) diet aids, or asthma, allergy, cough, cold or sinus preparations.
5. The blood-pressure-lowering effects of guanethidine may be decreased by this medication.
TELL YOUR DOCTOR if you are currently taking any of the medications listed above.

WARNINGS

● Tell your doctor about unusual or allergic reactions you have had to any medications, especially to dexbrompheniramine or to other antihistamines (such as azatadine, brompheniramine, carbinoxamine, chlorpheniramine, clemastine, cyproheptadine, dexchlorpheniramine, dimenhydrinate, dimethindene, diphenhydramine, diphen-

ylpyraline, doxylamine, hydroxyzine, promethazine, pyrilamine, trimeprazine, tripelennamine, or tripolidine); or
to pseudoephedrine or other adrenergic agents (such as albuterol, amphetamines, ephedrine, epinephrine, isoproterenol, metaproterenol, norepinephrine, phenylpropanolamine, and terbutaline).

● Tell your doctor if you now have, or if you have eve
had, diabetes mellitus (sugar diabetes), epilepsy, glaucoma, heart or blood vessel disease, hiatal hernia, high
blood pressure, myasthenia gravis, obstructed bladder or
intestinal tract, peptic ulcers, enlarged prostate gland, or
thyroid disease.

● Because this drug can reduce sweating and heat release
from the body, you should avoid excessive work and exercising in hot weather.

● This medication can cause drowsiness. Your ability to
perform tasks that require alertness, such as driving a car
or operating potentially dangerous machinery, may be decreased. Appropriate caution should therefore be taken.

● Be sure to tell your doctor if you are pregnant. The effects of this medication during pregnancy have not yet
been thoroughly studied in humans. Also, tell your doctor
if you are breastfeeding an infant. Small amounts of this
medication pass into breast milk and may cause unusual
excitement or irritability in nursing infants.

---

pseudoephedrine, tripolidine, guaifenesin, and codeine combination

BRAND NAMES (Manufacturers)
Actacin-C (Vangard)
Actamine-C (H.L. Moore)
Actifed-C (Burroughs Wellcome)
Allerfed C (Spencer-Mead)
Allerfrin with Codeine (Rugby)
Cophed-C (Coastal)
Dri-Phed with Codeine (Stayner)

Rofed C (Three P Products)
Triacin C (various manufacturers)
Trifed-C (Geneva Generics)
TYPE OF DRUG
Adrenergic (decongestant), antihistamine, expectorant, and cough suppressant
INGREDIENTS
pseudoephedrine as the hydrochloride salt, tripolidine as the hydrochloride salt, guaifenesin, and codeine
DOSAGE FORM
Oral syrup (30 mg pseudoephedrine, 2 mg tripolidine, 100 mg guaifenesin, and 10 mg codeine per 5 ml teaspoonful)
STORAGE
This medication should be stored at room temperature in a tightly closed container. This medication should never be frozen.

USES

This drug combination is used to provide symptomatic relief of coughs due to colds, minor upper respiratory infections, and allergy.

Pseudoephedrine belongs to a group of drugs known as adrenergic agents (decongestants). They act by constricting blood vessels in the nasal passages, thereby reducing swelling and congestion.

Tripolidine belongs to a group of drugs known as antihistamines (antihistamines block the action of histamine, a chemical released by the body during an allergic reaction). It is used to relieve or prevent symptoms of allergy.

Guaifenesin is an expectorant, which loosens bronchial secretions.

Codeine is a narcotic cough suppressant, which acts at the cough reflex center in the brain.

TREATMENT

To avoid stomach upset, you can take this medication with food or with a full glass of milk or water (unless your doctor directs you to do otherwise).

The oral syrup form of this medication should be measured carefully, with a specially designed, 5 ml measuring spoon. An ordinary kitchen teaspoon is not accurate enough.

If you miss a dose of this medication, take the missed dose as soon as possible, unless it is almost time for your next dose. In that case, don't take the missed dose at all; just return to your regular dosing schedule. Do not double the next dose.

SIDE EFFECTS

Minor. Blurred vision; constipation; diarrhea; difficult or painful urination; dizziness; dry mouth, throat, or nose; irritability; loss of appetite; confusion; nausea; restlessness; ringing or buzzing in the ears; rash; stomach upset; and unusual increase in sweating. These side effects should disappear in several days, as your body adjusts to the medication.

If you are constipated, increase the amount of fiber in your diet (raw vegetables, fruits, salads, bran, and whole-grain breads), and drink more water (unless your doctor tells you not to do so).

Chew sugarless gum, or suck on ice chips or a piece of hard candy, to reduce mouth dryness.

This medication can cause increased sensitivity to sunlight. It is therefore important to avoid prolonged exposure to sunlight and sunlamps. Wear protective clothing, and use an effective sunscreen.

If you feel dizzy or light-headed, sit or lie down awhile; get up from a sitting or lying position slowly, and be careful on stairs.

In order to avoid difficulty falling asleep, check with your doctor to see if you can take the last dose of this medication several hours before bedtime each day.

Major. Tell your doctor about any side effects that are persistent or particularly bothersome. IT IS ESPECIALLY IMPORTANT TO TELL YOUR DOCTOR about unusual bleeding or bruising; chest pain; feeling faint; headaches; palpitations; severe abdominal pain; or sore throat.

INTERACTIONS

This drug combination can interact with several other types of medication.

1. Concurrent use of it with other central nervous system depressants (drugs that slow the activity of the nervous system), such as barbiturates, benzodiazepine tranquilizers, muscle relaxants, narcotics, pain medications, phenothiazine tranquilizers, and alcohol, or with tricyclic antidepressants can cause extreme drowsiness.

2. Monoamine oxidase (MAO) inhibitors (isocarboxazid, pargyline, phenelzine, tranylcypromine) and tricyclic antidepressants can increase the side effects of this medication.

3. The blood-pressure-lowering effects of guanethidine, methyldopa, and reserpine may be decreased by this medication.

4. The side effects of the decongestant component of this medication may be increased by digoxin or over-the-counter (non-prescription) allergy, asthma, cough, cold, diet, or sinus preparations.

TELL YOUR DOCTOR if you are currently taking any of the medications listed above.

WARNINGS

• Tell your doctor about unusual or allergic reactions you have had to any medications, especially to tripolidine or other antihistamines (such as azatadine, brompheniramine, carbinoxamine, clemastine, cyproheptadine, chlorpheniramine, dexbrompheniramine, dimenhydrinate, dimethindene, diphenhydramine, diphenylpyraline, doxylamine, hydroxyzine, promethazine, pyrilamine, trimeprazine, tripelennamine); to pseudoephedrine or other adrenergic agents (such as albuterol, amphetamines, ephedrine, epinephrine, isoproterenol, metaproterenol, norepinephrine, phenylephrine, phenylpropanolamine, and terbutaline); to guaifenesin; or to codeine or any other narcotic cough suppressant or pain medication.

• Tell your doctor if you now have, or if you have ever had, asthma, brain disease, blockage of the urinary or digestive tracts, diabetes mellitus (sugar diabetes), colitis, gallbladder disease, glaucoma, heart or blood vessel disease, high blood pressure, kidney disease, liver disease, lung disease, peptic ulcers, enlarged prostate gland, or thyroid disease.

● This medication can cause drowsiness. Your ability to perform tasks that require alertness, such as driving a car or operating potentially dangerous machinery, may be decreased. Appropriate caution should therefore be taken.

● While you are taking this medication, drink at least eight glasses of water a day to help loosen bronchial secretions.

● Because this product contains codeine, it has the potential for abuse, and must be used with caution. Usually, it should not be taken on a regular schedule for longer than ten days at a time. Tolerance develops quickly; do not increase the dosage or stop taking the drug abruptly, unless you first consult your doctor. If you have been taking large amounts of this medication, or if you have been taking it for long periods of time, you may experience a withdrawal reaction (muscle aches, diarrhea, gooseflesh, runny nose, nausea, vomiting, shivering, trembling, stomach cramps, sleep disorders, irritability, weakness, yawning, and sweating) when you stop taking it. Your doctor may therefore want to reduce the dosage gradually.

● Before having surgery or any other medical or dental treatment, be sure to tell your doctor or dentist that you are taking this medication.

● Be sure to tell your doctor if you are pregnant. The effects of this medication during the early stages of pregnancy have not yet been thoroughly studied in humans. However, codeine, used regularly during the later stages of pregnancy, may lead to addiction of the fetus, resulting in withdrawal symptoms (irritability, excessive crying, tremors, fever, vomiting, diarrhea, sneezing, and yawning) in the newborn infant. Also, tell your doctor if you are breast-feeding an infant. Small amounts of this medication pass into breast milk and may cause unusual excitement or irritability in nursing infants.

Pseudo-Mal—see pseudoephedrine and
   dexbrompheniramine combination

Purebrom Compound T.D.—see
phenylpropanolamine, phenylephrine, and
brompheniramine combination

Puretane Expectorant—see phenylephrine,
phenylpropanolamine, brompheniramine, and
guaifenesin combination

Purodigin—see digitoxin

Pylora—see atropine, scopolamine, hyoscyamine, and
phenobarbital combination

Pyridamole—see dipyridamole

Pyridiate—see phenazopyridine

Pyridium—see phenazopyridine

QuadraHist—see phenylpropanolamine,
phenylephrine, chlorpheniramine, and
phenyltoloxamine combination

Questran—see cholestyramine

Quibron—see theophylline and guaifenesin
combination

Quibron-T—see theophylline

Quinaglute Dura-Tabs—see quinidine

Quinatime—see quinidine

---

quinethazone

BRAND NAME (Manufacturer)
Hydromox (Lederle)
TYPE OF DRUG
Diuretic (water pill) and anti-hypertensive

INGREDIENT
quinethazone
DOSAGE FORM
Tablets (50 mg)
STORAGE
This medication should be stored at room temperature in a tightly closed container.

USES
Quinethazone is prescribed to treat high blood pressure. It is also used to reduce fluid accumulation in the body caused by conditions such as heart failure, cirrhosis of the liver, kidney disease, and the long-term use of some medications. This medication reduces fluid accumulation by increasing the elimination of sodium and water through the kidneys.

TREATMENT
To decrease stomach irritation, you can take quinethazone with a glass of milk or with a meal (unless your doctor directs you to do otherwise). Try to take it at the same time every day. Avoid taking a dose after 6:00 P.M.—this will prevent you from having to get up during the night to urinate.

If you miss a dose of this medication, take the missed dose as soon as possible, unless it is almost time for the next dose. In that case, do not take the missed dose at all; just wait until the next scheduled dose. Do not double the dose.

This medication does not cure high blood pressure, but it will help to control the condition, as long as you continue to take it.

SIDE EFFECTS
Minor. Constipation; cramps; diarrhea; dizziness; drowsiness; headache; heartburn, itching; loss of appetite; nausea; restlessness; upset stomach; and vomiting. As your body adjusts to the medication, these side effects should disappear.

This medication can cause increased sensitivity to sunlight. It is therefore important to avoid prolonged exposure to sunlight and sunlamps. Wear protective clothing, and use an effective sunscreen.

To avoid dizziness or light-headedness when you stand, contract and relax the muscles of your legs for a few moments before rising. Do this by pushing one foot against the floor while raising the other foot slightly, alternating feet so that you are "pumping" your legs in a pedaling motion.

Major. Tell your doctor about any side effects that are persistent or particularly bothersome. IT IS ESPECIALLY IMPORTANT TO TELL YOUR DOCTOR about any unusual bleeding or bruising; blurred vision; confusion; difficulty breathing; dry mouth; excessive thirst; fever; joint pain; mood changes; muscle spasms; palpitations; skin rash; sore throat; tingling in the fingers or toes; excessive weakness; or yellowing of the eyes or skin.

INTERACTIONS

Quinethazone interacts with other types of medication.

1. It may decrease the effectiveness of oral anti-coagulants, anti-gout medications, insulin, oral anti-diabetic medicines, and methenamine.

2. Fenfluramine can increase the blood-pressure-lowering effects of quinethazone (which can be dangerous).

3. Indomethacin can decrease the blood-pressure-lowering effects (thereby counteracting the desired effects) of quinethazone.

4. Cholestyramine and colestipol decrease the absorption of this medication from the gastrointestinal tract, decreasing its effectiveness. Quinethazone should therefore be taken one hour before, or four hours after, a dose of cholestyramine or colestipol (if you have also been prescribed one of these medications).

5. Quinethazone may increase the side effects of amphotericin B, calcium, cortisone-like steroids (such as cortisone, dexamethasone, hydrocortisone, prednisone, prednisolone), digoxin, digitalis, lithium, quinidine, sulfonamide antibiotics, or vitamin D.

BE SURE TO TELL YOUR DOCTOR if you are taking any of the medicines listed above.

WARNINGS

• Tell your doctor about unusual or allergic reactions you have had to any medications, especially to diuretics, oral anti-diabetic medications, or sulfonamide antibiotics.

● Before you start taking quinethazone, tell your doctor if you now have. or if you have ever had, kidney disease or problems with urination, diabetes mellitus (sugar diabetes), gout, liver disease, asthma, pancreas disease, or systemic lupus erythematosus (SLE).

● Quinethazone can cause potassium loss. Signs of potassium loss include dry mouth, thirst, weakness, muscle pain or cramps, nausea, and vomiting. If you experience any of these symptoms, call your doctor. To help avoid potassium loss, take this drug with a glass of fresh or frozen orange juice or cranberry juice, or eat a banana every day. The use of a salt substitute also helps to prevent potassium loss. Do not change your diet, however, before discussing it with your doctor. Too much potassium can also be dangerous. Your doctor may want you to have blood tests performed periodically, in order to monitor your potassium levels.

● Limit your intake of alcoholic beverages while taking this medication, in order to prevent dizziness and lightheadedness.

● Do not take any over-the-counter (non-prescription) medications for weight control, or for allergy, asthma, cough, cold, or sinus problems, unless your doctor directs you to do so.

● To prevent dehydration (severe water loss) while taking this medication, check with your doctor if you have any illness that causes severe or continuous nausea, vomiting, or diarrhea.

● This medication can raise blood sugar in diabetic patients. Therefore, blood sugar levels should be carefully monitored by blood or urine tests when this medication is started.

● Be sure to tell your doctor if you are pregnant. This drug is able to cross the placenta. Studies in humans have not yet been completed, but adverse effects have been observed on the fetuses of animals who were given large doses of this drug during pregnancy. Also, tell your doctor if you are breastfeeding an infant. Small amounts of this drug can pass into breast milk, so caution is warranted.

Quinidex Extentabs—see quinidine

quinidine

BRAND NAMES (Manufacturers)
Cardioquin (Purdue Frederick)
Cin-Quin (Rowell)
Duraquin (Parke-Davis)
Quinaglute Dura-Tabs (Berlex)
Quinatime (Bolar)
Quinidex Extentabs (Robins)
Quinora (Key)
Quin-Release (Major)
SK-Quinidine Sulfate (Smith Kline & French)

TYPE OF DRUG
Anti-arrhythmic

INGREDIENT
quinidine as the sulfate, gluconate, or polygalacturonate
  salt

DOSAGE FORMS
Tablets (100 mg, 200 mg, 275 mg, and 300 mg)
Sustained-release tablets (300 mg, 324 mg, and 330 mg)
Capsules (200 mg and 300 mg)

STORAGE
Quinidine tablets and capsules should be stored at room
temperature, in tightly closed, light-resistant containers.

USES
Quinidine is used to treat heart arrhythmias. It corrects irregular heartbeats and helps to achieve a more normal
rhythm.

TREATMENT
To increase absorption of the drug, you should take quinidine on an empty stomach with a full glass of water, one
hour before or two hours after a meal. To lessen stomach
upset, however, ask your doctor if you can take it with food
or milk.

Try to take it at the same time(s) each day. Quinidine
works best when the amount of drug in your bloodstream
is kept constant. This medication should therefore be
taken at evenly spaced intervals, day and night. For example, if you are to take quinidine four times per day, the
doses should be spaced six hours apart.

The sustained-release tablets should be swallowed whole. Breaking, chewing, or crushing these tablets destroys their sustained-release activity, and possibly increases the side effects.

If you miss a dose of this medication and remember within two hours, take the missed dose, then return to your regular dosing schedule. If more than two hours have passed (four hours for the sustained-release tablets), do not take the missed dose; just return to your regular dosing schedule. Do not double the next dose.

SIDE EFFECTS

Minor. Abdominal pain; bitter taste in mouth; confusion; cramping; diarrhea; flushing; loss of appetite; nausea; restlessness; and vomiting. These side effects should disappear in several weeks, as your body adjusts to the medication.

Major. Tell your doctor about any side effects that are persistent or particularly bothersome. IT IS ESPECIALLY IMPORTANT TO TELL YOUR DOCTOR about unusual bleeding or bruising; blurred vision; difficulty breathing; dizziness; fainting; fever; headache; light-headedness; palpitations; ringing in the ears; or sore throat.

INTERACTIONS

Quinidine interacts with several foods and medications.
1. It can increase the effects of warfarin, which can lead to bleeding complications.
2. Acetazolamide, thiazide diuretics (water pills), sodium bicarbonate, antacids, and citrus fruit juices can increase the blood levels and side effects of quinidine.
3. Nifedipine, phenobarbital, phenytoin, and rifampin can decrease blood quinidine levels.
4. The combination of quinidine and phenothiazine tranquilizers, reserpine, or other anti-arrhythmic agents can lead to side effects on the heart.
5. Quinidine can increase the blood levels of digoxin, leading to serious side effects.
Before starting to take quinidine, BE SURE TO TELL YOUR DOCTOR if you are already taking any of the medications listed above.

WARNINGS

● Tell your doctor about unusual or allergic reactions you have had to any medications, especially to quinidine or quinine.

● Be sure to tell your doctor if you now have, or if you have ever had, heart block, hypokalemia (low blood levels of potassium), kidney disease, liver disease, lung disease, myasthenia gravis, psoriasis, or thyroid disease.

● Although many quinidine products are on the market, they are not all bioequivalent; that is, they may not all be absorbed into the bloodstream at the same rate or have the same overall pharmacologic activity. Don't change brands of this drug without consulting your doctor or pharmacist to make sure you are receiving an identically functioning product.

● Do not take any over-the-counter (non-prescription) asthma, allergy, sinus, cough, cold, or diet product unless you first check with your doctor or pharmacist.

● If this drug makes you dizzy or light-headed, do not take part in any activity that requires alertness, such as driving a car or operating dangerous equipment.

● Before having any surgery or other medical or dental treatment, be sure to tell your doctor or dentist that you are taking quinidine.

● Do not stop taking this drug without first consulting your doctor. Stopping quinidine abruptly may cause a serious change in the activity of your heart. Your doctor may therefore want to reduce your dosage gradually.

● Be sure to tell your doctor if you are pregnant. Although this drug appears to be safe, extensive studies in pregnant women have not yet been completed. Also, tell your doctor if you are breastfeeding an infant. Small amounts of quinidine pass into breast milk.

Quinora—see quinidine

Quin-Release—see quinidine

Racet-1%—see hydrocortisone and iodochlorhydroxyquin combination (topical)

Racet SE—see hydrocortisone (topical)

ranitidine

BRAND NAME (Manufacturer)
Zantac (Glaxo)
TYPE OF DRUG
Gastric acid secretion inhibitor (decreases stomach acid)
INGREDIENT
ranitidine as the hydrochloride salt
DOSAGE FORM
Tablets (150 mg)
STORAGE
Ranitidine should be stored at room temperature in a tightly closed, light-resistant container.

USES

Ranitidine is used to treat duodenal and gastric ulcers. It is also used in the long-term treatment of excessive stomach acid secretion, and in the prevention of recurrent ulcers. Ranitidine works by blocking the effects of histamine on the stomach, thereby reducing stomach acid secretion.

TREATMENT

You can take ranitidine either on an empty stomach or with food or milk.

Antacids can block the absorption of ranitidine. If you are taking antacids as well as ranitidine, at least one hour should separate doses of the two medications.

If you miss a dose of this medication, take the missed dose as soon as possible, unless it is almost time for the next dose. In that case, do not take the missed dose at all; just return to your regular dosing schedule. Do not double the next dose.

SIDE EFFECTS

Minor. Constipation; diarrhea; dizziness; headache; nausea; and stomach upset. These side effects should disappear in several days, as your body adjusts to the medication.

If you feel dizzy, sit or lie down awhile; get up slowly, and be careful on stairs.

Major. Tell your doctor about any side effects that are persistent or particularly bothersome. IT IS ESPECIALLY IMPORTANT TO TELL YOUR DOCTOR about unusual bleeding or bruising; confusion; decreased sexual ability; or weakness.

INTERACTIONS
The potential for ranitidine interacting with any other medication is small.

WARNINGS
• Tell your doctor about unusual or allergic reactions you have had to any medications, especially to ranitidine.
• Tell your doctor if you now have, or if you have ever had, kidney or liver disease.
• Ranitidine should be taken continuously for as long as your doctor prescribes. Stopping therapy early may be a cause of ineffective therapy.
• Cigarette smoking may block the beneficial effects of ranitidine.
• If this drug makes you dizzy, do not take part in any activity that requires alertness, such as driving a car or operating potentially dangerous equipment.
• Be sure to tell your doctor if you are pregnant. Ranitidine appears to be safe during pregnancy; however, extensive testing has not yet been completed. Also, tell your doctor if you are breastfeeding an infant. Small amounts of ranitidine pass into breast milk.

Rau-Sed—see reserpine

Rectacort—see hydrocortisone, benzyl benzoate, bismuth resorcin compound, bismuth subgallate, and Peruvian balsam combination (topical)

Reglan—see metoclopramide

Rela—see carisoprodol

Relaxadon—see atropine, scopolamine, hyoscyamine, and phenobarbital combination

Releserp-5—see reserpine

Renese—see polythiazide

Renoquid—see sulfonamides

Repen-VK—see penicillin VK

Reposans-10—see chlordiazepoxide

Resaid T.D.—see phenylpropanolamine and chlorpheniramine combination

Reserjen—see reserpine

---

reserpine

BRAND NAMES (Manufacturers)
Lemiserp (Lemmon)
Rau-Sed (Squibb)
Releserp-5 (Scott-Alison)
Reserjen (Jenkins)
reserpine (various manufacturers)
Reserpoid (Upjohn)
Sandril (Lilly)
Serpalan (Lannett)
Serpanray (Panray)
Serpasil (Ciba)
Serpate (Vale)
SK-Reserpine (Smith Kline & French)
Zepine (Foy)
TYPE OF DRUG
Anti-hypertensive
INGREDIENT
reserpine
DOSAGE FORMS
Tablets (0.1 mg, 0.25 mg, 0.5 mg, and 1 mg)
Sustained-release capsules (0.5 mg)
STORAGE
Reserpine should be stored at room temperature in tightly closed, light-resistant containers.

USES

Reserpine is used to treat high blood pressure. It works by depleting certain chemicals from the nervous system that are responsible for maintaining high blood pressure.

TREATMENT

In order to avoid stomach irritation, you can take reserpine with food or with a full glass of water or milk (unless your doctor directs you to do otherwise). Try to take reserpine at the same time(s) each day, in order to become accustomed to taking it.

The sustained-release form of this medication should be swallowed whole. Chewing, crushing, or breaking these capsules destroys their sustained-release activity, and possibly increases the side effects.

Reserpine does not cure hypertension, but it will help to control the condition, as long as you continue to take it.

If you miss a dose of this medication, take the missed dose as soon as possible, unless it is almost time for the next dose. In that case, do not take the missed dose at all; just return to your regular dosing schedule. Do not double the next dose.

SIDE EFFECTS

Minor. Abdominal pain; constipation; decrease in sexual desire; diarrhea; dizziness; dry mouth; headache; impotence; itching; loss of appetite; muscle aches; nasal congestion; nausea; nosebleeds; tremors; vomiting; and weight gain. These side effects should disappear in several weeks, as your body adjusts to the medication.

If you feel dizzy, sit or lie down awhile; get up slowly, and be careful on stairs.

To relieve mouth dryness, chew sugarless gum, or suck on ice chips or a piece of hard candy.

Major. Tell your doctor about any side effects that are persistent or particularly bothersome. IT IS ESPECIALLY IMPORTANT TO TELL YOUR DOCTOR about anxiety; black, tarry stools; unusual bleeding or bruising; chest pain; depression; difficulty urinating; drowsiness; enlarged breasts (in both sexes); fainting; fatigue; hearing loss; nervousness; nightmares; palpitations; rapid weight gain (three to five pounds within a week); rash; shortness of breath; or weakness.

INTERACTIONS

Reserpine interacts with several other types of medication.
1. Concurrent use of reserpine with central nervous system depressants (drugs that slow the activity of the brain and spinal cord), such as alcohol, antihistamines, barbiturates, benzodiazepine tranquilizers, muscle relaxants, narcotics, pain medications, phenothiazine tranquilizers, and sleeping medications, or with tricyclic anti-depressants can cause extreme drowsiness.
2. Reserpine can increase the side effects of digoxin and quinidine, and can decrease the effectiveness of levodopa.
3. Methotrimeprazine can increase the blood-pressure-lowering effects of reserpine, which can be dangerous.
4. Tricyclic anti-depressants can decrease the blood-pressure-lowering effects of reserpine.
5. Concurrent use of reserpine and monoamine oxidase (MAO) inhibitors can lead to severe side effects.
Before starting reserpine, BE SURE TO TELL YOUR DOCTOR if you are already taking any of the medications listed above.

WARNINGS

● Tell your doctor about unusual or allergic reactions you have had to medications, especially to reserpine or to any rauwolfia alkaloids.
● Before starting to take this medication, be sure to tell your doctor if you now have, or if you have ever had, arrhythmias; epilepsy; gallstones or gallbladder disease; heart disease; kidney disease; lung disease; mental depression; Parkinson's disease; peptic ulcers; pheochromocytoma; or ulcerative colitis.
● Reserpine should not be used within two weeks of electroshock therapy.
● If this drug makes you dizzy or drowsy, avoid tasks that require alertness, such as driving a car or operating potentially dangerous equipment.
● Before taking any over-the-counter (non-prescription) cough, cold, sinus, asthma, allergy, or diet medication, consult your doctor or pharmacist. Some of these products may increase your blood pressure.

- Reserpine may cause cancer in rats; it has not been shown conclusively to cause cancer in people.
- Be sure to tell your doctor if you are pregnant. Reserpine has been reported to cause birth defects in infants whose mothers received the drug during pregnancy. Also tell your doctor if you are breastfeeding an infant. Reserpine can pass into breast milk and cause side effects in the nursing infant.

Reserpoid—see reserpine

Respbid—see theophylline

Restoril—see temazepam

Retet—see tetracycline

Retin-A—see tretinoin

R-HCTZ-H—see hydralazine, hydrochlorothiazide, and reserpine combination

Rhinafed-EX—see pseudoephedrine and chlorpheniramine combination

Rhinolar-Ex 12—see phenylpropanolamine and chlorpheniramine combination

Rifadin—see rifampin

---

rifampin

BRAND NAMES (Manufacturers)
Rifadin (Merrell Dow)
Rimactane (Ciba)
TYPE OF DRUG
Antibiotic (infection fighter)
INGREDIENT
rifampin
DOSAGE FORM
Capsules (150 mg and 300 mg)

STORAGE
Rifampin should be stored at room temperature in a tightly closed, light-resistant container.

USES
Rifampin is an antibiotic that is used to treat tuberculosis and to prevent meningococcal meningitis. Rifampin works by preventing the growth and multiplication of susceptible bacteria. It is not effective against viruses, parasites, or fungi.

TREATMENT
Rifampin should be taken with a full glass of water on an empty stomach, one hour before or two hours after a meal. If this medication causes stomach irritation, however, ask your doctor to see if you can take it with food.

Try not to miss any doses of this medication. If you do miss a dose, take it as soon as possible, unless it is almost time for your next dose. In that case, do not take the missed dose at all; just return to your regular dosing schedule. Do not double the next dose.

It is important to continue to take this medication for the entire time prescribed by your doctor (which may be months to years), even if the symptoms disappear before the end of that period. If you stop taking the drug too soon, resistant bacteria are given a chance to continue growing, and your infection could recur.

SIDE EFFECTS
Minor. Diarrhea; dizziness; drowsiness; gas; headache; heartburn; loss of appetite; nausea; stomach irritation; and vomiting. These side effects should disappear in several days, as your body adjusts to the medication.

If you feel dizzy, sit or lie down awhile; get up slowly, and be careful on stairs.

Major. Tell your doctor about any side effects that are persistent or particularly bothersome. IT IS ESPECIALLY IMPORTANT TO TELL YOUR DOCTOR about confusion; difficult or painful urination; fatigue; fever; flushing; itching; muscle weakness; numbness; skin rash; uncoordinated movements; visual disturbances; or yellowing of the eyes or skin.

INTERACTIONS

Rifampin interacts with several other types of medication.
1. Concurrent use with p-aminosalicylic acid may decrease the blood levels and effectiveness of rifampin.
2. Rifampin can decrease the blood levels and effectiveness of metoprolol, propranolol, quinidine, adrenocorticosteroids (cortisone-like medicines), oral contraceptives, progestins, clofibrate, methadone, oral anti-coagulants (blood thinners, such as warfarin), oral anti-diabetic medicines, barbiturates, benzodiazepine tranquilizers, dapsone, digitoxin, and trimethoprim.
3. Concurrent use of rifampin with alcohol or isoniazid can lead to an increased risk of liver damage.
Before starting to take rifampin, BE SURE TO TELL YOUR DOCTOR if you are already taking any of the medications listed above.

WARNINGS

• Tell your doctor about unusual or allergic reactions you have had to any medication, especially to rifampin.
• Before starting to take this medication, be sure to tell your doctor if you now have, or if you have ever had, problems with alcohol or liver disease.
• Rifampin has been prescribed for your current infection only. Another infection later on, or one that someone else has, may require a different medicine. You should not give your medicine to other people, or use it for other infections, unless your doctor specifically directs you to do so.
• If this drug makes you dizzy or drowsy, do not take part in any activity that requires alertness, such as driving a car or operating potentially dangerous equipment.
• Rifampin can cause reddish-orange to reddish-brown discoloration of your urine, feces, saliva, sputum, sweat, and tears. This is a harmless effect. The drug may also permanently discolor soft contact lenses. You might want to stop wearing them while you are taking this medication. Discuss this with your ophthalmologist.
• Do not stop taking this medication unless you first check with your doctor. Stopping the drug and restarting it at a later time can lead to an increase in side effects.
• Be sure to tell your doctor if you are pregnant. Although rifampin appears to be safe in humans, birth de-

fects have been reported in animals whose mothers received large doses of the drug during pregnancy. Also, tell your doctor if you are breastfeeding an infant. Small amounts of rifampin pass into breast milk.

Rimactane—see rifampin

Rinade-BID—see pseudoephedrine and chlorpheniramine combination

Ritalin—see methylphenidate

Ritalin-SR—see methylphenidate

RMS Uniserts—see morphine

Robaxin—see methocarbamol

Robicillin VK—see penicillin VK

Robimycin—see erythromycin

Robitet Robicaps—see tetracycline

Rocaltrol—see calcitriol

Rofed C—see pseudoephedrine, tripolidine, guaifenesin, and codeine combination

Rondec—see pseudoephedrine and carbinoxamine combination

Rotane Expectorant—see phenylephrine, phenylpropanolamine, brompheniramine, and guaifenesin combination

Roxanol—see morphine

RP-Mycin—see erythromycin

Rufen—see ibuprofen

Rum-K—see potassium chloride

Saluron—see hydroflumethiazide

Sandimmune—see cyclosporine

Sandril—see reserpine

Sanorex—see mazindol

Sarisol—see butabarbital

S.A.S.-500—see sulfasalazine

Satric—see metronidazole

Scabene—see lindane

---

secobarbital

BRAND NAMES (Manufacturers)
secobarbital sodium (various manufacturers)
Seconal (Lilly)
TYPE OF DRUG
Sedative/hypnotic (sleeping aid)
INGREDIENT
secobarbital as the sodium salt
DOSAGE FORMS
Tablets (100 mg)
Capsules (50 mg and 100 mg)
Oral elixir (22 mg per 5 ml teaspoonful)
Suppositories (30 mg, 60 mg, 120 mg, and 200 mg)
STORAGE
Secobarbital tablets, capsules, and oral elixir should be
stored at room temperature in tightly closed containers.
The suppositories should be stored in the refrigerator.
Secobarbital should never be frozen.

USES
This medication belongs to a group of drugs known as barbiturates, which are central nervous system depressants

(drugs that slow the activity of the brain and spinal cord). It is used as a sleeping aid in the treatment of insomnia.

TREATMENT

You can take secobarbital at bedtime. The tablets, capsules, or oral elixir can be taken with water, food, or milk.

Each dose of the oral elixir should be measured carefully, with a specially designed, 5 ml measuring spoon. An ordinary kitchen teaspoon is not accurate enough. The elixir can be taken straight or mixed with water, milk, or fruit juice.

To insert the suppository form of this medication, first unwrap it and moisten it slightly with water (if the suppository is too soft, run cold water over it or refrigerate it for 30 minutes before you unwrap it). Lie down on your left side with your right knee bent. Push the suppository well into the rectum with your finger. Try to avoid having a bowel movement for at least an hour.

You should not use this drug as a sleeping aid for more than two weeks. With prolonged use, secobarbital loses its ability to produce and maintain sleep.

SIDE EFFECTS

Minor. Constipation; diarrhea; dizziness; drowsiness; headache; a "hangover" feeling; muscle or joint pain; nausea; stomach upset; and vomiting. These side effects should disappear in several days, as your body adjusts to the medication.

If you feel dizzy or light headed, sit or lie down awhile, get up slowly, and be careful on stairs.

To relieve constipation, increase the amount of fiber in your diet (bran, salads, fresh fruits and vegetables, and whole-grain breads), exercise, and drink more water (unless your doctor directs you to do otherwise).

Major. Tell your doctor about any side effects that are persistent or particularly bothersome. IT IS ESPECIALLY IMPORTANT TO TELL YOUR DOCTOR about unusual bleeding or bruising; chest tightness; confusion; depression; difficulty breathing; excitation; fatigue; feeling faint; hives or itching; loss of coordination; skin rash; slurred speech; sore throat; unusual weakness; or yellowing of the eyes or skin.

INTERACTIONS

Secobarbital interacts with other types of medication.

1. Concurrent use of it with other central nervous system depressants (such as antihistamines, benzodiazepine tranquilizers, muscle relaxants, narcotics, pain medications, phenothiazine tranquilizers, or alcohol) or with tricyclic anti-depressants can cause extreme drowsiness.

2. Valproic acid, chloramphenicol, and monoamine oxidase (MAO) inhibitors can prolong the effects of secobarbital.

3. Secobarbital can decrease the blood levels and effectiveness of oral anti-coagulants (blood thinners, such as warfarin), digoxin, tricyclic anti-depressants, cortisone-like medicines, doxycycline, quinidine, estrogens, birth control pills, phenytoin, acetaminophen, and carbamazepine.

4. The combination of secobarbital and furosemide can cause low blood pressure and fainting.

5. Secobarbital can increase the side effects of cyclophosphamide or large doses of acetaminophen.

Before starting secobarbital, BE SURE TO TELL YOUR DOCTOR if you are already taking any of the medications listed above.

WARNINGS

• Tell your doctor about unusual or allergic reactions you have had to any medications, especially to secobarbital or to other barbiturates (such as amobarbital, butabarbital, mephobarbital, metharbital, pentobarbital, phenobarbital, or primidone).

• Before starting to take this medication, be sure to tell your doctor if you now have, or if you have ever had, acute or chronic (long-term) pain; Addison's disease (an underactive adrenal gland); diabetes mellitus (sugar diabetes); kidney disease; liver disease; lung disease; mental depression; porphyria; or thyroid disease.

• If this medication makes you dizzy or drowsy during the day, do not take part in any activity that requires alertness, such as driving a car or operating potentially dangerous equipment.

• Secobarbital has the potential for abuse and must be used with caution. Tolerance develops quickly; do not increase the dosage or stop taking this drug unless you first consult your doctor. If you have been taking secobarbital for a long time or have been taking large doses, you may experience anxiety, muscle twitching, tremors, weakness, dizziness, nausea, vomiting, insomnia, or blurred vision when you stop taking it. To avoid this reaction, your doctor may want to reduce your dosage gradually.

● Be sure to tell your doctor if you are pregnant. Barbiturates cross the placenta, and there has been an association between birth defects and the use of this class of drugs during pregnancy. Such drugs may also lead to bleeding complications in the newborn. The risks should be discussed with your doctor. In addition, if secobarbital is used for long periods during the last three months of pregnancy, there is a chance that the infant will be born addicted to the medication, and will experience a withdrawal reaction (convulsions and irritability) at birth. Also, tell your doctor if you are breastfeeding an infant. Small amounts of secobarbital pass into breast milk and may cause drowsiness and breathing problems in nursing infants.

secobarbital sodium—see secobarbital

Seconal—see secobarbital

Sedabamate—see meprobamate

Sedadrops—see phenobarbital

Seds—see atropine, scopolamine, hyoscyamine, and phenobarbital combination

Semitard—see insulin

Septra—see sulfametnoxazole and trimethoprim combination

Septra DS—see sultamethoxazole and trimethoprim combination

Ser-A-Gen—see hydralazine, hydrochlorothiazide, and reserpine combination

Seralazide—see hydralazine, hydrochlorothiazide, and reserpine combination

Ser-Ap-Es—see hydralazine, hydrochlorothiazide, and reserpine combination

Serax—see oxazepam

Sereen—see chlordiazepoxide

Serentil—see mesoridazine

Ser Hydra Zine—see hydralazine, hydrochlorothiazide, and reserpine combination

Serophene—see clomiphene

Serpalan—see reserpine

Serpanray—see reserpine

Serpasil—see reserpine

Serpate—see reserpine

Simron—see iron supplements

Sinemet—see levodopa and carbidopa combination

Sinequan—see doxepin

Sinocon—see phenylpropanolamine, phenylephrine, chlorpheniramine, and phenyltoloxamine combination

SK-65—see propoxyphene

SK-65 APAP—see acetaminophen and propoxyphene combination

SK-65 Compound—see aspirin, caffeine, and propoxyphene combination

SK-Amitriptyline—see amitriptyline

SK-Ampicillin—see ampicillin

SK-APAP with Codeine—see acetaminophen and codeine combination

SK-Bamate—see meprobamate

SK-Chloral Hydrate—see chloral hydrate

SK-Chlorothiazide—see chlorothiazide

SK-Dexamethasone—see dexamethasone (systemic)

SK-Digoxin—see digoxin

SK-Diphenoxylate—see diphenoxylate and atropine

SK-Erythromycin—see erythromycin

SK-Furosemide—see furosemide

SK-Hydrochlorothiazide—see hydrochlorothiazide

SK-Lygen—see chlordiazepoxide

SK-Methocarbamol—see methocarbamol

SK-Oxycodone with Acetaminophen—see acetaminophen and oxycodone combination

SK-Oxycodone with Aspirin—see aspirin and oxycodone combination

SK-Penicillin—see penicillin VK

SK-Penicillin G—see penicillin G

SK-Phenobarbital—see phenobarbital

SK-Potassium Chloride—see potassium chloride

SK-Pramine—see imipramine

SK-Prednisone—see prednisone (systemic)

SK-Probenecid—see probenecid

SK-Propantheline Bromide—see propantheline

SK-Quinidine Sulfate—see quinidine

SK-Reserpine—see reserpine

SK-Soxazole—see sulfonamides

SK-Terpin Hydrate with Codeine—see terpin hydrate and codeine combination

SK-Tetracycline—see tetracycline

SK-Tolbutamide—see tolbutamide

Slo-bid Gyrocaps—see theophylline

Slo-Phyllin—see theophylline

Slo-Phyllin GG—see theophylline and guaifenesin combination

Slow-Fe—see iron supplements

Slow-K—see potassium chloride

Slyn-LL—see phendimetrazine

SMZ-TMP—see sulfamethoxazole and trimethoprim combination

---

sodium fluoride

BRAND NAMES (Manufacturers)
Fluoral (CooperCare)

Fluorigard (Colgate)
Fluorineed (Hanlon)
Fluorinse (CooperCare)
Fluoritab (Fluoritab)
Flura (Kirkman)
Flura-Drops (Kirkman)
Flura-Loz (Kirkman)
Karidium (Lorvic)
Karigel (Lorvic)
Kari-Rinse (Lorvic)
Luride (Hoyt)
Luride Lozi-Tabs (Hoyt)
Pediaflor (Rosa)
Phos-Flur (Hoyt)
Point-Two (Hoyt)
sodium fluoride (various manufacturers)
Thera-Flur (Hoyt)

TYPE OF DRUG

Fluoride supplement

INGREDIENT

fluoride as the sodium salt

DOSAGE FORMS

Tablets (0.25 mg, 0.5 mg, and 1 mg)
Oral drops (0.125 mg and 0.25 mg per drop and 0.5 mg per ml)
Oral rinse (0.02% and 0.09%)
Oral paste (2.3%)
Oral gel (0.5%)

STORAGE

Sodium fluoride tablets, drops, rinse, and paste should be stored at room temperature in tightly closed, plastic containers. This medication should never be frozen. Sodium fluoride drops, gel, and rinse should not be mixed or stored in glass containers (fluoride causes etching of glass); plastic containers should be used.

USES

Sodium fluoride is used as a dietary supplement for the prevention of dental caries (cavities) in children. It is intended for use in areas where community water supplies are not supplemented with fluoride. It acts to strengthen the chemical structure of teeth and bones and to help teeth resist the "acid attack" of cavity-producing bacteria. It is also being used in the treatment of osteoporosis.

TREATMENT

In order to avoid stomach irritation, you should take sodium fluoride tablets or drops after a meal (unless your doctor directs you to do otherwise).

The tablets can be allowed to dissolve in the mouth, or they can be chewed, swallowed whole, added to drinking water or fruit juice, or added to the water used to prepare infant formula or other food.

Each dose of the oral drops should be measured carefully, with the dropper provided. The dose can then be swallowed undiluted or mixed with fluids or food.

Sodium fluoride should not be taken with milk or other dairy products; these foods can decrease the gastrointestinal absorption of fluoride.

Sodium fluoride rinse, gel, and paste are most effective when used immediately after brushing your teeth, just before bedtime. You should apply the rinse, gel, or paste according to the directions included in the package. Rinse around and between your teeth for one minute, then spit out any excess liquid or paste. Do not swallow, unless your doctor directs you to do so.

In order to obtain maximum benefit from these products, you should not eat, drink, smoke, or rinse your mouth for at least 15 to 30 minutes after application.

If you miss a dose of this medication, take the missed dose as soon as possible, unless it is almost time for the next dose. In that case, do not take the missed dose at all; just return to your regular dosing schedule. Do not double the next dose.

SIDE EFFECTS

Minor. Headache; stomach upset; and weakness. These side effects should disappear in several days, as your body adjusts to the medication.

Major. Tell your doctor about any side effects that are persistent or particularly bothersome. IT IS ESPECIALLY IMPORTANT TO TELL YOUR DOCTOR about bloody or black, tarry stools; bone pain; constipation; discoloration of the teeth; skin rash; vomiting; or weight loss.

INTERACTIONS

Sodium fluoride does not interact with other medications, if it is used according to directions.

WARNINGS

● Tell your doctor about unusual or allergic reactions you have had to medications, especially to any fluoride-containing products.
● Before starting to take this medication, be sure to tell your doctor if you now have, or if you have ever had, mottling of the teeth or thyroid disease.
● Some of these products contain F.D. & C. Yellow Dye No. 5 (tartrazine), which can cause allergic-type symptoms (shortness of breath, rash, fainting) in certain susceptible individuals.
● This product should not be used for children under two years of age if the fluoride content of drinking water is 0.3 parts per million or more. It should not be used for children over two years of age if the fluoride content of drinking water is 0.7 parts per million or more. If you are unsure of the fluoride content of your drinking water, ask your doctor, or call your county health department.
● Be sure to tell your doctor if you are pregnant. Although sodium fluoride appears to be safe during pregnancy, extensive studies in humans have not yet been completed. It is not known whether this drug can help prevent caries in the infants of mothers who receive it during pregnancy. Also, tell your doctor if you are breastfeeding an infant. Sodium fluoride passes into breast milk.

Sodium Sulamyd—see sodium sulfacetamide (ophthalmic)

---

sodium sulfacetamide (ophthalmic)

BRAND NAMES (Manufacturers)
AK-Sulf (Akorn)
Bleph-10 (Allergan)
Cetamide (Alcon)

Isopto Cetamide (Alcon)
Ophthacet (Vortech)
Sodium Sulamyd (Schering)
sodium sulfacetamide (various manufacturers)
Sulf-10 (Smith Miller & Patch)
Sulfacel-15 (BioProducts)
Sulten-10 (Muro)

TYPE OF DRUG
Ophthalmic antibiotic

INGREDIENT
sodium sulfacetamide

DOSAGE FORMS
Ophthalmic drops (10% and 30%)
Ophthalmic ointment (10%)

STORAGE
Sodium sulfacetamide drops and ointment should be stored at room temperature in tightly closed containers. This medication should never be frozen. If the eye drops discolor or turn brown, they should be discarded. A change in color demonstrates a loss of potency.

USES
Sodium sulfacetamide is used to treat bacterial eye infections and corneal ulcers. Sodium sulfacetamide is an antibiotic that is effective against a wide range of bacteria. It acts by preventing production of the nutrients that are required for growth of the infecting bacteria. This medication is not effective against infections caused by viruses or fungi.

TREATMENT
Wash your hands with soap and water before applying this medication. In order to avoid contamination of the eye drops or ointment, be careful not to touch the dropper or the ointment tip, or let them touch your eyes; and DO NOT wipe off or rinse the dropper after use.

To apply the drops, tilt your head back and pull down the lower eyelid with one hand to make a pouch below the eye. Drop the prescribed amount of medicine into this pouch and slowly close your eyes. Try not to blink. Keep your eyes closed and place one finger at the corner of the eye, next to your nose, applying a slight pressure for a minute or two (this is done to prevent loss of medication into the nose and throat canal). Then wipe away the excess with a clean tissue.

To apply the ointment, tilt the head back, pull down the lower lid to form a pouch below the eye, and squeeze a small amount of ointment (approximately 1/8 to 1/4 inch) in a line along the pouch. Close the eyes, and place your finger at the corner of the eye next to your nose for a minute or two. Do not rub your eyes. Wipe off excess ointment.

Since this medication is somewhat difficult to apply, you may want to have someone else apply the drops or ointment for you.

It is important to continue to take this medication for the entire time prescribed by your doctor—even if the symptoms disappear before the end of that period. If you stop applying the drug too soon, resistant bacteria are given a chance to continue growing, and the infection could recur.

If you miss a dose of this medication, apply the missed dose as soon as possible, unless it is almost time for your next dose. In that case, do not apply the missed dose at all; just return to your regular dosing schedule. DO NOT use twice as much medication at the next dose.

SIDE EFFECTS

Minor. Sodium sulfacetamide may cause blurred vision, or burning or stinging in the eyes, immediately after it is applied (especially the 30% solution). This should last only a few minutes.

Major. Tell your doctor about any side effects that are persistent or particularly bothersome. IT IS ESPECIALLY IMPORTANT TO TELL YOUR DOCTOR about signs of irritation in the eyes (such as redness, swelling, or itching) that last more than several minutes; chills; fever; itching; or difficulty breathing. Also, if your symptoms of infection seem to be getting worse rather than improving, you should contact your doctor.

INTERACTIONS

Sodium sulfacetamide is incompatible with silver preparations.

WARNINGS

• Tell your doctor about unusual or allergic reactions you have had to medications, especially to sodium sulfacetamide or to any other sulfa medication (diuretics, oral antidiabetic medication, or sulfonamide antibiotics).

• Sodium sulfacetamide may cause eye sensitivity to bright light; wearing sunglasses may lessen this problem.

• This medication has been prescribed for your current infection only. Another infection later on, or one that someone else has, may require a different medicine. You should not give your medicine to other people, or use it for other infections, unless your doctor specifically directs you to do so.

• In order to allow your eye infection to clear, do not apply makeup to the affected eye.

• If there is no change in your condition two or three days after starting to take this medication, contact your doctor. The medication may not be effective for your particular infection.

• Be sure to tell your doctor if you are pregnant. No problems have yet been reported with this drug during pregnancy in humans; however, if large amounts of this drug are applied for prolonged periods, some of it may be absorbed into the bloodstream. Birth defects have been observed in the fetuses of animals who received large oral doses of this type of drug during pregnancy. Also, tell your doctor if you are breastfeeding an infant. If this drug is absorbed, small amounts may pass into the breast milk and may temporarily alter the bacteria in the intestinal tract of the nursing infant, resulting in diarrhea.

Solfoton—see phenobarbital

Soma—see carisoprodol

Somophyllin—see aminophylline

Somophyllin-T—see theophylline

Soprodol—see carisoprodol

Sorate—see isosorbide dinitrate

Sorbide T.D.—see isosorbide dinitrate

Sorbitrate—see isosorbide dinitrate

Sorbitrate SA—see isosorbide dinitrate

Spalix—see atropine, scopolamine, hyoscyamine, and phenobarbital combination

Scancap No. 1—see dextroamphetamine

Sparine—see promazine

Spasaid—see atropine, scopolamine, hyoscyamine, and phenobarbital combination

Spaslin—see atropine, scopolamine, hyoscyamine, and phenobarbital combination

Spasmolin—see atropine, scopolamine, hyoscyamine, and phenobarbital combination

Spasmophen—see atropine, scopolamine, hyoscyamine, and phenobarbital combination

Spasquid—see atropine, scopolamine, hyoscyamine, and phenobarbital combination

Spiractone—see spironolactone

Spironazide—see spironolactone and hydrochlorothiazide combination

spironolactone

BRAND NAMES (Manufacturers)
Alatone (Major)
Aldactone (Searle)
Spiractone (Three P Products)
spironolactone (various manufacturers)

TYPE OF DRUG
Diuretic (water pill) and anti-hypertensive
INGREDIENT
spironolactone
DOSAGE FORM
Tablets (25 mg, 50 mg, and 100 mg)
STORAGE
Spironolactone should be stored at room temperature in a tightly closed, light-resistant container.

USES
Spironolactone is prescribed to treat high blood pressure. It is also used to reduce fluid accumulation in the body caused by conditions such as heart failure, cirrhosis of the liver, kidney disease, and the long-term use of some medications. Spironolactone reduces fluid accumulation by increasing the elimination of sodium and water through the kidneys. It may be used in combination with other diuretics to prevent potassium loss. Since spironolactone blocks the effects of a chemical (aldosterone) released from the adrenal gland, it can also be used to diagnose and treat an overactive adrenal gland.

TREATMENT
To decrease stomach irritation, you can take spironolactone with a glass of milk or with a meal (unless your doctor directs you to do otherwise). Try to take it at the same time every day. Avoid taking a dose after 6:00 P.M.—this will prevent you from having to get up during the night to urinate.

This medication does not cure high blood pressure, but it will help to control the condition, as long as you continue to take it.

If you miss a dose of this medication, take the missed dose as soon as possible, unless it is almost time for the next one. In that case, do not take the missed dose at all; just wait until the next scheduled dose. Do not double the dose.

SIDE EFFECTS
Minor. Cramping; diarrhea; dizziness; drowsiness; dry mouth; headache; increased urination; nausea; rash; rest-

lessness; vomiting; and weakness. As your body adjusts to the medication, these side effects should disappear.

Dry mouth can be relieved by sucking on ice chips or a piece of hard candy, or by chewing sugarless gum.

To avoid dizziness or light-headedness when you stand, contract and relax the muscles of your legs for a few moments before rising. Do this by pushing one foot against the floor while raising the other foot slightly, alternating feet so that you are "pumping" your legs in a pedaling motion.

Major. Tell your doctor about any side effects that are persistent or particularly bothersome. IT IS ESPECIALLY IMPORTANT TO TELL YOUR DOCTOR about anxiety; clumsiness; confusion; stomach cramps; deepened voice (in women); enlarged breasts (in both sexes); fever; impotence; increased hair growth; irregular heartbeat; menstrual disturbances; post-menopausal bleeding; rapid weight gain (three to five pounds within a week); tingling in the fingers or toes; or uncoordinated movements.

INTERACTIONS

Spironolactone interacts with several foods and medications.

1. Concurrent use of it with amiloride, triamterene, potassium salts, low-salt milk, salt substitutes, captopril, or laxatives can cause serious side effects from hyperkalemia (high levels of potassium in the blood).

2. Spironolactone may increase the side effects of lithium, digoxin, digitoxin, and ammonium chloride.

3. The effectiveness of oral anti-coagulants (blood thinners, such as warfarin) may be decreased by this medication.

4. Aspirin may decrease the diuretic effects of spironolactone.

Before starting to take spironolactone, BE SURE TO TELL YOUR DOCTOR if you are already taking any of the medications listed above.

WARNINGS

• Tell your doctor about unusual or allergic reactions you have had to medications, especially to any diuretics.

• Tell your doctor if you now have, or if you have ever

had, kidney or urination problems, heart disease, hyperkalemia (high blood levels of potassium), liver disease, menstrual abnormalities, breast enlargement, or diabetes mellitus (sugar diabetes).

● Spironolactone can cause hyperkalemia. Signs of hyperkalemia include palpitations; confusion; numbness or tingling in the hands, feet or lips; anxiety; or unusual tiredness or weakness. In order to avoid this problem, do not alter your diet or use salt substitutes unless your doctor tells you to do so.

● Spironolactone has been shown to cause cancer in rats when administered in large doses. This effect has not been observed in humans.

● There are several "generic brands" of this drug. Consult your pharmacist about these items; some of them are not equivalent to the brand name medications.

● Limit your intake of alcoholic beverages in order to prevent dizziness and light-headedness while taking this medication.

● Do not take any over-the-counter (non-prescription) medication for weight control, or for allergy, asthma, cough, cold, or sinus problems, unless you first check with your doctor. Some of these products can increase blood pressure.

● To prevent severe water loss (dehydration) while taking this medication, check with your doctor if you have any illness that causes severe or continuous nausea, vomiting, or diarrhea.

● Be sure to tell your doctor if you are pregnant. This drug crosses the placenta. Studies in humans have not been completed, but adverse effects have been observed on the fetuses of animals who were given large doses of this drug during pregnancy. Also, tell your doctor if you are breastfeeding an infant. Small amounts of this drug pass into breast milk.

spironolactone and hydrochlorothiazide combination

BRAND NAMES (Manufacturers)
Alazide (Major)
Aldactazide (Searle)
Spironazide (Henry Schein)
spironolactone and hydrochlorothiazide (various manufacturers)
Spirozide (Rugby)
TYPE OF DRUG
Diuretic (water pill) and anti-hypertensive
INGREDIENTS
spironolactone and hydrochlorothiazide
DOSAGE FORM
Tablets (25 mg spironolactone and 25 mg hydrochlorothiazide; 50 mg spironolactone and 50 mg hydrochlorothiazide)
STORAGE
Spironolactone and hydrochlorothiazide should be stored at room temperature in a tightly closed, light-resistant container.

USES

Spironolactone and hydrochlorothiazide combination is prescribed to treat high blood pressure. It is also used to reduce fluid acccumulation in the body caused by conditions such as heart failure, cirrhosis of the liver, kidney disease, and the long-term use of some medications. This medication reduces fluid accumulation by increasing the elimination of sodium and water through the kidneys. Spironolactone is combined with hydrochlorothiazide to prevent potassium loss from the body.

TREATMENT

To decrease stomach irritation, you can take this medication with a glass of milk or with a meal (unless your doctor directs you to do otherwise). Try to take it at the same time every day. Avoid taking a dose after 6:00 P.M.—this will prevent you from having to get up during the night to urinate.

This medication does not cure high blood pressure, but it will help to control the condition, as long as you continue to take it.

If you miss a dose of this medication, take the missed dose as soon as possible, unless it is almost time for the next one. In that case, do not take the missed dose at all; just wait until the next scheduled dose. Do not double the dose.

SIDE EFFECTS

Minor. Confusion; constipation; cramping; diarrhea; dizziness; headache; increased urination; loss of appetite; lack of energy; light-headedness; nausea; rash; restlessness; unusual sweating; and vomiting. These side effects should disappear in several days, as your body adjusts to this medication.

This medication can cause increased sensitivity to sunlight. It is therefore important to avoid prolonged exposure to sunlight and sunlamps. Wear protective clothing, and use an effective sunscreen.

To avoid dizziness or light-headedness when you stand, contract and relax the muscles of your legs for a few moments before rising. Do this by pushing one foot against the floor while raising the other foot slightly, alternating feet so that you are "pumping" your legs in a pedaling motion.

Major. Tell your doctor about any side effects that are persistent or particularly bothersome. IT IS ESPECIALLY IMPORTANT TO TELL YOUR DOCTOR about unusual bleeding or bruising; breast tenderness or enlargement (in both sexes); blurred vision; clumsiness; confusion; deepening of the voice (in women); drowsiness; increased hairiness; impotence; irregular menstrual periods or vaginal bleeding; joint pain; mood changes; muscle cramps; numbness or tingling in the hands, feet, or lips; palpitations; rash; sore throat and fever; swelling of the legs or ankles; abnormal thirst or dry mouth; unusual tiredness or weakness; rapid weight gain (three to five pounds within a week); or yellowing of the eyes or skin.

INTERACTIONS

Spironolactone and hydrochlorothiazide combination interacts with several foods and medications.

1. Concurrent use of it with triamterene, amiloride, potassium salts, low-salt milk, salt substitutes, captopril, or laxatives can cause serious side effects from hyperkalemia (high levels of potassium in the blood).

2. This drug may decrease the effectiveness of oral anticoagulants, anti-gout medications, insulin, oral anti-diabetic medicines, and methenamine.

3. Fenfluramine may increase the blood-pressure-lowering effects of this drug.

4. Indomethacin and aspirin may decrease the blood-pressure-lowering effects of this medication.

5. Cholestyramine and colestipol can decrease the absorption of this medication from the gastrointestinal tract. Therefore, spironolactone and hydrochlorothiazide should be taken one hour before or four hours after a dose of cholestyramine or colestipol (if you have also been prescribed one of these medications).

6. Spironolactone and hydrochlorothiazide may increase the side effects of amphotericin B, ammonium chloride, calcium, cortisone-like steroids (such as cortisone, dexamethasone, hydrocortisone, prednisone, prednisolone), digoxin, digitalis, lithium, quinidine, sulfonamide, antibiotics, and vitamin D.

BE SURE TO TELL YOUR DOCTOR if you are already taking any of the medicines listed above.

WARNINGS

• Tell your doctor about unusual or allergic reactions you have had to any medications, especially to spironolactone or other diuretics (water pills), to oral anti-diabetic medications, or to sulfonamide antibiotics.

• Before you start taking spironolactone and hydrochlorothiazide, tell your doctor if you now have, or if you have ever had, kidney disease or problems with urination, diabetes mellitus (sugar diabetes), gout, liver disease, asthma, pancreas disease, systemic lupus erythematosus (SLE), hyperkalemia, menstrual abnormalities, breast enlargement, acidosis, or hypercalcemia.

• This drug can occasionally cause potassium loss from the body. Signs of potassium loss include dry mouth; muscle pain or cramps; thirst; nausea; vomiting; or weakness. If you experience any of these symptoms, call your doctor.

• Spironolactone can cause hyperkalemia. Signs of hyperkalemia include anxiety; confusion; numbness or tingling in the hands, feet, or lips; palpitations; or unusual tiredness or weakness. In order to avoid this problem, do not alter your diet and do not use salt substitutes unless you first consult your doctor.

• Spironolactone has been shown to cause cancer in rats when administered in large doses. This effect has not been observed in humans.

• There are several "generic brands" of this drug. Consult your pharmacist about these items. Some of them are not equivalent to the brand name medications.

• Limit your intake of alcoholic beverages in order to prevent dizziness and light-headedness while taking this medication.

• Do not take any over-the-counter (non-prescription) medication for weight control, or for allergy, asthma, cough, cold, or sinus problems, unless you first check with your doctor. Some of these products can increase blood pressure.

• To prevent severe water loss (dehydration) while taking this medication, check with your doctor if you have any illness that causes severe nausea, vomiting, or diarrhea.

• This medication can raise blood sugar levels in diabetic patients. Therefore, blood sugar should be monitored carefully with blood or urine tests when this medication is started.

• Be sure to tell your doctor if you are pregnant. This drug crosses the placenta. Although studies in humans have not yet been completed, adverse effects have been observed on the fetuses of animals who were given large doses of this drug during pregnancy. Also, tell your doctor if you are breastfeeding an infant. Small amounts of this medication pass into breast milk.

Spirozide—see spironolactone and hydrochlorothiazide combination

Sprx-1—see phendimetrazine

S-P-T—see thyroid hormone

Statobex—see phendimetrazine

Stelazine—see trifluoperazine

Sterane—see prednisolone (systemic)

Sterapred—see prednisone (systemic)

StuartNatal 1 + 1—see vitamins, prenatal

Sub-Quin—see procainamide

---

sucralfate

BRAND NAME (Manufacturer)
Carafate (Marion)
TYPE OF DRUG
Anti-ulcer
INGREDIENT
sucralfate
DOSAGE FORM
Tablets (1 gram)
STORAGE
Sucralfate should be stored at room temperature, in a tightly closed container.

USES

Sucralfate is used for the short-term treatment of ulcers. This medication binds to the surface of the ulcer, thereby protecting it from stomach acid and promoting healing.

TREATMENT

In order to obtain the maximum benefits from this drug, you should swallow it whole, with a full glass of water. Take it on an empty stomach, one hour before or two hours after a meal.

Do not take an antacid within 30 minutes of a dose of sucralfate. Antacids decrease the binding of sucralfate to the ulcer.

Continue to take sucralfate for the full length of time prescribed by your doctor, even if your symptoms disappear. Your ulcer may not yet be healed.

If you miss a dose of this medication, take the missed dose as soon as possible, unless it is almost time for the next dose. In that case do not take the missed dose at all; just return to your regular dosing schedule. Do not double the next dose.

SIDE EFFECTS

Minor. Back pain; constipation; diarrhea; dizziness; drowsiness; dry mouth; indigestion; itching; nausea; rash; and stomach pain. These side effects should disappear in several days, as your body adjusts to the medication.

If you feel dizzy, sit or lie down awhile; get up slowly, and be careful on stairs.

To relieve mouth dryness, chew sugarless gum, or suck on ice chips or a piece of hard candy.

Major. Tell your doctor about any side effects that are persistent or particularly bothersome. Also, if your condition does not improve or seems to be getting worse, you should contact your doctor.

INTERACTIONS

Sucralfate may prevent the absorption of tetracycline and fat-soluble vitamins (vitamins A, D, E, and K) from the gastrointestinal tract. BE SURE TO TELL YOUR DOCTOR if you are already taking tetracycline or vitamins.

WARNINGS

• Tell your doctor about unusual or allergic reactions you have had to any medications, especially to sucralfate.

• If sucralfate makes you dizzy or drowsy, avoid tasks that require alertness, such as driving a car or operating potentially dangerous equipment.

• Be sure to tell your doctor if you are pregnant. Although sucralfate appears to be safe, extensive studies in pregnant women have not yet been completed. Also, tell your doctor if you are breastfeeding an infant. It is not known whether or not sucralfate passes into breast milk.

Suldiazo—see sulfisoxazole and phenazopyridine combination

Sulf-10—see sodium sulfacetamide (ophthalmic)

Sulfacel-15—see sodium sulfacetamide (ophthalmic)

sulfacytine—see sulfonamides

sulfadiazine—see sulfonamides

Sulfadyne—see sulfasalazine

Sulfa-Gyn—see sulfathiazole, sulfacetamide, and sulfabenzamide combination

Sulfaloid—see sulfonamides

sulfamethiazole—see sulfonamides

sulfamethizole—see sulfonamides

sulfamethoxazole—see sulfonamides

---

sulfamethoxazole and phenazopyridine combination

BRAND NAME (Manufacturer)
Azo Gantanol (Roche)
TYPE OF DRUG
Antibiotic (infection fighter) and urinary tract analgesic (pain reliever)
INGREDIENTS
sulfamethoxazole and phenazopyridine as the hydrochloride salt

DOSAGE FORM

Tablets (500 mg sulfamethoxazole and 100 mg phenazopyridine)

STORAGE

These tablets should be stored at room temperature in a tightly closed, light-resistant container.

USES

This medication is used to treat painful infections of the urinary tract.

Sulfamethoxazole is a sulfonamide antibiotic. It acts by preventing production of the nutrients that are required for growth of the infecting bacteria. Phenazopyridine is excreted in the urine, where it exerts a topical analgesic effect on the urinary tract. This medication is not useful for any pain other than that of the urinary tract.

TREATMENT

It is best to take this medication with a full glass of water on an empty stomach, either one hour before or two hours after a meal. However, if it causes stomach upset, check with your doctor to see if you can take it with food or milk.

This medication works best when the level of medicine in your blood and urine is kept constant. It is best therefore to take the doses at evenly spaced intervals, day and night. For example, if you are to take four doses a day, the doses should be spaced six hours apart.

If you miss a dose of this medication, take the missed dose immediately. However, if you do not remember to take the missed dose until it is almost time for your next dose, take the missed dose immediately, and space the following dose about halfway through the regular interval between doses (wait about three hours, if you are taking four doses a day). Then return to your regular dosing schedule. Try not to skip any doses.

It is important to continue to take this medication for the entire time prescribed by your doctor (usually seven to 14 days), even if the symptoms disappear before the end of that period. If you stop taking the drug too soon, resistant bacteria are given a chance to continue growing, and the infection could recur.

SIDE EFFECTS

Minor. Abdominal pain; depression; diarrhea; dizziness; dry mouth; headache; indigestion; insomnia; loss of appetite; nausea; and vomiting. These side effects should disappear in several days, as your body adjusts to the medication.

If you feel dizzy, sit or lie down awhile; get up slowly, and be careful on stairs.

Sucking on ice chips or a piece of hard candy, or chewing sugarless gum, helps to relieve mouth dryness.

Sulfamethoxazole can cause increased sensitivity to sunlight. It is therefore important to avoid prolonged exposure to sunlight and sunlamps. Wear protective clothing and sunglasses, and use an effective sunscreen. However, a sunscreen containing para-aminobenzoic acid (PABA) interferes with the anti-bacterial activity of this medication, and should NOT be used.

Phenazopyridine causes your urine to become orange-red in color. This is not harmful. However, it may stain your clothing. The urine will return to its normal color soon after the drug is discontinued.

Major. Tell your doctor about any side effects that are persistent or particularly bothersome. IT IS ESPECIALLY IMPORTANT TO TELL YOUR DOCTOR about aching joints and muscles; back pain; unusual bleeding or bruising; bloating; chest pain; chills; confusion; convulsions; difficulty breathing; difficulty urinating; fever; hallucinations; hives; itching; loss of coordination; rash; ringing in the ears; sore throat; yellowing of the eyes or skin; or swollen ankles. Also, if your symptoms of infection seem to be getting worse rather than improving, you should contact your doctor.

INTERACTIONS

Sulfamethoxazole and phenazopyridine combination interacts with several other types of medication.

1. Sulfamethoxazole can increase the blood levels of active oral anti-coagulants (blood thinners, such as warfarin), oral anti-diabetic agents, methotrexate, oxyphenbutazone, phenylbutazone, and phenytoin, which can lead to serious side effects.

1014 sulfamethoxazole and phenazopyridine combination

2. Methenamine can increase the side effects to the kidneys caused by sulfamethoxazole.
3. Probenecid and sulfinpyrazone can increase the blood levels of sulfamethoxazole, which can lead to an increase in side effects.
BE SURE TO TELL YOUR DOCTOR if you are already taking any of the medications listed above.

WARNINGS

● Tell your doctor about unusual or allergic reactions you have had to medications, especially to phenazopyridine, sulfamethoxazole, or to any other sulfa drug (sulfonamide antibiotics, diuretics, dapsone, sulfoxone, oral anti-diabetic medications, or acetazolamide).
● Tell your doctor if you now have, or if you have ever had, glucose-6-phosphate dehydrogenase (G6PD) deficiency; kidney disease; liver disease; or porphyria.
● This medication has been prescribed for your current infection only. Another infection later on, or one that someone else has, may require a different medicine. You should not give your medicine to other people, or use it for other infections, unless your doctor specifically directs you to do so.
● This medication should be taken with lots of water, or orange or cranberry juice, in order to avoid the possibility of kidney stone formation.
● If this drug makes you dizzy, do not take part in any activity that requires alertness, such as driving a car or operating potentially dangerous equipment.
● Diabetic patients using this medication (phenazopyridine) may get delayed reactions or false-positive readings for sugar or ketones with urine tests. Clinitest is not affected by this medication, but the other urine sugar tests are.
● If there is no improvement in your condition several days after starting this medication, check with your doctor. This medication may not be effective against the bacteria causing your infection.
● Before having any surgery or other medical or dental treatment, be sure to tell your doctor or dentist that you are taking this medication.

• Be sure to tell your doctor if you are pregnant. Small amounts of sulfamethoxazole cross the placenta. Although this medication appears to be safe during pregnancy, extensive studies in humans have not yet been completed. Also, tell your doctor if you are breastfeeding an infant. Small amounts of this medication pass into breast milk and may temporarily alter the bacteria in the intestinal tract of the nursing infant, resulting in diarrhea. This medication should not be used in an infant less than two months of age (in order to avoid side effects involving the liver).

---

sulfamethoxazole and trimethoprim combination

BRAND NAMES (Manufacturers)
Bactrim (Roche)
Bactrim DS (Roche)
Bethaprim SS (Major)
Cotrim (Lemmon)
Septra (Burroughs Wellcome)
Septra DS (Burroughs Wellcome)
SMZ-TMP (Biocraft)
sulfamethoxazole and trimethoprim (various manufacturers)
Sulfatrim (various manufacturers)

TYPE OF DRUG
Antibiotic (infection fighter)

INGREDIENTS
sulfamethoxazole and trimethoprim

DOSAGE FORMS
Tablets (400 mg sulfamethoxazole and 80 mg trimethoprim)
Double-strength (DS) tablets (800 mg sulfamethoxazole and 160 mg trimethoprim)
Oral suspension (200 mg sulfamethoxazole and 40 mg trimethoprim per 5 ml teaspoonful)

STORAGE

Sulfamethoxazole and trimethoprim tablets and oral suspension should be stored at room temperature in tightly closed, light-resistant containers. The oral suspension does not need to be refrigerated. This medication should never be frozen.

USES

Sulfamethoxazole and trimethoprim combination is used to treat a broad range of infections, including urinary tract infections, certain respiratory and gastrointestinal infections, and otitis media (middle ear infections). Sulfamethoxazole and trimethoprim act by preventing production of the nutrients that are required for growth of the infecting bacteria.

TREATMENT

It is best to take this medication with a full glass of water on an empty stomach, either one hour before or two hours after a meal. However, if it causes stomach upset, check with your doctor to see if you can take it with food or milk.

The oral suspension form of this medication should be shaken well, just before measuring each dose. The contents tend to settle on the bottom of the bottle, so it is necessary to shake the container to evenly distribute the ingredients and equalize the doses. Each dose should then be measured carefully, with a specially designed, 5 ml measuring spoon. An ordinary kitchen teaspoon is not accurate enough.

This medication works best when the level of medicine in your bloodstream (and urine) is kept constant. It is best therefore to take the doses at evenly spaced intervals, day and night. For example, if you are to take two doses a day, the doses should be spaced 12 hours apart.

Try not to skip any doses.

If you miss a dose of this medication, take the missed dose immediately. However, if you do not remember to take the missed dose until it is almost time for your next dose, take the missed dose immediately, and space the following dose about halfway through the regular interval between doses (wait about six hours, if you are taking two doses a day). Then return to your regular dosing schedule.

It is important to continue to take this medication for the entire time prescribed by your doctor (usually seven to 14 days), even if the symptoms disappear before the end of that period. If you stop taking the drug too soon, resistant bacteria are given a chance to continue growing, and the infection could recur.

SIDE EFFECTS

Minor. Abdominal pain; diarrhea; dizziness; headache; loss of appetite; nausea; sore mouth; swollen or inflamed tongue; and vomiting. These side effects should disappear in several days, as your body adjusts to the medication.

If you feel dizzy, sit or lie down awhile; get up slowly, and be careful on stairs.

Sulfamethoxazole can cause increased sensitivity to sunlight. It is therefore important to avoid prolonged exposure to sunlight and sunlamps. Wear protective clothing and sunglasses, and use an effective sunscreen. However, a sunscreen containing para-aminobenzoic acid (PABA) interferes with the anti-bacterial activity of this medication, and should NOT be used.

Major. Tell your doctor about any side effects that are persistent or particularly bothersome. IT IS ESPECIALLY IMPORTANT TO TELL YOUR DOCTOR about unusual bleeding or bruising; convulsions; difficulty breathing; difficulty urinating; fever; hallucinations; itching; joint pain; rash; ringing in the ears; sore throat; swollen ankles; tingling in the hands or feet; unusual fatigue; or yellowing of the eyes or skin. Also, if your symptoms of infection seem to be getting worse rather than improving, you should contact your doctor.

INTERACTIONS

This combination medication interacts with several other types of medication.

1. Sulfamethoxazole can increase the blood levels of active oral anti-coagulants (blood thinners, such as warfarin), oral anti-diabetic agents, methotrexate, oxyphenbutazone, phenylbutazone, and phenytoin, which can lead to serious side effects.

2. Methenamine can increase the side effects to the kidneys caused by sulfamethoxazole.

3. Probenecid and sulfinpyrazone can increase the blood levels of sulfamethoxazole, which can lead to an increase in side effects.

4. Rifampin can increase the elimination of trimethoprim from the body, decreasing its anti-bacterial effects.

5. Concurrent use of trimethoprim with anti-neoplastic agents (anti-cancer drugs) can increase the risk of developing blood disorders.

6. Trimethoprim can decrease the elimination of phenytoin from the body, and increase the chance of side effects. BE SURE TO TELL YOUR DOCTOR if you are already taking any of the medications listed above.

WARNINGS

• Tell your doctor about unusual or allergic reactions you have had to any medications, especially to trimethoprim, sulfamethoxazole, or other sulfa drugs (sulfonamide antibiotic, diuretics, dapsone, sulfoxone, or oral anti-diabetic medications), or to acetazolamide.

• Tell your doctor if you now have, or if you have ever had, glucose-6-phosphate dehydrogenase (G6PD) deficiency; kidney disease; liver disease; porphyria; or megaloblastic anemia (folate-deficiency anemia).

• This medication has been prescribed for your current infection only. Another infection later on, or one that someone else has, may require a different medicine. You should not give your medicine to other people, or use it for other infections, unless your doctor specifically directs you to do so.

• This medication should be taken with lots of water, or orange or cranberry juice, in order to avoid the possibility of kidney stone formation.

• If this drug makes you dizzy, do not take part in any activity that requires alertness, such as driving a car or operating potentially dangerous equipment.

• If there is no improvement in your condition several days after starting to take this medication, check with your doctor. This medication may not be effective against the bacteria causing your infection.

• Before having any surgery or other medical or dental treatment, be sure to tell your doctor or dentist that you are taking this medication.

• Be sure to tell your doctor if you are pregnant. Small amounts of sulfamethoxazole and trimethoprim cross the placenta. Although these drugs appear to be safe during pregnancy, extensive studies in humans have not yet been completed. Trimethoprim has been shown to cause birth defects in the offspring of animals who received very large doses during pregnancy. Tell your doctor if you are breast-feeding an infant. Small amounts of sulfamethoxazole pass into breast milk and may temporarily alter the bacteria in the intestinal tract of the nursing infant, resulting in diarrhea. Also, small amounts of trimethoprim pass into breast milk, and there is a chance that it may cause anemia in the nursing infant. This combination medication should not be used in an infant less than two months of age (to avoid side effects involving the liver).

---

sulfasalazine

BRAND NAMES (Manufacturers)
Azulfidine (Pharmacia)
Azulfidine EN-tabs (Pharmacia)
S.A.S.-500 (Rowell)
Sulfadyne (Three P Products)
sulfasalazine (various manufacturers)
TYPE OF DRUG
Sulfonamide anti-inflammatory
INGREDIENT
sulfasalazine
DOSAGE FORMS
Tablets (500 mg)
Enteric-coated tablets (500 mg)
Oral suspension (250 mg per 5 ml teaspoonful)
STORAGE
Sulfasalazine tablets and suspension should be stored at room temperature in tightly closed containers. This medication should never be frozen.

USES

This medication is used to treat inflammatory bowel disease (regional enteritis or ulcerative colitis). In the intestine, salfasalazine is converted to 5-aminosalicylic acid, an aspirin-like drug, which acts to relieve inflammation.

TREATMENT

In order to avoid stomach irritation, you should take sulfasalazine with a full glass of water, with food, or after meals (unless your doctor directs you to do otherwise).

The enteric-coated tablets should be swallowed whole. The enteric coating is added to lessen stomach irritation. Chewing, breaking, or crushing these tablets destroys the coating.

The suspension form of this medication should be shaken well, just before measuring each dose. The contents tend to settle on the bottom of the bottle, so it is necessary to shake the container to evenly distribute the ingredients and equalize the doses. Each dose should then be measured carefully, with a specially designed, 5 ml measuring spoon. An ordinary kitchen teaspoon is not accurate enough.

If you miss a dose of this medication, take the missed dose as soon as possible, unless it is almost time for the next dose. In that case, do not take the missed dose at all; just return to your regular dosing schedule. Do not double the next dose.

SIDE EFFECTS

Minor. Diarrhea; dizziness; drowsiness; headache; insomnia; loss of appetite; nausea; stomach upset; and vomiting. These side effects should disappear in several days, as your body adjusts to the medication.

If you feel dizzy, sit or lie down awhile; get up slowly, and be careful on stairs.

This medication can increase your sensitivity to sunlight. You should therefore avoid prolonged exposure to sunlight and sunlamps. Wear protective clothing and sunglasses, and use an effective sunscreen.

Sulfasalazine can cause your urine to change to an orange-yellow color. This is a harmless effect.

Major. Tell your doctor about any side effects that are per-

sistent or particularly bothersome. IT IS ESPECIALLY IM-
PORTANT TO TELL YOUR DOCTOR about unusual
bleeding or bruising; convulsions; depression; difficult or
painful urination; fever; hallucinations; hearing loss; joint
pain; mouth sores; rash; ringing in the ears; sore throat;
tingling sensations; or yellowing of the eyes or skin.

INTERACTIONS

Sulfasalazine interacts with other types of medication.
1. It can increase the side effects of oral anti-coagulants
(blood thinners, such as warfarin), oral anti-diabetic
agents, methotrexate, phenytoin, oxphenbutazone, phenylbutazone, and sulfinpyrazone.
2. The blood levels and effectiveness of digoxin and folic
acid are decreased by concurrent use of sulfasalazine.
3. Probenecid can increase the blood levels and side effects of sulfasalazine.
Before starting to take sulfasalazine, BE SURE TO TELL
YOUR DOCTOR if you are already taking any of the medications listed above.

WARNINGS

• Tell your doctor about unusual or allergic reactions you
have had to medications, especially to sulfasalazine, aspirin or other salicylates, or to any sulfa or sulfonamide drug
(diuretics, oral anti-diabetic medications, acetazolamide,
sulfoxone, or dapsone).
• Before starting to take this medication, be sure to tell
your doctor if you now have, or if you have ever had, blood
disorders, blockage of the urinary tract or intestine, glu-
cose-6-phosphate dehydrogenase (G6PD) deficiency, kidney disease, liver disease, or porphyria.
• To help prevent the formation of kidney stones, try to
drink at least 8 to 12 glasses of water or fruit juice each day
while you are taking this medication (unless your doctor
directs you to do otherwise).
• Before having any surgery or other medical or dental
treatment, be sure to tell your doctor or dentist that you are
taking sulfasalazine.
• If your condition does not improve within a month or
two after starting to take sulfasalazine, check with your
doctor. It may be necessary to change your medication.

• Be sure to tell your doctor if you are pregnant. Although sulfasalazine appears to be safe during most of pregnancy, extensive studies in humans have not yet been completed. There is also concern that if this drug is taken during the ninth month of pregnancy, it may cause liver or brain disorders in the newborn infant. Also, tell your doctor if you are breastfeeding an infant. Small amounts of sulfasalazine pass into breast milk.

---

sulfathiazole, sulfacetamide, and sulfabenzamide combination

BRAND NAMES (Manufacturers)
Sulfa-Gyn (Mayrand)
Sultrin Triple Sulfa (Ortho)
Triple Sulfa (vaginal) (various manufacturers)
Trysul (Savage)
TYPE OF DRUG
Antibiotic (infection fighter)
INGREDIENTS
sulfathiazole, sulfacetamide, and sulfabenzamide
DOSAGE FORMS
Vaginal tablets (172.5 mg sulfathiazole, 143.75 mg sulfacetamide, and 184 mg sulfabenzamide)
Vaginal cream (3.42% sulfathiazole, 2.86% sulfacetamide, and 3.7% sulfabenzamide)
STORAGE
This medication should be stored at room temperature in tightly closed, light-resistant containers. It should never be frozen.

USES

Sulfathiazole, sulfacetamide, and sulfabenzamide are sulfonamide antibiotics used to treat vaginal infections. Sulfonamides work by blocking the production of essential nutrients, which kills the bacteria responsible for the infection.

TREATMENT

This product is packaged with instructions and an applicator. Read the instructions carefully before inserting the vaginal cream or tablets. Wash the applicator with warm water and soap, and thoroughly dry it after each use.

It is important to continue to take this medication for the entire time prescribed by your doctor, even if your symptoms disappear before the end of that period. If you stop taking the drug too soon, resistant bacteria are given a chance to continue growing, and your infection could recur.

If you miss a dose of this medication, insert the missed dose as soon as possible, unless it is almost time for the next dose. In that case, do not insert the missed dose at all; just return to your regular dosing schedule. Do not double the next dose.

SIDE EFFECTS

Minor. This medication can cause a mild, temporary burning or stinging sensation after the first few applications. As your body adjusts to the drug, these side effects should disappear.

Major. Tell your doctor about any side effects that are persistent or particularly bothersome. IT IS ESPECIALLY IMPORTANT TO TELL YOUR DOCTOR about itching, rash, swelling, redness, or any other signs of irritation that weren't present before you started taking this medication.

INTERACTIONS

This medication does not interact with other medications, if it is used according to directions.

WARNINGS

● Tell your doctor about unusual or allergic reactions you have had to medications, especially to sulfathiazole, sulfacetamide, or sulfabenzamide, or to any other sulfonamide antibiotics, diuretics (water pills), oral anti-diabetic medicines, dapsone, sulfone, or sulfoxone.

● Before starting to take this medication, be sure to tell your doctor if you now have, or if you have ever had, kidney disease.

- You should not use tampons while using this medication.
- During sexual intercourse, it is a good idea for your partner to wear a condom to prevent re-infection. Ask your doctor if it is necessary for your partner to be treated at the same time as you.
- This medication has been prescribed for your current infection only. Another infection later on, or one that someone else has, may require a different medicine. You should not give your medicine to other people, or use it for other infections, unless your doctor specifically directs you to do so.
- If the symptoms of your infection do not begin to improve within several days after starting to take this medication, CHECK WITH YOUR DOCTOR. This medication may not be effective for your infection.
- If you are pregnant, CHECK WITH YOUR DOCTOR to see if you should continue to use this medication.

Sulfatrim—see sulfamethoxazole and trimethoprim combination

---

sulfinpyrazone

BRAND NAME (Manufacturer)
Anturane (Ciba)
TYPE OF DRUG
Anti-gout and anti-platelet
INGREDIENT
sulfinpyrazone
DOSAGE FORMS
Tablets (100 mg)
Capsules (200 mg)
STORAGE
Sulfinpyrazone tablets and capsules should be stored at room temperature, in tightly closed containers.

USES
Sulfinpyrazone is used to treat gout. It acts by increasing

the elimination of uric acid (the chemical responsible for gout) by the kidneys. It is also used to prevent further heart attacks in patients who have had a recent attack. It prevents the formation of certain types of blood clots.

TREATMENT

In order to prevent stomach irritation, you should take sulfinpyrazone with food, milk, or antacids (unless your doctor directs you to do otherwise).

This medication does not cure gout, but it will help to control blood uric acid levels, as long as you continue to take it.

If you miss a dose of this medication, take the missed dose as soon as possible, unless it is almost time for your next dose. In that case, do not take the missed dose at all; just return to your regular dosing schedule. Do not double the next dose.

SIDE EFFECTS

Minor. Diarrhea; nausea; stomach upset; and vomiting. These side effects should disappear in several days, as your body adjusts to the medication.

Major. Tell your doctor about any side effects that are persistent or particularly bothersome. IT IS ESPECIALLY IMPORTANT TO TELL YOUR DOCTOR about back pain; bloody or black, tarry stools; convulsions; difficult or painful urination; fever; sore throat; skin rash; or unusual bleeding or bruising.

INTERACTIONS

Sulfinpyrazone interacts with several other types of medication.

1. Aspirin can increase uric acid levels, thereby decreasing the therapeutic effects of sulfinpyrazone.

2. Sulfinpyrazone can increase the side effects of sulfonamide antibiotics, oral anti-diabetic medications, oral anticoagulants (blood thinners, such as warfarin), and nitrofurantoin.

3. Alcohol, pyrazinamide, and diuretics (water pills) can increase the blood levels of uric acid, thereby decreasing the effectiveness of sulfinpyrazone.

Before starting to take this medication, BE SURE TO TELL
YOUR DOCTOR if you are already taking any of the medications listed above.

WARNINGS

• Tell your doctor about unusual or allergic reactions you
have had to any medications, especially to sulfinpyrazone,
dipyrone, oxyphenbutazone, or phenylbutazone.
• Before starting to take this medication, be sure to tell
your doctor if you now have, or if you have ever had, blood
disorders; kidney disease; peptic ulcers; or stomach or intestinal inflammation.
• Before taking any over-the-counter (non-prescription)
medication, check the label to see if it contains aspirin.
Aspirin can decrease the effectiveness of sulfinpyrazone.
• Sulfinpyrazone is not an analgesic (pain reliever) and
does not relieve an acute gout attack. It is used to prevent
future gout attacks.
• In order to prevent the formation of kidney stones, try
to drink at least 8 to 12 glasses of water or fruit juice each
day while taking this medication (unless your doctor directs you to do otherwise).
• Before having any surgery or other medical or dental
treatment, be sure to tell your doctor or dentist that you are
taking this medication. Treatment with sulfinpyrazone is
usually discontinued several days prior to surgery, to prevent bleeding complications.
• Be sure to tell your doctor if you are pregnant. Although this medication appears to be safe during pregnancy, extensive studies in humans have not yet been
completed. Also, tell your doctor if you are breastfeeding
an infant. It is not known whether or not sulfinpyrazone
passes into breast milk.

sulfisoxazole and
phenazopyridine combination

BRAND NAMES (Manufacturers)
Azo Gantrisin (Roche)

Azo-Sulfisoxazole (various manufacturers)
Azo-Sulfizin (Tutag)
Suldiazo (Kay)
TYPE OF DRUG
Antibiotic (infection fighter) and urinary tract analgesic
(pain reliever)
INGREDIENTS
sulfisoxazole and phenazopyridine as the hydrochloride
salt
DOSAGE FORM
Tablets (500 mg sulfisoxazole and 50 mg phenazopyridine)
STORAGE
Sulfisoxazole and phenazopyridine tablets should be
stored at room temperature in a tightly closed, light-resistant container.

USES
Sulfisoxazole and phenazopyridine combination is used
to treat painful infections of the urinary tract. Sulfisoxazole
is a sulfonamide antibiotic, which acts by preventing production of nutrients that are required for growth of the infecting bacteria. Phenazopyridine is excreted in the urine,
where it exerts a topical analgesic effect on the urinary
tract. This medication is not useful for any pain other than
that of the urinary tract.

TREATMENT
It is best to take this medication with a full glass of water
on an empty stomach, either one hour before or two hours
after a meal. However, if it causes stomach upset, check
with your doctor to see if you can take it with food or milk.
 This medication works best when the level of medication in your blood and urine is kept constant. It is best
therefore to take the doses at evenly spaced intervals, day
and night. For example, if you are to take four doses a day,
the doses should be spaced six hours apart.
 If you miss a dose of this medication, take the missed
dose immediately. However, if you do not remember to
take the missed dose until it is almost time for your next
dose, take the missed dose immediately and space the fol-

lowing dose about halfway through the regular interval between doses (wait about three hours, if you are taking four doses a day). Then return to your regular dosing schedule. Try not to skip any doses.

It is important to continue to take this medication for the entire time prescribed by your doctor (usually seven to 14 days), even if your symptoms disappear before the end of that period. If you stop taking the drug too soon, resistant bacteria are given a chance to continue growing, and the infection could recur.

SIDE EFFECTS

Minor. Abdominal pain; depression; diarrhea; dizziness; dry mouth; headache; indigestion; insomnia; loss of appetite; nausea; and vomiting. These side effects should disappear in several days, as your body adjusts to the medication.

If you feel dizzy, sit or lie down awhile; get up slowly, and be careful on stairs.

Sulfisoxazole can cause increased sensitivity to sunlight. It is therefore important to avoid prolonged exposure to sunlight and sunlamps. Wear protective clothing and sunglasses, and use an effective sunscreen. However, a sunscreen containing para-aminobenzoic acid (PABA) interferes with the anti-bacterial activity of this medication, and should NOT be used.

Phenazopyridine causes your urine to become orange-red in color. This is not harmful; however, it may stain your clothing. The urine will return to its normal color soon after the drug is discontinued.

Major. Tell your doctor about any side effects that are persistent or particularly bothersome. IT IS ESPECIALLY IMPORTANT TO TELL YOUR DOCTOR about aching joints and muscles; back pain; bloating; chest pain; chills; confusion; convulsions; difficulty breathing; difficulty urinating; fever; hallucinations; hives; itching; loss of coordination; rash; ringing in the ears; sore throat; swollen ankles; unusual bleeding or bruising; or yellowing of the eyes or skin. Also, if your symptoms of infection seem to be getting worse rather than improving, you should contact your doctor.

INTERACTIONS

This combination medication interacts with other drugs.
1. Sulfisoxazole can increase the blood levels of active oral anti-coagulants (blood thinners, such as warfarin), oral anti-diabetic agents, methotrexate, oxyphenbutazone, phenylbutazone, and phenytoin, which can lead to serious side effects.
2. Methenamine can increase the side effects to the kidneys caused by sulfisoxazole.
3. Probenecid and sulfinpyrazone can increase the blood levels of sulfisoxazole, which can lead to an increase of side effects.
Before starting to take this medication, BE SURE TO TELL YOUR DOCTOR if you are already taking any of the drugs listed above.

WARNINGS

● Tell your doctor about unusual or allergic reactions you have had to medications, especially to phenazopyridine or sulfisoxazole, or to any other sulfa drug (sulfonamide antibiotics, diuretics, dapsone, sulfoxone, oral anti-diabetic medications, or acetazolamide).
● Tell your doctor if you now have, or if you have ever had, glucose-6-phosphate dehydrogenase (G6PD) deficiency; kidney disease; liver disease; or porphyria.
● This medication has been prescribed for your current infection only. Another infection later on, or one that someone else has, may require a different medicine. You should not give your medicine to other people, or use it for other infections, unless your doctor specifically directs you to do so.
● This medication should be taken with lots of water, or orange or cranberry juice, in order to avoid the possibility of kidney stone formation.
● If this drug makes you dizzy, do not take part in any activity that requires alertness, such as driving a car or operating potentially dangerous equipment.
● Diabetic patients using this medication (phenazopyridine) may get delayed reactions or false-positive readings for sugar or ketones with urine tests. Clinitest is not affected by this medication, but other urine sugar tests are.

● If there is no improvement in your condition several days after starting to take this medication, check with your doctor. This medication may not be effective against the bacteria causing your infection.

● Before having any surgery or other medical or dental treatment, be sure to tell your doctor or dentist that you are taking this medication.

● Be sure to tell your doctor if you are pregnant. Small amounts of sulfisoxazole cross the placenta. Although this medication appears to be safe during pregnancy, extensive studies in humans have not been completed. Also, tell your doctor if you are breastfeeding an infant. Small amounts of this medication pass into breast milk and may temporarily alter the bacteria in the intestinal tract of a nursing infant, resulting in diarrhea. This medication should not be used in an infant less than two months of age (in order to avoid side effects involving the liver).

Sulfizin—see sulfonamides

---

sulfonamides

BRAND NAMES (Manufacturers)
Gantanol (Roche)
Gantanol DS (Roche)
Gantrisin (Roche)
Lipo-Gantrisin (Roche)
Microsul (Star)
Microsulfon (CMC)
multiple sulfonamides (various manufacturers)
Neotrizine (Lilly)
Proklar (O'Neal)
Renoquid (Parke-Davis)
SK-Soxazole (Smith Kline & French)
sulfacytine (various manufacturers)
sulfadiazine (various manufacturers)
Sulfaloid (O'Neal)
sulfamethiazole (various manufacturers)
sulfamethoxazole (various manufacturers)
Sulfizin (Reid-Provident)

Terfonyl (Squibb)
Thiosulfil (Ayerst)
Thiosulfil Forte (Ayerst)
Triple Sulfa (systemic) (various manufacturers)
Urifon (Amid)
Urobak (Shionogi USA)

TYPE OF DRUG

Anti-infective (infection fighter)

INGREDIENTS AND DOSAGE FORMS

sulfacytine (Renoquid)
Tablets (250 mg)
sulfadiazine (Microsulfon)
Tablets (500 mg)
sulfamethizole (Microsul, Proklar, Thiosulfil, Thiosulfil
    Forte, Urifon)
Tablets (250 mg, 500 mg, and 1,000 mg)
sulfamethoxazole (Gantanol, Gantanol DS, Urobak)
Tablets (500 mg and 1,000 mg)
Suspension (500 mg per 5 ml teaspoonful)
sulfisoxazole (Gantrisin, Lipo-Gantrisin, SK-Soxazole,
    Sulfizin)
Tablets (500 mg)
Syrup (500 mg per 5 ml teaspoonful)
Pediatric suspension (500 mg per 5 ml teaspoonful)
Emulsion, long-acting (1,000 mg per 5 ml teaspoonful)
multiple sulfonamides (Neotrizine, Sulfaloid, Terfonyl,
    Triple Sulfa)
Tablets (167 mg sulfadiazine, 167 mg sulfamerazine, and
    167 mg sulfamethazine)
Suspension (167 mg sulfadiazine, 167 mg sulfamerazine,
    and 167 mg sulfamethazine per 5 ml teaspoonful)

STORAGE

Keep these medications in their original containers, and
store them at room temperature.

USES

Sulfonamides are a family of related drugs that have activity against a large number of bacteria. This group of medications is often used to treat urinary tract infections, as
well as other infections. These medications destroy the
bacteria responsible for the infection.

TREATMENT

Sulfonamides should be taken with a full glass of water on an empty stomach (either one hour before or two hours after a meal). Several additional glasses of water should also be taken every day (unless your doctor directs you to do otherwise). Drinking extra water helps to prevent kidney damage.

Sulfonamides work best when the level of the medicine in your bloodstream is kept constant. It is therefore best to take the doses at evenly spaced intervals, day and night. For example, if you are to take four doses a day, the doses should be spaced about six hours apart.

If you have been prescribed the liquid suspension or emulsion form of this medication, be sure to shake the bottle well. The contents tend to settle on the bottom of the bottle, so it is necessary to shake the container to evenly distribute the ingredients and equalize the doses. Be sure to use specially marked droppers or spoons to accurately measure the correct amount of liquid. Household teaspoons vary in size and may not give you the correct dosage.

If you miss a dose, take the missed dose as soon as possible, unless it is almost time for your next dose. In that case, if you are taking two doses a day, space the missed dose and the next dose five to six hours apart; if you're taking three or more doses a day, space the missed dose and the next dose two to four hours apart, or double the next dose. Then return to your regular dosing schedule.

It is very important to continue to take this medication for the entire time prescribed by your doctor (usually ten days), even if the symptoms disappear before the end of that period. If you stop taking the drug too soon, resistant bacteria are given a chance to continue growing, and your infection could recur.

SIDE EFFECTS

Minor. Diarrhea; dizziness; headache; loss of appetite; nausea; and vomiting. As your body adjusts to the medication, these side effects usually disappear. This medication can cause discoloration of the urine, which is harmless.

These drugs can increase your sensitivity to sunlight. In order to avoid this side effect, limit your exposure to sunlight and sunlamps. Wear protective clothing and sun-glasses; and use an effective sunscreen, but not one that contains para-aminobenzoic acid (PABA). PABA interferes with the anti-bacterial activity of this medication.

Major. Tell your doctor about any side effects that are persistent or particularly bothersome. IT IS ESPECIALLY IMPORTANT TO TO TELL YOUR DOCTOR about aching of joints and muscles; blood in the urine; difficulty swallowing; itching; lower back pain; pain while urinating; pale skin; redness, blistering, or peeling of the skin; skin rash; sore throat and fever; swelling of the front part of the neck; unusual bleeding or bruising; unusual tiredness; or yellowing of the eyes or skin. Also, if your symptoms of infection seem to be getting worse rather than improving, you should contact your doctor.

INTERACTIONS

Sulfonamides interact with several types of drugs.

1. Aminobenzoic acid can decrease the effectiveness of the sulfonamides.

2. The activity and side effects of anti-coagulants (blood thinners, such as warfarin), oral anti-diabetic medications, methotrexate, aspirin, phenytoin, and thiopental may be increased when sulfonamides are also taken.

3. Oxyphenbutazone, phenylbutazone, methenamine, probenecid, and sulfinpyrazone can increase the toxicity of the sulfonamides.

BE SURE TO TELL YOUR DOCTOR if you are already taking any of these medications.

WARNINGS

● Before starting to take this medication, tell your doctor about any unusual or allergic reactions you have had to drugs, especially to furosemide, thiazide diuretics (water pills), dapsone, sulfoxone, oral anti-diabetic medication, or oral glaucoma medication.

● Tell your doctor if you now have, or if you have ever had, glucose-6-phosphate dehydrogenase (G6PD) deficiency, liver disease, porphyria, or kidney disease.

● Before having any surgery or other medical or dental treatment, be sure to tell your doctor or dentist that you are taking a sulfonamide.

• This medication has been prescribed for your current infection only. Another infection later on, or one that someone else has, may require a different medicine. You should not give your medicine to other people or use it for other infections, unless your doctor specifically directs you to do so.

• Be sure to tell your doctor if you are pregnant. This medication, if given to a woman late in pregnancy, can be toxic to the infant. Also, tell your doctor if you are breast-feeding an infant. Sulfonamides can pass into breast milk and may cause side effects in a small number of nursing infants—those who have glucose-6-phosphate dehydrogenase (G6PD) deficiency. In addition, you should not give sulfonamides to an infant less than one month of age, unless your doctor specifically directs you to do so.

---

sulindac

BRAND NAME (Manufacturer)
Clinoril (Merck Sharp & Dohme)
TYPE OF DRUG
Non-steroidal anti-inflammatory analgesic (pain reliever)
INGREDIENT
sulindac
DOSAGE FORM
Tablets (150 mg and 200 mg)
STORAGE
This medication should be stored in a closed container at room temperature, away from heat and direct sunlight.

USES
Sulindac is used to treat the inflammation (pain, swelling, and stiffness) of certain types of arthritis, gout, bursitis, and tendinitis.

TREATMENT
You should take this medication on an empty stomach 30 to 60 minutes before meals or two hours after meals, so that it gets into your bloodstream quickly. However, to decrease stomach irritation, your doctor may want you to

take the medicine with food or antacids.

If you are taking sulindac to relieve arthritis, you must take it regularly, as directed by your doctor. It may take up to three weeks for you to feel the full benefits of this medication. Sulindac does not cure arthritis, but it will help to control the condition, as long as you continue to take it

It is important to take sulindac on schedule and not to miss any doses. If you do miss a dose, take it as soon as possible, unless it is almost time for your next dose. In that case, don't take the missed dose at all; just return to your regular dosing schedule. Do not double the next dose.

SIDE EFFECTS

Minor. Bloating; constipation; diarrhea; difficulty sleeping; dizziness; drowsiness; headache; heartburn; indigestion; light-headedness; loss of appetite; nausea; nervousness; soreness of the mouth; unusual sweating; and vomiting. As your body adjusts to the drug, these side effects should disappear.

If you become dizzy, sit or lie down awhile; and be careful on stairs.

Acetaminophen may be helpful in relieving headaches.
Major. If any side effects are persistent or particularly bothersome, you should report them to your doctor. IT IS ESPECIALLY IMPORTANT TO TELL YOUR DOCTOR about bloody or black, tarry stools; blurred vision; confusion; depression; difficulty breathing, or wheezing; difficulty hearing; difficult or painful urination; pounding heartbeat; ringing or buzzing in the ears; skin rash, hives, or itching; stomach pain; swelling of the feet; tightness in the chest; unexplained sore throat and fever; unusual bleeding or bruising; unusual fatigue or weakness; unusual weight gain; or yellowing of the eyes or skin.

INTERACTIONS

Sulindac interacts with several types of medication.
1. Anti-coagulants (blood thinners, such as warfarin) can lead to an increase in bleeding complications.
2. Aspirin, salicylates, or other anti-inflammation medication can cause an increase in stomach irritation.
3. Sulindac can increase the amount of probenecid in the bloodstream when the drugs are taken concurrently.

BE SURE TO TELL YOUR DOCTOR if you are already taking any of the medications listed above.

WARNINGS

● Tell your doctor if you have ever had unusual or allergic reactions to sulindac or any of the other chemically related drugs (including aspirin, other salicylates, diflunisal, fenoprofen, ibuprofen, meclofenamate, mefenamic acid, naproxen, oxyphenbutazone, phenylbutazone, piroxicam, indomethacin, tolmetin, and zomepirac).

● Tell your doctor if you now have, or if you have ever had, bleeding problems; colitis, stomach ulcers, or other stomach problems; epilepsy; heart disease; high blood pressure; asthma; kidney disease; liver disease; mental illness; or Parkinson's disease.

● If sulindac makes you dizzy or drowsy, do not take part in any activity that requires alertness, such as driving a car or operating potentially dangerous equipment.

● Because this drug can prolong your bleeding time, it is important to tell your doctor or dentist that you are taking this drug, before having any surgery or other medical or dental treatment.

● Stomach problems are more likely to occur if you take aspirin regularly or drink alcoholic beverages while being treated with this medication. These should therefore be avoided (unless your doctor directs you to do otherwise).

● Be sure to tell your doctor if you are pregnant. Studies in humans have not yet been completed, but unwanted effects have been shown on the development of bones and organs in the offspring of animals who received sulindac during pregnancy. If taken late in pregnancy, this type of drug can also prolong labor. Also, tell your doctor if you are breastfeeding an infant. Small amounts of sulindac can pass into breast milk.

Sulten-10—see sodium sulfacetamide (ophthalmic)

Sultrin Triple Sulfa—see sulfathiazole, sulfacetamide, and sulfabenzamide combination

Sumox—see amoxicillin

Sumycin—see tetracycline

Supen—see ampicillin

Suprazine—see trifluoperazine

Surmontil—see trimipramine

Susano—see atropine, scopolamine, hyoscyamine, and phenobarbital combination

Sustaire—see theophylline

Symmetrel—see amantadine

Synacort—see hydrocortisone (topical)

Synalar—see fluocinolone (topical)

Synalar-HP—see fluocinolone (topical)

Synalgos-DC—see aspirin, caffeine, dihydrocodeine, and promethazine combination

Synemol—see fluocinolone (topical)

Synkayvite—see vitamin K

Synthroid—see levothyroxine

Tagamet—see cimetidine

Tagatap—see phenylpropanolamine, phenylephrine, and brompheniramine combination

Talwin NX—see pentazocine

Tamine Expectorant—see phenylephrine, phenylpropanolamine, brompheniramine, and guaifenesin combination

Tamine SR—see phenylpropanolamine, phenylephrine, and brompheniramine combination

---

tamoxifen

BRAND NAME (Manufacturer)
Nolvadex (Stuart)
TYPE OF DRUG
Anti-estrogen and anti-neoplastic (anti-cancer drug)
INGREDIENT
tamoxifen as the citrate salt
DOSAGE FORM
Tablets (10 mg)
STORAGE
Tamoxifen should be stored at room temperature in a tightly closed, light-resistant container.

USES
This medication is used to treat advanced breast cancer in post-menopausal women. Tamoxifen is a non-steroidal anti-estrogen drug. It is unclear how tamoxifen works, but it may block estrogen binding to breast tissue, thereby slowing tumor growth.

TREATMENT
Tamoxifen can be taken either on an empty stomach or with food or milk, as directed by your doctor.

If you miss a dose of this medication, take the missed dose as soon as possible, unless it is almost time for the next dose. In that case, do not take the missed dose at all; just return to your regular dosing schedule. Do not double the next dose.

SIDE EFFECTS
Minor. Dizziness; food distaste; headache; hot flashes; light-headedness; nausea; and vomiting. These side effects should disappear in several weeks, as your body adjusts to the medication.

If you feel dizzy or light-headed, sit or lie down awhile; get up slowly, and be careful on stairs.

It is important to continue taking this medication despite any nausea or vomiting that may occur.

You may experience an increase in bone and tumor pain when tamoxifen is first started. The pain generally subsides rapidly, but may require the temporary use of analgesics (pain relievers).

Major. Tell your doctor about any side effects that are persistent or particularly bothersome. IT IS ESPECIALLY IMPORTANT TO TELL YOUR DOCTOR about blurred vision; chills; depression; fever; rapid weight gain (three to five pounds within a week); rash; sore throat; unusual weakness; or vaginal bleeding or discharge.

INTERACTIONS

Tamoxifen does not interact with other medications, as long as it is used according to directions.

WARNINGS

● Tell your doctor about unusual or allergic reactions you have had to any medications, especially to tamoxifen.

● Before starting to take this medication, be sure to tell your doctor if you now have, or if you have ever had, blood disorders or visual disturbances.

Taractan—see chlorprothixene

Tavist—see clemastine

Tavist-1—see clemastine

T. D. Alermine—see chlorpheniramine

Teebaconin—see isoniazid

Tegamide—see trimethobenzamide

Tegopen—see cloxacillin

Tegretol—see carbamazepine

Telechlor S.R.—see chlorpheniramine

temazepam

BRAND NAME (Manufacturer)
Restoril (Sandoz)
TYPE OF DRUG
Sedative/hypnotic (sleeping aid)
INGREDIENT
temazepam
DOSAGE FORM
Capsules (15 mg and 30 mg)
STORAGE
This medication should be stored at room temperature in a tightly closed, light-resistant container.

USES
Temazepam is prescribed to treat insomnia, including problems with falling asleep, waking during the night, and early morning wakefulness. It is not clear exactly how this medicine works, but it may relieve insomnia by acting as a depressant of the central nervous system.

TREATMENT
This medicine should be taken 30 to 60 minutes before bedtime. It can be taken with food or a full glass of water if stomach upset occurs. Do not take this medication with a dose of antacids, since they may retard its absorption from the gastrointestinal tract.

If you are taking this medication regularly and you miss a dose, take the missed dose immediately, if you remember within an hour of the scheduled time. If more than an hour has passed, skip the dose you missed and wait for the next scheduled time. Do not double the dose.

SIDE EFFECTS
Minor. Bitter taste in mouth; constipation; depression; diarrhea; dizziness; drowsiness (after a night's sleep); dry mouth; fatigue; flushing; headache; heartburn; excess saliva; loss of appetite; nausea; nervousness; sweating; and vomiting. As your body adjusts to the medicine, these side effects should disappear.

If you feel dizzy, sit or lie down awhile; get up slowly, and be careful on stairs.

Major. Tell your doctor about any side effects that are persistent or particularly bothersome. IT IS ESPECIALLY IMPORTANT TO TELL YOUR DOCTOR about blurred or double vision; chest pain; difficulty urinating; fainting; falling; fever; joint pain; hallucinations; mouth sores; nightmares; palpitations; rash; severe depression; shortness of breath; slurred speech; sore throat; uncoordinated movements; unusual excitement; unusual tiredness; or yellowing of the eyes or skin.

INTERACTIONS

Temazepam interacts with a number of other medications.
1. To prevent over-sedation, this drug should not be taken with alcohol, other sedative drugs, or central nervous system depressants (such as antihistamines, barbiturates, muscle relaxants, pain medicines, narcotics, medicines for seizures, phenothiazine tranquilizers), or with anti-depressants.
2. Temazepam may decrease the effectiveness or carbamazepine, levodopa, and oral anti-coagulants (blood thinners), and may increase the effects of phenytoin.
3. Disulfiram and isoniazid can increase the blood levels of temazepam, which can lead to toxic effects.
4. Concurrent use of rifampin may decrease the effectiveness of temazepam.
If you are currently taking any of the medications listed above, CONSULT YOUR DOCTOR about their use.

WARNINGS

● Tell your doctor about unusual or allergic reactions you have had to any medications, especially to temazepam or other benzodiazepine tranquilizers (such as alprazolam, chlordiazepoxide, clorazepate, diazepam, flurazepam, halazepam, lorazepam, oxazepam, prazepam, and triazolam).
● Tell your doctor if you now have, or if you have ever had, liver disease, kidney disease, epilepsy, lung disease, myasthenia gravis, porphyria, mental depression, or mental illness.
● This medicine can cause drowsiness. Avoid tasks that require alertness, such as driving a car or operating potentially dangerous machinery.

- Temazepam has the potential for abuse and must be used with caution. Tolerance may develop quickly; do not increase the dosage without first consulting your doctor. It is also important not to stop taking this drug suddenly if you have been taking it in large amounts, or if you have used it for several weeks. Your doctor may want to reduce the dosage gradually.

- This is a safe drug when used properly. When it is combined with other sedative drugs or alcohol, however, serious side effects may develop.

- Be sure to tell your doctor if you are pregnant. This type of medicine may increase the chance of birth defects if it is taken during the first three months of pregnancy. In addition, too much use of this medicine during the last six months of pregnancy may result in addiction of the fetus, leading to withdrawal side effects in the newborn. Also, use of this medicine during the last weeks of pregnancy may cause drowsiness, slowed heartbeat, and breathing difficulties in the infant. Tell your doctor if you are breastfeeding an infant. This medicine can pass into breast milk and cause drowsiness, slowed heartbeat, and breathing difficulties in nursing infants.

Tenormin—see atenolol

Tenstan—see aspirin, caffeine, and butalbital combination

Tenuate—see diethylpropion

Tenuate Dospan—see diethylpropion

Tepanil—see diethylpropion

Tepanil Ten-Tab—see diethylpropion

terbutaline

BRAND NAMES (Manufacturers)
Brethine (Geigy)
Bricanyl (Merrell·Dow)

TYPE OF DRUG
Bronchodilator
INGREDIENT
terbutaline as the sulfate salt
DOSAGE FORM
Tablets (2.5 mg and 5 mg)
STORAGE
Terbutaline tablets should be stored at room temperature in a tightly closed, light-resistant container.

USES

Terbutaline is used to relieve wheezing and shortness of breath caused by lung diseases such as asthma, bronchitis, and emphysema. This drug acts directly on the muscles of the bronchi (breathing tubes) to relieve bronchospasm (muscle contractions of the bronchi), which in turn reduces airway resistance, and allows air to move more freely to and from the lungs—making breathing easier.

TREATMENT

In order to lessen stomach upset, you can take terbutaline with food (unless your doctor directs you to do otherwise).

If you miss a dose of this medication and it is within an hour of the missed dose, take it when you remember, then follow your regular dosing schedule for the next dose. If you miss the dose by more than an hour or so, just wait until the next scheduled dose. Do not double the dose.

SIDE EFFECTS

Minor. Anxiety; dizziness; headache; flushing; irritability; insomnia; loss of appetite; muscle cramps; nausea; nervousness; restlessness; sweating; tremors; vomiting; and weakness. These side effects should disappear in several days, as your body adjusts to the medication.

In order to avoid difficulty falling asleep, check with your doctor to see if you can take the last dose of this medication several hours before bedtime each day.

If you feel dizzy, sit or lie down awhile; get up from a sitting or lying position slowly, and be careful on stairs.
Major. Tell your doctor about any side effects that are persistent or particularly bothersome. IT IS ESPECIALLY IM-

PORTANT TO TELL YOUR DOCTOR about chest pain; difficult or painful urination; or palpitations.

INTERACTIONS

Terbutaline interacts with several other types of medication.

1. The beta-blockers (atenolol, metoprolol, nadolol, pindolol, propranolol, timolol) antagonize (act against) this medication, decreasing its effectiveness.

2. Monoamine oxidase (MAO) inhibitors; tricyclic antidepressants; antihistamines; levothyroxine; and over-the-counter (non-prescription) cough, cold, allergy, asthma, diet, and sinus medications may increase the side effects of terbutaline.

3. There may be a change in the dosage requirements of insulin or oral anti-diabetic medications when terbutaline is started.

4. The blood-pressure-lowering effects of guanethidine may be decreased by this medication.

TELL YOUR DOCTOR if you are already taking any of the medications listed above.

WARNINGS

• Tell your doctor about unusual or allergic reactions you have had to medications, especially to terbutaline or any related drug (albuterol, amphetamines, ephedrine, epinephrine, isoproterenol, norepinephrine, phenylephrine, phenylpropanolamine, pseudoephedrine, or metaproterenol).

• Tell your doctor if you now have, or if you have ever had, diabetes, glaucoma, high blood pressure, epilepsy, heart disease, enlarged prostate gland, or thyroid disease.

• This medication can cause dizziness. Your ability to perform tasks that require alertness, such as driving a car or operating potentially dangerous machinery, may be decreased. Appropriate caution should therefore be taken.

• Before having any surgery or other medical or dental treatment, be sure to tell your doctor or dentist that you are taking this medication.

• Do not exceed the recommended dosage of this medication; excessive use may lead to an increase in side effects or a loss of effectiveness. Contact your doctor if you do not respond to the usual dose of this medication. It may be a sign of worsening asthma, which may require additional therapy.

● Be sure to tell your doctor if you are pregnant. The effects of this medication during pregnancy have not yet been thoroughly studied in humans. Also, tell your doctor if you are breastfeeding an infant. Small amounts of terbutaline pass into breast milk.

Terfonyl—see sulfonamides

---

terpin hydrate and codeine combination

BRAND NAMES (Manufacturers)
SK-Terpin Hydrate with Codeine (Smith Kline & French)
terpin hydrate with codeine (various manufacturers)
TYPE OF DRUG
Expectorant and cough suppressant
INGREDIENTS
terpin hydrate, codeine, and alcohol
DOSAGE FORM
Oral elixir (85 mg terpin hydrate and 10 mg codeine per 5
  ml teaspoonful, with 40% alcohol)
STORAGE
Terpin hydrate and codeine elixir should be stored at room temperature, in a tightly closed container. This medication should never be frozen. If crystals form in the bottle, they can be dissolved by warming the closed container in warm water, then gently shaking it.

USES
This medication is used to relieve coughs due to colds. Terpin hydrate is an expectorant, which loosens lung secretions. Codeine is a cough suppressant, which acts on the cough center in the brain.

TREATMENT
You can take terpin hydrate and codeine elixir either on an empty stomach or, to avoid stomach irritation, with food

or milk (as directed by your doctor).

Each dose should be measured carefully, with a specially designed, 5 ml measuring spoon. An ordinary kitchen teaspoon is not accurate enough.

To help loosen the mucus in the lungs, you should drink a glass of water after each dose.

If you miss a dose of this medication, take the missed one as soon as possible, unless it is almost time for the next dose. In that case, do not take the missed dose at all; just return to your regular dosing schedule. Do not double the next dose.

SIDE EFFECTS

Minor. Constipation; dizziness; drowsiness; nausea; restlessness; stomach upset; vomiting; and weakness. These side effects should disappear in several days, as your body adjusts to the medication.

If you feel dizzy, sit or lie down awhile; change positions slowly, and be careful on stairs.

If you are constipated, increase the amount of fiber in your diet (raw vegetables, fruits, salads, bran, and whole-grain breads), and drink more water (unless your doctor directs you to do otherwise).

Major. Tell your doctor about any side effects that are persistent or particularly bothersome. IT IS ESPECIALLY IMPORTANT TO TELL YOUR DOCTOR about blurred vision; cold, clammy skin; confusion; convulsions; difficulty breathing; or fainting.

INTERACTIONS

Terpin hydrate and codeine combination interacts with a number of other medications.

1. Concurrent use of it with other central nervous system depressants (drugs that slow the activity of the brain and spinal cord), such as alcohol, barbiturates, benzodiazepine tranquilizers, muscle relaxants, other narcotics, pain medications, phenothiazine tranquilizers, and sleeping medications, or with tricyclic anti-depressants can lead to extreme drowsiness.

2. Use of a monoamine oxidase (MAO) inhibitor within 14 days of terpin hydrate and codeine can lead to serious side effects.

BE SURE TO TELL YOUR DOCTOR if you are already taking any of the medications listed above.

WARNINGS

● Tell your doctor about unusual or allergic reactions you have had to any medications, especially to terpin hydrate or codeine, or to other narcotics (such as hydrocodone, hydromorphone, meperidine, methadone, opium, oxycodone, propoxyphene, and pentazocine).

● Before starting to take this medication, be sure to tell your doctor if you now have, or if you have ever had, asthma; brain disease; epilepsy; gallstones or gallbladder disease; gastrointestinal diseases; heart disease; kidney disease; liver disease; lung disease; mental disorders; enlarged prostate gland; or thyroid disease.

● If this drug makes you dizzy or drowsy, do not take part in activities that require alertness, such as driving a car or operating potentially dangerous equipment.

● While you are taking this medication, drink at least eight glasses of water a day (to help loosen lung secretions).

● Because this product contains codeine, it has the potential for abuse, and must be used with caution. Tolerance may develop quickly; therefore, you should not use it in higher doses, or for longer periods, than recommended by your doctor. If you have been taking it for longer than several weeks, do not stop taking it until you first check with your doctor. Stopping the drug abruptly can lead to a withdrawal reaction (body aches, diarrhea, gooseflesh, vomiting, restlessness, runny nose, sneezing, yawning, sweating, or trembling). Your doctor may therefore want to reduce your dosage gradually.

● Be sure to tell your doctor if you are pregnant. Alcohol has been shown to cause birth defects when taken during pregnancy. In addition, large amounts of codeine taken during pregnancy can lead to addiction in the developing fetus, resulting in withdrawal reactions in the newborn infant. Also, tell your doctor if you are breastfeeding an infant. Codeine and alcohol pass into breast milk and can cause extreme drowsiness in the nursing infant.

Terramycin—see oxytetracycline

Testred—see methyltestosterone

Tetra-C—see tetracycline

Tetracaps—see tetracycline

---

tetracycline

BRAND NAMES (Manufacturers)
Achromycin V (Lederle)
Cycline-250 (Scrip)
Cyclopar (Parke-Davis)
Deltamycin (Trimen)
Nor-Tet (Vortech)
Panmycin (Upjohn)
Retet (Reid-Provident)
Robitet Robicaps (Robins)
SK-Tetracycline (Smith Kline & French)
Sumycin (Squibb)
Tetra-C (Century)
Tetracaps (Circle)
tetracycline hydrochloride (various manufacturers)
Tetracyn (Pfipharmecs)
Tetralan (Lannett)
Tetram (Dunhall)
TYPE OF DRUG
Antibiotic (infection fighter)
INGREDIENT
tetracycline as the hydrochloride salt
DOSAGE FORMS
Tablets (250 mg and 500 mg)
Capsules (100 mg, 250 mg, and 500 mg)
Oral suspension (125 mg per 5 ml teaspoonful)
STORAGE
Tetracycline tablets, capsules, and oral suspension should be stored at room temperature in tightly closed, light-resistant containers. Any unused portion of the suspension should be discarded after 14 days, because the drug loses its potency after that period. This medication should never be frozen.

USES

Tetracycline is used to treat acne and a wide variety of bacterial infections. It acts by inhibiting the growth of bacteria. Bacteria may be partly responsible for the development of acne lesions. Tetracycline kills susceptible bacteria, but is is not effective against viruses or fungi.

TREATMENT

Ideally, this medication should be taken on an empty stomach, one hour before or two hours after a meal. It should be taken with a full glass of water in order to avoid irritating the throat or esophagus (swallowing tube). If this drug causes stomach upset, however, you can take it with food (unless your doctor directs you to do otherwise).

Avoid consuming any dairy products (milk, cheese, etc.) within two hours of any dose of this drug. Avoid taking antacids and laxatives that contain aluminum, calcium, or magnesium within an hour or two of a dose. Avoid taking any medication containing iron within three hours of a dose. These products chemically bind tetracycline in the stomach and gastrointestinal tract, preventing the drug from being absorbed into the body.

The oral suspension form of this medication should be shaken well just before measuring each dose. The contents tend to settle on the bottom of the bottle, so it is necessary to shake the container to evenly distribute the ingredients and equalize the doses. Each dose should then be measured carefully, with a specially designed, 5 ml measuring spoon. An ordinary kitchen teaspoon is not accurate enough. The oral suspension form of this medication should not be mixed with any other substance, unless your doctor directs you to do so.

Tetracycline works best when the level of medicine in your bloodstream is kept constant. It is best therefore to take the doses at evenly spaced intervals, day and night. For example, if you are to take four doses a day, the doses should be spaced six hours apart.

If you miss a dose of this medication, take the missed dose immediately. However, if you do not remember to take the missed dose until it is almost time for your next dose, take it; then space the following dose about halfway through the regular interval between doses. Then return to your regular dosing schedule. Try not to skip any doses.

It is important to continue to take this medication for the entire time prescribed by your doctor, even if the symptoms disappear before the end of that period. If you stop taking the drug too soon, resistant bacteria are given a chance to continue growing, and the infection could recur.

SIDE EFFECTS

Minor. Diarrhea; discoloration of the nails; dizziness; loss of appetite; nausea; stomach cramps and upset; and vomiting. These side effects should disappear in several days, as your body adjusts to the medication.

Tetracycline can increase your sensitivity to sunlight. In order to avoid this side effect, limit your exposure to sunlight and sunlamps. Wear protective clothing and sunglasses, and use an effective sunscreen.

Major. Tell your doctor about any side effects that are persistent or particularly bothersome. IT IS ESPECIALLY IMPORTANT TO TELL YOUR DOCTOR about unusual bleeding or bruising; darkened tongue; difficulty breathing; joint pain; mouth irritation; rash; rectal or vaginal itching; sore throat and fever; or yellowing of the eyes or skin. Also, if your symptoms of infection seem to be getting worse rather than improving, you should contact your doctor.

INTERACTIONS

Tetracycline interacts with several other types of medication.

1. It can increase the absorption of digoxin, which may lead to digoxin toxicity.

2. The gastrointestinal side effects (nausea, vomiting, stomach upset) of theophylline may be increased by tetracycline.

3. The dosage of oral anti-coagulants (blood thinners, such as warfarin) may need to be adjusted when this medication is started.

4. Tetracycline may decrease the effectiveness of oral contraceptives (birth control pills)—pregnancy could result. You should therefore use another form of birth control while taking tetracycline. Discuss this with your doctor.

TELL YOUR DOCTOR if you are currently taking any of the medications listed above.

WARNINGS

● Tell your doctor about unusual or allergic reactions you have had to any medications, especially to tetracycline or to oxytetracycline, doxycycline, or minocycline.

● Tell your doctor if you now have, or if you have ever had, kidney or liver disease.

● Tetracycline can affect tests for syphilis; tell your doctor you are taking this medication if you are also being treated for this disease.

● Make sure that your prescription for this medication is marked with the drug's expiration date. The drug should be discarded after the expiration date. If tetracycline is used after it has expired, serious side effects (especially to the kidneys) could result.

● This medication has been prescribed for your current infection only. Another infection later on, or one that someone else has, may require a different medicine. You should not give your medicine to other people, or use it for other infections, unless your doctor specifically directs you to do so.

● Be sure to tell your doctor if you are pregnant or if you are breastfeeding an infant. Tetracycline crosses the placenta and passes into breast milk. If used during their development, this drug can cause permanent discoloration of the teeth and can inhibit tooth and bone growth. In addition, it should not be used for infants or for children less than eight years of age.

tetracycline hydrochloride—see tetracycline

Tetracyn—see tetracycline

Tetralan—see tetracycline

Tetram—see tetracycline

Tetramine—see oxytetracycline

Texacort—see hydrocortisone (topical)

T-Gesic Forte—see acetaminophen and hydrocodone combination

Thalitone—see chlorthalidone

Theo-24—see theophylline

Theobid—see theophylline

Theobron—see theophylline

Theoclear—see theophylline

Theocolate—see theophylline and guaifenesin combination

Theo-Dur—see theophylline

Theolair—see theophylline

Theolate—see theophylline and guaifenesin combination

Theo-Lix—see theophylline

Theolixir—see theophylline

Theon—see theophylline

Theophyl—see theophylline

---

theophylline

BRAND NAMES (Manufacturers)
Aerolate (Fleming)
Aquaphylline (Ferndale)
Asmalix (Century)
Bronkodyl (Breon)
Constant-T (Geigy)
Duraphyl (McNeil)

Elixicon (Berlex)
Elixomin (Cenci)
Elixophylline (Berlex)
LaBID (Norwich Eaton)
Lanophyllin (Lannett)
Liquaphylline (Paddock)
Lixolin (Mallard)
Lodrane (Poythress)
Quibron-T (Mead Johnson)
Respbid (Boehringer Ingelheim)
Slo-bid Gyrocaps (Rorer)
Slo-Phyllin (Rorer)
Somophyllin-T (Fisons)
Sustaire (Roerig)
Theo-24 (Searle)
Theobid (Glaxo)
Theobron (Upsher-Smith)
Theoclear (Central)
Theo-Dur (Key)
Theolair (Riker)
Theo-Lix (Vale)
Theolixir (Ulmer)
Theon (Bock)
Theophyl (McNeil)
theophylline (various manufacturers)
Theospan (Laser)
Theostat (Laser)
Theo-Time (Major)
Theovent (Schering)
Uniphyl (Purdue Frederick)

TYPE OF DRUG

Bronchodilator

INGREDIENT

theophylline

DOSAGE FORMS

Tablets (100 mg, 125 mg, 200 mg, 225 mg, 250 mg, and
   300 mg)
Chewable tablets (100 mg)
Capsules (50 mg, 100 mg, 200 mg, and 250 mg)
Sustained-release tablets and capsules (50 mg, 65 mg, 75
   mg, 100 mg, 125 mg, 130 mg, 200 mg, 250 mg, 260
   mg, and 300 mg)

Oral liquid (80 mg, 112.5 mg, 150 mg, 160 mg, and 300 mg per 15 ml tablespoonful)

Oral suspension (300 mg per 15 ml tablespoonful)

STORAGE

Theophylline tablets, capsules, liquid, and suspension should be stored at room temperature in tightly closed containers. This medication should never be frozen.

USES

Theophylline is prescribed to treat breathing problems (wheezing and shortness of breath) caused by asthma, bronchitis, or emphysema. It relaxes the muscles of the bronchial airways (breathing tubes), which opens the air passages to the lungs, and allows air to move in and out more easily.

TREATMENT

Theophylline should be taken on an empty stomach, 30 to 60 minutes before a meal, or two hours after a meal. If this medication causes stomach irritation, however, you can take it with food or with a full glass of water or milk (unless your doctor directs you to do otherwise).

Anti-diarrhea medications prevent the absorption of theophylline from the gastrointestinal tract. Therefore, at least one hour should separate doses of one of these medications and theophylline.

The sustained-release tablets and capsules should be swallowed whole. Chewing, crushing, or crumbling the tablets or capsules destroys their sustained-release activity, and possibly increases the side effects. If the tablet is scored for breaking, you can break it along these lines. If the capsules are too large to swallow, they can be opened and the contents mixed with jam, jelly, or applesauce. The mixture should then be swallowed without chewing.

If you are using the suspension form of this medication, the bottle should be shaken well before measuring each dose. The contents tend to settle on the bottom of the bottle. It must therefore be shaken in order to evenly distribute the medication and equalize the doses. Each dose of the oral liquid or suspension should be measured carefully, with a specially designed, 5 ml measuring spoon or a cup designed for that purpose. Ordinary kitchen spoons are not accurate enough.

Theophylline works best when the level of the medicine in your bloodstream is kept constant. It is best therefore to take it at evenly spaced intervals, day and night. For example, if you are to take four doses a day, the doses should be spaced six hours apart.

Try not to miss any doses of this medication. If you do miss a dose, take the missed dose as soon as possible, unless it is almost time for the next dose. In that case, do not take the missed dose at all; just return to your regular dosing schedule. Do not double the next dose.

SIDE EFFECTS

Minor. Diarrhea; dizziness; flushing; headache; heartburn; increased urination; insomnia; irritability; loss of appetite; nausea; nervousness; stomach pain; and vomiting. These side effects should disappear in several days, as your body adjusts to the medication.

If you feel dizzy or light-headed, sit or lie down awhile; get up slowly, and be careful on stairs.

Major. Tell your doctor about any side effects that are persistent or particularly bothersome. IT IS ESPECIALLY IMPORTANT TO TELL YOUR DOCTOR about black, tarry stools; confusion; convulsions; difficulty breathing; fainting; muscle twitches; palpitations; rash; severe abdominal pain; or unusual weakness.

INTERACTIONS

Theophylline interacts with other types of medication.

1. It can increase the effects (diuresis) of furosemide.

2. Reserpine, in combination with theophylline, can cause a rapid heart rate.

3. Beta-blockers (atenolol, metoprolol, nadolol, pindolol, propranolol, timolol) can decrease the effectiveness of theophylline.

4. Theophylline can increase the side effects of over-the-counter (non-prescription) sinus, cough, cold, asthma, allergy, and diet products; digoxin; and oral anti-coagulants (blood thinners, such as warfarin).

5. It can decrease the effectiveness of phenytoin and lithium.

6. Phenobarbital can increase the elimination of theophylline from the body, decreasing its effectiveness.

7. Cimetidine, erythromycin, troleandomycin, allopurinol, and thiabendazole can decrease the elimination of theophylline from the body and increase its side effects. Before you start to take this medication, BE SURE TO TELL YOUR DOCTOR if you are already taking any of the medications listed above.

WARNINGS

- Tell your doctor about any unusual or allergic reactions you have had to medications, especially to theophylline, aminophylline, caffeine, dyphylline, oxtriphylline, or theobromine.
- Tell your doctor if you now have, or if you have ever had, an enlarged prostate gland, fibrocystic breast disease, heart disease, kidney disease, low or high blood pressure, liver disease, stomach ulcers, or thyroid disease.
- Cigarette or marijuana smoking may affect this drug's action. BE SURE TO TELL YOUR DOCTOR if you smoke. Also, do not suddenly stop smoking without informing your doctor.
- High fever, diarrhea, the flu, and influenza vaccinations can affect the action of this drug. Therefore, tell your doctor about episodes of high fever or prolonged diarrhea. Before having any vaccinations, especially those to prevent the flu, BE SURE TO TELL YOUR DOCTOR that you are taking this medication.
- Avoid drinking large amounts of caffeine-containing beverages (coffee, cocoa, tea, cola drinks), and avoid eating large amounts of chocolate. These products may increase the side effects of theophylline.
- Do not change your diet without first consulting your doctor. Char-broiled foods or a high-protein, low-carbohydrate diet may affect the action of this drug.
- Before having any surgery or other medical or dental treatment, be sure to tell your doctor or dentist that you are taking this medication.
- Before taking any over-the-counter (non-prescription) asthma, allergy, cough, cold, sinus, or diet product, ask your doctor or pharmacist. These products may add to the side effects of theophylline.
- Be sure to tell your doctor if you are pregnant. Al-

though theophylline appears to be safe during pregnancy, extensive studies have not yet been completed. Birth defects have been observed in the offspring of animals who received large doses of this drug during pregnancy. Also, tell your doctor if you are breastfeeding an infant. Small amounts of theophylline pass into breast milk and may cause irritability, fretfulness, or insomnia in nursing infants.

theophylline and guaifenesin combination

BRAND NAMES (Manufacturers)
Bronchial (Geneva Generics)
Glyceryl-T (Rugby)
Lanophyllin-GG (Lannett)
Quibron (Mead Johnson)
Slo Phyllin GG (Rorer)
Theocolate (Bay)
Theolate (various manufacturers)
TYPE OF DRUG
Bronchodilator and expectorant
INGREDIENTS
theophylline and guaifenesin
DOSAGE FORMS
Capsules (150 mg theophylline and 90 mg guaifenesin; 300 mg theophylline and 180 mg guaifenesin)
Oral liquid (150 theophylline and 90 mg guaifenesin per 15 ml tablespoonful)
STORAGE
Theophylline and guaifenesin capsules and oral liquid should be stored at room temperature in tightly closed containers. This medication should never be frozen.

USES
This medication is prescribed to treat breathing problems (wheezing and shortness of breath) caused by asthma, bronchitis, or emphysema. Theophylline relaxes the smooth muscles of the bronchial airways (breathing tubes), which opens up the air passages, allowing air to

move more easily to and from the lungs. Guaifenesin is an expectorant that loosens lung secretions.

TREATMENT

Theophylline and guaifenesin should be taken on an empty stomach, 30 to 60 minutes before a meal, or two hours after a meal. If this medication causes stomach irritation, however, you can take it with food or with a full glass of water or milk (unless your doctor directs you to do otherwise).

Anti-diarrhea medications prevent the absorption of theophylline. Therefore, at least one hour should separate doses of these two types of medication.

The dose of the oral liquid should be measured carefully, with a specially designed, 5 ml measuring spoon or a cup designed for that purpose. An ordinary kitchen spoon is not accurate enough.

Theophylline works best when the level of medicine in your bloodstream is kept constant. It is best therefore to take the doses at evenly spaced intervals, day and night. For example, if you are to take four doses a day, the doses should be spaced six hours apart.

Try not to miss any doses of this medication. If you do miss a dose, take the missed dose as soon as possible, unless it is almost time for the next dose. In that case, do not take the missed dose at all; just return to your regular dosing schedule. Do not double the next dose.

SIDE EFFECTS

Minor. Diarrhea; dizziness; flushing; headache; heartburn; increased urination; insomnia; irritability; loss of appetite; nausea; nervousness; paleness; stomach pain; and vomiting. These side effects should disappear in several days, as your body adjusts to the medication.

If you feel dizzy or light-headed, sit or lie down awhile; get up slowly, and be careful on stairs.

Major. Tell your doctor about any side effects that are persistent or particularly bothersome. IT IS ESPECIALLY IMPORTANT TO TELL YOUR DOCTOR about black, tarry stools; confusion; convulsions; difficulty breathing; fainting; muscle twitches; palpitations; rash; severe abdominal pain; or unusual weakness.

INTERACTIONS

Theophylline interacts with other types of medication.

1. It can increase the effects (diuresis) of furosemide.

2. Reserpine, in combination with theophylline, can cause a rapid heart rate.

3. Beta-blockers (atenolol, metoprolol, nadolol, pindolol, propranolol, timolol) can decrease the effectiveness of theophylline.

4. Theophylline can increase the side effects of over-the-counter (non-prescription) sinus, cough, cold, asthma, allergy, and diet products; digoxin; and oral anti-coagulants (blood thinners, such as warfarin).

5. It can decrease the effectiveness of phenytoin and lithium.

6. Phenobarbital can increase the elimination of theophylline from the body, decreasing its effectiveness.

7. Cimetidine, erythromycin, troleandomycin, allopurinol, and thiabendazole can decrease the elimination of theophylline from the body and increase its side effects.

Before starting to take this medication, BE SURE TO TELL YOUR DOCTOR if you are already taking any of the medications listed above.

WARNINGS

● Tell your doctor about unusual or allergic reactions you have had to any medications, especially to theophylline, aminophylline, caffeine, dyphylline, oxtriphylline, theobromine, or guaifenesin.

● Tell your doctor if you now have, or if you have ever had, an enlarged prostate gland; fibrocystic breast disease; heart disease; kidney disease; low or high blood pressure; liver disease; stomach ulcers; or thyroid disease.

● Cigarette or marijuana smoking may affect this drug's action. BE SURE TO TELL YOUR DOCTOR if you smoke. Also, do not suddenly stop smoking without informing your doctor.

● High fever, diarrhea, the flu, or an influenza vaccination can also affect the action of this drug. You should tell your doctor about episodes of high fever or prolonged diarrhea. Before having any vaccinations, especially those to prevent the flu, BE SURE TO TELL YOUR DOCTOR that you are taking this medication.

● Avoid drinking large amounts of caffeine-containing beverages (coffee, cocoa, tea, cola drinks), and avoid eating large amounts of chocolate. These products may increase the side effects of theophylline.

● While you are taking this medication, drink at least eight glasses of water a day, to help loosen bronchial secretions (unless your doctor directs you to do otherwise).

● Do not change your diet without first consulting your doctor. Char-broiled foods or a high-protein, low-carbohydrate diet can affect the action of this drug.

● Before having any surgery or other medical or dental treatment, be sure to tell your doctor or dentist that you are taking this medication.

● Be sure to tell your doctor if you are pregnant. Although theophylline appears to be safe during pregnancy, extensive studies in humans have not yet been completed. Birth defects have been observed in the offspring of animals who received large doses of this drug during pregnancy. Also, tell your doctor if you are breastfeeding an infant. Small amounts of theophylline pass into breast milk and may cause irritability, fretfulness, and insomnia in nursing infants.

Theospan—see theophylline

Theostat—see theophylline

Theo-Time—see theophylline

Theovent—see theophylline

Thera-Flur—see sodium fluoride

Thianal—see hydrochlorothiazide

---

thioridazine

BRAND NAMES (Manufacturers)
Mellaril (Sandoz)
Millazine (Major)
thioridazine hydrochloride (various manufacturers)

TYPE OF DRUG
Phenothiazine tranquilizer
INGREDIENT
thioridazine as the hydrochloride salt
DOSAGE FORMS
Tablets (10 mg, 25 mg, 50 mg, 100 mg, 150 mg, and 200 mg)
Oral concentrate (30 mg and 100 mg per ml)
Oral suspension (25 mg and 100 mg per 5 ml teaspoonful)
STORAGE
The tablet form of this medication should be stored at room temperature in a tightly closed, light-resistant container. The oral concentrate and the oral suspension forms of this medication should be stored in the refrigerator in tightly closed, light-resistant containers. If the oral concentrate or suspension turns to a slight yellow color, the medicine is still effective and can be used. However, if they change color markedly or have particles floating in them, they should not be used, but discarded down the sink. This medication should never be frozen.

USES

Thioridazine is prescribed to treat the symptoms of certain types of mental illness, such as emotional symptoms of psychosis, the manic phase of manic-depressive illness, and severe behavioral problems in children. This medication is thought to relieve the symptoms of mental illness by blocking certain chemicals involved with nerve transmission in the brain. Thioridazine may also be used to treat anxiety.

TREATMENT

In order to avoid stomach irritation, you can take this medication with a meal or with a glass of water or milk (unless your doctor directs you to do otherwise).

Antacids and anti-diarrhea medicine may decrease the absorption of this medication from the gastrointestinal tract. Therefore, at least one hour should separate doses of one of these medicines and thioridazine.

The oral suspension form of this medication should be shaken well, just before measuring each dose. The contents tend to settle on the bottom of the bottle, so it is necessary to shake the container to evenly distribute the ingredients and equalize the doses. Each dose should then be measured carefully, with a specially designed 5 ml measuring spoon. An ordinary kitchen teaspoon is not accurate enough.

The oral concentrate form of this medication should be measured carefully with the dropper provided, then added to 4 ounces ($1/2$ cup) or more of water, milk, juice, or a carbonated beverage, or to applesauce or pudding, immediately prior to administration. To prevent possible loss of effectiveness, the medication should not be diluted in tea, coffee, or apple juice.

If you miss a dose of this medication, take the missed dose as soon as possible, then return to your regular dosing schedule. If it is almost time for the next dose, however, skip the one you missed and return to your regular schedule. Do not double the dose (unless your doctor directs you to do so).

The full effects of this medication for the control of emotional or mental symptoms may not become apparent for two weeks after you start to take it.

SIDE EFFECTS

Minor. Blurred vision; constipation; decreased sweating; diarrhea; discoloration of the urine to red, pink, or redbrown; dizziness; drooling; drowsiness; dry mouth; fatigue; jitteriness; menstrual irregularities; nasal congestion; restlessness; tremors; vomiting; and weight gain. As your body adjusts to the medication, these side effects should disappear.

If you are constipated, increase the amount of fiber in your diet (raw vegetables, fruits, salads, bran, and wholegrain breads), and drink more water (unless your doctor directs you to do otherwise).

Chew sugarless gum, or suck on ice chips or a piece of hard candy, to reduce mouth dryness.

This medication can cause increased sensitivity to sunlight. It is therefore important to avoid prolonged exposure to sunlight and sunlamps. Wear protective clothing, and use an effective sunscreen.

To avoid dizziness or light-headedness when you stand,

contract and relax the muscles of your legs for a few moments before rising. Do this by pushing one foot against the floor while raising the other foot slightly, alternating feet so that you are "pumping" your legs in a pedaling motion.

Major. Tell your doctor about any side effects that are persistent or particularly bothersome. IT IS ESPECIALLY IMPORTANT TO TELL YOUR DOCTOR about unusual bleeding or bruising; breast enlargement (in both sexes); chest pain; convulsions; darkened skin; difficulty swallowing or breathing; fainting; fever; impotence; involuntary movements of the face, mouth, jaw, or tongue; palpitations; rash; sleep disorders; sore throat; uncoordinated movements; visual disturbances; or yellowing of the eyes or skin.

INTERACTIONS

Thioridazine interacts with other types of medication.

1. It can cause extreme drowsiness when combined with alcohol or other central nervous system depressants (drugs that slow the activity of the nervous system), such as barbiturates, benzodiazepine tranquilizers, muscle relaxants, narcotics, and pain medications, or with tricyclic anti-depressants.

2. Thioridazine can decrease the effectiveness of amphetamines, guanethidine, anti-convulsants, and levodopa.

3. The side effects of epinephrine, monoamine oxidase (MAO) inhibitors, propranolol, phenytoin, and tricyclic anti-depressants may be increased when combined with this medication.

4. Lithium may increase the side effects and decrease the effectiveness of this medication.

Before starting to take thioridazine, BE SURE TO TELL YOUR DOCTOR if you are already taking any of the medications listed above.

WARNINGS

• Tell your doctor about unusual or allergic reactions you have had to any medications, especially to thioridazine or any other phenothiazine tranquilizers (such as acetophenazine, carphenazine, chlorpromazine, fluphenazine, mesoridazine, perphenazine, piperacetazine, prochlorperazine, promazine, trifluoperazine, and triflupromazine), or to loxapine.

• Tell your doctor if you now have, or if you have ever had, any blood disease, bone marrow disease, brain disease, breast cancer, blockage in the urinary or digestive tracts, alcoholism, drug-induced depression, epilepsy, severe high or low blood pressure, diabetes mellitus (sugar diabetes), glaucoma, heart or circulatory disease, liver disease, lung disease, Parkinson's disease, peptic ulcers, or an enlarged prostate gland.

• Tell your doctor about any recent exposure to a pesticide or an insecticide. Thioridazine may increase the side effects from the exposure.

• To prevent over-sedation, avoid drinking alcoholic beverages while taking this medication.

• If this medication makes you dizzy or drowsy, do not take part in any activity that requires alertness, such as driving a car or operating potentially dangerous equipment. Be careful on stairs, and avoid getting up suddenly from a lying or sitting position.

• Prior to having surgery or other medical or dental treatment, be sure your doctor or dentist knows that you are taking thioridazine.

• Some of the side effects caused by this drug can be prevented by taking an anti-parkinson drug. Discuss this with your doctor.

• This type of medication has been reported to cause certain tumors in rats. This effect has not been shown to occur in humans.

• This medication can decrease sweating and heat release from the body. You should therefore avoid getting overheated (strenuous exercise in hot weather; hot baths, showers, and saunas).

• Do not stop taking this medication suddenly. If the drug is stopped abruptly you may experience nausea, vomiting, stomach upset, headache, increased heart rate, insomnia, tremulousness, or a worsening of your condition. Your doctor may want to reduce the dosage gradually.

• If you are planning to have a myelogram, or any procedure in which dye will be injected into your spinal cord, tell your doctor that you are taking this medication.

• Avoid spilling the oral concentrate or suspension form

of this medication on your skin or clothing; they may cause redness and irritation of the skin.

• While taking this medication, do not take any over-the-counter (non-prescription) medication for weight control, or for cough, cold, allergy, asthma, or sinus problems, unless you first check with your doctor. The combination of these medications with thioridazine may cause high blood pressure.

• Your doctor may want to schedule you for an eye examination if you take thioridazine for longer than a year. Prolonged use of this drug can cause visual disturbances.

• Be sure to tell your doctor if you are pregnant. Small amounts of this medication cross the placenta. Although there are reports of safe use of this drug during pregnancy, there are also reports of liver disease and tremors in newborn infants whose mothers received this type of medication close to term. Also, tell your doctor if you are breastfeeding an infant. Small amounts of this medication pass into breast milk and may cause unwanted effects in nursing infants.

thioridazine hydrochloride—see thioridazine

Thiosulfil—see sulfonamides

Thiosulfil Forte—see sulfonamides

thiothixene

BRAND NAME (Manufacturer)
Navane (Roerig)
TYPE OF DRUG
Anti-psychotic
INGREDIENT
thiothixene as the hydrochloride salt
DOSAGE FORMS
Capsules (1 mg, 2 mg, 5 mg, 10 mg, and 20 mg)
Oral concentrate (5 mg per ml)
STORAGE
Thiothixene capsules should be stored at room temperature in a tightly closed, light-resistant container. The oral

concentrate should be stored in the refrigerator in a tightly closed, light-resistant container. This medication should never be frozen.

USES

Thiothixene is prescribed to treat the symptoms of certain types of mental illness, such as emotional symptoms of psychosis. It is thought to relieve the symptoms of mental illness by blocking certain chemicals involved with nerve transmission in the brain.

TREATMENT

To avoid stomach irritation, you can take the capsule form of thiothixene with a meal or with a glass of water or milk (unless your doctor directs you to do otherwise).

The oral concentrate form of this medication should be measured carefully with the dropper provided, then added to four ounces ($1/2$ cup) or more of water, milk, juice, or a carbonated beverage, or to applesauce or pudding, immediately prior to administration. To prevent possible loss of effectiveness, the medication should not be diluted in tea, coffee, or apple juice.

Antacids and anti-diarrhea medicine decrease the absorption of this medication from the gastrointestinal tract. Therefore, at least one hour should separate doses of one of these medicines and thiothixene.

If you miss a dose of this medication, take the missed dose as soon as possible, then return to your regular dosing schedule. If it is almost time for the next dose, however, skip the one you missed and return to your regular schedule. Do not double the dose unless your doctor directs you to do so.

The full effects of this medication for the control of emotional or mental symptoms may not become apparent for two weeks after you start to take it.

SIDE EFFECTS

Minor. Blurred vision; constipation; decreased sweating; diarrhea; discoloration of the urine to red, pink, or red-brown; dizziness; drooling; drowsiness; dry mouth; fatigue; jitteriness; menstrual irregularities; nasal congestion; restlessness; tremors; vomiting; and weight gain. As your body adjusts to the medication, these side effects should disappear.

If you are constipated, increase the amount of fiber in your diet (raw vegetables, fruits, salads, bran, and whole-grain breads), and drink more water (unless your doctor directs you to do otherwise).

To reduce mouth dryness, chew sugarless gum, or suck on ice chips or a piece of hard candy.

This medication can cause increased sensitivity to sunlight. It is therefore important to avoid prolonged exposure to sunlight and sunlamps. Wear protective clothing, and use an effective sunscreen.

To avoid dizziness or light-headedness when you stand, contract and relax the muscles of your legs for a few moments before rising. Do this by pushing one foot against the floor while raising the other foot slightly, alternating feet so that you are "pumping" your legs in a pedaling motion.

Major. Tell your doctor about any side effects that are persistent or particularly bothersome. IT IS ESPECIALLY IMPORTANT TO TELL YOUR DOCTOR about unusual bleeding or bruising; breast enlargement (in both sexes); chest pain; convulsions; darkened skin; difficulty swallowing or breathing; fainting; fever; impotence; involuntary movements of the face, mouth, jaw, or tongue; palpitations; rash; sleep disorders; sore throat; uncoordinated movements; visual disturbances; or yellowing of the eyes or skin.

INTERACTIONS

Thiothixene interacts with other types of medication.

1. It can cause extreme drowsiness when combined with alcohol or other central nervous system depressants (drugs that slow the activity of the nervous system), such as barbiturates, benzodiazepine tranquilizers, muscle relaxants, narcotics, and pain medications, or with tricyclic anti-depressants.

2. Thiothixene can decrease the effectiveness of amphetamines, guanethidine, anti-convulsants, and levodopa

3. The side effects of epinephrine, monoamine oxidase (MAO) inhibitors, and tricyclic anti-depressants may be increased when combined with this medication.

4. Lithium may increase the side effects and decrease the effectiveness of thiothixene.

BE SURE TO TELL YOUR DOCTOR if you are already taking any of the medications listed above.

WARNINGS

• Tell your doctor about any unusual or allergic reactions you have had to medications, especially to thiothixene, chlorprothixene, or any phenothiazine tranquilizer.

• Tell your doctor if you now have, or if you have ever had, any blood disease, bone marrow disease, brain disease, breast cancer, blockage in the urinary or digestive tract, alcoholism, drug-induced depression, epilepsy, severe high or low blood pressure, diabetes mellitus (sugar diabetes), glaucoma, heart or circulatory disease, liver disease, lung disease, Parkinson's disease, peptic ulcers, or an enlarged prostate gland.

• Avoid drinking alcoholic beverages while taking this medication, in order to prevent over-sedation.

• If this medication makes you dizzy or drowsy, do not take part in any activity that requires alertness, such as driving a car or operating potentially dangerous equipment. Be careful on stairs, and avoid getting up suddenly from a lying or sitting position.

• Before having any surgery or other medical or dental treatment, be sure to tell your doctor or dentist that you are taking this medication.

• Some of the side effects caused by this drug can be prevented by taking an anti-parkinson drug. Discuss this with your doctor.

• This type of medication has been reported to cause certain tumors in rats. This effect has not been shown to occur in humans.

• This medication can decrease sweating and heat release from the body. You should therefore avoid getting overheated (strenuous exercise in hot weather; hot baths, showers, and saunas).

• Do not stop taking this medication suddenly. If the drug is stopped abruptly you may experience nausea, vomiting, stomach upset, headache, increased heart rate, insomnia, tremulousness, or worsening of your condition. Your doctor may want to reduce the dosage gradually.

- If you are planning to have a myelogram, or any procedure in which dye is injected into the spinal cord, tell your doctor that you are taking this medication.
- Avoid spilling the oral concentrate form of this medication on your skin or clothing; it can cause redness and irritation of the skin.
- While taking this medication, do not take any over-the-counter (non-prescription) medication for weight control, or for cough, cold, allergy, asthma, or sinus problems, unless you first check with your doctor. The combination of these medications may cause high blood pressure.
- Be sure to tell your doctor if you are pregnant. Small amounts of this medication cross the placenta. Although there are reports of safe use of this drug during pregnancy, there are also reports of liver disease and tremors in newborn infants whose mothers received this type of medication close to term. Also, tell your doctor if you are breastfeeding an infant. Small amounts of this medication pass into breast milk and may cause unwanted effects in nursing infants.

Thiuretic—see hydrochlorothiazide

Thorazine—see chlorpromazine

Thorazine Spansules—see chlorpromazine

Thor-Prom—see chlorpromazine

Thyrar—see thyroid hormone

---

thyroid hormone

BRAND NAMES (Manufacturers)
Armour Thyroid (Armour)
S-P-T (Fleming)
Thyrar (Armour)
Thyroid Strong (Marion)
Thyroid USP (various manufacturers)
Thyro-Teric (Mallard)
Westhroid (Western Research)

TYPE OF DRUG
Thyroid hormone
INGREDIENT
thyroid hormone
DOSAGE FORMS
Tablets (16 mg, 32 mg, 65 mg, 97 mg, 130 mg, 195 mg, 260 mg, and 325 mg)
Enteric-coated tablets (32 mg, 65 mg, 130 mg, and 195 mg)
Sugar-coated tablets (32 mg, 65 mg, 130 mg, and 195 mg)
Capsules (65 mg, 130 mg, 195 mg, and 325 mg)
   Note that 16 mg = $^{1}/_{4}$ grain (gr); 32 mg = $^{1}/_{2}$ gr; 65 mg = 1 gr; 97 mg = $1^{1}/_{2}$ gr; 130 mg = 2 gr; 195 mg = 3 gr; 260 mg = 4 gr; and 325 mg = 5 gr.
STORAGE
Thyroid hormone should be stored at room temperature in a tightly closed, light-resistant container.

USES

This medication is prescribed to replace natural thyroid hormones that are absent because of a disorder of the thyroid gland. This product is obtained from the thyroid glands of cows or pigs.

TREATMENT

Thyroid hormone tablets should be taken on an empty stomach with a full glass of water. If this medication upsets your stomach, check with your doctor to see if you can take it with food or milk.

   In order to get used to taking this medication, try to take it at the same time each day. Try not to miss any doses. If you do miss a dose of this medication, take it as soon as you remember, unless it is almost time for the next dose. In that case, do not take the missed dose at all; just return to your regular dosing schedule. Do not double the next dose. If you miss more than one or two doses of this medication, check with your doctor.

SIDE EFFECTS

Minor. Constipation; dry, puffy skin; fatigue; headache; listlessness; muscle aches; and weight gain. These side effects should disappear in several days, as your body adjusts to the medication.

To relieve constipation, increase the amount of fiber in your diet (bran, fresh fruits and vegetables, salads, and whole-grain breads), and drink more water (unless your doctor directs you to do otherwise).

Major. Tell your doctor about any side effects that are persistent or particularly bothersome. Most of the major side effects associated with this drug are the result of too large a dose. The dosage of this medication may need to be adjusted if you experience any of the following side effects: chest pain; diarrhea; fever; heat intolerance; insomnia; irritability; leg cramps; menstrual irregularities; nervousness; palpitations; shortness of breath; sweating; trembling; or weight loss. CHECK WITH YOUR DOCTOR.

INTERACTIONS

Thyroid hormone interacts with several other types of medication.

1. Dosing requirements for insulin or oral anti-diabetic agents may change when this medication is used.

2. The effects of oral anti-coagulants (blood thinners, such as warfarin) may be increased by thyroid hormone, which could lead to bleeding complications.

3. Cholestyramine and colestipol chemically bind thyroid hormone in the gastrointestinal tract, preventing its absorption. Therefore, at least four hours should separate doses of thyroid hormone and one of these medications (if you have also been prescribed one of these medications).

4. Estrogens (oral contraceptives) may change your dosing requirements for thyroid hormone.

5. The side effects of digoxin may be increased by thyroid hormone.

6. Phenobarbital may decrease the effectiveness of thyroid hormone.

7. Phenytoin, tricyclic anti-depressants, and over-the-counter (non-prescription) allergy, asthma, cough, cold, sinus, or diet medications may increase the side effects of thyroid hormone.

BE SURE TO TELL YOUR DOCTOR if you are already taking any of the medications listed above.

WARNINGS

• Tell your doctor about any unusual or allergic reactions you have had to medications, especially to thyroid hormone or to beef or pork products.

• Tell your doctor if you now have, or if you have ever had, angina pectoris; diabetes mellitus (sugar diabetes); heart disease; high blood pressure; kidney disease; or an underactive adrenal or pituitary gland.

• If you have an underactive thyroid gland, you may need to take this medication for life. You should not stop taking it unless you first check with your doctor.

• Before having surgery or any other medical or dental treatment, be sure to tell your doctor or dentist that you are taking thyroid hormone.

• Over-the-counter (non-prescription) allergy, asthma, cough, cold, sinus, and diet medications can increase the side effects of thyroid hormone. Therefore, check with your doctor or pharmacist before taking ANY of these products.

• Although many thyroid products are on the market, they are not all bioequivalent; that is, they may not all be absorbed into the bloodstream at the same rate or have the same overall activity. DON'T CHANGE BRANDS of this drug without first consulting your doctor or pharmacist to make sure you are receiving an equivalent product.

• Be sure to tell your doctor if you are pregnant. Thyroid hormone does not readily cross the placenta, and the drug appears to be safe during pregnancy. However, your dosing requirements of thyroid hormone may change during pregnancy. Also, tell your doctor if you are breastfeeding an infant. Small amounts of thyroid hormone pass into breast milk.

Thyroid Strong—see thyroid hormone

Thyroid USP—see thyroid hormone

Thyro-Teric—see thyroid hormone

Tigan—see trimethobenzamide

timolol (ophthalmic)

BRAND NAME (Manufacturer)
Timoptic (Merck Sharp & Dohme)
TYPE OF DRUG
Anti-glaucoma ophthalmic solution
INGREDIENT
timolol as the maleate salt
DOSAGE FORM
Ophthalmic drops (0.25% and 0.5%)
STORAGE
Timolol ophthalmic drops should be stored at room temperature in a tightly closed container. This medication should never be frozen. If this medication discolors or turns brown, it should be discarded—a color change demonstrates a loss of potency.

USES

Timolol ophthalmic is used to reduce pressure in the eye caused by glaucoma or other eye conditions. This medication belongs to a group of drugs known as beta-blockers. When applied to the eye, timolol reduces pressure within the eye by decreasing eye fluid (aqueous humor) production, and perhaps by increasing the outflow of fluid from the eye.

TREATMENT

Wash your hands with soap and water before applying this medication. In order to avoid contamination of the eye drops, be careful not to touch the dropper, or let it touch your eye; do not wipe off or rinse the dropper after use.

To apply the drops, tilt your head back and pull down your lower eyelid with one hand, to make a pouch below the eye. Drop the prescribed amount of medicine into this pouch and slowly close your eyes. Try not to blink. Keep your eyes closed, and place one finger at the corner of the eye next to your nose for a minute or two, applying a slight pressure (this is done to prevent loss of medication into the nose and throat canal). Then wipe away any excess with a clean tissue. Since applying the medication is somewhat difficult to do, you may want to have someone else apply the drops for you.

If you miss a dose of this medication, apply the missed dose as soon as possible, then return to your regular dosing schedule. However, if it is almost time for the next dose, skip the dose you missed. If the medication is only used once a day, and you don't remember until the next day, skip the missed dose. Do not double the next dose.

SIDE EFFECTS

Minor. When you first apply this medication, it may sting your eyes. This should stop in a few minutes.

Major. Tell your doctor about any side effects that are persistent or particularly bothersome. IT IS ESPECIALLY IMPORTANT TO TELL YOUR DOCTOR about irritation of the eye that lasts more than a few minutes after application; itching; skin rash; or hives. Major side effects are rare when this product is used correctly. However, rare occurrences of anxiety, bronchospasm, confusion, depression, dizziness, drowsiness, generalized rash, indigestion, loss of appetite, nausea, weakness, and a slight reduction of the resting heart rate have been observed in some users of this drug. If you have any of these symptoms, contact your doctor.

INTERACTIONS

Timolol ophthalmic may increase the side effects of reserpine and oral beta-blockers. Before starting to take timolol, TELL YOUR DOCTOR if you are already taking any of these medications.

WARNINGS

• Tell your doctor about unusual or allergic reactions you have had to medications, especially to timolol or to any other beta-blocker (atenolol, metoprolol, nadolol, pindolol, or propranolol).

• Tell your doctor if you now have, or if you have ever had, asthma, diabetes mellitus (sugar diabetes), heart disease, or myasthenia gravis.

• Be sure to tell your doctor if you are pregnant. Small amounts of timolol may be absorbed into the bloodstream. Although studies in humans have not yet been completed, birth defects have been observed in the fetuses of animals who were given large oral doses of this type of drug during pregnancy. Also, tell your doctor if you are breastfeeding an infant. If this drug reaches the bloodstream and passes into the breast milk, it can cause a slowed heart rate in the nursing infant.

timolol (systemic)

BRAND NAME (Manufacturer)
Blocadren (Merck Sharp & Dohme)
TYPE OF DRUG
Beta-adrenergic blocking agent
INGREDIENT
timolol maleate
DOSAGE FORM
Tablets (5 mg, 10 mg, and 20 mg)
STORAGE
Timolol should be stored at room temperature in a tightly closed, light-resistant container.

USES
Timolol is used to treat high blood pressure and to prevent additional heart attacks in heart attack patients. It belongs to a group of medicines known as beta-adrenergic blocking agents or, more commonly, beta-blockers. These drugs work by controlling nerve impulses along certain nerve pathways.

TREATMENT
Timolol can be taken with a glass of water, with meals, immediately following meals, or on an empty stomach, depending on your doctor's instructions. Try to take the medication at the same time(s) each day.

Try not to miss any doses of this medicine. If you do miss a dose, take the missed dose as soon as possible. However, if the next scheduled dose is within eight hours (if you are taking this medicine only once a day) or within four hours (if you are taking this medicine more than once a day), do not take the missed dose at all; just return to your regular dosing schedule. Do not double the next dose.

It is important to remember that timolol does not cure

high blood pressure, but it will help to control the condition, as long as you continue to take it.

SIDE EFFECTS

Minor. Anxiety; cold hands or feet (due to decreased blood circulation to skin, fingers, and toes); constipation; decreased sexual ability; diarrhea; difficulty sleeping; drowsiness; dryness of the eyes, mouth, and skin; headache; nausea; nervousness; numbness or tingling of the fingers or toes; stomach discomfort; tiredness; or weakness. These side effects should disappear during treatment, as your body adjusts to the medicine.

If you are extra-sensitive to the cold, be sure to dress warmly during cold weather.

Plain, non-medicated eye drops (artificial tears) may help to relieve eye dryness.

Sucking on ice chips or chewing sugarless gum helps to relieve mouth and throat dryness.

Major. Tell your doctor about any side effects that are persistent or particularly bothersome. IT IS ESPECIALLY IMPORTANT TO TELL YOUR DOCTOR about confusion; depression; difficulty breathing, or wheezing; dizziness; fever and sore throat; hair loss; hallucinations; lightheadedness; nightmares; rapid weight gain (three to five pounds within a week); reduced alertness; skin rash; swelling; or unusual bleeding or bruising.

INTERACTIONS

Timolol interacts with a number of other types of medication.

1. Indomethacin has been shown to decrease the blood-pressure-lowering effects of the beta-blockers. This may also happen with aspirin or other salicylates.

2. Concurrent use of beta-blockers and calcium channel blockers (diltiazem, nifedipine, and verapamil) can lead to heart failure or very low blood pressure.

3. Cimetidine can increase the blood concentrations of timolol, which can result in greater side effects.

4. Side effects may also be increased when beta-blockers are taken with clonidine, digoxin, epinephrine, phenylephrine, phenylpropanolamine, phenothiazine tranquilizers, reserpine, or monoamine oxidase (MAO) inhibitors.

At least 14 days should separate the use of a beta-blocker and an MAO inhibitor.

5. Beta-blockers may antagonize (work against) the effects of theophylline, aminophylline, albuterol, metaproterenol, and terbutaline.

6. Beta-blockers can also interact with insulin or oral anti-diabetic agents—raising or lowering blood sugar levels or masking the symptoms of low blood sugar.

BE SURE TO TELL YOUR DOCTOR if you are currently taking any of the medicines listed above.

WARNINGS

• Before starting to take this medication, it is important to tell your doctor if you have ever had unusual or allergic reactions to any beta-blocker (atenolol, metoprolol, nadolol, pindolol, propranolol, and timolol).

• Tell your doctor if you now have, or if you have ever had, allergies, asthma, hay fever, eczema, slow heartbeat, bronchitis, diabetes mellitus (sugar diabetes), emphysema, heart or blood vessel disease, kidney disease, liver disease, thyroid disease, or poor circulation in the fingers or toes.

• You may want to check your pulse while taking this medication. If your pulse is much slower than your usual rate (or if it is less than 50 beats per minute), check with your doctor. A pulse rate that is too slow may cause circulation problems.

• This medicine may affect your body's response to exercise. Be sure you discuss with your doctor how much exercise is safe for you, taking into account your medical condition.

• It is important that you do not stop taking this medicine without first checking with your doctor. Some conditions may become worse when the medicine is stopped suddenly, and the danger of a heart attack is increased in some patients. Your doctor may want you to gradually reduce the amount of medicine you take, before stopping completely. Make sure that you have enough medicine on hand to last through vacations and holidays.

• Before having any kind of surgery or other medical or dental treatment, tell your doctor or dentist that you are taking this medication. Often, this medication will be dis-

continued 48 hours prior to any major surgery.
- Timolol can cause dizziness, drowsiness, light-headedness; or decreased alertness. Therefore, exercise caution while driving a car or using any potentially dangerous machinery.
- While taking this medicine, do not use any over-the-counter (non-prescription) allergy, asthma, cough, cold, sinus, or diet preparations, unless you first check with your pharmacist or doctor. Some of these medicines can result in high blood pressure and slow heartbeat when taken at the same time as timolol.
- Be sure to tell your doctor if you are pregnant. Animal studies have shown that some beta-blockers can cause problems in pregnancy when used at very high doses. Adequate studies have not yet been completed in humans, but there has been some association between beta-blockers used during pregnancy and low birth rate, as well as breathing problems and slow heart rate in newborn infants. However, other reports have shown no effects on newborn infants. Also, tell your doctor if you are breast-feeding an infant. Small amounts of timolol may pass into breast milk.

Timoptic—see timolol (ophthalmic)

Tipramine—see imipramine

Tofranil—see imipramine

Tofranil-PM—see imipramine

---

tolazamide

BRAND NAME (Manufacturer)
Tolinase (Upjohn)
TYPE OF DRUG
Oral anti-diabetic
INGREDIENT
tolazamide
DOSAGE FORM
Tablets (100 mg, 250 mg, and 500 mg)

STORAGE

This medication should be stored at room temperature, in a tightly closed container.

USES

Tolazamide is used for the treatment of diabetes mellitus (sugar diabetes) that appears in adulthood and cannot be managed by control of diet alone. This type of diabetes is known as noninsulin-dependent diabetes (sometimes called maturity-onset or Type II diabetes). Tolazamide lowers blood sugar by increasing the release of insulin from the pancreas.

TREATMENT

In order for this medication to work correctly, it must be taken as directed by your doctor. It is best to take this medicine at the same time each day, in order to maintain a constant blood sugar level. It is therefore important to try not to miss any doses of tolazamide. If you do miss a dose, take it as soon as possible, unless it is almost time for the next dose. In that case, do not take the missed dose at all; just return to your regular dosing schedule. Do not double the next dose. Tell your doctor if you feel any side effects from missing a dose of this drug.

SIDE EFFECTS

Minor. Diarrhea; headache; heartburn; loss of appetite; nausea; stomach pain; stomach discomfort; or vomiting. These side effects usually disappear during treatment, as your body adjusts to the medicine.

Major. Tell your doctor about any side effects that are persistent or particularly bothersome. IT IS ESPECIALLY IMPORTANT TO TELL YOUR DOCTOR about dark urine; fatigue; itching of the skin; light-colored stools; sore throat and fever; unusual bleeding or bruising; or yellowing of the eyes or skin.

INTERACTIONS

Tolazamide interacts with a number of other medications.
1. Chloramphenicol; guanethidine; insulin; monoamine oxidase (MAO) inhibitors; oxyphenbutazone; oxytetracycline; phenylbutazone; probenecid; aspirin or other sali-

cylates; and sulfonamide antibiotics, when combined with tolazamide, can lower blood sugar levels—sometimes to dangerously low levels.

2. Thyroid hormones; dextrothyroxine; epinephrine; phenytoin; thiazide diuretics (water pills); and cortisone-like medications (such as dexamethasone, hydrocortisone, and prednisone), combined with tolazamide, can actually increase blood sugar—just what you are trying to avoid.

3. Oral anti-diabetic medications can increase the effects of warfarin, which can lead to bleeding complications.

4. Beta-blocking medications (atenolol, metoprolol, nadolol, pindolol, propranolol, and timolol) combined with tolazamide can result in either high or low blood sugar levels. Beta-blockers can also mask the symptoms of low blood sugar, which can be dangerous.

BE SURE TO TELL YOUR DOCTOR if you are already taking any of the medications listed above.

WARNINGS

● It is important to tell your doctor if you have ever had unusual or allergic reactions to this medicine or to any sulfa medication [sulfonamide antibiotics, diuretics (water pills), or other oral anti-diabetics].

● It is also important to tell your doctor if you now have, or if you have ever had, kidney disease, liver disease, severe infections, or thyroid disease.

● Avoid drinking alcoholic beverages while taking this medication (unless otherwise directed by your doctor). Some patients who take this medicine suffer nausea; vomiting; dizziness; stomach pain; pounding headache; sweating; and redness of the face and skin, when they drink alcohol. Also, large amounts of alcohol can lower blood sugar to dangerously low levels.

● It is important to follow the special diet that your doctor gave you. This is an important part of controlling your blood sugar, and is necessary in order for this medicine to work properly.

● Before having any surgery or other medical or dental treatment, be sure to tell your doctor or dentist that you are taking this medication.

● Test for sugar in your urine as directed by your doctor. It is a convenient way to determine whether or not your dia-

betes is being controlled by this medicine.
- Tolazamide may increase your sensitivity to sunlight. It is therefore important to use caution during exposure to the sun. You may want to wear protective clothing and sunglasses. Use an effective sunscreen and avoid exposure to sunlamps.
- Eat or drink something containing sugar right away if you experience any symptoms of low blood sugar (such as anxiety; chills; cold sweats; cool or pale skin; drowsiness; excessive hunger; headache; nausea; nervousness; rapid heartbeat; shakiness; or unusual tiredness or weakness). It is important that your family and friends know the symptoms of low blood sugar and what to do if they observe any of these symptoms in you.

Check with your doctor—even if these symptoms are corrected by the sugar, it is important to contact your doctor as soon as possible. The blood-sugar-lowering effects of this medicine can last for hours, and your symptoms may return during this period. Good sources of sugar are orange juice, corn syrup, honey, sugar cubes, and table sugar. You are at greatest risk of developing low blood sugar if you skip or delay meals, exercise more than usual, cannot eat because of nausea or vomiting, or drink large amounts of alcohol.
- Diabetics who are taking oral anti-diabetic medication may need to be switched to insulin if they develop diabetic coma, have a severe infection, are scheduled for major surgery, or become pregnant.
- Be sure to tell your doctor if you are pregnant. Your dosing requirements for tolazamide may change during pregnancy. Although studies in humans have not been completed, adverse effects have been observed on the fetuses of animals who received this type of drug during pregnancy. Also, tell your doctor if you are breastfeeding an infant. Small amounts of tolazamide may pass into breast milk.

tolbutamide

BRAND NAMES (Manufacturers)
Oramide (Major)

Orinase (Upjohn)
SK-Tolbutamide (Smith Kline & French)
tolbutamide (various manufacturers)
TYPE OF DRUG
Oral anti-diabetic
INGREDIENT
tolbutamide
DOSAGE FORM
Tablets (250 mg and 500 mg)
STORAGE
This medication should be stored at room temperature in
a tightly closed container.

USES

Tolbutamide is used for the treatment of diabetes mellitus
(sugar diabetes) that appears in adulthood and cannot be
managed by control of diet alone. This type of diabetes is
known as noninsulin-dependent diabetes (sometimes
called maturity-onset or Type II diabetes). Tolbutamide
lowers blood sugar by increasing the release of insulin
from the pancreas.

TREATMENT

In order for this medication to work correctly, it must be
taken as directed by your doctor. It is best to take this medicine at the same time(s) each day, in order to maintain a
constant blood sugar level. It is therefore important to try
not to miss any doses of tolbutamide. If you do miss a
dose, take it as soon as possible, unless it is almost time for
the next dose. In that case, do not take the missed dose at
all; just return to your regular dosing schedule. Do not
double the next dose. Tell your doctor if you feel any side
effects from missing a dose of this drug.

SIDE EFFECTS

Minor. Diarrhea; headache; heartburn; loss of appetite;
nausea; stomach pain; stomach discomfort; or vomiting.
These side effects usually disappear during treatment, as
your body adjusts to the medicine.
Major. Tell your doctor about any side effects that are persistent or particularly bothersome. IT IS ESPECIALLY IM-
PORTANT TO TELL YOUR DOCTOR about dark urine;

fatigue; itching of the skin; light-colored stools; sore throat and fever; unusual bleeding or bruising; or yellowing of the eyes or skin.

INTERACTIONS

Tolbutamide interacts with a number of other medications.

1. Chloramphenicol; guanethidine; insulin; monoamine oxidase (MAO) inhibitors; oxyphenbutazone; oxytetracycline; phenylbutazone; probenecid; aspirin or other salicylates; and sulfonamide antibiotics, when combined with tolbutamide, can lower blood sugar levels—sometimes to dangerously low levels.

2. Thyroid hormones; dextrothyroxine; epinephrine; phenytoin; thiazide diuretics (water pills); and cortisone-like medications (such as dexamethasone, hydrocortisone, and prednisone), combined with tolbutamide, can actually increase blood sugar levels—just what you are trying to avoid.

3. Oral anti-diabetic medications can increase the effects of blood thinners, such as warfarin, which can lead to bleeding complications.

4. Beta-blocking medications (atenolol, metoprolol, nadolol, pindolol, propranolol, and timolol) combined with tolbutamide can result in either high or low blood sugar levels. Beta-blockers can also mask the symptoms of low blood sugar, which can be dangerous.

BE SURE TO TELL YOUR DOCTOR if you are already taking any of the medications listed above.

WARNINGS

● It is important to tell your doctor if you have ever had unusual or allergic reactions to this medicine or to any sulfa medication [sulfonamide antibiotics, diuretics (water pills), or other oral anti-diabetics].

● It is also important to tell your doctor if you now have, or if you have ever had, kidney disease, liver disease, severe infection, or thyroid disease.

● Avoid drinking alcoholic beverages while taking this medication (unless otherwise directed by your doctor). Some patients who take this medicine suffer nausea; vomiting; dizziness; stomach pain; pounding headache;

sweating; and redness of the face and skin when they drink alcohol. Also, large amounts of alcohol can lower blood sugar to dangerously low levels.

• It is important to follow the special diet that your doctor gave you. This is an important part of controlling your blood sugar, and is necessary in order for this medicine to work properly.

• Before having any kind of surgery or other medical or dental treatment, be sure to tell your doctor or dentist that you are taking this medicine.

• Test for sugar in your urine as directed by your doctor. It is a convenient way to determine whether or not your diabetes is being controlled by this medicine.

• Tolbutamide may increase your sensitivity to sunlight. It is therefore important to use caution during exposure to the sun. You may want to wear protective clothing and sunglasses. Use an effective sunscreen and avoid exposure to sunlamps.

• Eat or drink something containing sugar right away if you experience any symptoms of low blood sugar (such as anxiety; chills; cold sweats; cool or pale skin; drowsiness; excessive hunger; headache; nausea; nervousness; rapid heartbeat; shakiness; or unusual tiredness or weakness). It is important that your family and friends know the symptoms of low blood sugar and what to do if they observe any of these symptoms in you.

Check with your doctor—even if these symptoms are corrected by the sugar, it is important to contact your doctor as soon as possible. The blood-sugar-lowering effects of this medicine can last for hours, and your symptoms may return during this period. Good sources of sugar are orange juice, corn syrup, honey, sugar cubes, and table sugar. You are at greatest risk of developing low blood sugar if you skip or delay meals, exercise more than usual, cannot eat because of nausea or vomiting, or drink large amounts of alcohol.

• Diabetics who are taking oral anti-diabetic medication may need to be switched to insulin if they develop diabetic coma, have a severe infection, are scheduled for major surgery, or become pregnant.

• Be sure to tell your doctor if you are pregnant. Your dosing requirements for tolbutamide may change during pregnancy. Although studies in humans have not yet been completed, adverse effects have been observed on the fetuses of animals who received this drug during pregnancy. Also, tell your doctor if you are breastfeeding an infant. Small amounts of tolbutamide may pass into breast milk.

Tolectin—see tolmetin

Tolectin DS—see tolmetin

Tolinase—see tolazamide

---

tolmetin

BRAND NAMES (Manufacturers)
Tolectin (McNeil)
Tolectin DS (McNeil)
TYPE OF DRUG
Non-steroidal anti-inflammatory analgesic (pain reliever)
INGREDIENT
tolmetin as the sodium salt
DOSAGE FORMS
Tablets (200 mg)
Capsules (400 mg)
STORAGE
This medication should be stored in tightly closed containers at room temperature, away from heat and direct sunlight.

USES
Tolmetin is used to treat the inflammation (pain, swelling, and stiffness) of certain types of arthritis, gout, bursitis, and tendinitis.

TREATMENT
You should take this medication on an empty stomach 30 to 60 minutes before meals or two hours after meals, so that it gets into your bloodstream quickly. However, to decrease stomach irritation, your doctor may want you to take the medicine with food or antacids.

If you are taking tolmetin to relieve arthritis, you must

take it regularly, as directed by your doctor. It may take up to two weeks before you feel the full benefits of this medication. Tolmetin does not cure arthritis, but it will help to control the condition, as long as you continue to take it.

It is important to take tolmetin on schedule and not to miss any doses. It you do miss a dose, take it as soon as possible, unless it is almost time for your next dose. In that case, don't take the missed dose at all; just return to your regular dosing schedule. Do not double the next dose.

SIDE EFFECTS

Minor. Bloating; constipation; diarrhea; difficulty sleeping; dizziness; drowsiness; headache; heartburn; indigestion; light-headedness; loss of appetite; nausea; nervousness; soreness of the mouth; unusual sweating; or vomiting. As your body adjusts to the drug, these side effects should disappear.

If you become dizzy, sit or lie down awhile; and be careful on stairs.

Acetaminophen may be helpful in relieving any headaches.

Major. Tell your doctor about any side effects that are persistent or particularly bothersome. IT IS ESPECIALLY IMPORTANT TO TELL YOUR DOCTOR about bloody or black, tarry stools; blurred vision; confusion; depression; difficult or painful urination; difficulty breathing, or wheezing; difficulty hearing; pounding heartbeat; ringing or buzzing in the ears; skin rash, hives, or itching; stomach pain; swelling of the feet; tightness in the chest; unexplained sore throat and fever; unusual bleeding or bruising; unusual fatigue or weakness; unusual weight gain; or yellowing of the eyes or skin.

INTERACTIONS

Tolmetin interacts with several types of medications.
1. Anti-coagulants (blood thinners, such as warfarin) in combination with tolmetin can lead to an increase in bleeding complications.
2. Aspirin, salicylates, or other anti-inflammation medications can increase the stomach irritation caused by tolmetin.
BE SURE TO TELL YOUR DOCTOR if you are already tak-

ing any of the medications listed above.

WARNINGS

• Before you take this medication, it is important to tell your doctor if you have ever had unusual or allergic reactions to tolmetin or any of the other chemically related drugs (including aspirin, other salicylates, diflunisal, fenoprofen, ibuprofen, meclofenamate, mefenamic acid, naproxen, oxyphenbutazone, phenylbutazone, piroxicam, sulindac, indomethacin, and zomepirac).

• Tell your doctor if you now have, or if you have ever had, bleeding problems; colitis, stomach ulcers, or other stomach problems; epilepsy; heart disease; high blood pressure; asthma; kidney disease; liver disease; mental illness; or Parkinson's disease.

• If this drug makes you dizzy or drowsy, do not take part in any activity that requires alertness, such as driving a car or operating potentially dangerous equipment.

• Because this drug can prolong your bleeding time, it is important to tell your doctor or dentist that you are taking this drug, before having any surgery or other medical or dental treatment.

• Stomach problems are more likely to occur if you take aspirin regularly or drink alcohol while being treated with this medication. These should therefore be avoided (unless your doctor directs you to do otherwise).

• Be sure to tell your doctor if you are pregnant. Studies in humans have not yet been completed, but unwanted effects have been reported on the offspring of animals who received this type of medication during pregnancy. If taken late in pregnancy, tolmetin can also prolong labor. Also, tell your doctor if you are breastfeeding an infant. Small amounts of tolmetin can pass into breast milk.

Topsyn—see fluocinonide (topical)

Totacillin—see ampicillin

Tranmep—see meprobamate

Transderm-Nitro—see nitroglycerin (topical)

Tranxene—see clorazepate

Tranxene SD—see clorazepate

Trates Granucaps—see nitroglycerin (systemic)

---

trazodone

BRAND NAME (Manufacturer)
Desyrel (Mead Johnson)
TYPE OF DRUG
Anti-depressant (mood elevator)
INGREDIENT
trazodone
DOSAGE FORM
Tablets (50 mg and 100 mg)
STORAGE
Trazodone tablets should be stored at room temperature in a tightly closed, light-resistant container.

USES
Trazodone is used to relieve the symptoms of mental depression. It is thought to relieve depression by increasing the concentration of certain chemicals involved with nerve transmission in the brain.

TREATMENT
Trazodone should be taken exactly as your doctor prescribes. It can be taken with water, milk, or food to lessen the chance of stomach irritation (unless your doctor tells you to do otherwise).

If you miss a dose of this medication, take the missed dose as soon as possible, then return to your regular dosing schedule. If, however, the dose you missed was a once-a-day bedtime dose, do not take that dose in the morning; check with your doctor instead. If the dose is taken in the morning, it may cause some unwanted side effects. Never double the dose.

The benefits of therapy with this medication may not become apparent for two to four weeks.

SIDE EFFECTS

Minor. Blurred vision; constipation; diarrhea; dizziness; drowsiness; dry mouth; gas; headache; heartburn; light-headedness; nausea; sleep disorders; vomiting; and weight gain or loss. These side effects should disappear in several days, as your body adjusts to the medication.

Dry mouth can be relieved by chewing sugarless gum, or by sucking on ice chips or a piece of hard candy.

To relieve constipation, increase the amount of fiber in your diet (bran, salads, fresh fruits and vegetables, whole-grain breads), exercise, and drink more water (unless your doctor directs you to do otherwise).

To avoid dizziness and light-headedness when you stand, contract and relax the muscles of your legs for a few moments before rising. Do this by pushing one foot against the floor while raising the other foot slightly, alternating feet so that you are "pumping" your legs in a pedaling motion.

This medication may cause increased sensitivity to sunlight. You should therefore avoid prolonged exposure to sunlight and sunlamps. Wear protective clothing and sunglasses, and use an effective sunscreen.

Major. Tell your doctor about any side effects that are persistent or particularly bothersome. IT IS ESPECIALLY IMPORTANT TO TELL YOUR DOCTOR about unusual bleeding or bruising; chest tightness; confusion; difficult or painful urination; hallucinations; loss of coordination; mood changes; muscle aches or pains; palpitations; rash; ringing in the ears; shortness of breath; tingling in the fingers or toes; tremors; or unusual tiredness or weakness.

INTERACTIONS

Trazodone interacts with several other types of medication.

1. Extreme drowsiness can occur when trazodone is taken with central nervous system depressants (drugs that slow the activity of the nervous system), including alcohol, antihistamines, barbiturates, benzodiazepine tranquilizers, muscle relaxants, narcotics, pain medications, phenothiazine tranquilizers, and sleeping medications.

2. The concurrent use of trazodone and monoamine oxidase (MAO) inhibitors should be undertaken very carefully, because the combination can result in fever, convulsions, or high blood pressure.

3. Trazodone may increase the blood levels of digoxin and phenytoin, which can lead to increased side effects.

4. The blood-pressure-lowering effects of anti-hypertensive medication may be increased by trazodone, which can be dangerous.

BE SURE TO TELL YOUR DOCTOR if you are already taking any of the medications listed above.

WARNINGS

● Tell your doctor if you have had unusual or allergic reactions to any medications, especially to trazodone.

● Tell your doctor if you now have, or if you have ever had, electroshock therapy; a problem with alcoholism; heart disease; a recent heart attack; kidney disease; or liver disease.

● If this drug makes you dizzy or drowsy, do not take part in any activity that requires alertness, such as driving a car or operating potentially dangerous equipment.

● Before having any surgery or other medical or dental treatment, be sure to tell your doctor or dentist that you are taking this medication.

● Do not stop taking this drug suddenly. Stopping this medication abruptly may cause nausea, headache, stomach upset, fatigue, or worsening of your condition. Your doctor may therefore want to reduce the dosage gradually.

● The effects of this medication may last as long as seven days after you've stopped taking it, so continue to observe all precautions during this period.

● Be sure to tell your doctor if you are pregnant. Problems in humans have not been reported; however, studies have shown side effects on the fetuses of animals who were given this medication in large doses during pregnancy. Also, tell your doctor if you are breastfeeding an infant. Small amounts of this drug pass into breast milk and may cause unwanted effects, such as irritability or sleeping problems, in nursing infants.

Tremin—see trihexyphenidyl

tretinoin

BRAND NAME (Manufacturer)
Retin-A (Ortho)
TYPE OF DRUG
Acne preparation
INGREDIENT
tretinoin (retinoic acid; vitamin A acid)
DOSAGE FORMS
Cream (0.05% and 0.1%)
Gel (0.01% and 0.025%)
Liquid (0.05%)
STORAGE
Tretinoin cream, gel, and liquid should be stored at room temperature in tightly closed, light-resistant containers. This medication should never be frozen.

USES

Tretinoin is used topically (on the skin) to treat acne vulgaris. It appears to work by increasing the turnover (death and replacement) of skin cells.

TREATMENT

This product is packaged with instructions for the patient. Read them carefully before applying tretinoin.

Wash your skin with a mild or hypoallergenic soap and warm water. Pat dry with a clean towel. Then wait about 30 minutes before applying tretinoin cream, gel, or liquid. The medication should be applied once a day, just before going to bed. Apply it only to the skin where the acne lesions appear, unless you are directed to do otherwise by your doctor. Be sure to cover the entire affected area LIGHTLY. You may use a fingertip, gauze pad, or cotton swab to apply the liquid. To avoid applying too much medication, be careful not to oversaturate the gauze pad or cotton swab. To avoid contamination, use a gauze pad or cotton swab only once, then throw it away.

During the early weeks of treatment with this drug, there may be an apparent increase in skin lesions. This is usually not a reason to discontinue its use. However, your doctor may want to change the concentration of the drug. Benefits may be noted within two to three weeks, although more than six weeks may be required before definite benefits are observed.

If you miss a dose of this medication, apply the missed dose as soon as possible, then go back to your regular dosing schedule. However, if you don't remember until the following day, do not apply the missed dose at all; just return to your regular dosing schedule.

SIDE EFFECTS

Minor. Immediately after applying tretinoin, you may experience a sensation of warmth, a mild stinging sensation, or a redness of the skin. After a few days, some peeling of the skin is to be expected. You may also find that you have a heightened sensitivity to sunlight, wind, or cold. If this drug does increase your sensitivity to sunlight, avoid prolonged exposure to sunlight and sunlamps. Wear protective clothing, and use an effective sunscreen.

Major. Tell your doctor about any side effects that are persistent or particularly bothersome. IT IS ESPECIALLY IMPORTANT TO TELL YOUR DOCTOR about blistering, crusting, redness, severe burning, swelling, or a marked darkening or lightening of the skin.

INTERACTIONS

Tretinoin interacts with several other products:

1. Abrasive or medicated soaps or cleaners;

2. Other acne preparations (particularly peeling agents containing sulfur, resorcinol, benzoyl peroxide, or salicylic acid);

3. Cosmetics that have a strong drying effect; and

4. Locally applied products containing high amounts of alcohol, spices, or lime.

These products should be used with caution, since they can increase the irritation caused by tretinoin.

WARNINGS

• Tell your doctor about unusual or allergic reactions you have had to any medications, especially to tretinoin or vitamin A.

• Before starting to take this medication, be sure to tell your doctor if you have eczema.

• This medication should not be used if you are sunburned; it may increase the irritation.

• Tretinoin should be kept away from the eyes, the mouth, the angles of the nose, open cuts, and mucous membranes; it can severely irritate these sensitive areas.

• Avoid washing your face too often while using tretinoin. Be sure to use a mild or bland soap.

• Normal use of non-medicated cosmetics is permissible, but the skin should be cleaned thoroughly before tretinoin is applied.

Triacin C—see pseudoephedrine, tripolidine, guaifenesin, and codeine combination

---

triamcinolone (systemic)

BRAND NAMES (Manufacturers)
Aristocort (Lederle)
Kenacort (Squibb)
triamcinolone (various manufacturers)
TYPE OF DRUG
Adrenocorticosteroid hormone
INGREDIENT
triamcinolone
DOSAGE FORMS
Tablets (1 mg, 2 mg, 4 mg, 8 mg, and 16 mg)
Oral syrup (2 mg and 4 mg per 5 ml teaspoonful as the diacetate salt)
STORAGE
Triamcinolone tablets and oral syrup should be stored at room temperature in tightly closed containers.

USES

Your adrenal glands naturally produce certain cortisone-like chemicals. These chemicals are involved in various regulatory processes in the body (such as maintenance of fluid balance, temperature, and reactions to inflammation). Triamcinolone belongs to a group of drugs known as adrenocorticosteroids (or cortisone-like medications). It is used to treat a variety of disorders, including endocrine and rheumatic disorders; asthma; blood diseases; certain cancers; eye disorders; gastrointestinal disturbances such as ulcerative colitis; respiratory diseases; and inflammations such as arthritis, dermatitis, and poison ivy. How this drug acts to relieve these disorders is not completely understood.

TREATMENT

In order to prevent stomach irritation, you can take triamcinolone with food or milk (unless your doctor directs you to do otherwise).

To help avoid potassium loss while using this drug, take your dose with a glass of fresh or frozen orange juice, or eat a banana each day. The use of a salt substitute also helps prevent potassium loss. Check with your doctor.

If you are taking only one dose of this medication each day, try to take it before 9:00 A.M. This will mimic the body's normal production of this type of chemical.

The oral syrup form of this medication should be measured carefully, with a specially designed, 5 ml measuring spoon. A kitchen teaspoon is not accurate enough.

It is important to try not to miss any doses of triamcinolone. If you do miss a dose of this medication:
1. If you are taking it more than once a day, take the missed dose as soon as possible; then return to your regular dosing schedule. If it is already time for the next dose, double the dose.
2. If you are taking this medication once a day, take the dose you missed as soon as possible, unless you don't remember until the next day. In that case do not take the missed dose at all; just follow your regular dosing schedule. Do not double the next dose.
3. If you are taking this drug every other day, take it as soon as you remember. If you missed the scheduled dose by a whole day, take it when you remember, then skip a day before you take the next dose. Do not double the dose.
If you miss more than one dose, CONTACT YOUR DOCTOR.

SIDE EFFECTS

Minor. Dizziness; false sense of well-being; increased appetite; increased sweating; indigestion; menstrual irregularities; muscle weakness; nausea; reddening of the skin on the face; restlessness; sleep disorders; thinning of the skin; and weight gain. These side effects should disappear in several days, as your body adjusts to the medication.

Major. Tell your doctor about any side effects that are persistent or particularly bothersome. IT IS ESPECIALLY IMPORTANT TO TELL YOUR DOCTOR about abdominal enlargement; abdominal pain; acne or other skin problems; back or rib pain; bloody or black, tarry stools; blurred vision; unusual bruising or bleeding; convulsions; difficulty breathing; eye pain; fatigue; fever and sore throat; growth impairment (in children); headaches; impaired healing of wounds; increased thirst and urination; mental depression; mood changes; muscle wasting; muscle weakness; nightmares; rapid weight gain (three to five pounds within a week); rash; or unusual weakness.

INTERACTIONS

Triamcinolone interacts with other types of medication.

1. Alcohol, aspirin, and anti-inflammation medications (such as diflunisal, ibuprofen, indomethacin, mefenamic acid, meclofenamate, naproxen, piroxicam, sulindac, and tolmetin) aggravate the stomach problems that are common with use of this medication.

2. A change in the dosage requirements of oral anti-coagulants, oral anti-diabetic drugs, or insulin may be necessary when this medication is started or stopped.

3. The loss of potassium caused by triamcinolone can lead to serious side effects in individuals taking digoxin. Thiazide diuretics (water pills) can increase the potassium loss caused by triamcinolone.

4. Phenobarbital, phenytoin, rifampin, and ephedrine can increase the elimination of triamcinolone from the body, thereby decreasing its effectiveness.

5. Oral contraceptives and estrogen-containing drugs may decrease the elimination of this drug from the body, which can lead to an increase in side effects.

6. Triamcinolone can increase the elimination of aspirin and isoniazid from the body, thereby decreasing the effectiveness of these two medications.

7. Cholestyramine and colestipol can chemically bind this medication in the stomach and gastrointestinal tract, preventing its absorption.

TELL YOUR DOCTOR if you are currently taking any of the medications listed above.

WARNINGS

• Tell your doctor about unusual or allergic reactions you have had to any medications, especially to triamcinolone or other adrenocorticosteroids (such as betamethasone, cortisone, dexamethasone, fluprednisolone, hydrocortisone, methylprednisolone, paramethasone, prednisolone, or prednisone).

• Tell your doctor if you now have, or if you have ever had, bone disease; diabetes mellitus (sugar diabetes); emotional instability; glaucoma; fungal infections; heart disease; high blood pressure; high cholesterol levels; myasthenia gravis; peptic ulcers; osteoporosis; thyroid disease; tuberculosis; severe ulcerative colitis; kidney disease; or liver disease.

• If you are using this medication for longer than a week, you may need to receive higher doses if you are subjected to stress, such as serious infections, injury, or surgery. Discuss this with your doctor.

• If you have been taking this drug for more than a week, do not stop taking it suddenly. If it is stopped abruptly, you may experience abdominal or back pain, difficulty breathing, dizziness, fainting, fever, muscle or joint pain, nausea, vomiting, or extreme weakness. Your doctor may therefore want to reduce the dosage gradually. Never increase the dosage or take the drug for longer than the prescribed time, unless you first consult your doctor.

• While you are taking this drug, you should not be vaccinated or immunized. This medication decreases the effectiveness of vaccines and can lead to overwhelming infection if a live virus is administered.

• Before having any surgery or other medical or dental treatment, be sure to tell your doctor or dentist that you are taking this medication.

• Because this drug can cause glaucoma and cataracts with long-term use, your doctor may want you to have your eyes examined by an ophthalmologist periodically during treatment.

• If you are taking this medication for prolonged periods, you should wear or carry an identification card or notice stating that you are taking an adrenocorticosteroid.

● This medication can raise blood sugar levels in diabetic patients. Blood sugar should therefore be monitored carefully with blood or urine tests when this medication is started.

● Some of these products contain F.D. & C. Yellow Dye No. 5 (tartrazine), which can cause allergic-type reactions (difficulty breathing, wheezing, rash, or fainting) in certain susceptible individuals.

● Be sure to tell your doctor if you are pregnant. This drug crosses the placenta. Although studies in humans have not yet been completed, birth defects have been observed in the fetuses of animals who were given large doses of this type of drug during pregnancy. Also, tell your doctor if you are breastfeeding an infant. Small amounts of this drug pass into breast milk, and may cause growth suppression or a decrease in natural adrenocorticosteroid production in the nursing infant.

triamcinolone (topical)

BRAND NAMES (Manufacturers)
Aristocort (Lederle)
Aristocort A (Lederle)
Flutex (Syosset)
Kenac (NMC)
Kenalog (Squibb)
Kenalog-H (Squibb)
triamcinolone acetonide (various manufacturers)
Trymex (Savage)
TYPE OF DRUG
Adrenocorticosteroid hormone
INGREDIENT
triamcinolone as the acetonide salt
DOSAGE FORMS
Ointment (0.025%, 0.1%, and 0.5%)
Cream (0.025%, 0.1%, and 0.5%)
Lotion (0.025% and 0.1%)
Aerosol (two seconds of spray delivers approximately 0.2 mg of drug)

STORAGE

Triamcinolone ointment, cream, and lotion should be stored at room temperature in tightly closed containers. This medication should never be frozen.

The spray form (foam) of this medication is packed under pressure. It should not be stored near heat or an open flame, or in direct sunlight; and the container should never be punctured.

USES

Your adrenal glands naturally produce certain cortisone-like chemicals. These chemicals are involved in various regulatory processes in the body (such as fluid balance, temperature, and reactions to inflammation). Triamcinolone belongs to a group of drugs known as adrenocortico-steroids (or cortisone-like medications). It is used to relieve the skin inflammation (redness, swelling, itching, and discomfort) associated with conditions such as dermatitis, eczema, and poison ivy. How this drug acts to relieve these disorders is not completely understood.

TREATMENT

Before applying this medication, wash your hands. Then, unless your doctor gives you different instructions, gently wash the area of the skin where the medication is to be applied. With a clean towel, pat the area almost dry; it should be slightly damp when you put the medicine on.

If you are using the lotion form of this medication, shake it well before pouring out the medicine. The contents tend to settle on the bottom of the bottle, so it is necessary to shake the container to evenly distribute the ingredients and equalize the doses.

Apply a small amount of the medication to the affected area in a thin layer. Do not bandage the area unless your doctor tells you to do so. If you are to apply an occlusive dressing (like kitchen plastic wrap), be sure you understand the instructions.

If you are using the aerosol spray form of this medication, shake the can in order to disperse the medication evenly. Hold the can upright, six to eight inches from the area to be sprayed, and spray the area for one to three seconds. DO NOT SMOKE while you are using the aerosol spray; the contents are under pressure and may explode when exposed to heat or flames.

If you miss a dose of this medication, apply the dose as soon as possible, unless it is almost time for the next application. In that case, do not apply the missed dose; just return to your regular dosing schedule. Do not put twice as much medication on your skin at the next application.

SIDE EFFECTS

Minor. Acne; burning sensation; skin dryness; irritation of the affected area; itching; and rash.

If the affected area is extremely dry or scaling, the skin may be moistened by soaking in water or by applying water with a clean cloth before applying the medication. The ointment form is probably better for dry skin.

A mild, temporary stinging sensation may occur after this medication is applied. If this persists, contact your doctor.

Major. Tell your doctor about any side effects that are persistent or particularly bothersome. IT IS ESPECIALLY IMPORTANT TO TELL YOUR DOCTOR about blistering; increased hair growth; loss of skin color; secondary infection in the area being treated; or thinning of the skin with easy bruising.

INTERACTIONS

This medication does not interact with other medications, as long as it is used according to directions.

WARNINGS

• Tell your doctor about unusual or allergic reactions you have had to any medications, especially to triamcinolone or other adrenocorticosteroids (such as amcinonide, beta-methasone, clocortolone, cortisone, desonide, desoximetasone, dexamethasone, diflorasone, flumethasone, fluocinolone, fluocinonide, fluorometholone, flurandrenolide, halcinonide, hydrocortisone, methylprednisolone, prednisolone, or prednisone).

• Tell your doctor if you now have, or if you have ever had, blood vessel disease, chicken pox, diabetes mellitus (sugar diabetes), fungal infection, peptic ulcers, shingles, tuberculosis, tuberculosis of the skin, vaccinia, or any other type of infection, especially at the site currently being treated.

● If irritation develops while using this drug, immediately discontinue its use and notify your doctor.

● This product is not for use in the eyes or mucous membranes. Exposure of this medication to the eye may result in ocular (to the eye) side effects.

● Do not use this product with an occlusive wrap unless your doctor directs you to do so. Systemic absorption of this drug is increased if extensive areas of the body are treated, particularly if occlusive bandages are used. If it is necessary for you to use this drug under a wrap, follow your doctor's instructions exactly; do not leave the wrap in place longer than specified.

● If you are using this medication on a child's diaper area, do not put tight-fitting diapers or plastic pants on the child. This may lead to increased systemic absorption of the drug and a possible increase in side effects.

● In order to avoid freezing skin tissue when using the aerosol form of triamcinolone, make sure that you do not spray for more than three seconds; and hold the container at least six inches away.

● When using the aerosol form of this medication on the face, cover your eyes, and do not inhale the spray (in order to prevent side effects).

● Be sure to tell your doctor if you are pregnant. If large amounts of triamcinolone are applied for prolonged periods, some of it will be absorbed and may cross the placenta. Although studies in humans have not yet been completed, birth defects have been observed in the fetuses of animals who were given large oral doses of this type of drug during pregnancy. Also, tell your doctor if·you are breastfeeding an infant. If absorbed through the skin, small amounts of triamcinolone pass into breast milk, and may cause growth suppression or a decrease in natural adrenocorticosteroid production in the nursing infant.

triamcinolone acetonide—see triamcinolone (topical)

triamcinolone, neomycin, gramicidin, and nystatin combination—see triamcinolone, neomycin, nystatin, and gramicidin combination (topical)

triamcinolone, neomycin, nystatin, and gramicidin combination (topical)

BRAND NAMES (Manufacturers)
Mycolog (Squibb)
Myco Triacet (various manufacturers)
Mytrex (Savage)
NGT (Geneva Generics)
Nysolone (Spencer-Mead)
triamcinolone, neomycin, gramicidin, and nystatin (various manufacturers)
Tri-Statin (Rugby)

TYPE OF DRUG
Adrenocorticosteroid and anti-infective

INGREDIENTS
triamcinolone as the acetonide salt, neomycin as the sulfate salt, nystatin, and gramicidin

DOSAGE FORMS
Cream (0.1% triamcinolone, 2.5 mg neomycin, 100,000 units nystatin, and 0.25 mg gramicidin per gram)
Ointment (0.1% triamcinolone, 2.5 mg neomycin, 100,000 units nystatin, and 0.25 mg gramicidin per gram)

STORAGE
The cream and ointment should be stored at room temperature in tightly closed containers. This medication should never be frozen.

USES

Your adrenal glands naturally produce certain cortisone-like chemicals. These chemicals are involved in various regulatory processes in the body (such as fluid balance, temperature, and reactions to inflammation). Triamcinolone belongs to a group of drugs known as adrenocorticosteroids (or cortisone-like medications). It is used to relieve the skin inflammation (redness, swelling, itching, and discomfort) associated with conditions such as dermatitis, eczema, and poison ivy. How this drug acts to relieve these disorders is not completely understood. Neomycin and gramicidin are antibiotics, which act to prevent the growth and multiplication of infecting bacteria. Nystatin is an antiinfective agent that is active against the fungus *Candida albicans*.

TREATMENT

Before applying this medication, wash your hands. Then, unless your doctor gives you different instructions, gently wash the area of skin where the medication is to be applied. With a clean towel, pat the area almost dry; it should be slightly damp when you put the medication on.

Apply a small amount of this medication to the affected area in a thin layer. Do not bandage the area unless your doctor tells you to do so. If you are to apply an occlusive dressing (like kitchen plastic wrap), be sure you understand the instructions.

If you miss a dose of this medication, apply the dose as soon as possible, unless it is almost time for the next application. In that case, do not apply the missed dose; just return to your regular dosing schedule. Do not put twice as much of the medication on your skin at the next application.

SIDE EFFECTS

Minor. Acne; burning sensation; irritation of the affected area; itching; rash; and skin dryness.

If the affected area is extremely dry or scaling, the skin may be moistened by soaking in water or by applying water with a clean cloth before applying the medication. The ointment form is probably better for dry skin.

A mild, temporary stinging sensation may occur after this medication is applied. If this persists, contact your doctor.

Major. Tell your doctor about any side effects that are persistent or particularly bothersome. IT IS ESPECIALLY IMPORTANT TO TELL YOUR DOCTOR about blistering; increased hair growth; loss of skin color; secondary infection in the area being treated; or thinning of the skin with easy bruising. Also, if your symptoms of infection seem to be getting worse rather than improving, you should contact your doctor.

INTERACTIONS

This medication does not interact with other medications, as long as it is used according to directions.

WARNINGS

• Tell your doctor about unusual or allergic reactions you have had to any medications, especially to triamcinolone or other adrenocorticosteroids (such as amcinonide, betamethasone, clocortolone, desonide, desoximetasone, cortisone, dexamethasone, diflorasone, flumethasone, fluocinolone, fluocinonide, fluorometholone, flurandrenolide, halcinonide, hydrocortisone, methylprednisolone, prednisolone, or prednisone); neomycin; nystatin; or gramicidin.

• Tell your doctor if you now have, or if you have ever had, circulation problems, or viral or fungal infections of the skin (in addition to the *Candida* infection).

• If irritation develops while you are using this drug, immediately discontinue its use and notify your doctor.

• This product is not for use in the eyes, nor should it be used in the external ear canal of people with perforated eardrums. Exposure of this medication to the eye may result in ocular (to the eye) side effects.

• Do not use this product with an occlusive wrap unless your doctor directs you to do so. Systemic absorption of this drug is increased when extensive areas of the body are treated, particularly if occlusive bandages are used. If it is necessary for you to use this drug under a wrap, follow your doctor's instructions exactly; do not leave the wrap in place longer than specified.

• If you are using this medication on a child's diaper area, do not put tight-fitting diapers or plastic pants on the child. This may lead to increased systemic absorption of the drug and a possible increase in side effects.

• Be sure to tell your doctor if you are pregnant. If large amounts of this drug are applied for prolonged periods, some of it will be absorbed and may cross the placenta. Although studies in humans have not yet been completed, birth defects have been observed in the fetuses of animals who were given large oral doses of this type of drug during pregnancy. Also, tell your doctor if you are breastfeeding an infant. If absorbed through the skin, small amounts of this medication pass into breast milk, and may cause growth suppression or a decrease in natural adrenocorticosteroid production in the nursing infant.

---

triamterene

BRAND NAME (Manufacturer)
Dyrenium (Smith Kline & French)
TYPE OF DRUG
Diuretic (water pill) and anti-hypertensive
INGREDIENT
triamterene
DOSAGE FORM
Capsules (50 mg and 100 mg)
STORAGE
Triamterene should be stored at room temperature in a tightly closed, light-resistant container.

USES

Triamterene is prescribed to treat high blood pressure. It is also used to reduce fluid accumulation in the body caused by conditions such as heart failure, cirrhosis of the liver, kidney disease, and the long-term use of some medications. Triamterene reduces fluid accumulation by increasing the elimination of sodium and water through the kidneys. It may also be used in combination with other diuretics to prevent potassium loss.

TREATMENT

To decrease stomach irritation, you can take triamterene with a glass of milk or with a meal (unless your doctor directs you to do otherwise). Try to take it at the same time(s) every day. Avoid taking a dose after 6:00 P.M.—this will prevent you from having to get up during the night to urinate.

This medication does not cure high blood pressure, but it will help to control the condition, as long as you continue to take it.

If you miss a dose of this medication, take the missed dose as soon as possible, unless it is almost time for the next one. In that case, do not take the missed dose at all; just wait until the next scheduled dose. Do not double the dose.

SIDE EFFECTS

Minor. Diarrhea; dizziness; drowsiness; dry mouth; head-ache; increased thirst; nausea; tiredness; upset stomach; and vomiting. As your body adjusts to triamterene, these side effects should disappear.

Triamterene may cause the urine to turn bluish in color; this is harmless.

Dry mouth can be relieved by sucking on ice chips or a piece of hard candy, or by chewing sugarless gum.

This medication can cause increased sensitivity to sunlight. It is therefore important to avoid prolonged exposure to sunlight and sunlamps. Wear protective clothing, and use an effective sunscreen.

To avoid dizziness or light-headedness when you stand, contract and relax the muscles of your legs for a few moments before rising. Do this by pushing one foot against the floor while raising the other foot slightly, alternating feet so that you are "pumping" your legs in a pedaling motion.

Major. Tell your doctor about any side effects that are persistent or particularly bothersome. IT IS ESPECIALLY IMPORTANT TO TELL YOUR DOCTOR about anxiety; back or flank (side) pain; confusion; cracking at the corners of the mouth; difficulty breathing; extreme weakness; fever; mouth sores; painful urination; rash; a red or inflamed tongue; sore throat; or unusual bleeding or bruising

INTERACTIONS

Triamterene interacts with several foods and medications.
1. Concurrent use of it with spironolactone, amiloride, potassium salts, low-salt milk, salt substitutes, captopril, or laxatives can cause serious side effects from hyperkalemia (high levels of potassium in the blood).
2. Triamterene may decrease the effectiveness of anti-gout medications, insulin, and oral anti-diabetic medications.
3. It may increase the side effects of lithium.

4. Indomethacin may decrease the diuretic effects of triamterene.

BE SURE TO TELL YOUR DOCTOR if you are already taking any of the medications listed above.

WARNINGS

● Before starting to take triamterene, be sure to tell your doctor if you have ever had unusual or allergic reactions to medications, especially to any diuretics.

● Tell your doctor if you now have, or if you have ever had, kidney disease, kidney stones, or urination problems; hyperkalemia; diabetes mellitus (sugar diabetes); liver disease; acidosis; or gout.

● Triamterene can cause hyperkalemia (high blood levels of potassium). Signs of hyperkalemia include palpitations; confusion; numbness or tingling in the hands, feet, or lips; anxiety; or unusual tiredness or weakness. In order to avoid this problem, do not alter your diet and do not use salt substitutes unless your doctor tells you to do so.

● Limit your intake of alcoholic beverages while taking this medication, in order to prevent dizziness and light-headedness.

● Do not take any over-the-counter (non-prescription) medication for weight control, or for allergy, asthma, cough, cold, or sinus problems, unless you first check with your doctor. Some of these products can lead to an increase in blood pressure.

● To prevent severe water loss (dehydration) while taking this medication, check with your doctor if you have any illness that causes severe or continuous nausea, vomiting, or diarrhea.

● Triamterene may interfere with certain blood level determinations of quinidine (an anti-arrhythmia, heart medication). Be sure to tell your doctor that you are taking triamterene, if you are also taking quinidine.

● Be sure to tell your doctor if you are pregnant. This drug crosses the placenta. Although studies in humans have not yet been completed, adverse effects have been reported on the fetuses of animals who received large doses of this drug during pregnancy. Also, tell your doctor if you are breastfeeding an infant. Small amounts of triamterene pass into breast milk.

triamterene and hydrochlorothiazide combination

BRAND NAME (Manufacturer)
Dyazide (Smith Kline & French)
TYPE OF DRUG
Diuretic (water pill) and anti-hypertensive
INGREDIENTS
triamterene and hydrochlorothiazide
DOSAGE FORM
Capsules (50 mg triamterene and 25 mg
  hydrochlorothiazide)
STORAGE
Triamterene and hydrochlorothiazide should be stored at
room temperature in a tightly closed, light-resistant con-
tainer.

USES

Triamterene and hydrochlorothiazide combination is prescribed to treat high blood pressure. It is also used to reduce fluid accumulation in the body caused by conditions
such as heart failure, cirrhosis of the liver, kidney disease,
and the long-term use of some medications. It reduces
fluid accumulation by increasing the elimination of sodium and water through the kidneys. Triamterene is combined with hydrochlorothiazide to prevent potassium loss
from the body.

TREATMENT

To decrease stomach irritation, you can take this medication with a glass of milk or with a meal (unless your doctor
directs you to do otherwise). Try to take it at the same time
every day. Avoid taking a dose after 6:00 P.M.—this will prevent you from having to get up during the night to urinate.

This medication does not cure high blood pressure, but
it will help to control the condition, as long as you continue to take it.

If you miss a dose of this medication, take the missed
dose as soon as possible, unless it is almost time for the

next one. In that case, do not take the missed dose at all;
just wait until the next scheduled dose. Do not double the
dose.

SIDE EFFECTS

Minor. Constipation; cramps; diarrhea; dizziness;
drowsiness; dry mouth; headache; itching; loss of appetite; nausea; restlessness; upset stomach; vomiting. As
your body adjusts to this medication, these side effects
should disappear.

This medication can cause increased sensitivity to sunlight. It is therefore important to avoid prolonged exposure
to sunlight and sunlamps. Wear protective clothing, and
use an effective sunscreen.

To avoid dizziness or light-headedness when you stand,
contract and relax the muscles of your legs for a few moments before rising. Do this by pushing one foot against
the floor while raising the other foot slightly, alternating
feet so that you are "pumping" your legs in a pedaling motion.

To relieve mouth dryness, suck on ice chips or a piece of
hard candy, or chew sugarless gum.

Triamterene can cause the urine to turn to a bluish color;
this is a harmless side effect.

Major. Tell your doctor about any side effects that are persistent or particularly bothersome. IT IS ESPECIALLY IM-
PORTANT TO TELL YOUR DOCTOR about unusual
bleeding or bruising; back or flank (side) pain; cracking at
the corners of the mouth; difficulty urinating; difficulty
breathing; fatigue; mood changes; muscle cramps or
spasms; palpitations; rash; red or inflamed tongue; sore
throat; tingling in the fingers or toes; weakness; or yellowing of the eyes or skin.

INTERACTIONS

Triamterene and hydrochlorothiazide combination interacts with several foods and medications.

1. Concurrent use of it with spironolactone, amiloride,
potassium salts, low-salt milk, salt substitutes, captopril, or
laxatives can cause serious side effects from hyperkalemia
(high levels of potassium in the blood).

2. This drug may decrease the effectiveness of oral anti-coagulants, anti-gout medications, insulin, oral anti-diabetic medicines, and methenamine.

3. Fenfluramine may increase the blood-pressure-lowering effects of this drug (which can be dangerous).

4. Indomethacin may decrease the effectiveness of this medication.

5. Cholestyramine and colestipol can decrease the absorption of this medication from the gastrointestinal tract. Therefore, triamterene and hydrochlorothiazide should be taken one hour before or four hours after a dose of cholestyramine or colestipol (if you have also been prescribed one of these medications).

6. This medication may increase the side effects of amphotericin B, calcium, cortisone-like steroids (such as cortisone, dexamethasone, hydrocortisone, prednisone, prednisolone), digoxin, digitalis, lithium, quinidine, sulfonamide antibiotics, and vitamin D.

BE SURE TO TELL YOUR DOCTOR if you are already taking any of the medications listed above.

WARNINGS

• Tell your doctor about unusual or allergic reactions you have had to medications, especially to triamterene or any other diuretic (water pills), or to oral anti-diabetic medicines or sulfonamide antibiotics.

• Before you start to take triamterene and hydrochlorothiazide, tell your doctor if you now have, or if you have ever had, kidney disease or problems with urination; diabetes mellitus (sugar diabetes); gout; liver disease; asthma; pancreas disease; systemic lupus erythematosus (SLE); anemia; blood diseases; hypercalcemia; or hyperkalemia.

• This drug can occasionally cause potassium loss from the body. Signs of potassium loss include dry mouth; thirst; weakness; muscle pain or cramps; nausea; and vomiting. If you experience any of these symptoms, call your doctor.

• Triamterene can cause hyperkalemia (high levels of potassium in the blood). Signs of hyperkalemia include palpitations; confusion; numbness or tingling in the hands,

feet, or lips; anxiety; or unusual tiredness or weakness. In
order to avoid this problem, do not alter your diet and do
not use salt substitutes unless you first consult your doctor.

● Triamterene may interfere with certain blood level determinations of quinidine (an anti-arrythmia, heart medication). Be sure to tell your doctor that you are taking
triamterene and hydrochlorothiazide if you are also taking
quinidine.

● Limit your intake of alcoholic beverages while taking
this medication, in order to prevent dizziness and light-
headedness.

● Do not take any over-the-counter (non-prescription)
medication for weight control, or for allergy, asthma,
cough, cold, or sinus problems, unless you first check
with your doctor. Some of these products can lead to an
increase in blood pressure.

● To prevent severe water loss (dehydration) while taking
this medication, check with your doctor if you have any illness that causes severe nausea, vomiting, or diarrhea.

● This medication can raise blood sugar levels in diabetic
patients. Therefore, blood sugar should be monitored
carefully with blood or urine tests when this medication is
started.

● Be sure to tell your doctor if you are pregnant. This
drug crosses the placenta. Although studies in humans
have not yet been completed, adverse effects have been
observed on the fetuses of animals who received large
doses of this type of drug during pregnancy. Also, tell your
doctor if you are breastfeeding an infant. Small amounts of
this drug pass into breast milk.

Triavil—see perphenazine and amitriptyline
    combination

---

triazolam

BRAND NAME (Manufacturer)
Halcion (Upjohn)
TYPE OF DRUG
Sedative/hypnotic (sleeping aid)

INGREDIENT
triazolam
DOSAGE FORM
Tablets (0.25 mg and 0.5 mg)
STORAGE
This medication should be stored at room temperature in a tightly closed, light-resistant container.

USES
Triazolam is prescribed to treat insomnia, including problems with falling asleep, waking during the night, and early morning wakefulness. It is not clear exactly how this medicine works, but it may relieve insomnia by acting as a depressant of the central nervous system.

TREATMENT
This medicine should be taken 30 to 60 minutes before bedtime. It can be taken with a full glass of water or with food, if stomach upset occurs. Do not take this medication with a dose of antacids, since they may retard its absorption.

If you are taking this medication regularly and you miss a dose, take the missed dose immediately, if you remember within an hour of the scheduled time. If more than an hour has passed, skip the dose you missed and wait for the next scheduled dose. Do not double the dose.

SIDE EFFECTS
Minor. Bitter taste in mouth; constipation; depression; diarrhea; dizziness; drowsiness (after a night's sleep); dry mouth; fatigue; flushing; headache; heartburn; excess saliva; loss of appetite; nausea; nervousness; sweating; and vomiting. As your body adjusts to the medication, these side effects should disappear.

Dry mouth can be relieved by chewing sugarless gum or by sucking on ice chips.

If you feel dizzy, sit or lie down awhile; get up slowly, and be careful on stairs.

Major. Tell your doctor about any side effects that are persistent or particularly bothersome. IT IS ESPECIALLY IMPORTANT TO TELL YOUR DOCTOR about blurred or double vision; chest pain; difficulty urinating; fainting; falling; fever; joint pain; hallucinations; mouth sores; nightmares; palpitations; rash; severe depression; shortness of breath; slurred speech; sore throat; uncoordinated movements; unusual excitement; unusual tiredness; or yellowing of the eyes or skin.

INTERACTIONS

Triazolam interacts with a number of other medications.
1. To prevent over-sedation, it should not be taken with alcohol, other sedative drugs, or central nervous system depressants such as antihistamines, barbiturates, muscle relaxants, pain medicines, narcotics, medicines for seizures, or phenothiazine tranquilizers; or with anti-depressants.
2. Triazolam may decrease the effectiveness of carbamazepine, levodopa, and oral anti-coagulants (blood thinners, such as warfarin); and may increase the side effects of phenytoin.
3. Disulfiram, isoniazid, and cimetidine can increase the blood levels of triazolam, which can lead to toxic effects.
4. Concurrent use of rifampin may decrease the effectiveness of triazolam.
If you are already taking any of the medications listed above, CONSULT YOUR DOCTOR about their use.

WARNINGS

• Tell your doctor about any unusual or allergic reactions you have had to medications, especially to triazolam or other benzodiazepine tranquilizers (such as alprazolam, chlordiazepoxide, clorazepate, diazepam, flurazepam, halazepam, lorazepam, oxazepam, prazepam, or temazepam).
• Tell your doctor if you now have, or if you have ever had, liver disease, kidney disease, epilepsy, lung disease, myasthenia gravis, porphyria, mental depression, or mental illness.
• This medicine can cause drowsiness. Avoid tasks that require mental alertness, such as driving a car or operating potentially dangerous machinery.
• Triazolam has the potential for abuse and must be used with caution. Tolerance may develop quickly; do not in-

crease the dosage without first consulting your doctor. It is also important not to stop taking this drug suddenly if you have been taking it in large amounts, or if you have used it for several weeks. Your doctor may want to reduce the dosage gradually.

● This is a safe drug when used properly. When it is combined with other sedative drugs or with alcohol, however, serious side effects can develop.

● Be sure to tell your doctor if you are pregnant. This type of medicine may increase the chance of birth defects if it is taken during the first three months of pregnancy. In addition, too much use of this medicine during the last six months of pregnancy may lead to addiction of the fetus, resulting in withdrawal side effects in the newborn. Also, use of this medicine during the last weeks of pregnancy may cause drowsiness, slowed heartbeat, and breathing difficulties in the infant. Tell your doctor if you are breastfeeding an infant. This medicine can pass into breast milk and cause drowsiness, slowed heartbeat, and breathing difficulties in nursing infants.

Tri-Bay-Flor—see vitamins A, D, and C with fluoride

Trichlorex—see trichlormethiazide

---

trichlormethiazide

BRAND NAMES (Manufacturers)
Aquazide (Western Research)
Diurese (American Urologicals)
Metahydrin (Merrell Dow)
Mono-Press (T.E. Williams)
Naqua (Schering)
Niazide (Major)
Trichlorex (Lannett)
trichlormethiazide (various manufacturers)
TYPE OF DRUG
Diuretic (water pill) and anti-hypertensive
INGREDIENT
trichlormethiazide

DOSAGE FORM
Tablets (2 mg and 4 mg)
STORAGE
This medication should be stored at room temperature in a tightly closed container.

USES

Trichlormethiazide is prescribed to treat high blood pressure. It is also used to reduce fluid accumulation in the body caused by conditions such as heart failure, cirrhosis of the liver, kidney disease, and the long-term use of some medications. This medication reduces fluid accumulation by increasing the elimination of sodium and water through the kidneys.

TREATMENT

To decrease stomach irritation, you can take this medication with a glass of milk or with a meal (unless your doctor directs you to do otherwise). Try to take it at the same time every day. Avoid taking a dose after 6:00 P.M.—this will prevent you from having to get up during the night to urinate.

If you miss a dose of this medication, take the missed dose as soon as possible, unless it is almost time for the next dose. In that case, do not take the missed dose at all; just wait until the next scheduled dose. Do not double the dose.

This medication does not cure high blood pressure, but it will help to control the condition, as long as you continue to take it.

SIDE EFFECTS

Minor. Constipation; cramps; diarrhea; dizziness; drowsiness; headache; heartburn; itching; loss of appetite; nausea; restlessness; upset stomach; vomiting. As your body adjusts to the medication, these side effects should disappear.

This medication can cause increased sensitivity to sunlight. It is therefore important to avoid prolonged exposure to sunlight and sunlamps. Wear protective clothing, and use an effective sunscreen.

To avoid dizziness or light-headedness when you stand, contract and relax the muscles of your legs for a few moments before rising. Do this by pushing one foot against the floor while raising the other foot slightly, alternating feet so that you are "pumping" your legs in a pedaling motion.

Major. Tell your doctor about any side effects that are persistent or particularly bothersome. IT IS ESPECIALLY IMPORTANT TO TELL YOUR DOCTOR about unusual bleeding or bruising; blurred vision; confusion; difficulty breathing; dry mouth; excessive thirst; fever; joint pain; mood changes; muscle spasms; palpitations; skin rash; sore throat; tingling in the fingers or toes; excessive weakness; or yellowing of the eyes or skin.

INTERACTIONS

Trichlormethiazide interacts with several other types of medication.

1. It may decrease the effectiveness of oral anti-coagulants, anti-gout medications, insulin, oral anti-diabetic medicines, and methenamine.

2. Fenfluramine can increase the blood-pressure-lowering effects of trichlormethiazide (which can be dangerous).

3. Indomethacin can decrease the blood-pressure-lowering effects (thereby counteracting the desired effects) of trichlormethiazide.

4. Cholestyramine and colestipol decrease the absorption of this medication from the gastrointestinal tract. Trichlormethiazide should therefore be taken one hour before, or four hours after, a dose of cholestyramine or colestipol (if you have also been prescribed one of these medications).

5. Trichlormethiazide may increase the side effects of amphotericin B, calcium, cortisone-like steroids (such as cortisone, dexamethasone, hydrocortisone, prednisone, prednisolone), digoxin, digitalis, lithium, quinidine, sulfonamide antibiotics, and vitamin D.

BE SURE TO TELL YOUR DOCTOR if you are already taking any of the medications listed above.

WARNINGS

● Tell your doctor about unusual or allergic reactions you have had to any medications, especially to diuretics, oral anti-diabetic medications, or sulfonamide antibiotics.

• Before you start taking trichlormethiazide, tell your doctor if you now have, or if you have ever had, kidney disease or problems with urination, diabetes mellitus (sugar diabetes), gout, liver disease, asthma, pancreas disease, or systemic lupus erythematosus (SLE).

• Trichlormethiazide can cause potassium loss. Signs of potassium loss include dry mouth, thirst, weakness, muscle pain or cramps, nausea, and vomiting. If you experience any of these symptoms, call your doctor. To help avoid potassium loss, take this drug with a glass of fresh or frozen orange or cranberry juice, or eat a banana every day. The use of a salt substitute also helps to prevent potassium loss. Do not change your diet, however, before discussing it with your doctor. Too much potassium can also be dangerous. Your doctor may want you to have blood tests performed periodically, in order to monitor your potassium levels.

• Limit your intake of alcoholic beverages while taking this medication, in order to prevent dizziness and lightheadedness.

• If you have high blood pressure, do not take any over-the-counter (non-prescription) medications for weight control or for allergy, asthma, cough, cold, or sinus problems, unless your doctor directs you to do so.

• To prevent dehydration (severe water loss) while taking this medication, check with your doctor if you have any illness that causes severe nausea, vomiting, or diarrhea.

• This medication can raise blood sugar levels in diabetic patients. Therefore, blood sugar should be carefully monitored by blood or urine tests when this medication is started.

• Some of these products contain F.D. & C. Yellow Dye No. 5 (tartrazine), which can cause allergic-type reactions (difficulty breathing, wheezing, rash, or fainting) in certain susceptible individuals.

• Be sure to tell your doctor if you are pregnant. This drug is able to cross the placenta. Although studies in humans have not been completed, adverse effects have been observed on the fetuses of animals who received large doses of this type of drug during pregnancy. Also, tell your doctor if you are breastfeeding an infant. Although problems in humans have not been reported, small amounts of

this drug can pass into breast milk, so caution is war
ranted

Trifed-C—see pseudoephedrine, tripolidine,
   guaifenesin, and codeine combination

---

trifluoperazine

BRAND NAMES (Manufacturers)
Stelazine (Smith Kline & French)
Suprazine (Major)
trifluoperazine (various manufacturers)
TYPE OF DRUG
Phenothiazine tranquilizer
INGREDIENT
trifluoperazine as the hydrochloride salt
DOSAGE FORMS
Tablets (1 mg, 2 mg, 5 mg, and 10 mg)
Oral concentrate (100 mg per ml)
STORAGE
The tablet form of this medication should be stored at
room temperature in a tightly closed, light-resistant con-
tainer. The oral concentrate form of this medication should
be stored in the refrigerator in a tightly closed, light-resis-
tant container. If the oral concentrate turns to a slight yellow color, the medicine is still effective and can be used.
However, if it changes color markedly, or has particles
floating in it, it should not be used, but discarded down
the sink. This medication should never be frozen.

USES

Trifluoperazine is prescribed to treat the symptoms of certain types of mental illness, such as emotional symptoms
of psychosis, the manic phase of manic-depressive illness,
and severe behavioral problems in children. This medication is thought to relieve the symptoms of mental illness by
blocking certain chemicals involved with nerve transmission in the brain.

TREATMENT

In order to avoid stomach irritation, you can take the tablet form of this medication with a meal or with a glass of water or milk (unless your doctor directs you to do otherwise).

The oral concentrate form of this medication should be measured carefully with the dropper provided, then added to 4 ounces ($^1/_2$ cup) or more of water, milk, juice, or a carbonated beverage, or to applesauce or pudding, immediately prior to administration. To prevent possible loss of effectiveness, the medication should not be diluted with tea, coffee, or apple juice.

Antacids and anti-diarrhea medicine may decrease the absorption of this medication from the gastrointestinal tract. Therefore, at least one hour should separate doses of one of these medicines and trifluoperazine.

If you miss a dose of this medication, take the missed dose as soon as possible and return to your regular dosing schedule. If it is almost time for the next dose, however, skip the one you missed and return to your regular schedule. Do not double the dose (unless your doctor directs you to do so).

The full effects of this medication for the control of emotional or mental symptoms may not become apparent for two weeks after you start to take it.

SIDE EFFECTS

Minor. Blurred vision; constipation; decreased sweating; diarrhea; discoloration of the urine to red, pink, or red-brown; dizziness; drooling; drowsiness; dry mouth; fatigue; jitteriness; menstrual irregularities; nasal congestion; restlessness; tremors; vomiting; and weight gain. As your body adjusts to the medication, these side effects should disappear.

If you are constipated, increase the amount of fiber in your diet (raw vegetables, fruits, salads, bran, and whole-grain breads), and drink more water (unless your doctor directs you to do otherwise).

Chew sugarless gum, or suck on ice chips or a piece of hard candy, to reduce mouth dryness.

This medication can cause increased sensitivity to sunlight. It is therefore important to avoid prolonged exposure to sunlight and sunlamps. Wear protective clothing, and use an effective sunscreen.

To avoid dizziness or light-headedness when you stand, contract and relax the muscles of your legs for a few moments before rising. Do this by pushing one foot against the floor while raising the other foot slightly, alternating feet so that you are "pumping" your legs in a pedaling motion.

Major. Tell your doctor about any side effects that are persistent or particularly bothersome. IT IS ESPECIALLY IMPORTANT TO TELL YOUR DOCTOR about any unusual bleeding or bruising; breast enlargement (in both sexes); chest pain; convulsions; darkened skin; difficulty swallowing or breathing; fainting; fever; impotence; involuntary movements of the face, mouth, jaw, or tongue; palpitations; rash; sleep disorders; sore throat; uncoordinated movements; visual disturbances; or yellowing of the eyes or skin.

INTERACTIONS

Trifluoperazine interacts with several other types of medication.

1. It can cause extreme drowsiness when combined with alcohol or other central nervous system depressants (drugs that slow the activity of the nervous system), such as barbiturates, benzodiazepine tranquilizers, muscle relaxants, narcotics, and pain medications; or with tricyclic anti-depressants.

2. Trifluoperazine can decrease the effectiveness of amphetamines, guanethidine, anti-convulsants, and levodopa.

3. The side effects of epinephrine, monoamine oxidase (MAO) inhibitors, propranolol, phenytoin, and tricyclic anti-depressants may be increased when combined with this medication.

4. Lithium may increase the side effects and decrease the effectiveness of this medication.

Before starting to take trifluoperazine, BE SURE TO TELL YOUR DOCTOR if you are already taking any of the medications listed above.

WARNINGS

• Tell your doctor about any unusual or allergic reactions you have had to medications, especially to trifluoperazine

or other phenothiazine tranquilizers (such as acetophenazine, carphenazine, chlorpromazine, fluphenazine, mesoridazine, perphenazine, piperacetazine, prochlorperazine, promazine, thioridazine, and triflupromazine), or to
loxapine.

● Tell your doctor if you now have, or if you have ever
had, any blood disease, bone marrow disease, brain disease, breast cancer, blockage of the urinary or digestive
tract, alcoholism, drug-induced depression, epilepsy, severe high or low blood pressure, diabetes mellitus (sugar
diabetes), glaucoma, heart or circulatory disease, liver disease, lung disease, Parkinson's disease, peptic ulcers, or
an enlarged prostate gland.

● Tell your doctor about any recent exposure to a pesticide or an insecticide. Trifluoperazine may increase the
side effects from the exposure.

● To prevent over-sedation, avoid drinking alcoholic beverages while taking this medication.

● If this medication makes you dizzy or drowsy, do not
take part in any activity that requires alertness, such as
driving a car or operating potentially dangerous equipment. Be careful on stairs, and avoid getting up suddenly
from a lying or sitting position.

● Prior to having surgery or any other medical or dental
treatment, be sure to tell your doctor or dentist that you are
taking this medication.

● Some of the side effects caused by this drug can be prevented by taking an anti-parkinson drug. Discuss this with
your doctor.

● This type of medication has been reported to cause certain tumors in rats. This effect has not been shown to occur in humans.

● This medication can decrease sweating and heat release from the body. You should therefore avoid getting
overheated (strenuous exercise in hot weather; hot baths,
showers, and saunas).

● Do not stop taking this medication suddenly. If the drug
is stopped abruptly, you may experience nausea, vomiting,
stomach upset, headache, increased heart rate, insomnia,
tremulousness, or a worsening of your condition. Your
doctor may want to reduce the dosage gradually.

● If you are planning to have a myelogram, or any procedure in which dye will be injected into your spinal cord, tell your doctor that you are taking this medication.

• Avoid spilling the oral concentrate form of this medication on your skin or clothing; it may cause redness and irritation of the skin.

• While taking this medication, do not take any over-the-counter (non-prescription) medication for weight control, or for cough, cold, allergy, asthma, or sinus problems, unless you first check with your doctor. The combination of these medications with trifluoperazine may cause high blood pressure.

• Be sure to tell your doctor if you are pregnant. Small amounts of this medication cross the placenta. Although there are reports of safe use of this drug during pregnancy, there are also reports of liver disease and tremors in newborn infants whose mothers received this medication close to term. Also, tell your doctor if you are breastfeeding an infant. Small amounts of this medication pass into breast milk, and may cause unwanted effects in nursing infants.

trifluoperazine hydrochloride—see trifluoperazine

---

triflupromazine

BRAND NAME (Manufacturer)
Vesprin (Squibb)
TYPE OF DRUG
Phenothiazine tranquilizer
INGREDIENT
triflupromazine as the hydrochloride salt
DOSAGE FORM
Oral suspension (50 mg per 5 ml teaspoonful)
STORAGE
This medication should be stored in the refrigerator in a tightly closed, light-resistant container. It should never be frozen.

USES

Triflupromazine is prescribed to treat the symptoms of certain types of mental illness, such as emotional symptoms of psychosis, the manic phase of manic-depressive illness, and severe behavioral problems in children. This medication is thought to relieve the symptoms of mental illness by blocking certain chemicals involved with nerve transmission in the brain. Triflupromazine may also be used to treat anxiety, nausea, and vomiting (this medication works at the vomiting center in the brain, to relieve nausea and vomiting).

TREATMENT

In order to avoid stomach irritation, you can take this medication with a meal or with a glass of water or milk (unless your doctor directs you to do otherwise).

To ensure accurate dosage of triflupromazine, be sure to shake the bottle well to evenly disperse the medication. Then, measure the oral suspension carefully with a specially designed, 5 ml measuring spoon. An ordinary kitchen teaspoon is not accurate enough.

Antacids and anti-diarrhea medicine may decrease the absorption of this medication from the gastrointestinal tract. Therefore, at least one hour should separate doses of one of these medicines and triflupromazine.

If you miss a dose of this medication, take the missed dose as soon as possible and return to your regular dosing schedule. If it is almost time for the next dose, however, skip the one you missed and return to your regular schedule. Do not double the dose (unless your doctor directs you to do so).

The full effects of this medication for the control of emotional or mental symptoms may not become apparent for two weeks after you start to take it.

SIDE EFFECTS

Minor. Blurred vision; constipation; decreased sweating; diarrhea; discoloration of the urine to red, pink, or red-brown; dizziness; drooling; drowsiness; dry mouth; fatigue; jitteriness; menstrual irregularities; nasal congestion; restlessness; tremors; vomiting; and weight gain. As your body adjusts to the medication, these side effects should disappear.

If you are constipated, increase the amount of fiber in your diet (raw vegetables, fruits, salads, bran, and whole-grain breads), and drink more water (unless your doctor directs you to do otherwise).

Chew sugarless gum, or suck on ice chips or a piece of hard candy, to reduce mouth dryness.

This medication can cause increased sensitivity to sunlight. It is therefore important to avoid prolonged exposure to sunlight and sunlamps. Wear protective clothing, and use an effective sunscreen.

To avoid dizziness or light-headedness when you stand, contract and relax the muscles of your legs for a few moments before rising. Do this by pushing one foot against the floor while raising the other foot slightly, alternating feet so that you are "pumping" your legs in a pedaling motion.

Major. Tell your doctor about any side effects that are persistent or particularly bothersome. IT IS ESPECIALLY IMPORTANT TO TELL YOUR DOCTOR about any unusual bleeding or bruising; breast enlargement (in both sexes); chest pain; convulsions; darkened skin; difficulty swallowing or breathing; fainting; fever; impotence; involuntary movements of the face, mouth, jaw, or tongue; palpitations; rash; sleep disorders; sore throat; uncoordinated movements; visual disturbances; or yellowing of the eyes or skin.

INTERACTIONS

Triflupromazine interacts with several other types of medication.

1. It can cause extreme drowsiness when combined with alcohol or other central nervous system depressants (drugs that slow the activity of the nervous system), such as barbiturates, benzodiazepine tranquilizers, muscle relaxants, narcotics, or pain medications; or with tricyclic anti-depressants.

2. Triflupromazine can decrease the effectiveness of amphetamines, guanethidine, anti-convulsants, and levodopa.

3. The side effects of epinephrine, monoamine oxidase (MAO) inhibitors, propranolol, phenytoin, and tricyclic anti-depressants may be increased when combined with this medication.

4. Lithium may increase the side effects and decrease the effectiveness of this medication.

Before starting to take triflupromazine, BE SURE TO TELL YOUR DOCTOR if you are already taking any of the medications listed above.

WARNINGS

• Tell your doctor about any unusual or allergic reactions you have had to medications, especially to triflupromazine or other phenothiazine tranquilizers (such as acetophenazine, carphenazine, chlorpromazine, fluphenazine, mesoridazine, perphenazine, piperacetazine, prochlorperazine, promazine, thioridazine, and trifluoperazine), or to loxapine.

• Tell your doctor if you now have, or if you have ever had, any blood disease, bone marrow disease, brain disease, breast cancer, blockage of the urinary or digestive tract, alcoholism, drug-induced depression, epilepsy, severe high or low blood pressure, diabetes mellitus (sugar diabetes), glaucoma, heart or circulatory disease, liver disease, lung disease, Parkinson's disease, peptic ulcers, or an enlarged prostate gland.

• Tell your doctor about any recent exposure to a pesticide or an insecticide. Triflupromazine may increase the side effects from the exposure.

• To prevent over-sedation, avoid drinking alcoholic beverages while taking this medication.

• If this medication makes you dizzy or drowsy, do not take part in any activity that requires alertness, such as driving a car or operating potentially dangerous equipment. Be careful on stairs, and avoid getting up suddenly from a lying or sitting position.

• Prior to having surgery or any other medical or dental treatment, be sure to tell your doctor or dentist that you are taking this medication.

• Some of the side effects caused by this drug can be prevented by taking an anti-parkinson drug. Discuss this with your doctor.

• This type of medication has been reported to cause certain tumors in rats. This effect has not been shown to occur in humans.

• This medication can decrease sweating and heat release from the body. You should therefore avoid getting overheated (strenuous exercise in hot weather; hot baths, showers, and saunas).

• Do not stop taking this medication suddenly. If the drug is stopped abruptly, you may experience nausea, vomiting, stomach upset, headache, increased heart rate, insomnia, tremulousness, or a worsening of your condition. Your doctor may want to reduce the dosage gradually.

• If you are planning to have a myelogram, or any procedure in which dye will be injected into your spinal cord, be sure to tell your doctor that you are taking this medication.

• Avoid spilling this medication on your skin or clothing; it may cause redness and irritation of the skin.

• While taking this medicine, do not use any over-the-counter (non-prescription) medication for weight control, or for cough, cold, allergy, asthma, or sinus problems, unless you first check with your doctor. The combination of these medications with triflupromazine may cause high blood pressure.

• Be sure to tell your doctor if you are pregnant. Small amounts of this medication cross the placenta. Although there are reports of safe use of this drug during pregnancy, there are also reports of liver disease and tremors in newborn infants whose mothers received this type of medication close to term. Also, tell your doctor if you are breastfeeding an infant. Small amounts of this medication pass into breast milk, and may cause unwanted effects in nursing infants.

Trigot—see ergoloid mesylates

Trihexane—see trihexyphenidyl

Trihexidyl—see trihexyphenidyl

Trihexy—see trihexyphenidyl

trihexyphenidyl

BRAND NAMES (Manufacturers)
Aphen (Major)

Artane (Lederle)
Artane Sequels (Lederle)
Tremin (Schering)
Trihexane (Rugby)
Trihexidyl (Henry Schein)
Trihexy (Geneva Generics)
trihexyphenidyl hydrochloride (various manufacturers)
TYPE OF DRUG
Anti-parkinson
INGREDIENT
trihexyphenidyl as the hydrochloride salt
DOSAGE FORMS
Tablets (2 mg and 5 mg)
Sustained-release capsules (5 mg)
Oral elixir (2 mg per 5 ml teaspoonful, with 5% alcohol)
STORAGE
Trihexyphenidyl tablets, capsules, and oral elixir should
be stored at room temperature in tightly closed containers.
This medication should never be frozen.

USES

Trihexyphenidyl is used to treat the symptoms of Parkinson's disease or to control the side effects of phenothiazine tranquilizers. It is not clearly understood how this
medication works, but it is thought to act by balancing certain chemicals in the brain.

TREATMENT

In order to reduce stomach irritation, you should take trihexyphenidyl with food, or just after a meal.

Antacids and anti-diarrhea medicines prevent the absorption of this medication, so at least one hour should
separate doses of trihexyphenidyl and one of these medicines.

The oral elixir form of this medication should be measured carefully, with a specially designed, 5 ml measuring
spoon. An ordinary kitchen teaspoon is not accurate
enough.

The sustained-release capsules should be swallowed
whole. Chewing, crushing, or breaking the capsules destroys their sustained-release activity, and possibly increases the side effects.

If you miss a dose of this medication, take the missed dose as soon as possible, unless it is within two hours of the next dose (for the tablets or oral elixir), or within eight hours of the next dose (for the sustained-release capsules). In that case, don't take the missed dose at all; just return to your regular dosing schedule. Do not double the next dose.

SIDE EFFECTS

Minor. Bloating; blurred vision; constipation; dizziness; drowsiness; dry mouth, throat, and nose; false sense of well-being; headache; increased sensitivity of the eyes to light; muscle cramps; nausea; nervousness; reduced sweating; and weakness. These side effects should disappear in several days, as your body adjusts to the medication.

If you are constipated, increase the amount of fiber in your diet (fresh fruits and vegetables, salads, bran, whole-grain breads), exercise, and drink more water (unless your doctor directs you to do otherwise).

Chew sugarless gum, or suck on ice chips or a piece of hard candy, to reduce mouth dryness.

Wear sunglasses if your eyes become sensitive to light.

To avoid dizziness and light-headedness when you stand, contract and relax the muscles of your legs for a few moments before rising. Do this by pushing one foot against the floor while raising the other foot slightly, alternating feet so that you are "pumping" your legs in a pedaling motion.

Major. Tell your doctor about any side effects that are persistant or particularly bothersome. IT IS ESPECIALLY IMPORTANT TO TELL YOUR DOCTOR about depression; difficulty urinating; hallucinations; involuntary muscle movements; numbness or tingling of the fingers or toes; palpitations; or unusual excitement.

INTERACTIONS

Trihexyphenidyl interacts with other types of medication.

1. It can cause extreme drowsiness when combined with alcohol or other central nervous system depressants (drugs that slow the activity of the nervous system), such as antihistamines, barbiturates, benzodiazepine tranquilizers, muscle relaxants, narcotics, and pain medications; or with tricyclic anti-depressants.

2. Amantadine, antihistamines, haloperidol, monoamine oxidase (MAO) inhibitors, phenothiazine tranquilizers, procainamide, quinidine, and tricyclic anti-depressants can increase the side effects of trihexyphenidyl.

3. Trihexyphenidyl can increase the elimination of chlorpromazine from the body, and decrease its effectiveness.

BE SURE TO TELL YOUR DOCTOR if you are already taking any of the medications listed above.

WARNINGS

● Tell your doctor about unusual or allergic reactions you have had to any medications, especially to trihexyphenidyl.

● Tell your doctor if you now have, or if you have ever had, achalasia, glaucoma, heart disease, myasthenia gravis, blockage of the intestinal or urinary tract, enlarged prostate gland, stomach ulcers, or thyroid disease.

● If this medication makes you dizzy or drowsy, do not take part in any activity that requires alertness, such as driving a car or operating potentially dangerous equipment. Be careful on stairs; and avoid getting up from a lying or sitting position suddenly.

● This medication can decrease sweating and heat release from the body. You should therefore avoid getting overheated (strenuous exercise in hot weather; hot baths, showers, or saunas).

● Be sure to tell your doctor if you are pregnant. Although trihexyphenidyl appears to be safe during pregnancy, extensive studies have not yet been completed. Also, tell your doctor if you are breastfeeding an infant. Small amounts of this medication may pass into breast milk.

trihexyphenidyl hydrochloride—see trihexyphenidyl

Tri-Hydroserpine—see hydralazine,
    hydrochlorothiazide, and reserpine combination

Trilafon—see perphenazine

Trilafon Repetabs—see perphenazine

Trimcaps—see phendimetrazine

---

trimethobenzamide

BRAND NAMES (Manufacturers)
Tegamide (G & W)
Tigan (Beecham)
trimethobenzamide (various manufacturers)
TYPE OF DRUG
Anti-emetic (anti-nauseant)
INGREDIENT
trimethobenzamide as the hydrochloride salt
DOSAGE FORMS
Capsules (100 mg and 250 mg)
Suppositories (100 mg and 200 mg)
STORAGE
Trimethobenzamide capsules and suppositories should be stored at room temperature in tightly closed containers.

USES

Trimethobenzamide is used to control nausea and vomiting. It is thought to act directly on the vomiting center in the brain.

TREATMENT

Trimethobenzamide capsules can be taken with a full glass of water.

The suppository form of this medication should be inserted into the rectum (if the suppository is too soft to insert, run it under cold water or put it in the refrigerator for 30 minutes). To insert it, remove the foil wrapper; moisten the suppository with a little water; then lie down on your left side with your right knee bent. Push the suppository up into your rectum with your finger. Remain lying down for a few minutes. Try to avoid having a bowel movement for an hour or longer, to allow the drug time to be absorbed.

If you miss a dose of this medication, take the missed dose as soon as possible, unless it is almost time for the next dose. In that case, do not take the missed dose at all; just return to your regular dosing schedule. Do not double the next dose.

SIDE EFFECTS

Minor. Diarrhea; dizziness; drowsiness; headache; and muscle cramps. These side effects should disappear in several days, as your body adjusts to the medication.

If you feel dizzy or light-headed, sit or lie down awhile; get up slowly, and be careful on stairs.

Major. Tell your doctor about any side effects that are persistent or particularly bothersome. IT IS ESPECIALLY IMPORTANT TO TELL YOUR DOCTOR about back pain; unusual bleeding or bruising; blurred vision; convulsions; depression; disorientation; mouth sores; rash; tremors; unusual hand or face movements; or yellowing of the eyes or skin.

INTERACTIONS

Concurrent use of trimethobenzamide with central nervous system depressants (drugs that slow the activity of the nervous system), such as alcohol, antihistamines, barbiturates, benzodiazepine tranquilizers, muscle relaxants, narcotics, pain medications, phenothiazine tranquilizers and sleeping medications, or with tricyclic anti-depressants can cause extreme drowsiness.

BE SURE TO TELL YOUR DOCTOR if you are already taking one of these medications.

WARNINGS

• Tell your doctor about unusual or allergic reactions you have had to any medications, especially to trimethobenzamide (or to benzocaine if you are using the suppository form).

• Before starting to take this medication, be sure to tell your doctor if you now have, or if you have ever had, acute fever, dehydration, electrolyte imbalance, encephalitis, enteritis, intestinal infection, or viral infections.

• If this drug makes you dizzy or drowsy, do not take part in any activity that requires alertness, such as driving a car or operating potentially dangerous equipment.

• Be sure to tell your doctor if you are pregnant. Although this drug appears to be safe, extensive studies in pregnant women have not yet been completed. Also, tell your doctor if you are breastfeeding an infant. It is not known whether or not trimethobenzamide passes into breast milk.

trimethoprim

BRAND NAMES (Manufacturers)
Proloprim (Burroughs Wellcome)
trimethoprim (various manufacturers)
Trimpex (Roche)
TYPE OF DRUG
Antibiotic (infection fighter)
INGREDIENT
trimethoprim
DOSAGE FORM
Tablets (100 mg and 200 mg)
STORAGE
Trimethoprim tablets should be stored in a dry place at room temperature, in a light-resistant container.

USES

This antibiotic is used in the treatment of uncomplicated urinary tract infections. It acts by preventing production of the nutrients that are required for the growth of the infecting bacteria. Trimethoprim kills a wide range of bacteria, but it is not effective against viruses or fungi.

TREATMENT

You can take trimethoprim tablets on an empty stomach or, to avoid stomach upset, with food or milk.

This medication works best when the level of the medicine in your urine is kept constant. It is best therefore to take the doses at evenly spaced intervals, day and night. For example, if you are to take two doses a day, the doses should be spaced 12 hours apart.

If you miss a dose of this medication, take the missed dose immediately. However, if you do not remember to take the missed dose until it is almost time for your next dose, space the missed dose and the following dose about ten to 12 hours apart (if you take one dose a day), or five to six hours apart (if you are taking two doses a day). Then return to your regular dosing schedule. Try not to skip any doses.

It is important to continue to take this medication for the entire time prescribed by your doctor (usually seven to 14 days), even if the symptoms disappear before the end of that period. If you stop taking the drug too soon, resistant bacteria are given a chance to continue growing, and the infection could recur.

SIDE EFFECTS

Minor. Abdominal pain; diarrhea; headache; loss of appetite; nausea; swollen or inflamed tongue; unusual taste in the mouth; vomiting. These side effects should disappear in several days, as your body adjusts to the medication.

Major. Tell your doctor about any side effects that are persistent or particularly bothersome. IT IS ESPECIALLY IMPORTANT TO TELL YOUR DOCTOR about unusual bleeding or bruising; itching; skin rash; sore throat and fever; unusual fatigue; or unusually pale skin. Also, if your symptoms of infection seem to be getting worse rather than improving, you should contact your doctor.

INTERACTIONS

Trimethoprim interacts with several other medications.

1. Rifampin can increase the elimination of trimethoprim from the body and decrease its anti-bacterial effectiveness.

2. Concurrent use of trimethoprim with anti-neoplastic agents (anti-cancer drugs) can increase the risk of developing blood disorders.

3. Trimethoprim can decrease the elimination of phenytoin from the body and increase the chance of side effects. Before starting to take this medication, BE SURE TO TELL YOUR DOCTOR if you are already taking any of the medications listed above.

WARNINGS

• Tell your doctor about unusual or allergic reactions you have had to any medications, especially to trimethoprim.

• Tell your doctor if you now have, or if you have ever

had, megaloblastic anemia (folate-deficiency anemia), kidney disease, or liver disease.
• This medication has been prescribed for your current infection only. Another infection later on, or one that someone else has, may require a different medicine. You should not give your medicine to other people, or use it for other infections, unless your doctor specifically directs you to do so.
• If there is no improvement in your condition several days after starting this medication, check with your doctor. Trimethoprim may not be effective against the bacteria causing your infection.
• Before having any surgery or other medical or dental treatment, be sure to tell your doctor or dentist that you are taking this medication.
• Be sure to tell your doctor if you are pregnant. Although there are reports of safe use of trimethoprim during pregnancy, extensive studies in humans have not yet been completed. In addition, this medication has been shown to cause birth defects in the offspring of animals who received very large doses of it during pregnancy. Also, tell your doctor if you are breastfeeding an infant. Small amounts of trimethoprim pass into breast milk, and there is a chance that it may cause anemia in the nursing infant.

trimipramine

BRAND NAME (Manufacturer)
Surmontil (Ives)
TYPE OF DRUG
Tricyclic anti-depressant (mood elevator)
INGREDIENT
trimipramine as the maleate salt
DOSAGE FORM
Capsules (25 mg, 50 mg, and 100 mg)
STORAGE
This medication should be stored at room temperature in a tightly closed container.

USES
Trimipramine is used to relieve the symptoms of mental

depression. This medication belongs to a group of drugs referred to as the tricyclic anti-depressants. These medicines are thought to relieve depression by increasing the concentration of certain chemicals necessary for nerve transmission in the brain.

TREATMENT

This medication should be taken exactly as your doctor prescribes. You can take it with water or with food to lessen the chance of stomach irritation, unless your doctor tells you to do otherwise.

If you miss a dose of this medication, take the missed dose as soon as possible, then return to your regular dosing schedule. However, if the dose you missed was a once-a-day bedtime dose, do not take that dose in the morning; check with your doctor instead. If the dose is taken in the morning, it may cause some unwanted side effects. Never double the dose.

The effects of therapy with this medication may not become apparent for two or three weeks.

SIDE EFFECTS

Minor. Agitation; anxiety; blurred vision; confusion; constipation; cramps; diarrhea; dizziness; drowsiness; dry mouth; fatigue; heartburn; insomnia; loss of appetite; nausea; peculiar tastes in the mouth; restlessness; sweating; vomiting; weakness; and weight gain or loss. As your body adjusts to the medication, these side effects should disappear.

Dry mouth can be relieved by chewing sugarless gum, or by sucking on ice chips or a piece of hard candy.

To relieve constipation, increase the amount of fiber (bran, salad, fruits, whole-grain breads, and fresh vegetables) in your diet, and drink more water (unless your doctor directs you to do otherwise).

To avoid dizziness or light-headedness when you stand, contract and relax the muscles of your legs for a few moments before rising. Do this by pushing one foot against the floor while raising the other foot slightly, alternating feet so that you are "pumping" your legs in a pedaling motion.

This medication may cause increased sensitivity to sunlight. You should therefore avoid prolonged exposure to sunlight and sunlamps. Wear protective clothing, and use an effective sunscreen.

Major. Tell your doctor about any side effects that are persistent or are particularly bothersome. IT IS ESPECIALLY IMPORTANT TO TELL YOUR DOCTOR about chest pain; convulsions; difficulty urinating; enlarged or painful breasts (in both sexes); fainting; fever; hair loss; hallucinations; headaches; impotence; mood changes; mouth sores; nervousness; nightmares; numbness in the fingers or toes; palpitations; rapid weight gain (three to five pounds within a week); ringing in the ears; seizures; skin rash; sleep disorders; sore throat; tremors; uncoordinated movements or balance problems; unusual bleeding or bruising; or yellowing of the eyes or skin.

INTERACTIONS

Trimipramine interacts with other types of medication.

1. Extreme drowsiness can occur when this medicine is taken with central nervous system depressants (medicines that slow the activity of the nervous system), including alcohol, antihistamines, barbiturates, benzodiazepine tranquilizers, muscle relaxants, narcotics, pain medications, phenothiazine tranquilizers, and sleeping medications, or with other tricyclic anti-depressants.

2. Trimipramine may decrease the effectiveness of anti-seizure medications, and may block the blood-pressure-lowering effects of clonidine and guanethidine.

3. Oral contraceptives (estrogens) can increase the side effects and reduce the effectiveness of the tricyclic anti-depressants (including trimipramine).

4. Tricyclic anti-depressants may increase the side effects of thyroid medication and over-the-counter (non-prescription) cough, cold, allergy, asthma, sinus, and diet medications.

5. The concurrent use of tricyclic anti-depressants and monoamine oxidase (MAO) inhibitors should be undertaken very carefully, because the combination may result in fever, convulsions, or high blood pressure.

Before starting to take trimipramine, BE SURE TO TELL YOUR DOCTOR if you are already taking any of the medications listed above.

WARNINGS

- Tell your doctor if you have had unusual or allergic reactions to any medications, especially to trimipramine or other tricyclic anti-depressants (such as amitriptyline, imipramine, doxepin, amoxapine, protriptyline, desipramine, maprotiline, and nortriptyline).
- Tell your doctor if you now have, or if you have ever had, asthma, high blood pressure, liver or kidney disease, heart disease, a recent heart attack, circulatory disease, stomach problems, intestinal problems, alcoholism, difficulty urinating, enlarged prostate gland, epilepsy, glaucoma, thyroid disease, mental illness, or electroshock therapy.
- If this drug makes you dizzy or drowsy, do not take part in any activity that requires alertness, such as driving a car or operating potentially dangerous equipment.
- Before having any surgery or other medical or dental treatment, be sure to tell your doctor or dentist that you are taking this medication.
- Do not stop taking this drug suddenly. Stopping it abruptly can cause nausea, headache, stomach upset, fatigue, or a worsening of your condition. Your doctor may want to reduce the dosage gradually.
- The effects of this medication may last as long as seven days after you have stopped taking it, so continue to observe all precautions during that period.
- Be sure to tell your doctor if you are pregnant. Problems in humans have not been reported; however, studies have shown side effects in the fetuses of animals who were given large doses of this medication during pregnancy. Also, tell your doctor if you are breastfeeding an infant. Small amounts of this drug can pass into breast milk and may cause unwanted effects, such as irritability or sleeping problems, in nursing infants.

Trimox—see amoxicillin

Trimpex—see trimethoprim

Trimstat—see phendimetrazine

Trimtabs—see phendimetrazine

Trinalin Repetabs—see pseudoephedrine and azatadine combination

Tri-Phen-Chlor—see phenylpropanolamine, phenylephrine, chlorpheniramine, and phenyltoloxamine combination

Triphen Expectorant—see phenylephrine, phenylpropanolamine, brompheniramine, and guaifenesin combination

Triple Sulfa (systemic)—see sulfonamides

Triple Sulfa (vaginal)—see sulfathiazole, sulfacetamide, and sulfabenzamide combination

Tri-Statin—see triamcinolone, neomycin, nystatin, and gramicidin combination (topical)

Tri-Vi-Flor—see vitamins A, D, and C with fluoride

Tri-Vitamin with Fluoride Drops—see vitamins A, D, and C with fluoride

Truphylline—see aminophylline

Trymegen—see chlorpheniramine

Trymex—see triamcinolone (topical)

Trysul—see sulfathiazole, sulfacetamide, and sulfabenzamide combination

Tudencon—see phenylpropanolamine, phenylephrine, chlorpheniramine, and phenyltoloxamine combination

Tuss-Ade—see phenylpropanolamine and caramiphen combination

Tuss-Allergine Modified T.D.—see phenylpropanolamine and caramiphen combination

Tussionex—see phenyltoloxamine and hydrocodone combination

Tuss-Ornade—see phenylpropanolamine and caramiphen combination

Tusstat—see diphenhydramine

Tuzon—see chlorzoxazone and acetaminophen combination

Tylenol with Codeine—see acetaminophen and codeine combination

Tylox—see acetaminophen and oxycodone combination

Ty-Tab—see acetaminophen and codeine combination

Ulcort—see hydrocortisone (topical)

Ultracef—see cefadroxil

Ultratard—see insulin

Unifast Unicelles—see phentermine

Unipen—see nafcillin

Uniphyl—see theophylline

Unipres—see hydralazine, hydrochlorothiazide, and reserpine combination

Urecholine—see bethanechol

Urex—see methenamine

Urifon—see sulfonamides

Uri-Tet—see oxytetracycline

Urobak—see sulfonamides

Uticillin VK—see penicillin VK

Utimox—see amoxicillin

Valdrene—see diphenhydramine

Valisone—see betamethasone valerate (topical)

Valium—see diazepam

---

valproic acid

BRAND NAMES (Manufacturers)
Depakene (Abbott)
Depakote (Abbott)
  Note: Divalproex sodium, sold under the brand name
Depakote, is chemically and therapeutically similar to
valproic acid. It has been formulated as an enteric-coated
tablet in order to prolong its effects and to decrease stom-
ach irritation.
TYPE OF DRUG
Anti-convulsant
INGREDIENT
valproic acid or valproate as the sodium salt
DOSAGE FORMS
Capsules (250 mg)
Enteric-coated tablets (500 mg)
Oral syrup (250 mg per 5 ml teaspoonful)
STORAGE
Valproic acid should be stored at room temperature, in
tightly closed containers. This medication should never be
frozen.

USES
Valproic acid is used to treat various seizure disorders. It
prevents seizures or convulsions by increasing concentrations of a certain chemical (gamma amino butyric acid) in
the brain.

TREATMENT

In order to avoid stomach irritation, you should take valproic acid with food or milk (unless your doctor directs you to do otherwise).

The capsules or enteric-coated tablets should be swallowed whole. Chewing or opening the capsules before swallowing releases their contents, which may cause irritation of the mouth and throat.

Each dose of valproic acid oral syrup should be measured carefully, with a specially designed, 5 ml measuring spoon. An ordinary kitchen teaspoon is not accurate enough.

Valproic acid works best when the level of the medicine in the bloodstream is kept constant. It is best therefore to take the doses at evenly spaced intervals, day and night. For example, if you are to take four doses a day, the doses should be spaced six hours apart.

It is important to try not to miss any doses of this medication. If you do miss a dose, take it as soon as you remember, if it is within six hours of the scheduled time. If more than six hours have passed, do not take the missed dose at all; just return to your regular dosing schedule. Do not double the next dose. If you miss two or more consecutive doses, contact your doctor as soon as possible.

SIDE EFFECTS

Minor. Constipation; diarrhea; dizziness; drowsiness; hair loss; headache; increased or decreased appetite; insomnia; nausea; stomach upset; vomiting; and weight gain or loss. These side effects should disappear in several days, as your body adjusts to the medication.

To relieve constipation, increase the amount of fiber in your diet (bran, salads, fresh fruits and vegetables, and whole-grain breads), exercise, and drink more water (unless your doctor directs you to do otherwise).

If you feel dizzy, sit or lie down awhile; get up slowly, and be careful on stairs.

Major. Tell your doctor about any side effects that are persistent or particularly bothersome. IT IS ESPECIALLY IMPORTANT TO TELL YOUR DOCTOR about unusual bleeding or bruising; blurred vision; cramps; depression;

loss of coordination; menstrual disorders; mental disorders; skin rash; tremors; weakness; or yellowing of the eyes or skin.

INTERACTIONS

Valproic acid interacts with other types of medication.

1. Concurrent use of it with other central nervous system depressants (drugs that slow the activity of the brain and spinal cord), such as alcohol, antihistamines, barbiturates, muscle relaxants, narcotics, pain medications, phenothiazine tranquilizers, and sleeping medications, or with tricyclic anti-depressants can lead to extreme drowsiness.

2. Valproic acid can lead to bleeding complications when combined with oral anti-coagulants (blood thinners, such as warfarin), aspirin, dipyridamole, or sulfinpyrazone.

3. Valproic acid can increase the blood levels and side effects of phenobarbital and primidone.

4. The combination of valproic acid and clonazepam or phenytoin can lead to an increase in seizure activity.

BE SURE TO TELL YOUR DOCTOR if you are already taking any of the medications listed above.

WARNINGS

• Tell your doctor about unusual or allergic reactions you have had to any medications, especially to valproic acid, sodium valproate, or divalproex sodium.

• Before starting to take this medication, be sure to tell your doctor if you now have, or if you have ever had, blood disorders, kidney disease, or liver disease.

• If this drug makes you dizzy or drowsy, do not take part in any activity that requires alertness, such as driving a car or operating potentially dangerous equipment.

• Before having any surgery or other medical or dental treatment, be sure to tell your doctor or dentist that you are taking this medication.

• Do not stop taking this medication unless you first check with your doctor. Stopping the drug abruptly may lead to a worsening of your condition. Your doctor may want to reduce your dosage gradually or start you on another medication when valproic acid is discontinued. Make sure you have enough medication on hand to last through holidays and vacations.

● Diabetic patients should know that valproic acid can interfere with urine tests for ketones. You should therefore check with your doctor before adjusting your insulin dose.

● Be sure to tell your doctor if you are pregnant. Valproic acid has been shown to cause birth defects in the offspring of animals who received large doses of the drug during pregnancy. It has also been associated with spinal cord birth defects in humans, when used during the first three months of pregnancy. The risks and benefits of treatment should be discussed with your doctor. Also, tell your doctor if you are breastfeeding an infant. Small amounts of valproic acid pass into breast milk.

Valrelease—see diazepam

Vamate—see hydroxyzine

Vanatal—see atropine, scopolamine, hyoscyamine, and phenobarbital combination

Vasal Granucaps—see papaverine

Vaso-80 Unicelles—see pentaerythritol tetranitrate

Vasocap—see papaverine

Vasodilan—see isoxsuprine

Vasospan—see papaverine

V-Cillin K—see penicillin VK

Veetids—see penicillin VK

Velosef—see cephradine

Velosulin—see insulin

Veltane—see brompheniramine

Ventolin—see albuterol

Veracillin—see dicloxacillin

---

verapamil

BRAND NAMES (Manufacturers)
Calan (Searle)
Isoptin (Knoll)
TYPE OF DRUG
Anti-anginal (calcium channel blocker)
INGREDIENT
verapamil as the hydrochloride salt
DOSAGE FORM
Tablets (80 mg and 120 mg)
STORAGE
Verapamil should be stored at room temperature, in a
tightly closed container.

USES

Verapamil is used to treat angina pectoris (chest pain). It
belongs to a group of drugs known as calcium channel
blockers. It is not clearly understood how verapamil
works, but it is thought to increase the blood supply to the
heart.

TREATMENT

You should take verapamil on an empty stomach with a
full glass of water, one hour before or two hours after a
meal (unless your doctor directs you to do otherwise).

If you miss a dose of this medication, take the missed
dose as soon as possible, unless it is almost time for the
next dose. In that case, do not take the missed dose at all;
just return to your regular dosing schedule. Do not double
the next dose.

SIDE EFFECTS

Minor. Abdominal pain; blurred vision; constipation;
headache; sleeplessness; loss of balance; muscle cramps;
nausea; sweating; and tremors. These side effects should
disappear in several days, as your body adjusts to the medication.
Major. Tell your doctor about any side effects that are per-

sistent or particularly bothersome. IT IS ESPECIALLY IM-PORTANT TO TELL YOUR DOCTOR about changes in menstruation; confusion; depression; fainting; fatigue; hair loss; itching; palpitations; rapid weight gain (three to five pounds within a week); shortness of breath; swelling of the hands or feet; or unusual weakness.

INTERACTIONS

Verapamil interacts with several other types of medication.
1. The concurrent use of alcohol and verapamil can cause a severe drop in blood pressure, and fainting.
2. Beta-blockers (atenolol, metoprolol, nadalol, pindolol, propranolol, and timolol) and digoxin should be used cautiously with verapamil, because side effects to the heart may be increased.
3. Disopyramide should not be taken within 48 hours of verapamil; the combination could lead to heart failure.
Before starting to take verapamil, BE SURE TO TELL YOUR DOCTOR if you are already taking any of the medications listed above.

WARNINGS

• Tell your doctor about unusual or allergic reactions you have had to any medications, especially to verapamil.
• Before starting to take this medication, be sure to tell your doctor if you now have, or if you have ever had, any type of heart disease, kidney disease, liver disease, low blood pressure, or a slowed heartbeat.
• Your doctor may want you to check your pulse regularly while you are taking this medication. If your heart rate drops below 50 beats per minute, contact your doctor.
• Verapamil is not effective for an attack of chest pain that has already started; it is used to prevent attacks from occurring.
• Do not stop taking this drug without first consulting your doctor. Stopping abruptly may lead to a worsening of your chest pain. Your doctor may therefore want to reduce your dosage gradually or have you switch to another medication when verapamil is discontinued.
• In order to prevent dizziness or fainting while taking this medication, try not to stand for long periods of time,

avoid drinking alcoholic beverages, and avoid getting overheated (strenuous exercise in hot weather; hot baths,
showers, and saunas).
● Be sure to tell your doctor if you are pregnant. Although verapamil appears to be safe, extensive studies in
pregnant women have not yet been completed. Also, tell
your doctor if you are breastfeeding an infant. Small
amounts of verapamil pass into breast milk.

Versapen—see hetacillin

Versapen-K—see hetacillin

Vesicholine—see bethanechol

Vesprin—see triflupromazine

Vibramycin—see doxycycline

Vibra Tabs—see doxycycline

Vicodin—see acetaminophen and hydrocodone
combination

Vi-Daylin-F—see vitamins, multiple, with fluoride

Vi-Daylin-F ADC Drops—see vitamins A, D, and C
with fluoride

Vioform-Hydrocortisone—see hydrocortisone and
iodochlorhydroxyquin combination (topical)

Viokase—see pancreatin

Virilon—see methyltestosterone

Visken—see pindolol

Vistaril—see hydroxyzine

vitamin D—see ergocalciferol (vitamin D)

vitamin K

BRAND NAMES (Manufacturers)
Menadione (Lilly)
Mephyton (Merck Sharp & Dohme)
Synkayvite (Roche)
TYPE OF DRUG
Vitamin K supplement
INGREDIENTS
menadione, menadiol sodium diphosphate, or phytona-
dione
DOSAGE FORM
Tablets (5 mg)
STORAGE
Vitamin K tablets should be stored at room temperature in
a tightly closed, light-resistant container.

USES
Vitamin K is required by the body to produce the blood
clots that are necessary for wound-healing and the day-to-
day repair of body tissues. Normally, bacteria present in
the gastrointestinal tract produce large quantities of the vitamin, which is then absorbed into the bloodstream.
Some vitamin K is also absorbed directly from the foods
we eat (leafy green vegetables, meats, and dairy products).
This medication is used as a supplement for those patients
who cannot, for various reasons (for example, gastrointestinal bypass, malnutrition, antibiotic therapy), absorb sufficient vitamin K from their gastrointestinal tracts. It
thereby prevents the blood clotting disorders that would
result from vitamin K deficiency.

TREATMENT
Vitamin K can be taken either on an empty stomach or, to
avoid stomach irritation, with food or milk (unless your
doctor directs you to do otherwise).
   If you miss a dose of this medication, take the missed
dose as soon as possible, unless it is almost time for the
next dose. In that case, do not take the missed dose at all;
just return to your regular dosing schedule. Do not double
the next dose. Tell your doctor about any missed doses.

SIDE EFFECTS

Minor. Headache; nausea; stomach upset; alterations in taste; and vomiting. These side effects should disappear in several days, as your body adjusts to the medication.

Major. Tell your doctor about any side effects that are persistent or particularly bothersome. IT IS ESPECIALLY IMPORTANT TO TELL YOUR DOCTOR about itching; shortness of breath; or skin rash.

INTERACTIONS

Vitamin K interacts with a number of other medications.

1. Antibiotics, quinine, quinidine, aspirin, oral anti-diabetic medications, cholestyramine, colestipol, and mineral oil can increase the dosage requirements of vitamin K.

2. Vitamin K can reduce the effectiveness of oral anti-coagulants (blood thinners, such as warfarin).

BE SURE TO TELL YOUR DOCTOR if you are already taking any of the medications listed above.

WARNINGS

● Tell your doctor about unusual or allergic reactions you have had to any medication, especially to vitamin K.

● Be sure to tell your doctor if you now have, or if you have ever had, glucose-6-phosphate dehydrogenase (G6PD) deficiency, or liver disease.

● Before having any surgery or other medical or dental treatment, be sure to tell your doctor or dentist that you are taking this medication.

● Be sure to tell your doctor if you are pregnant. Although vitamin K appears to be safe during pregnancy, extensive studies in humans have not yet been completed. Also, tell your doctor if you are breastfeeding an infant. It is not known whether or not vitamin K passes into breast milk.

vitamins A, D, and C with fluoride

BRAND NAMES (Manufacturers)

Tri-Bay-Flor (Bay)

Tri-Vi-Flor (Mead Johnson)
Tri-Vitamin with Fluoride Drops (Rugby)
Vi-Daylin-F ADC Drops (Ross)
TYPE OF DRUG
Multivitamin and fluoride supplement
INGREDIENTS
vitamin A, vitamin D, vitamin C, and fluoride
DOSAGE FORMS
Chewable tablets (2,500 IU [international units] vitamin A,
    400 IU vitamin D, 60 mg vitamin C, and 1 mg fluoride)
Oral drops (1,500 IU vitamin A, 400 IU vitamin D, 35 mg
    vitamin C, and 0.25 mg or 0.5 mg fluoride per ml)
STORAGE
The chewable tablets should be stored at room temperature in a tightly closed, light-resistant container. The oral drops should be stored at room temperature in the original plastic container (glass containers interact with and destroy the fluoride in the solution). A slight darkening in the color of the drops does not indicate a loss in potency of the vitamins or fluoride; the solution can still be used safely. This medication should never be frozen.

USES
Multivitamins with fluoride are used to protect against tooth decay and vitamin deficencies in children. Fluoride has been found to be helpful in preventing cavities.

TREATMENT
The tablets should be either chewed or crushed before being swallowed. To provide maximum protection, the tablets should be taken at bedtime, after the teeth have been brushed. Nothing should be eaten for at least 15 minutes after chewing the tablets, to allow the fluoride to work on the teeth.

The oral drop form of this medication can be taken directly, or can be mixed with cereal, juice, or other foods. The dose should be measured carefully, with the dropper provided.

Milk prevents the absorption of fluoride from the gastrointestinal tract. Therefore, this product should not be taken with milk or other dairy products.

If you miss a dose of this medication, take the missed

dose as soon as possible, unless it is almost time for the next dose. In that case, do not take the missed dose at all; just return to your regular dosing schedule. Do not double the next dose.

SIDE EFFECTS

Minor. This product seldom causes side effects, but can occasionally cause constipation; diarrhea; drowsiness; fatigue; loss of appetite; nausea; vomiting; and weakness. These side effects should disappear in several days, as your body adjusts to the medication.

Major. Tell your doctor about any side effects that are persistent or particularly bothersome. IT IS ESPECIALLY IMPORTANT TO TELL YOUR DOCTOR about bloody or black, tarry stools; difficulty swallowing; discoloration of the teeth; drooling; excitation; mouth sores; rash; stomach cramps; or tremors.

INTERACTIONS

This product does not interact with other medications, if it is used according to directions.

WARNINGS

• Tell your doctor about unusual or allergic reactions you have had to any medications, especially to vitamins or to fluoride.

• Tell your doctor if you now have, or if you have ever had, bone, heart, kidney, or thyroid disease.

• The chewable tablets should not be used if the fluoride content of your drinking water is 0.7 parts per million or more. The oral drops should not be used by infants less than two years of age, in areas where the drinking water contains 0.3 parts per million or more of fluoride. If you are unsure of the fluoride content of your drinking water, ask your doctor or call your County Health Department.

• You should NEVER refer to this medication as "candy" or "candy-flavored vitamins." Your child may take you literally and swallow too many.

vitamins, multiple, with fluoride

BRAND NAMES (Manufacturers)
Florvite (Everett)
Pedi-Vit with Fluoride Drops (Three P Products)
Poly-Vi-Flor (Mead Johnson)
Polyvite with Fluoride Drops (Geneva Generics)
Vi-Daylin-F (Ross)

TYPE OF DRUG
Multivitamin and fluoride supplement

INGREDIENTS
vitamins A, D, E, C, B_6, B_{12}, folic acid, riboflavin, niacin, fluoride, and thiamine

DOSAGE FORMS
Chewable tablets (2,500 IU [international units] vitamin A, 400 IU vitamin D, 15 IU vitamin E, 60 mg vitamin C, 0.3 mg folic acid, 1.05 mg thiamine, 1.2 mg riboflavin, 13.5 mg niacin, 1.05 mg vitamin B_6, 4.5 mcg vitamin B_{12}, and 0.5 mg or 1.0 mg fluoride)
Oral drops (1,500 IU vitamin A, 400 IU vitamin D, 5 IU vitamin E, 35 mg vitamin C, 0.5 mg thiamine, 0.6 mg riboflavin, 8 mg niacin, 0.4 mg vitamin B_6, 2 mcg vitamin B_{12}, and 0.25 mg or 0.5 mg fluoride per ml)

STORAGE
The chewable tablets should be stored at room temperature in a tightly closed, light-resistant container. The oral drops should be stored at room temperature in the original plastic container (glass containers interact with and destroy the fluoride in the solution). A slight darkening in the color of the drops does not indicate a loss in potency of the vitamins or fluoride; the solution can still be used safely. This medication should never be frozen.

USES
Multivitamins with fluoride are used to protect against tooth decay and vitamin deficiencies in children. Fluoride has been found to be helpful in preventing cavities.

TREATMENT
The tablets should be either chewed or crushed before be-

ing swallowed. To provide maximum protection, the tablets should be taken at bedtime, after the teeth have been brushed. Nothing should be eaten for at least 15 minutes after chewing the tablets, to allow the fluoride to work on the teeth.

The oral drop form of this medication can be taken directly, or can be mixed with cereal, juice, or other foods. The dose should be measured carefully, with the dropper provided.

Milk prevents the absorption of fluoride from the gastrointestinal tract. Therefore, this product should not be taken with milk or other dairy products.

If you miss a dose of this medication, take the missed dose as soon as possible, unless it is almost time for the next dose. In that case, do not take the missed dose at all; just return to your regular dosing schedule. Do not double the next dose.

SIDE EFFECTS

Minor. This product seldom causes side effects, but can occasionally cause constipation; diarrhea; drowsiness; fatigue; loss of appetite; nausea; vomiting; and weakness. These side effects should disappear in several days, as your body adjusts to the medication.

Major. Tell your doctor about any side effects that are persistent or particularly bothersome. IT IS ESPECIALLY IMPORTANT TO TELL YOUR DOCTOR about bloody or black, tarry stools; difficulty swallowing; discoloration of the teeth; drooling; excitation; mouth sores; rash; stomach cramps; or tremors.

INTERACTIONS

This product does not interact with other medications, if it is used according to directions.

WARNINGS

● Tell your doctor about unusual or allergic reactions you have had to any medications, especially to vitamins or to fluoride.

● Tell your doctor if you now have, or if you have ever had, bone, heart, kidney, or thyroid disease.

● The chewable tablets should not be used if the fluoride

content of your drinking water is 0.7 parts per million or more. The oral drops should not be used by infants less than two years of age, in areas where the drinking water contains 0.3 parts per million or more of fluoride. If you are unsure of the fluoride content of your drinking water, ask your doctor or call your County Health Department.

● You should NEVER refer to this medication as "candy" or "candy-flavored vitamins." Your child may take you literally and swallow too many.

vitamins, prenatal

BRAND NAME (Manufacturer)
StuartNatal 1 + 1 (Stuart)

TYPE OF DRUG
Multivitamin and mineral supplement

INGREDIENTS
calcium, iron, iodine, magnesium, folic acid, and vitamins A, D, E, B_1, B_2, B_3, B_6, B_{12}, and C

DOSAGE FORM
Tablets (200 mg calcium, 65 mg iron, 150 mcg iodine, 100 mg magnesium, 1.0 mg folic acid, 8,000 IU [international units] vitamin A, 400 IU vitamin D, 30 IU vitamin E, 2.55 mg vitamin B_1, 3 mg vitamin B_2, 20 mg vitamin B_3, 10 mg vitamin B_6, 12 mcg vitamin B_{12}, and 90 mg vitamin C)

STORAGE
These tablets should be stored at room temperature in a tightly closed, light-resistant container.

USES
This product is a multivitamin and mineral supplement for use during pregnancy and nursing.

TREATMENT
In order to avoid stomach irritation, you can take this product with food or with a full glass of water or milk.

If you miss a dose of this medication, take the missed dose as soon as possible, unless it is almost time for the next dose. In that case do not take the missed dose at all;

just return to your regular dosing schedule. Do not double the next dose.

SIDE EFFECTS

Minor. Constipation; diarrhea; nausea; stomach upset; and vomiting. These side effects should disappear in several days, as your body adjusts to the medication.

To relieve constipation, increase the amount of fiber in your diet (bran, salads, fresh fruits and vegetables, and whole-grain breads), exercise, and drink more water (unless your doctor directs you to do otherwise).

Black stools are a normal consequence of iron therapy, and should not present a problem.

Major. Tell your doctor about any side effects that are persistent or particularly bothersome. IT IS ESPECIALLY IMPORTANT TO TELL YOUR DOCTOR about bloody or tarry stools, or severe abdominal pain.

INTERACTIONS

This product prevents the absorption of tetracycline from the gastrointestinal tract. Therefore, at least two hours should separate doses of these two types of medications.

WARNINGS

- Tell your doctor about unusual or allergic reactions you have had to medications, especially to any vitamins, minerals, or iron.
- Be sure to tell your doctor if you now have, or if you have ever had, bone disease, liver disease, kidney disease, or stomach ulcers.
- Because this product may mask the symptoms of pernicious anemia, it should be used only under a doctor's supervision.

Vivactil—see protriptyline

Voxin-PG—see phenylpropanolamine and guaifenesin combination

Voxsuprine—see isoxsuprine

Vytone—see hydrocortisone and iodochlorhydroxyquin
   combination (topical)

---

warfarin

BRAND NAMES (Manufacturers)
Coufarin (Bolar)
Coumadin (Endo)
Panwarfin (Abbott)
TYPE OF DRUG
Anti-coagulant
INGREDIENT
warfarin as the sodium salt
DOSAGE FORM
Tablets (2 mg, 2.5 mg, 5 mg, 7.5 mg, and 10 mg)
STORAGE
Warfarin should be stored at room temperature in a tightly
closed, light-resistant container.

USES
Warfarin is used to prevent blood clot formation. It acts by
decreasing the production of blood clotting substances by
the liver.

TREATMENT
You can take warfarin with a full glass of water. In order to
become accustomed to taking this medication, try to take
it at the same time each day.
   If you miss a dose of this medication, take the missed
dose as soon as possible, unless it is almost time for the
next dose. In that case, do not take the missed dose at all;
just return to your regular dosing schedule. Do not double
the next dose. If you miss more than two doses in a row,
contact your doctor.

SIDE EFFECTS
Minor. Blurred vision; cramps; decreased appetite; diarrhea; and nausea. These side effects should disappear in
several days, as your body adjusts to the medication.
Major. Tell your doctor about any side effects that are persistent or particularly bothersome. IT IS ESPECIALLY IM-

PORTANT TO TELL YOUR DOCTOR about bloody or black, tarry stools; coughing up blood; fever; heavy bleeding from cuts; internal bleeding (signs of internal bleeding include abdominal pain or swelling, and vomiting up blood or coffee-ground-like material); loss of hair; mouth sores; nosebleeds; nausea; rash; red urine; severe bruising; severe headache; swelling of joints; unusually heavy menstrual bleeding; or yellowing of the eyes or skin.

INTERACTIONS

Warfarin interacts with several other types of medication.
1. Alcohol, allopurinol, anabolic steroids, antibiotics, chloral hydrate, chloramphenicol, cimetidine, clofibrate, danazol, disulfiram, glucagon, metronidazole, phenylbutazone, quinidine, salicylates, sulfinpyrazone, sulindac, thyroid hormones, and triclofos can increase the effects of warfarin, which can be dangerous.
2. Barbiturates, carbamazepine, cholestyramine, colestipol, estrogens, ethchlorvynol, glutethimide, griseofulvin, oral contraceptives, phenytoin, rifampin, and vitamin K can decrease the effectiveness of warfarin.
3. Adrenocorticosteroids (cortisone-like medications), anti-cancer drugs, dipyridamole, indomethacin, oxyphenbutazone, phenylbutazone, potassium, quinidine, quinine, and salicylates can increase the bleeding complications of warfarin.
4. Warfarin can increase the side effects of oral anti-diabetic agents and phenytoin.
Before starting to take warfarin, BE SURE TO TELL YOUR DOCTOR if you are already taking any of the medications listed above.

WARNINGS

• Tell your doctor about unusual or allergic reactions you have had to any medications, especially to warfarin.
• Before starting to take this medication, BE SURE TO TELL YOUR DOCTOR if you now have, or if you have ever had, any condition for which bleeding is an added risk—an aneurysm, blood disorders, cancer, diabetes mellitus (sugar diabetes), congestive heart failure, edema, endocarditis, high blood pressure, in-dwelling catheters, intestinal infections, kidney disease, liver disease, malnutrition,

menstrual difficulties, pericarditis, surgery, thyroid disease, tuberculosis, ulcers, vasculitis, or wounds and injuries.

● Before having any surgery or other medical or dental treatment, BE SURE TO TELL YOUR DOCTOR OR DENTIST THAT YOU ARE TAKING WARFARIN.

● Do not take any aspirin-containing products while you are on warfarin, unless you first check with your doctor. Aspirin can increase the risk of bleeding complications from warfarin.

● Avoid any kind of activity, such as contact sports, that might lead to a blow or other physical injury. Tell your doctor about any fall or blow that occurs. Warfarin can cause HEAVY bleeding from cuts.

● Use an electric razor for shaving to reduce the risk of cutting yourself, and be careful brushing your teeth.

● A number of factors can affect your body's response to warfarin, including travel, diet, the environment, and your physical state. This drug should therefore be monitored carefully.

● Do not stop taking warfarin without first consulting your doctor. If you stop taking this drug abruptly, you may experience blood clotting. Your doctor may therefore want to reduce your dosage gradually.

● Some of these products contain F.D. & C. Yellow Dye No. 5 (tartrazine), which can cause allergic-type symptoms (rash, shortness of breath, or fainting) in certain susceptible individuals.

● Be sure to tell your doctor if you are pregnant. Warfarin has been associated with birth defects and bleeding complications in fetuses. Also, tell your doctor if you are breastfeeding an infant. Small amounts of warfarin pass into breast milk.

Weh-less—see phendimetrazine

Weightrol—see phendimetrazine

Wellcovorin—see leucovorin

Westcort—see hydrocortisone (topical)

Westhroid—see thyroid hormone

Wigrettes—see ergotamine

Wilpowr—see phentermine

Wvamycin S—see erythromycin

Wygesic—see acetaminophen and propoxyphene
combination

Wymox—see amoxicillin

Wytensin—see guanabenz

Xanax—see alprazolam

Zantac—see ranitidine

Zarontin—see ethosuximide

Zaroxolyn—see metolazone

Zepine—see reserpine

Zide—see hydrochlorothiazide

Zorprin—see aspirin

Zovirax—see acyclovir

Zoxaphen—see chlorzoxazone and acetaminophen
combination

Zyloprim—see allopurinol

Canadian Brand Names

Following is a list of commonly prescribed Canadian brand name medications and their manufacturers. Also listed are the profile names under which you can find information about each brand name drug.

BRAND NAME (Manufacturer)	Profile
Accelerase® (Organon)	pancrelipase
Acet-Am® (Organon)	theophylline
Adalat® (Miles)	nifedipine
Algoverine® (Rougier)	phenylbutazone
Alloprin® (ICN)	allopurinol
Amersol® (Horner)	ibuprofen
Ampicin® (Bristol)	ampicillin
Anadol® (Row)	aspirin, caffeine, butalbital, and codeine combination
Anapolon® (Syntex)	oxymetholone
Antazone® (ICN)	sulfinpyrazone
Anturan® (Geigy)	sulfinpyrazone
Aparkane® (ICN)	trihexyphenidyl
Athrombin-K® (Purdue Frederick)	warfarin
Bactopen® (Beecham)	cloxacillin
Bensylate® (ICN)	benztropine
Bentylol® (Merrell)	dicyclomine
Benuryl® (ICN)	probenecid
Betaloc® (Astra)	metoprolol
Bonamine® (Pfizer)	meclizine

BRAND NAME (Manufacturer)	Profile
Canesten® (Miles)	clotrimazole (vaginal)
Carbolith® (ICN)	lithium
Cefracycline® (Frosst)	tetracycline
Ceporex® (Glaxo)	cephalexin
Chloronase® (Hoechst)	chlorpropamide
Claripex® (ICN)	clofibrate
Cloxilean® (Organon)	cloxacillin
Corium® (ICN)	chlordiazepoxide and clidinium combination
Coronex® (Ayerst)	isosorbide dinitrate
Corophyllin® (Beecham)	aminophylline
Dalacin C (Upjohn)	clindamycin
Depen® (Horner)	penicillamine
Detensol® (Desbergers)	propranolol
Dimelor® (Lilly)	acetohexamide
Diuchlor H (Medic)	hydrochlorothiazide
Dixarit® (Boehringer)	clonidine
Dopamet® (ICN)	methyldopa
Duretic® (Abbott)	methyclothiazide
Eltroxin® (Glaxo)	levothyroxine
E-Pam® (ICN)	diazepam
Erythromid® (Abbott)	erythromycin
Euglucon® (USV)	glyburide
Hip-Rex® (Riker)	methenamine
Indocid® (MSD)	indomethacin
Intrabutazone® (Organon)	phenylbutazone
Konakion® (Roche)	vitamin K
Kwellada® (R & C)	lindane
Largactil® (Rhône-Poulenc)	chlorpromazine
Levate® (ICN)	amitriptyline
Lidemol® (Syntex)	fluocinonide
Lithane® (Pfizer)	lithium
Lithizine® (Maney)	lithium
Loxapac® (Lederle)	loxapine
Maxeran® (Nordic)	metoclopramide
Mazepine® (ICN)	carbamazepine
Medicycline® (Medic)	tetracycline
Medilium® (Medic)	chlordiazepoxide
Medimet-250® (Medic)	methyldopa

BRAND NAME (Manufacturer)	Profile
Megacillin® (Frosst)	penicillin G
Meravil® (Medic)	amitriptyline
Meval® (Medic)	diazepam
Minestrin 1/20® (P.D.)	oral contraceptives
Min-Ovral® (Wyeth)	oral contraceptives
Mobenol® (Horner)	tolbutamide
Myclo® (Boehringer)	clotrimazole
Nadopen-V® (Nadeau)	penicillin VK
Natrimax® (Trianon)	hydrochlorothiazide
Natulan® (Roche)	procarbazine
Neo-Tetrine® (Neolab)	tetracycline
Neo-Tran® (Neolab)	meprobamate
Neo-Tric® (Neolab)	metronidazole
Neo-Zoline® (Neolab)	phenylbutazone
Nephronex® (Cortunon)	nitrofurantoin
Nitrostabilin® (A & H)	nitroglycerin
Nobesine® (Nadeau)	diethylpropion
Novamoxin® (Novopharm)	amoxicillin
Novobutamide® (Novopharm)	tolbutamide
Novobutazone® (Novopharm)	phenylbutazone
Novocloxin® (Novopharm)	cloxacillin
Novodipam® (Novopharm)	diazepam
Novodoparil® (Novopharm)	methyldopa and hydrochlorothiazide combination
Novofibrate® (Novopharm)	clofibrate
Novoflupam® (Novopharm)	flurazepam
Novoflurazine® (Novopharm)	trifluoperazine
Novofuran® (Novopharm)	nitrofurantoin
Novohexidyl® (Novopharm)	trihexyphenidyl
Novohydrazide® (Novopharm)	hydrochlorothiazide
Novolexin® (Novopharm)	cephalexin
Novomedopa® (Novopharm)	methyldopa
Novomepro® (Novopharm)	meprobamate
Novomethacin® (Novopharm)	indomethacin
Novonidazole® (Novopharm)	metronidazole
Novopoxide® (Novopharm)	chlordiazepoxide
Novopramine® (Novopharm)	imipramine
Novopranol® (Novopharm)	propranolol

BRAND NAME (Manufacturer)	Profile
Novopropamide® (Novopharm)	chlorpropamide
Novopropoxyn® (Novopharm)	propoxyphene
Novopurol® (Novopharm)	allopurinol
Novopyrazone® (Novopharm)	sulfinpyrazone
Novoridazine® (Novopharm)	thioridazine
Novosemide® (Novopharm)	furosemide
Novosoxazole® (Novopharm)	sulfisoxazole
Novotetra® (Novopharm)	tetracycline
Novothalidone® (Novopharm)	chlorthalidone
Novotriamzide® (Novopharm)	triamterene and hydrochlorothiazide combination
Novotrimel® (Novopharm)	sulfamethoxazole and trimethoprim combination
Novotriphyl® (Novopharm)	oxtriphylline
Novotriptyn® (Novopharm)	amitriptyline
Nyaderm (K-Line)	nystatin
Oestrilin® (Desbergers)	estrogens, conjugated
Orbenin® (Ayerst)	cloxacillin
Oxpam® (ICN)	oxazepam
Penbritin® (Ayerst)	ampicillin
Peptol® (Horner)	cimetidine
Pertofrane® (Geigy)	desipramine
Phelantin® (P.D.)	phenytoin
Phenazo® (ICN)	phenazopyridine
Ponderal® (Servier)	fenfluramine
Proavil® (Pro Doc)	perphenazine and amitriptyline combination
Procytox® (Horner)	cyclophosphamide
Propion® (Pro Doc)	diethylpropion
Purinol® (Horner)	allopurinol
PVF® (Frosst)	penicillin VK
Radiostol® (A & H)	calciferol
Regibon® (Medic)	diethylpropion
Reserfia® (Medic)	reserpine
Rimifon® (Roche)	isoniazid
Rival® (Riva)	diazepam

BRAND NAME (Manufacturer)	Profile
Rivotril® (Roche)	clonazepam
Rofact® (ICN)	rifampin
Roucol® (Rougier)	allopurinol
Rouphylline® (Rougier)	oxtriphylline
Rhythmodan® (Roussel)	disopyramide
Salazopyrin® (Pharmacia)	sulfasalazine
Solazine® (Horner)	trifluoperazine
Solium® (Horner)	chlordiazepoxide
Somnol® (Horner)	flurazepam
Som-Pam® (ICN)	flurazepam
Stabinol® (Horner)	chlorpropamide
Stemetil® (Rhône-Poulenc)	prochlorperazine
Stievaa® (Stiefel)	tretinoin
Stress-Pam® (Sabex)	diazepam
Sulcrate® (Nordic)	sucralfate
Terfluzine® (ICN)	trifluoperazine
Tertroxin® (Glaxo)	liothyronine
Triptil® (MSD)	protriptyline
Uridon® (ICN)	chlorthalidone
Uritol® (Horner)	furosemide
Urozide® (ICN)	hydrochlorothiazide
Vimicon® (Frosst)	cyproheptadine
Vivol® (Horner)	diazepam
Warfilone® (Frosst)	warfarin
Warnerin® (P.D.)	warfarin
Winpred® (ICN)	prednisone
Zynol® (Horner)	sulfinpyrazone

Please note that **meperidine** *is known as* **pethidine** *in Canada.*

Glossary

abuse, drug—the self-administration of any drugs (prescription, non-prescription, or illicit) for non-therapeutic purposes

achalasia—an obstruction that occurs in the lower esophagus (swallowing tube) that is thought to be due to loss of nerve function to the region; the obstruction may result in the retention of food in the upper esophagus

acne vulgaris—a disease that occurs primarily during puberty and adolescence. It is characterized by inflammatory eruptions over the face, back, and shoulders; the condition is due to overactive sebaceous glands and is probably affected by hormonal activity

addiction—the tendency to become dependent (physically and psychologically) upon certain drugs. If use of the drug is abruptly stopped, symptoms of distress and withdrawal can occur; there may also be an irresistible impulse to take the drug again

adrenal glands—two small structures located just above the kidneys; these glands manufacture, store, and release certain chemicals (including hormones) that are essential to maintaining normal body function

adrenergic—a substance that mimics the action of adrenalin (epinephrine); this body chemical is involved with processes such as regulating blood pressure and body temperature

adrenocorticosteroids—a class of drugs that mimic the activity of cortisol, a hormone that is released by the adrenal glands; drugs of this type are most often used to treat inflammations

agonist—a drug that increases the action of another drug or a naturally produced body chemical

allergy—an excessive sensitivity of body cells to a specific substance (antigen, allergen) that results in various types of reactions, including blood disorders, fainting, flushing, hives, rash, shortness of breath, or wheezing

amphetamine—a substance that acts as a central nervous system stimulant

anal—pertaining to the anus

analgesic—a drug that provides relief of pain

anorectal—pertaining to the region of the last few inches of the gastrointestinal tract (anus and rectum)

anorectic—a drug that diminishes appetite or causes an aversion to food

anus—the opening at the lower end of the digestive tract through which body wastes are extruded

antacid—a drug that neutralizes excess acidity, usually in the stomach

antagonist—a drug that decreases (acts against) the action of another drug or a naturally produced body chemical

anti-anginal—a drug that relieves or prevents the chest pain associated with angina pectoris; such a drug usually works by increasing the oxygen supply to the heart

antibiotic—a drug that destroys or prevents the growth of bacteria and/or fungi

anti-cholinergic—a drug that antagonizes (acts against) the activity of the parasympathetic (cholinergic) nervous system; drugs of this type are used to treat certain gastrointestinal and urinary tract disorders

anti-coagulant—a drug that prevents blood clot formation

anti-convulsant—a drug that prevents or stops seizures (convulsions)

anti-depressant—a drug that is used to prevent or treat depression

anti-diabetic—a drug that is used to increase blood insulin levels or to increase the utilization of insulin by body cells

anti-diarrheal—a drug that is used to prevent or treat diarrhea

anti-emetic—a drug that is used to treat or prevent nausea and vomiting

anti-fungal—a drug that is used to prevent or treat infections caused by a fungus organism

anti-hyperlipidemic—a drug that decreases blood lipid (fat) and/or cholesterol levels

anti-hypertensive—a drug that decreases blood pressure

anti-infective—a drug that is used to prevent or treat infections caused by a variety of organisms

anti-inflammatory—a drug that counteracts or suppresses inflammation

anti-manic—a drug used to prevent or treat the symptoms of mania (including symptoms such as excitement, confused speech patterns, exaltation, and unstable attention)

anti-nauseant—a drug that is used to prevent or treat nausea and vomiting

anti-psychotic—a drug that is used to prevent or treat the symptoms of psychosis (mental disorders)

anti-spasmodic—a drug that relieves spasms (violent, involuntary muscular contractions or sudden constrictions) of a passage or canal, such as the urinary or digestive tract

antitussive—a drug that is used to relieve coughing; may be narcotic

anti-viral—a drug that is used to prevent or treat infections caused by a virus

anuria—the total supression of urine production

anxiety—a feeling of apprehension, uncertainty, or fear, without apparent cause, usually accompanied by restlessness and gastrointestinal discomfort

barbiturate—a member of a group of drugs that have central nervous system-depressing properties; barbiturates are used to treat insomnia, anxiety, seizures, and drug withdrawal

beta-blocker—a group of drugs that prevent stimulation of certain nerve receptors (beta-adrenergic receptors), thereby decreasing the activity of the heart; such medications are used to treat arrythmia (heart beat irregularities), angina (chest pain), and hypertension (high blood pressure)

biliary tract—the gallbladder and biliary ducts; the structures involved in the production and secretion of bile (the body fluid that aids in the digestion of fats)

blood sugar—the concentration of sugar (glucose) in the bloodstream; the amount of blood sugar is usually tightly controlled by two hormones (insulin and glucagon). Any malfunctions of these hormones result in changes in blood sugar levels; knowledge of blood sugar levels is especially important to diabetic patients

bronchi—plural of bronchus. Refers to the smaller air passages (breathing tubes) that connect the trachea (windpipe) to the lungs; these air passages are usually surrounded by muscle and have mucous glands and cartilage in their walls

bronchodilator—a drug that relaxes the muscles of the bronchi and increases their diameter; such an action makes breathing easier for asthmatic patients

bronchospasm—a narrowing or constriction of the bronchi; this type of process occurs during an asthma attack, and occasionally during a severe allergic reaction

capsule—a solid dosage form in which the drug is enclosed in a soluble "shell" of gelatin; this container easily dissolves in the gastrointestinal tract, where the medication can then be absorbed

cardiac glycoside—a drug related to digitalis that is used to slow the heart rate and to increase the force of contraction of the heart muscle

central nervous system—the brain and spinal cord

contraceptive—a drug that prevents pregnancy

convulsions—uncontrollable and involuntary violent contractions of the muscles, usually due to an abnormality in brain function

decongestant—a drug that relieves congestion in the upper respiratory tract

dehydration—the depletion of body water

depressant—a drug that decreases the normal activity of a body system or function; for example, a central nervous system depressant reduces the activity of the brain and spinal cord

dialysis, kidney—a technique for separating and removing certain chemical substances (waste products) from the blood; kidney dialysis is used for patients whose kidneys have failed to perform this vital function

dilation—the enlargement or expansion of a cavity, canal, tube, blood vessel, or opening

diuretic—a drug that acts on the kidneys to increase the volume of urine produced; also called a water pill

dosage—the size, frequency, and number of doses of a drug to be taken

dose—the amount of a drug to be taken at any one time

drug abuse—see abuse, drug

edema—an accumulation of excessive amounts of body fluids; swelling

electrolyte—small particles in solution (usually salts, such as sodium chloride or potassium chloride) that are especially important to fluid balance in the body

elixir—a sweetened liquid, containing alcohol, that is used to dissolve active medicinal ingredients

emetic—a substance that causes vomiting

endocrine—pertaining to a ductless gland, which produces secretions (hormones) that are distributed in the body by way of the bloodstream

enteric-coated—a medicinal preparation (usually a tablet) that is specially covered to allow it to pass through the stomach unaltered, and to disintegrate in the intestines

enuresis—bed-wetting; involuntary passage of urine, usually occurring during sleep

enzyme—a protein secreted by cells that acts to speed up chemical reactions, while remaining itself unchanged in the process

expectorant—a drug used to increase the secretion of mucus, thus making it easier to "bring up" phlegm from the upper respiratory tract

fetus—a later stage in the development of an embryo in the womb; in humans this stage of development takes place between the eighth week after conception, and birth

gastric—pertaining to the stomach

gastrointestinal—pertaining to the stomach and intestines

g (gram)—a unit of weight in the metric system (500 grams is equal to a little over 1 pound)

generic—a non-proprietary drug name, usually describing the drug's chemical structure; such a name is not protected by trademark

hallucinations—perceptions of sights, sounds, smells, or tastes that do not exist; usually, such sensations arise from a disorder of the nervous system

histamine—a chemical substance produced by the body in especially large amounts during an allergic reaction; this chemical is responsible for many of the symptoms associated with an allergic reaction (flushing, rash, swelling, wheezing)

hormone—a chemical substance produced by a gland in one part of the body, then carried by the bloodstream to exert an effect elsewhere; substances of this type play a major role in regulating many body functions (for example, growth, blood pressure, temperature)

hypercalcemia—an abnormally high concentration of calcium in the bloodstream

hyperphosphatemia—an abnormally high concentration of phosphates in the bloodstream

hyperthermia—an unusually high fever (elevated body temperature)

hypnotic—a drug that produces sleep

hypocalcemia—an abnormally low concentration of calcium in the bloodstream

hypoparathyroidism—a condition due to the decrease or absence of the secretion of parathyroid hormones, usually resulting in hypocalcemia and severe muscle spasms

ileostomy—an opening, created by surgery, leading from the ileum (part of the small intestine) to the outside of the body, through which the intestinal contents can discharge

immunosuppressant—a drug that decreases the body's defensive response to foreign substances and tissues. An immunosuppressant is used to prevent the body's rejection of transplanted organs; a medication of this type may also be used to treat autoimmune diseases (conditions in which the body recognizes itself as foreign), such as rheumatoid arthritis

insomnia—prolonged and abnormal inability to obtain adequate sleep

intestinal—relating to the intestines (the part of the digestive tract connecting the stomach to the anus)

intramuscular—within the substance of a muscle; an intramuscular injection is made by placing the hypodermic needle directly into a muscle

intraocular—pertaining to the region within the eyeball

intravenous—within, or entering by way of, the veins

kidney dialysis—see dialysis, kidney

lipid—a fatty or waxy substance

mania—a psychiatric disorder characterized by excitement, excessive cheerfulness, increased activity, unstable attention, and rapid thought and speech

mcg (microgram)—a very small unit of measurement of weight (1 mcg = one millionth of a gram)

mEq (milliequivalent)—a unit of measure used in calculating concentrations of certain chemicals (for example, 1 mEq of potassium chloride = 75 mg)

metabolism—the sum of processes by which a particular substance (nutrient, drug, etc.) is either produced or broken down within the body

mg (milligram)—a small unit of measurement of weight (1 mg = one thousandth of a gram)

ml (milliliter)—a unit of measure of a liquid substance (5 ml = 1 teaspoon)

monoamine oxidase (MAO) inhibitor—a drug that antagonizes (acts against) the action of monoamine oxidase enzymes; MAO inhibitors thereby raise the concentration of certain chemicals in the brain, and are used as anti-depressants or anti-hypertensives

narcotic—a drug that in moderate doses dulls the senses, relieves pain, and produces sleep; this type of medication is addictive, so it must be used with caution

nebulization—the process of breaking up a liquid into a fine spray or vapor

nebulizer—an apparatus for changing a liquid solution into the form of a fine spray or vapor

ocular—pertaining to the eye

ophthalmic—pertaining to the eye

oral—relating to the mouth; medications that can be taken by mouth

otic—pertaining to the ear

over-the-counter (OTC)—a medication that can be obtained without a prescription

palpitations—strong and rapid heartbeats; they can usually be felt or perceived as a pounding or throbbing, and may or may not be irregular in rhythm

parenteral—introduction of medication into the body by ways other than by mouth; parenteral usually refers to the administration of nutrients or drugs through the veins

pediculocide—a preparation used to treat a person infested with lice

pill—a small, rounded mass, containing a medicinal substance, that is designed to be swallowed whole

placebo—a substance in the form of a medication that contains no pharmacologically active ingredients

placenta—the organ within the uterus (womb) that connects the fetus to the wall of the mother's uterus and allows the fetus to receive nutrients from the mother and to dispose of waste products

porphyria—a hereditary disorder of the metabolism of porphyrin (a natural pigment)

psychosis—a mental disorder characterized by defective or lost contact with reality

rectal—pertaining to the rectum—the terminal portion (approximately 5 inches) of the digestive tract

rheumatic—relating to or suffering from rheumatism; rheumatism is an indefinite term that is applied to various conditions characterized by pain or inflammation involving the joints or muscles

sedative—a drug that produces a quieting or calming effect

seizure—a sudden onset of a disease or of a certain symptom, such as a convulsion

side effect—an unwanted effect of drug therapy in addition to the desired therapeutic effect; side effects range from minor annoyances to harmful reactions

steroid—a large family of chemically related compounds, including some hormones; synthetic steroids are sometimes used to treat allergic or inflammatory reactions

subcutaneous—under the skin

sulfa drug—an anti-bacterial drug belonging to the chemical group of sulfonamides; oral anti-diabetic medications and dapsone also belong to this chemical group

suppository—a small, solid body, containing a drug, that is shaped for administration by insertion into the rectum or vagina

symptom—any subjective evidence of a disease or disorder (for example, pain)

tablet—a solid dosage form containing a medicinal substance. Tablets vary in shape, size, and weight; they usually contain inactive binders or fillers as well as the active ingredients

term—the normal time; the end of pregnancy

tetany—a disorder characterized by intermittent muscle spasms or contractions, which can be accompanied by tremors, pain, or tingling sensations; tetany is usually the result of a reduction in blood calcium levels

therapeutic—of, or relating to, the treatment of diseases or disorders by effective drugs, diet, surgery, or other methods

tolerance—the condition of requiring continually increasing dosages of a drug to obtain the same level of therapeutic effect, while at the same time developing an ever-increasing risk of side effects

topical—administration of a drug to or on the skin or mucous membranes

toxic—poisonous, harmful, potentially lethal

tranquilizer—a drug that calms, soothes, quiets, or pacifies, without altering clarity of mind or consciousness (when taken in normal doses)

tremulousness—trembling of parts of the body, especially the hands

vaccine—a medication containing weakened or killed organisms that stimulates the body to increase its defenses against that particular organism

vaginal—pertaining to the vagina

vasoconstrictor—a drug that narrows blood vessels, thereby decreasing blood flow and increasing blood pressure

vasodilator—a drug that causes widening of the blood vessels, thereby increasing blood flow and decreasing blood pressure

vitamin—a chemical, present in foods, that is necessary to normal body function

withdrawal—a group of unpleasant and occasionally life-threatening symptoms a person will experience if deprived of the accustomed dose of certain types of medications; a wide range of drugs may be associated with a withdrawal reaction, including narcotic analgesics, antidepressants, most sedative/hypnotics, and some antihypertensives

Drug Type Index

A

acne preparation
  isotretinoin, 587
  tretinoin, 1091

adrenergic
  methylphenidate, 682
  phenylephrine, phenylpropanolamine, brompheniramine, and guaifenesin
    combination, 847
  phenylephrine, potassium guaiacolsulfonate, promethazine, and codeine
    combination, 850
  phenylpropanolamine and caramiphen combination, 854
  phenylpropanolamine and chlorpheniramine combination, 857
  phenylpropanolamine and guaifenesin combination, 861
  phenylpropanolamine, phenylephrine, and brompheniramine combination,
    863
  phenylpropanolamine, phenylephrine, chlorpheniramine, and
    phenyltoloxamine combination, 867
  pseudoephedrine and azatadine combination, 953
  pseudoephedrine and carbinoxamine combination, 956
  pseudoephedrine and chlorpheniramine combination, 959
  pseudoephedrine and dexbrompheniramine combination, 964
  pseudoephedrine, tripolidine, guaifenesin, and codeine combination, 967

adrenocorticosteroid hormone
  betamethasone (systemic), 169
  betamethasone dipropionate (topical), 173
  betamethasone valerate (topical), 176
  cortisone (systemic), 315
  dexamethasone (systemic), 350
  fluocinolone (topical), 454
  fluocinonide (topical), 457
  flurandrenolide (topical), 465
  halcinonide (topical), 499
  hydrocortisone (systemic), 523
  hydrocortisone (topical), 527
  hydrocortisone and iodochlorhydroxyquin combination (topical), 532
  hydrocortisone, benzyl benzoate, bismuth resorcin compound, bismuth
    subgallate, and Peruvian balsam combination (topical), 536
  hydrocortisone, polymyxin B, and neomycin combination (otic), 539
  hydrocortisone, polymyxin B, neomycin, and bacitracin combination
    (ophthalmic), 542
  methylprednisolone (systemic), 686
  prednisolone (systemic), 896
  prednisone (systemic), 900
  triamcinolone (systemic), 1093
  triamcinolone (topical), 1097
  triamcinolone, neomycin, nystatin, and gramicidin combination (topical), 1101

amphetamine, 46
  amphetamine, 109
  dextroamphetamine, 357

methamphetamine, 660
anabolic hormone
    oxandrolone, 768
    oxymetholone, 778
analgesic, 47
    acetaminophen and codeine combination, 55
    acetaminophen and hydrocodone combination, 58
    acetaminophen and oxycodone combination, 62
    acetaminophen and propoxyphene combination, 65
    aspirin, 117
    aspirin and codeine combination, 121
    aspirin and oxycodone combination, 125
    aspirin, caffeine, and butalbital combination, 128
    aspirin, caffeine, butalbital, and codeine combination, 132
    aspirin, caffeine, dihydrocodeine, and promethazine combination, 136
    aspirin, caffeine, and propoxyphene combination, 140
    chlorzoxazone and acetaminophen combination, 270
    codeine, 307
    diflunisal, 376
    fenoprofen, 451
    hydromorphone, 549
    ibuprofen, 555
    indomethacin, 565
    meclofenamate, 634
    mefenamic acid, 638
    meperidine, 641
    meprobamate and aspirin combination, 646
    methadone, 657
    morphine, 714
    naproxen, 727
    orphenadrine, aspirin, and caffeine combination, 762
    pentazocine, 808
    phenazopyridine, 824
    phenylbutazone, 844
    piroxicam, 884
    propoxyphene, 937
    sulfamethoxazole and phenazopyridine combination, 1011
    sulfisoxazole and phenazopyridine combination, 1026
    sulindac, 1034
    tolmetin, 1085
androgen
    methyltestosterone, 690
anorectic
    diethylpropion, 370
    fenfluramine, 448
    mazindol, 628
    phendimetrazine, 826
    phenmetrazine, 833
    phentermine, 840
anti-alcoholic
    disulfiram, 401
anti-allergic, 49
    cromolyn sodium (inhalation), 320

cromolyn sodium (nasal), 322
See also antihistamine
anti-anginal, 35
diltiazem, 387
dipyridamole, 396
isosorbide dinitrate, 583
nifedipine, 736
nitroglycerin (systemic), 742
nitroglycerin (topical), 746
pentaerythritol tetranitrate, 806
verapamil, 1143
anti-anxiety
chlordiazepoxide, 236
chlordiazepoxide and amitriptyline combination, 239
chlordiazepoxide and clidinium combination, 243
clorazepate, 297
diazepam, 362
halazepam, 496
lorazepam, 617
meprobamate, 644
oxazepam, 770
prazepam, 890
See also sedative/hypnotic
anti-arrhythmic, 35
disopyramide, 398
procainamide, 911
quinidine, 976
anti-asthmatic
cromolyn sodium (inhalation), 320
antibiotic, 43
amoxicillin, 106
ampicillin, 112
carbenicillin, 207
cefaclor, 214
cefadroxil, 217
cephalexin, 220
cephradine, 223
chloramphenicol (systemic), 233
cinoxacin, 278
clindamycin (systemic), 282
clindamycin (topical), 285
cloxacillin, 304
cyclacillin, 324
dicloxacillin, 365
doxycycline, 408
erythromycin, 430
erythromycin and sulfisoxazole combination, 433
hetacillin, 508
hydrocortisone and iodochlorhydroxyquin combination (topical), 532
hydrocortisone, polymyxin B, and neomycin combination (otic), 539
hydrocortisone, polymyxin B, neomycin, and bacitracin combination
    (ophthalmic), 542

isoniazid, 580
methenamine, 664
metronidazole, 701
minocycline, 707
nafcillin, 722
nalidixic acid, 724
neomycin, bacitracin, polymyxin B, and gramicidin combination (ophthalmic),
    731
nitrofurantoin, 739
oxacillin, 765
oxytetracycline, 780
penicillin G, 800
penicillin VK, 803
rifampin, 984
sodium sulfacetamide (ophthalmic), 997
sulfamethoxazole and phenazopyridine combination, 1011
sulfamethoxazole and trimethoprim combination, 1015
sulfathiazole, sulfacetamide, and sulfabenzamide combination, 1022
sulfisoxazole and phenazopyridine combination, 1026
sulfonamides, 1030
tetracycline, 1048
triamcinolone, neomycin, nystatin, and gramicidin combination (topical), 1101
trimethoprim, 1131
anti-cancer
    See anti-neoplastic
anti-cholinergic, 40
    atropine, scopolamine, hyoscyamine, and phenobarbital combination, 147
    benztropine, 166
    chlordiazepoxide and clidinium combination, 243
    diphenoxylate and atropine, 393
    prochlorperazine and isopropamide combination, 922
    propantheline, 935
    trihexyphenidyl, 1125
    See also anti-spasmodic
anti-coagulant, 37
    heparin, 506
    warfarin, 1154
anti-convulsant, 47
    carbamazepine, 204
    clonazepam, 291
    ethosuximide, 445
    phenobarbital, 836
    phenytoin, 875
    primidone, 904
    valproic acid, 1139
anti-depressant
    amitriptyline, 95
    amoxapine, 103
    chlordiazepoxide and amitriptyline combination, 239
    desipramine, 346
    doxepin, 404
    imipramine, 558
    maprotiline, 625

nortriptyline, 750
perphenazine and amitriptyline combination, 819
phenelzine, 830
protriptyline, 949
trazodone, 1088
trimipramine, 1133
See also tricyclic anti-depressant; tetracyclic anti-depressant
anti-diabetic, 42
acetohexamide, 68
chlorpropamide, 259
glipizide, 477
glyburide, 482
insulin, 568
tolazamide, 1078
tolbutamide, 1081
anti-diarrheal, 41
diphenoxylate and atropine, 393
loperamide, 615
anti-emetic
meclizine, 631
metoclopramide, 692
prochlorperazine, 917
trimethobenzamide, 1129
anti-estrogen
tamoxifen, 1038
anti-fungal, 44
clotrimazole (topical), 300
clotrimazole (vaginal), 302
griseofulvin, 486
ketoconazole, 591
miconazole (vaginal), 704
nystatin, 754
anti-glaucoma, 39
epinephrine (ophthalmic), 414
pilocarpine (ophthalmic), 878
timolol (ophthalmic), 1073
anti-gout
allopurinol, 77
colchicine, 310
probenecid, 907
sulfinpyrazone, 1024
antihistamine
ammonium chloride, bromodiphenhydramine, diphenhydramine, codeine,
    and potassium guaiacolsulfonate combination, 99
azatadine, 151
brompheniramine, 184
carbinoxamine, 210
chlorpheniramine, 250
clemastine, 280
cyproheptadine, 340
dexchlorpheniramine, 354
diphenhydramine, 389
hydroxyzine, 552

phenylephrine, phenylpropanolamine, brompheniramine, and guaifenesin combination, 847
phenylephrine, potassium guaiacolsulfonate, promethazine, and codeine combination, 850
phenylpropanolamine and chlorpheniramine combination, 857
phenylpropanolamine, phenylephrine, and brompheniramine combination, 863
phenylpropanolamine, phenylephrine, chlorpheniramine, and phenyltoloxamine combination, 867
phenyltoloxamine and hydrocodone combination, 871
promethazine, potassium guaiacolsulfonate, and codeine combination, 931
pseudoephedrine and azatadine combination, 952
pseudoephedrine and carbinoxamine combination, 956
pseudoephedrine and chlorpheniramine combination, 959
pseudoephedrine and dexbrompheniramine combination, 964
pseudoephedrine, tripolidine, guaifenesin, and codeine combination, 967

anti-hyperlipidemic, 38
cholestyramine, 272
clofibrate, 287
colestipol, 312
gemfibrozil, 475
probucol, 909

anti-hypertensive, 36
amiloride, 85
amiloride and hydrochlorothiazide combination, 88
atenolol, 144
bendroflumethiazide, 159
benzthiazide, 163
bumetanide, 188
captopril, 201
chlorothiazide, 247
chlorthalidone, 266
clonidine, 294
cyclothiazide, 336
ethacrynic acid, 439
furosemide, 471
guanabenz, 488
guanadrel, 491
guanethidine, 493
hydralazine, 512
hydralazine, hydrochlorothiazide, and reserpine combination, 514
hydrochlorothiazide, 520
hydroflumethiazide, 546
indapamide, 562
methyclothiazide, 671
methyldopa, 674
methyldopa and hydrochlorothiazide combination, 678
metolazone, 694
minoxidil, 710
pargyline, 791
prazosin, 893
quinethazone, 972
reserpine, 981
spironolactone, 1001

spironolactone and hydrochlorothiazide combination, 1005
triamterene, 1104
triamterene and hydrochlorothiazide combination, 1107
trichlormethiazide, 1013
anti-infective, 43
  acyclovir, 72
  amantadine, 82
  hydrocortisone and iodochlorhydroxyquin combination (topical), 532
  lindane, 605
  metronidazole, 701
  sulfonamides, 1030
  triamcinolone, neomycin, nystatin, and gramicidin combination (topical), 1101
  See also antibiotic; anti-fungal
anti-inflammatory, 48
  sulfasalazine, 1019
  See also adrenocorticosteroid hormone; non-steroidal anti-inflammatory
    analgesic
anti-manic
  lithium, 610
anti-migraine
  ergotamine, 423
  ergotamine and caffeine combination, 426
anti-nauseant, 40
  See also anti-emetic
anti-neoplastic, 45
  busulfan, 191
  chlorambucil, 231
  cyclophosphamide, 332
  lomustine, 613
  methotrexate, 669
  mitotane, 712
  procarbazine, 914
  tamoxifen, 1038
anti-parasitic, 44
  lindane, 605
  metronidazole, 701
anti-parkinson, 47
  amantadine, 82
  benztropine, 166
  bromocriptine, 182
  levodopa, 596
  levodopa and carbidopa combination, 599
  trihexyphenidyl, 1125
anti-platelet
  sulfinpyrazone, 1024
anti-psychotic
  chlorprothixene, 262
  haloperidol, 501
  loxapine, 620
  thiothixene, 1065
  See also phenothiazine tranquilizers
anti-rheumatic
  penicillamine, 798

anti-spasmodic
dicyclomine, 367
diphenoxylate and atropine, 393
oxybutynin, 776
anti-tubercular
isoniazid, 580
rifampin, 984
antitussive, 48
See also adrenergic; antihistamine; cough suppressant
anti-ulcer, 40
cimetidine, 275
propantheline, 935
ranitidine, 979
sucralfate, 1009
anti-viral, 44
acyclovir, 72
amantadine, 82
appetite suppressant
See anorectic

B
benzodiazepine tranquilizer
alprazolam, 80
chlordiazepoxide, 236
clorazepate, 297
diazepam, 362
flurazepam, 468
halazepam, 496
lorazepam, 617
oxazepam, 770
prazepam, 890
temazepam, 1040
triazolam, 1110
beta-adrenergic blocking agent (beta-blocker), 38
atenolol, 144
metoprolol, 698
nadolol, 718
pindolol, 881
propranolol, 940
propranolol and hydrochlorothiazide combination, 944
timolol (ophthalmic), 1073
timolol (systemic), 1075
birth control pill
See oral contraceptives
bronchodilator, 49
albuterol, 74
aminophylline, 91
isoetharine, 577
metaproterenol, 654
oxtriphylline, 773
terbutaline, 1042
theophylline, 1085
theophylline and guaifenesin combination, 1057

C
calcium channel blocker, 39
   diltiazem, 387
   nifedipine, 736
   verapamil, 1143
cardiac glycoside, 37
   digitoxin, 379
   digoxin, 381
cephalosporin antibiotic
   cefaclor, 214
   cefadroxil, 217
   cephalexin, 220
   cephradine, 223
chelator
   penicillamine, 798
cholinergic
   bethanechol, 179
contraceptives
   See oral contraceptives
cough suppressant
   ammonium chloride, bromodiphenhydramine, diphenhydramine, codeine,
      and potassium guaiacolsulfonate combination, 99
   codeine, 307
   phenylephrine, potassium guaiacolsulfonate, promethazine, and codeine
      combination, 850
   phenylpropanolamine and caramiphen combination, 854
   phenyltoloxamine and hydrocodone combination, 871
   promethazine, potassium guaiacolsulfonate, and codeine combination, 931
   pseudoephedrine, tripolidine, guaifenesin, and codeine combination, 967
   terpin hydrate and codeine combination, 1043

D
decongestants, 49
   See also adrenergic; cough suppressant
digestive enzymes
   pancreatin, 784
   pancrelipase, 786
diuretic, 36
   amiloride, 85
   amiloride and hydrochlorothiazide combination, 88
   bendroflumethiazide, 159
   benzthiazide, 163
   bumetanide, 188
   chlorothiazide, 247
   chlorthalidone, 266
   cyclothiazide, 336
   ethacrynic acid, 439
   furosemide, 471
   hydralazine, hydrochlorothiazide, and reserpine combination, 514
   hydrochlorothiazide, 520
   hydroflumethiazide, 546
   indapamide, 562
   methyclothiazide, 671

methyldopa and hydrochlorothiazide combination, 678
metolazone, 694
propranolol and hydrochlorothiazide combination, 944
quinethazone, 972
spironolactone, 1001
spironolactone and hydrochlorothiazide combination, 1005
triamterene, 1104
triamterene and hydrochlorothiazide combination, 1107
trichlormethiazide, 1113
dopamine agonist
bromocriptine, 182
dopamine antagonist
metoclopramide, 692

E
emetic
ipecac, 573
estrogen, 42
diethylstilbestrol, 373
estrogens, conjugated, 437
ethinyl estradiol, 442
expectorant
ammonium chloride, bromodiphenhydramine, diphenhydramine, codeine,
and potassium guaiacolsulfonate combination, 99
phenylephrine, phenylpropanolamine, brompheniramine, and guaifenesin
combination, 847
phenylephrine, potassium guaiacolsulfonate, promethazine, and codeine
combination, 850
phenylpropanolamine and guaifenesin combination, 861
promethazine, potassium guaiacolsulfonate, and codeine combination, 931
pseudoephedrine, tripolidine, guaifenesin, and codeine combination, 967
terpine hydrate and codeine combination, 1045
theophylline and guaifenesin combination, 1057

F
fertility drug
clomiphene, 290
fluoride supplement
sodium fluoride, 994
folic acid analog
leucovorin, 594

G
gallstone dissolver
chenodiol, 226
gastric acid secretion inhibitor
cimetidine, 275
ranitidine, 979

H
hormone, 41
See also adrenocorticosteroid hormone; anabolic hormone; androgen;
antibiotic; estrogen; oral contraceptives; progesterone; thyroid hormone

I
immunosuppressant
> azathioprine, 154
> cyclophosphamide, 332
> cyclosporine, 334

M
mineral supplement
> iron supplements, 574
> potassium chloride, 888
> sodium fluoride, 994

monoamine oxidase (MAO) inhibitor
> pargyline, 791
> phenelzine, 830

multivitamin
> See vitamins

muscle relaxant
> baclofen, 156
> carisoprodol, 212
> chlorzoxazone and acetaminophen combination, 270
> cyclobenzaprine, 329
> dantrolene, 343
> methocarbamol, 667
> orphenadrine, aspirin, and caffeine combination, 762

N
non-steroidal anti-inflammatory analgesic
> aspirin, 117
> diflunisal, 376
> fenoprofen, 451
> ibuprofen, 555
> indomethacin, 565
> meclofenamate, 634
> mefenamic acid, 638
> naproxen, 727
> phenylbutazone, 844
> piroxicam, 884
> sulindac, 1034
> tolmetin, 1085

O
oral contraceptives, 43, 758

P
pediculocide, 44
> lindane, 605

phenothiazine tranquilizer
> chlorpromazine, 254
> fluphenazine, 460
> mesoridazine, 649
> perphenazine, 815
> perphenazine and amitriptyline combination, 819
> prochlorperazine, 917
> prochlorperazine and isopropamide combination, 922
> promazine, 926

thioridazine, 1060
trifluoperazine, 1117
triflupromazine, 1121
potassium replacement
potassium chloride, 888
progesterone
medroxyprogesterone, 636

S
scabicide, 44
lindane, 605
sedative/hypnotic, 45
alprazolam, 80
aspirin, caffeine, and butalbital combination, 128
aspirin, caffeine, butalbital, and codeine combination, 132
atropine, scopolamine, hyoscyamine, and phenobarbital combination, 147
butabarbital, 193
chloral hydrate, 228
chlordiazepoxide, 236
clorazepate, 297
diazepam, 362
diphenhydramine, 389
flurazepam, 468
glutethimide, 480
halazepam, 496
hydroxyzine, 552
lorazepam, 617
meprobamate, 644
meprobamate and aspirin combination, 646
oxazepam, 770
pentobarbital, 811
phenobarbital, 836
prazepam, 890
secobarbital, 988
temazepam, 1040
triazolam, 1110
sleeping aid
See sedative/hypnotic
steroids
See adrenocorticosteroid hormone
stimulant
pemoline, 796
stop smoking aid
nicotine gum, 734
sulfonamide anti-inflammatory
sulfasalazine, 1019

T
tetracyclic anti-depressant
maprotiline, 625
thyroid hormone, 41
levothyroxine, 602
liothyronine, 607
thyroid hormone, 1069

tranquilizer, 46
   See also anti-anxiety; phenothiazine tranquilizer; benzodiazepine tranquilizer;
      sedative/hypnotic
tricyclic anti-depressant
   amitriptyline, 95
   amoxapine, 103
   desipramine, 346
   doxepin, 404
   imipramine, 558
   nortriptyline, 750
   perphenazine and amitriptyline combination, 819
   protriptyline, 949
   trimipramine, 1133

U
uricosuric
   probenecid, 907
urinary tract analgesic
   phenazopyridine, 824
   sulfamethoxazole and phenazopyridine combination, 1011
   sulfisoxazole and phenazopyridine combination, 1026
uterine stimulant
   ergonovine, 421

V
vaginal medication
   clotrimazole (vaginal), 302
   miconazole (vaginal), 704
   nystatin, 754
vasoconstrictor
   ergotamine, 423
   ergotamine and caffeine combination, 426
vasodilator, 38
   cyclandelate, 327
   ergoloid mesylates, 419
   isoxsuprine, 588
   papaverine, 788
vitamin D
   ergocalciferol (vitamin D), 417
vitamin D analog
   calcifediol, 197
   calcitriol, 199
   dihydrotachysterol, 384
vitamin K supplement
   vitamin K, 1146
vitamin, 50
   calcifediol, 197
   calcitriol, 199
   dihydrotachysterol, 384
   ergocalciferol (vitamin D), 417
   leucovorin, 594
   vitamin K, 1146
   vitamins A, D, and C with fluoride, 1147
   vitamins, multiple, with fluoride, 1150
   vitamins, prenatal, 1152